Handbook of Clinical Pulmonology

Handbook of Clinical Pulmonology

Editor: Gabriella Goodwin

AMERICAN
MEDICAL PUBLISHERS
www.americanmedicalpublishers.com

AMERICAN
MEDICAL PUBLISHERS
www.americanmedicalpublishers.com

Cataloging-in-Publication Data

Handbook of clinical pulmonology / edited by Gabriella Goodwin.
p. cm.
Includes bibliographical references and index.
ISBN 979-8-88740-144-7
1. Lungs--Diseases. 2. Lungs--Diseases--Diagnosis. 3. Lungs--Diseases--Treatment.
4. Respiratory organs--Diseases. 5. Respiratory infections. I. Goodwin, Gabriella.
RC756 .H36 2023
616.24--dc23

American Medical Publishers,
41 Flatbush Avenue,
1st Floor, New York,
NY 11217, USA

ISBN 979-8-88740-144-7 (Hardback)

Contents

Preface

This book was inspired by the evolution of our times; to answer the curiosity of inquisitive minds. Many developments have occurred across the globe in the recent past which has transformed the progress in the field.

Pulmonology is a branch of medicine that specializes in the diseases involving the respiratory tract. It is concerned with the diagnosis and treatment of diseases of the lungs. These respiratory diseases include emphysema, asthma, pneumonia and tuberculosis. There are several clinical procedures that can be used for the diagnosis of pulmonary diseases, which includes blood tests, arterial blood gas tests, pulmonary function testing, bronchoscopy, CT scan, chest X-rays, etc. Surgical procedures can also be used to take a sample from inside the lung or chest to assist with the diagnosis. Spirometry is one of the diagnostic methods used to diagnose airflow obstruction. The treatment of pulmonary diseases involves medications which can either be inhaled or taken in oral form. Inhalers are used in the treatment of inflammatory lung conditions like chronic obstructive pulmonary disease or asthma. This book outlines the diagnosis and treatment of respiratory diseases in detail. It presents researches and studies performed by experts across the globe. The book is appropriate for medical students and professionals seeking detailed information in this area of medicine.

This book was developed from a mere concept to drafts to chapters and finally compiled together as a complete text to benefit the readers across all nations. To ensure the quality of the content we instilled two significant steps in our procedure. The first was to appoint an editorial team that would verify the data and statistics provided in the book and also select the most appropriate and valuable contributions from the plentiful contributions we received from authors worldwide. The next step was to appoint an expert of the topic as the Editor-in-Chief, who would head the project and finally make the necessary amendments and modifications to make the text reader-friendly. I was then commissioned to examine all the material to present the topics in the most comprehensible and productive format.

I would like to take this opportunity to thank all the contributing authors who were supportive enough to contribute their time and knowledge to this project. I also wish to convey my regards to my family who have been extremely supportive during the entire project.

Editor

1

Isolated Pauci-Immune Pulmonary Capillaritis Associated with Hydrocarbon Inhalation and Marijuana Smoking: An Unusual Case of Severe Hypoxemia

Jason S. Oh[1] **Uni Wong**[2] **Divyansh Bajaj**[3] **and Stella E. Hines**[4]

[1]*Wellstar Health System, Wellstar Pulmonary and Critical Care Medicine, Medical College of Georgia at Augusta University, Department of Medicine, Augusta, GA, USA*
[2]*Department of Medicine, Division of Gastroenterology, University of Maryland School of Medicine, Baltimore, MD, USA*
[3]*Department of Internal Medicine, Quinnipiac University Frank H. Netter MD School of Medicine/St. Vincent's Medical Center, Bridgeport, CT, USA*
[4]*Department of Medicine, Division of Occupational and Environmental Medicine and Division of Pulmonary & Critical Care Medicine, University of Maryland School of Medicine, Baltimore, MD, USA*

Correspondence should be addressed to Stella E. Hines; shines@som.umaryland.edu

Academic Editor: Daniel T. Merrick

We present a case report of a patient with Isolated pauci-immune pulmonary capillaritis (IPIPC). A 40-year-old male presented with acute onset severe hypoxemic respiratory failure. He had just returned home from work as a cabinetmaker, where he experienced inhalational exposure to hydrocarbons and solvents, and had smoked a marijuana cigarette. He was hypotensive, and his chest imaging showed bilateral dependent infiltrates. His hypoxemia made little improvement after conventional ventilator support and broad-spectrum antibacterial therapy and he was considered too unstable to tolerate diagnostic bronchoscopy with bronchoalveolar lavage. His laboratory evaluation initially showed microscopic hematuria which later cleared, but other tests including serologic autoimmune assessment were negative, and he did not have any traditional risk factors for vasculitis. A video-assisted thoracoscopic lung biopsy revealed diffuse alveolar hemorrhage with pulmonary capillaritis on histopathology. He was diagnosed with IPIPC and initiated on immunosuppressive therapy. He was soon liberated from mechanical ventilation and improved to hospital discharge. Diffuse alveolar hemorrhage from Goodpasture's Syndrome has manifested following inhalation of hydrocarbons and following smoking. This has not previously been reported with IPIPC. Given the lack of other findings and risk factors, his IPIPC was likely associated with occupational exposures to hydrocarbons as a cabinetmaker compounded by marijuana smoking.

1. Introduction

Isolated pauci-immune pulmonary capillaritis (IPIPC) is a rare clinical entity. It is a small vessel vasculitis limited to alveolar capillaries with the absence of systemic manifestations. In most cases, serological testing for antineutrophilic cytoplasmic antibodies (ANCA) is also negative. No specific etiology of the disease has yet, been identified. We present a case of IPIPC temporally associated with inhalation of hydrocarbons as a potential occupational trigger of insult coupled with marijuana smoking.

2. Case Report

A previously healthy 40-year-old Caucasian man was transferred to the intensive care unit with acute hypoxemic respiratory failure (AHRF). He was found unarousable by his wife about 1 hour after arriving home from his job at an industrial cabinet production facility. Emergency medical services brought him to an outside institution where they noted pink frothy secretions on intubation. His white blood cell count was 15,800/mm^3, hemoglobin 17.4 gm/dL, and platelets 252,000/μL. His bicarbonate was 16.8 mmol/L, blood

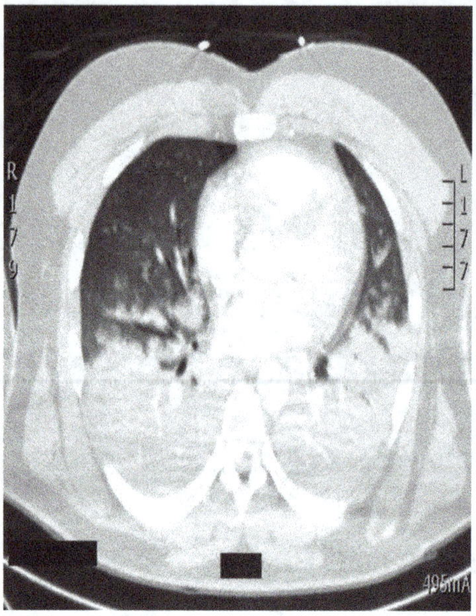

Figure 1: CT chest (axial view) demonstrating bilateral lung infiltrates, more prominent in the lower lobes.

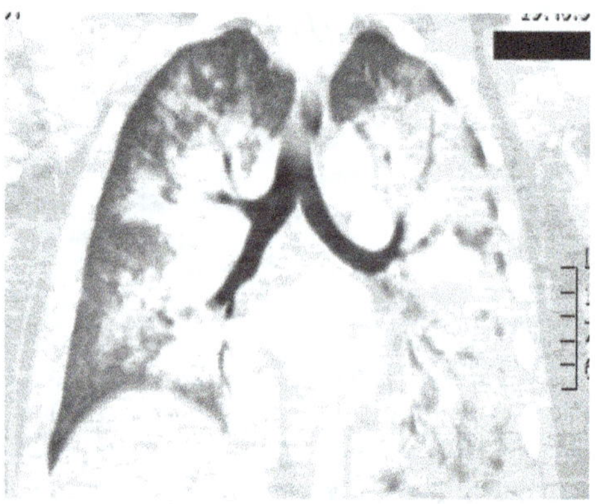

Figure 2: CT chest (coronal view) demonstrating bilateral diffuse lung infiltrates.

urea nitrogen (BUN) 15 mg/dL, creatinine (Cr) 1.8 mg/dL and glucose 371 mg/dL. An arterial blood gas (ABG) showed a pH of 6.99, $PaCO_2$ 68 mmHg and PaO_2 of 63 mmHg on an FiO_2 of 1.0 and PEEP of 10 cm H_2O. These findings suggested volume depletion with a combined metabolic and respiratory acidemia. Chest computed tomography (CT) angiography was negative for pulmonary embolism but showed bilateral dependent airspace opacities (Figures 1 and 2). Toxicological work-up revealed only tetrahydrocannabinol (THC). He was then transferred to our institution for further management.

Upon arrival, he remained hypoxemic and hypotensive. ABG showed a pH of 7.20, $PaCO_2$ of 52 mmHg and a PaO_2 was 53 mmHg on an FiO_2 1.0 and PEEP 15 cm H_2O. White blood cell count was 11,900/mm^3, hemoglobin 18.4 gm/dL, platelet 244,000/μL, BUN 13 mg/dL and Cr 1.23 mg/dL with normal electrolytes. Urine analysis (UA) showed >50 red blood cells (RBCs) per high-powered field and 1 + protein without active sediment or casts on microscopy. Liver and

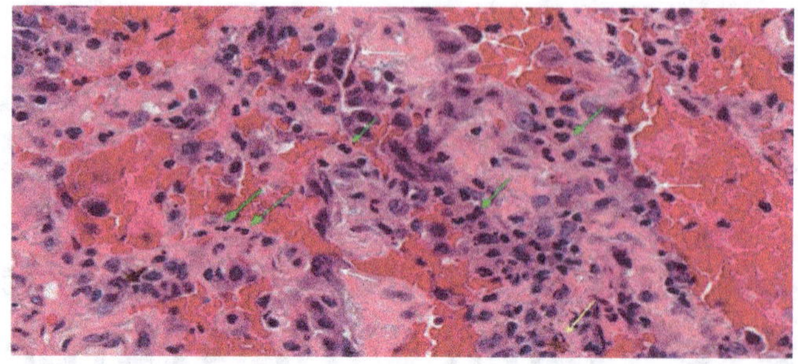

Figure 3: High magnification view showing intra-alveolar hemorrhage, widened septa containing neutrophils (green arrows) and occasional hemosiderin macrophages (yellow arrow). Pneumocytes (white arrows) show reactive changes indicative of acute lung injury (Hematoxylin-eosin ×400).

coagulation panels were normal. His lactate level was 4.0 mmol/L, later improving to 2.5 mmol/L.

The patient was considered clinically too tenuous to safely tolerate a diagnostic bronchoscopy with bronchoalveolar lavage, given the high FiO_2 and PEEP requirements. Infectious workup included endotracheal aspirate culture, blood cultures, urine culture, urine legionella antigen and serum cryptococcal antigen. All were negative, and the patient remained afebrile throughout hospitalization.

Electrocardiography did not suggest ischemia and saline-contrasted transthoracic echocardiography demonstrated no intracardiac shunt but suggested pulmonary hypertension with the right atrial pressure >15 mm Hg by inferior vena cava response to the sniff test. Antibacterial therapy consisted of piperacillin/tazobactam, vancomycin and azithromycin.

The differential diagnosis included a vasculitic pulmonary renal syndrome given the AHRF, frothy secretions despite normal cardiac function, and microscopic hematuria. Human immunodeficiency virus screening, antinuclear antibody, ANCA profile, anti-proteinase 3 and anti-myeloperoxidase antibodies were all negative. Hypercoagulability studies with antiphospholipid antibody, anticardiolipin antibody and dilute Russell Viper Venom test were also negative. His microscopic hematuria improved following hydration. The C-reactive protein level was 8.4 mg/dL and erythrocyte sedimentation rate 105 mm/hr.

Video-assisted thoracoscopic surgery (VATS) was performed for lung biopsy on hospital day 3 for severe hypoxemia despite antibiotics and lung protective ventilation and concern for vasculitis. Intraoperative bronchial wash with bacterial and fungal cultures as well as Pneumocystis jirovecii antigen, respiratory viral nucleic acid polymerase chain reaction (PCR) panel and acid-fast bacilli (AFB) smear with culture were negative.

Histology showed widespread intra-alveolar hemorrhage with organizing injury, hemosiderin-laden macrophages, scattered intra-arterial thrombi and diffuse perivascular neutrophilic infiltrates consistent with capillaritis in all lobes of the right lung. There were no eosinophilic or lymphocytic infiltrates, granulomas, or fibrotic areas. Immunofluorescence for complement and antibodies was also negative. AFB, fungal & bacterial cultures of the biopsy specimen were unremarkable (Figure 3).

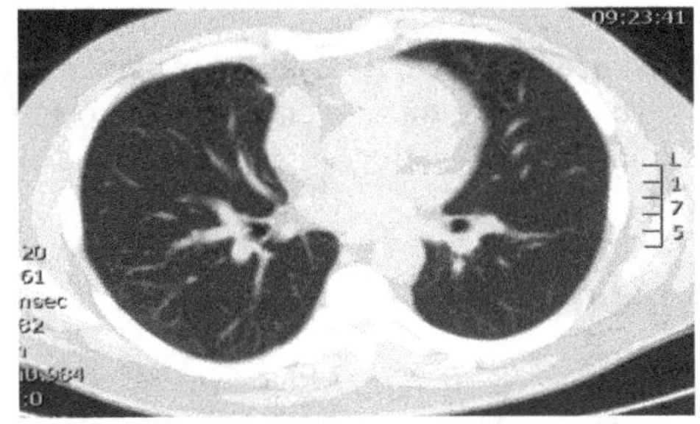

Figure 4: CT chest (axial view) demonstrating complete resolution of lung infiltrates, two months post discharge from the hospital.

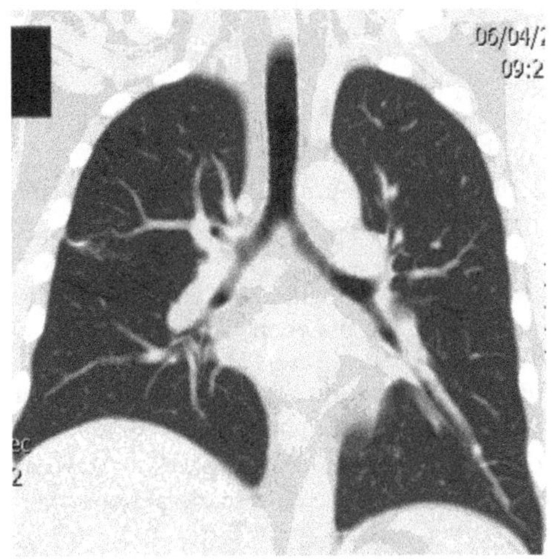

Figure 5: Coronal CT chest at lung window showing complete resolution of infiltrates, two months post discharge from the hospital.

With these unexpected results, an occupational medicine consultation was requested for possible exposure-related contributions to our patient's pulmonary vasculitis. Further history revealed that he had not changed clothes upon arrival home directly from work. Within the hour interval between his arrival and unresponsiveness, he had smoked a rolled marijuana cigarette. His workplace manufactured commercial cabinets out of pre-fabricated materials varying from wood products to polymer-based plastics. The patient's tasks included spraying volatile solvents, coatings and lacquers onto the cabinetry. Important components of the aerosolized materials included methyl acetate, methoxymethane, hexane, 2-methylpropane and propane. He did not work with any acid anhydrides. He sometimes, wore a paper, non-fit-tested mask during his work. The patient was chronically exposed to these aerosolized chemical agents for at least several years. He also used to smoke marijuana intermittently a few times every week, for several years.

Given the dense pulmonary vasculitis with severe AHRF, negative immune studies, and lack of evidence for extra-pulmonary vasculitis, the patient was diagnosed with isolated pauci-immune pulmonary capillaritis. Intravenous cyclophosphamide at 750 mg/m^2 and intravenous methylprednisolone 1,000 mg per day were initiated on day 8 of mechanical ventilation with rapid improvement in respiratory function and ventilator liberation the next day. CT imaging two months later revealed radiographic resolution of his disease (Figures 4 and 5).

3. Discussion

Diffuse alveolar hemorrhage (DAH) manifests with red blood cells (RBCs) scattered throughout the intra-alveolar space. The classic presentation of hemoptysis, bilateral diffuse infiltrates on chest radiograph, and anemia is uncommon, thus, making the diagnosis challenging. Bronchoscopy with bronchoalveolar lavage (BAL) showing increasing RBC counts on serial aliquots and the presence of hemosiderin [1] is diagnostic of DAH. Once confirmed, a good history and physical (H&P) with laboratory evaluation often reveals the etiology among many potential causes: infectious [2] precipitators of diffused alveolar damage, coagulation disorders, idiopathic pulmonary hemosiderosis and immune-related disorders such as the vasculitides. The etiology is important, as treatment can include corticosteroids, cytotoxic agents or immune-modulators.

Pulmonary capillaritis is a subset of vasculitis with damage to the alveolar microcirculation [1]. Renal or lung biopsy should be performed if the H&P with serologic testing is nondiagnostic when the BAL shows DAH. Renal biopsy is typically performed when suspecting a pulmonary-renal syndrome, such as granulomatosis with polyangiitis or Goodpasture's syndrome, as it is usually considered less invasive than lung biopsy [3]. Lung histological findings include intra-alveolar RBCs, erythrophagocytosis, hemosiderin-laden macrophages and neutrophilic infiltration of the interalveolar interstitium.

Although aspiration pneumonia was considered initially as a cause of his AHRF, the patient's presentation seemed inconsistent with a septic etiology given his lack of fever, his cool extremities and negative cultures. DAH from vasculitis seemed possible, but still unlikely given his lack of other systemic manifestations, negative serologies and abrupt onset of symptoms.

The initial high ventilator settings, his profession as a cabinetmaker and the lack of abnormal noninvasive diagnostic clues concerned us for a vasculitis or atypical pneumonitis that would be best diagnosed via surgical biopsy, instead of bronchoscopy with BAL. Renal biopsy was considered but felt to be of low yield given the normalization of his urinalysis and renal function without specific intervention.

Our suspicions were confirmed on VATS biopsy which showed DAH with pulmonary capillaritis. IPIPC is a rare entity in medical literature. In 1997, Jennings et al. described pauci-immune pulmonary capillaritis in eight out of twenty-nine patients with DAH and biopsy proven pulmonary capillaritis. We performed a search on PubMed and MEDLINE on key words of "pauci immune pulmonary capillaritis" and "diffuse alveolar hemorrhage" and identified eight case reports where pauci-immune pulmonary capillaritis resulted in DAH [4–11] and one where there was no evidence of DAH, only neutrophils in the interalveolar interstitium on histology [12].

Inhalation exposures have been associated with pulmonary hemorrhage syndromes [13, 14]. These include hydrocarbon exposures and smoking with pulmonary hemorrhage in Goodpasture's syndrome [15, 16]. A direct causal relationship has not yet been found; however, numerous studies demonstrate the association [17–27]. Direct damage to the alveolar-capillary interface is hypothesized to expose the vulnerable basement membrane to immune reactivity and development of Goodpasture's syndrome in susceptible individuals [28]. The culprit antigen is found in the collagen type IV component of the basement membrane. Exposure to hydrocarbons and smoking is thought to cause a conformational shift in the quaternary structure of one of the collagen hexamers [α 345NC1] to expose the antigen(s) [18].

A toxicological study demonstrated that systemic administration of hydrocarbon oil can induce vasculitis and DAH in mice within 2 weeks of exposure in a dose-dependent fashion [29]. The pathogenesis of DAH resulting from hydrocarbon oil was attributed to the infiltration of lung parenchyma by B1B cells, a specific subset of B cells. B1B cells act by producing large amounts of IgM antibody which has been implicated in triggering a complement-mediated inflammatory response. DAH from vasculitis is increasingly being treated with the B cell-depleting rituximab, which may be an optimal therapy for hydrocarbon-associated DAH [30]. The authors also found that oropharyngeal aspiration of even very low doses of hydrocarbon oil led to significant lung inflammation and minimal hemorrhage in mice. This may share similarities with human opportunities for hydrocarbon inhalational exposure.

While this patient did not meet criteria for Goodpasture's syndrome, perhaps there was a similar mechanism of injury. His lack of traditional risk factors for vasculitis or connective tissue disease makes an exposure injury more suspect, especially given the occupational inhalation exposure to volatile hydrocarbons followed by marijuana smoking. He had worked with several different volatile products.

The spray adhesive used to seal wood paneling to a polymer coating was composed of methyl acetate (25–35%), methoxymethane (15–25%), hexane (10–20%), 2-methylpropane (5–10%), and propane (5–10%) [31]. Our patient did not wear a respiratory protective device, but rather a non-fit-tested paper mask during work. This would not have prevented inhalational exposure to a gas or vapor. We hypothesize that his hydrocarbon exposure, combined with smoking, could have damaged his alveolar-capillary interface via a mechanism like that of Goodpasture's syndrome.

Jennings et al. reported that three of their eight patients with pauci-immune pulmonary capillaritis were also marijuana smokers [32]. The association between marijuana use and DAH has been demonstrated in several recent case reports [33–36]. A few studies have also implicated marijuana use in causing airway inflammation and parenchymal injury which could further contribute to the occurrence of vasculitis and DAH [37, 38]. Alternatively, the combustion of a previously inhaled hydrocarbon as one smokes tobacco or marijuana may serve as a trigger for vascular injury.

We hypothesize that our patient sustained small vessel injury from hydrocarbon exposure combined with marijuana smoking, resulting in IPIPC and severe hypoxemic respiratory failure. This potential association between hydrocarbon inhalational exposure and IPIPC is the first case that we know of in the literature. Additional studies further exploring this possible association are needed. As availability of recreational and medical marijuana continues to rise among working adults, recognition of this association is also needed in the medical community.

Acknowledgments

We would like to thank Dr. Allen Burke, MD, Professor, Department of Pathology, University of Maryland Medical Center for providing us with the histopathology images of the lung biopsy.

References

[1] A. R. Lara and M. I. Schwarz, "Diffuse alveolar hemorrhage," *Chest*, vol. 137, no. 5, pp. 1164–1171, 2010.

[2] E. Marchiori, G. Zanetti, and B. Hochhegger, "Diffuse alveolar hemorrhage in infectious diseases," *Chest*, vol. 139, no. 1, pp. 228–229, 2011.

[3] H. R. Collard and M. I. Schwarz, "Diffuse alveolar hemorrhage and rare infiltrative disorders of the lung," in *Murray and Nadel's Textbook of Respiratory Medicine*, V. C. M. R. Broaddus, J. D. Ernst, S. C. Lazarus, T. E. King, and J. F. Murray, Eds., p. 1207, Elsevier, Philadelphia, PA, 6th edition, 2016.

[4] P. R. Gupta, T. K. Khublani, S. Anupam Soni, A. Feroz, and A. K. Mehrotra, " Isolated pauci-immune pulmonary capillaritis," *Lung India*, vol. 32, no. 1, p. 56, 2015.

[5] A. S. Monteiro, G. Addor, D. H. Nigri, W. Torres, and C. A. B. Franco, "Diffuse alveolar hemorrhage resulting from pauci-immune pulmonary capillaritis," *Jornal de Pneumologia*, vol. 29, no. 4, pp. 217–220, 2003.

[6] G. Thompson, U. Specks, and R. Cartin-Ceba, "Isolated pauciimmune pulmonary capillaritis successfully treated with rituximab," *Chest*, vol. 147, no. 4, pp. 134–136, 2015.

[7] A. Athanasopoulou, A. Kavvada, C. Labrakis et al., "Isolated pauci-immune pulmonary capillaritis: rare case of diffuse alveolar hemorrhage," *Annals of Translational Medicine*, vol. 4, no. 22, Article ID AB038, 2016.

[8] M. Milić and M Miraš, "Diffuse alveolar hemorrhage in isolated pulmonary capillaritis–case report," *Serbian Archives for Complete Medicine*, vol. 142, no. 3-4, pp. 233–238, 2014.

[9] R. Gupta, W. Naji, A. Jindal, B. S. Patel, G. Mittal, and A. Labelle, "A rare case of isolated pauci-immune pulmonary capillaritis," *International Journal of Critical illness and Injury Science*, vol. 4, no. 4, pp. 319–320, 2014.

[10] C. Liak, A. Gupta, M. Joneja, and C. D'Arsigny, "Isolated pauci-immune pulmonary capillaritis presenting as diffuse alveolar hemorrhage," in *ATSA39 Autoimmune Lung Disease: Case Reports. American Thoracic Society International Conference Abstracts*, p. 1463, American Thoracic Society, Washington, 2017.

[11] R. Malik, J. Jaddaoui, and S. Beegle, "A case of idiopathic pauci immune pulmonary capillaritis (IPIPC)," in *A35 Case Reports in Autoimmune Lung Disease. American Thoracic Society International Conference Abstracts*, p. 1375, American Thoracic Society, Texas, 2016.

[12] D. M. Nierman, T. H. Kalb, M. H. Ornstein, and J. Gil, "A patient with antineutrophil cytoplasmic antibody-negative pulmonary

capillaritis and circulating primed neutrophils," *Arthritis & Rheumatism*, vol. 38, no. 12, pp. 1855–1858, 1995.

[13] L. Barregard, S. Enestrom, O. Ljunghusen, J. Wieslander, and P. Hultman, "A study of autoantibodies and circulating immune complexes in mercury-exposed chloralkali workers," *International Archives of Occupational and Environmental Health*, vol. 70, no. 2, pp. 101–106, 1997.

[14] P. Bernis, J. Hamels, A. Quoidbach, P. Mahieu, and P. Bouvy, "Remission of Goodpasture's syndrome after withdrawal of an unusual toxic," *Clinical Nephrology*, vol. 23, no. 6, pp. 312–317, 1985.

[15] T. Yamamoto and C. B. Wilson, "Binding of anti-basement membrane antibody to alveolar basement membrane after intratracheal gasoline instillation in rabbits," *The American Journal of Pathology*, vol. 126, no. 3, pp. 497–505, 1987.

[16] M. Donaghy and A. J. Rees, "Cigarette smoking and lung haemorrhage in glomerulonephritis caused by autoantibodies to glomerular basement membrane," *The Lancet*, vol. 2, no. 8364, pp. 1390–1393, 1983.

[17] G. J. Bombassei and A. A. Kaplan, "The association between hydrocarbon exposure and anti-glomerular basement membrane antibody-mediated disease (Goodpasture's syndrome)," *American Journal of Industrial Medicine*, vol. 21, no. 2, pp. 141–153, 1992.

[18] A. L. Chan, S. Louie, K. O. Leslie, M. M. Juarez, and T. E. Albertson, "Cutting edge issues in Goodpasture's disease," *Clinical Reviews in Allergy & Immunology*, vol. 41, no. 2, pp. 151–162, 2011.

[19] D. N. Churchill, A. Fine, and M. H. Gault, "Association between hydrocarbon exposure and glomerulonephritis. An appraisal of the evidence," *Nephron*, vol. 33, no. 3, pp. 169–172, 1983.

[20] F. Keller and H. Nekarda, "Fatal relapse in Goodpasture's syndrome 3 years after plasma exchange," *Respiration*, vol. 48, no. 1, pp. 62–66, 1985.

[21] A. Mutti, R. Alinovi, E. Bergamaschi et al., "Nephropathies and exposure to perchloroethylene in dry-cleaners," *Lancet*, vol. 340, no. 8813, pp. 189–93, 1992.

[22] A. M. Keogh, L. S. Ibels, D. H. Allen, J. P. Isbister, and M. C. Kennedy, "Exacerbation of Goodpasture's syndrome after inadvertent exposure to hydrocarbon fumes," *British Medical Journal*, vol. 288, no. 6412, p. 188, 1984.

[23] U. Ravnskov, "Acute glomerulonephritis and exposure to organic solvents in father and daughter," *Acta Medica Scandinavica*, vol. 205, no. 7, pp. 581–582, 1979.

[24] M. K. Shah, "Outcomes in patients with Goodpasture's syndrome and hydrocarbon exposure," *Renal Failure*, vol. 24, no. 5, pp. 545–555, 2002.

[25] B. Stengel, S. Cenee, J. C. Limasset et al., "Immunologic and renal markers among photogravure printers exposed to toluene," *Scandinavian Journal of Work, Environment & Health*, vol. 24, no. 4, pp. 276–284, 1998.

[26] A. Stevenson, M. Yaqoob, H. Mason, P. Pai, and G. M. Bell, "Biochemical markers of basement membrane disturbances and occupational exposure to hydrocarbons and mixed solvents," *Quarterly Journal of Medicine*, vol. 88, no. 1, pp. 23–28, 1995.

[27] G. J. Beirne and J. T. Brennan, "Glomerulonephritis associated with hydrocarbon solvents," *Archives of Environmental Health: An International Journal*, vol. 25, no. 5, pp. 365–369, 1972.

[28] D. J. Salant, "Immunopathogenesis of crescentic glomerulonephritis and lung purpura," *Kidney International*, vol. 32, no. 3, pp. 408–425, 1987.

[29] P. Prasad, *Mechanisms of Chemically-Induced Diffuse Pulmonary Hemorrhage*, UCLA, USA, 2017.

[30] M. Nasser and V. Cottin, "Alveolar hemorrhage in vasculitis (primary and secondary)," *Seminars in Respiratory and Critical Care Medicine*, vol. 39, no. 4, pp. 482–493, 2018.

[31] 3M United States, "3M United States," 2019, https://www.3m.com/3M/en_US/company-us/all-3m-products/~/3M-Hi-Strength-90-Spray-Adhesive/?N=5002385+3293242219&rt=rud.

[32] C. A. Jennings, T. E. King Jr, R. Tuder, R. M. Cherniack, and M. I. Schwarz, "Diffuse alveolar hemorrhage with underlying isolated, pauciimmune pulmonary capillaritis," *American Journal of Respiratory and Critical Care Medicine*, vol. 155, no. 3, pp. 1101–1109, 1997.

[33] M. I. Shafi, S. Liaquat, and D. Auckley, "Up in smoke: an unusual case of diffuse alveolar hemorrhage from marijuana," *Respiratory Medicine Case Reports*, vol. 25, pp. 22–24, 2018.

[34] Z. Moatemri, H. Zaibi, S. Dabboussi et al., "Alveolar haemorrhage following a cannabis water pipe," *Revue de Pneumologie Clinique*, vol. 72, no. 5, pp. 316–319, 2016.

[35] F. Grassin, M. Andre, B. Rallec, E. Combes, U. Vinsonneau, and N. Paleiron, "Fatal alveolar haemorrhage following a "bang" of cannabis," *Revue des Maladies Respiratoires*, vol. 28, no. 7, pp. 919–923, 2011.

[36] A. Loschner, A. Cihla, F. Jalali, and S. Ghamande, "Diffuse alveolar hemorrhage: add "greenhouse effect" to the growing list," *Chest*, vol. 140, no. 4, p. 149, 2011.

[37] M. D. Roth, A. Arora, S. H. Barsky, E. C. Kleerup, M. Simmons, and D. P. Tashkin, "Airway inflammation in young marijuana and tobacco smokers," *American Journal of Respiratory and Critical Care Medicine*, vol. 157, no. 3, pp. 928–937, 1998.

[38] T. A. Sarafian, J. A. M. Magallanes, H. Shau, D. Tashkin, and M. D. Roth, "Oxidative stress produced by marijuana smoke," *American Journal of Respiratory Cell and Molecular Biology*, vol. 20, no. 6, pp. 1286–1293, 1999.

2

Intrapleural Tenecteplase for Complicated Parapneumonic Pleural Effusion

Husain Kadhem[1] **Kannan Sridharan**[2] **and Naser Naser**[1]

[1]*Department of Internal Medicine, Salmaniya Medical Complex, Manama, Bahrain*
[2]*Department of Pharmacology & Therapeutics, College of Medicine & Medical Sciences, Arabian Gulf University, Manama, Bahrain*

Correspondence should be addressed to Husain Kadhem; hmj22@hotmail.com

Academic Editor: Akif Turna

Intrapleural thrombolytics have shown promising results in complicated parapneumonic pleural effusions reducing the need for surgical interventions. Until now, studies have evaluated primarily streptokinase, urokinase, and recently, alteplase. In this case series, we share our experience with tenecteplase—a tissue-specific plasminogen activator in 15 patients. We observed that tenecteplase is effective in 14/15 (93.3%) of our patients, and none of them had any bleeding episodes.

1. Introduction

Parapneumonic pleural effusion occurs in approximately 35-60% of patients with pneumonia [1]. Conventional management practice of chest tube drainage and antimicrobial drugs in complicated parapneumonic effusion is effective in three-fourths of the cases [2]. Surgical management through pulmonary decortication was observed with an overall mortality of 3% and postoperative complications in 39% of the patients [3]. Pleural infections predispose to increased deposition of plasminogen activator inhibitors 1 and 2, thereby increasing the intrapleural fibrin deposition resulting in loculations [4]. Intrapleural thrombolytics facilitate pleural fluid drainage in complicated and loculated effusions by breaking up the loculations. A Cochrane review that included studies with streptokinase, urokinase, and alteplase concluded a significantly reduced mortality and requirement of surgical intervention [5]. Until date, there is only one preliminary report available with the use of tenecteplase as intrapleural thrombolytic agent [6]. Tenecteplase, like alteplase, is a recombinant tissue plasminogen activator selective to tissue plasminogen, thus expected with lower incidences of adverse events such as bleeding, following the systemic administration [7]. We wish to share our experience in using tenecteplase for facilitating the pleural fluid drainage in 15 patients with parapneumonic effusions in the present case series.

2. Case Series

We encountered 15 patients with parapneumonic effusion with the median (range) age of 43 (33-72) years and except for one; all the study participants were males. Written consent was obtained from each study participant. The baseline characteristics of the study participants are listed in Table 1. All the included patients had exudative polymorphic pleural fluid on aspiration. Most of the study participants had shown elevated total white blood cell count and C-reactive protein levels. Three participants were detected with loculated pleural effusion in ultrasonogram while seven by computed tomography. Twelve patients had pleural catheter, while three had chest tube for draining the pleural fluid.

3. Description of the Interventions

Following the confirmation of pleural effusion, ultrasound was carried out to identify the biggest pocket for inserting the catheter under ultrasound guidance and with local anesthesia. Special pleural catheter was prepared by keeping the stylet inside the catheter. After administration of local

Table 1: Key characteristics of the study participants.

S. No.	Age; sex	Concomitant disorder	Baseline respiratory symptoms	Baseline total WBC count (count × 109/L)	Baseline CRP (mg/L)	Aspirated pleural fluid glucose (mmol/L)	Aspirated pleural fluid WBC count (cells/μL)	Neutrophil percentage in the pleural fluid (%)	Number of loculations as detected in USG	Number of loculations as detected in CT
1	41; M	None	F, P, D	11	305	Not available	790	82	2	3
2	54; M	Dyslipidemia	F, P, C, S	8	161	6.9	7890	70	1	2
3	33; M	None	P, C, S	16	241	6.8	1420	30	1	1
4	37; M	COVID-19	F, P, D	15	160	Not available	2100	50	1	Not done
5	37; M	None	F, P	14	Not available	2.6	8740	79	1	1
6	34; M	None	F, P, D	24	191	0.2	1306	NA	1	2
7	49; M	Diabetes	P	13	160	7.3	830	87	1	Not done
8	72; M	Liver transplantation and CVA	C, S, D	12	Not available	Not available	1610	80	1	2
9	40; Fe	None	F, P, D	13	Not available	1.1	21780	84	1	1
10	41; M	G6PD deficiency	F, P, D	11	180	0.2	2180	83	1	1
11	56; M	G6PD deficiency, diabetes	F, P, C, S, D	8.8	291	3.9	890	89	2	3
12	48; M	Diabetes, systemic hypertension	P, C, D	13.3	202	13.1	1580	65	1	2
13	68; M	Diabetes, IHD, atrial fibrillation	D	14	206	7.7	2160	88	1	1
14	71; M	Dyslipidemia, CVA	F, P, C, S, D	10	Not available	0.2	7210	90	1	1
15	64; M	None	D	16	Not available	2.2	520	61	2	3

M: male; Fe: female; COVID-19: coronavirus 2019 infection; CVA: cerebrovascular accident; IHD: ischemic heart disease; F: fever; P: chest pain; C: cough; D: dyspnea; USG: ultrasonogram; CT: computed tomography.

Table 2: Details regarding the intervention (tenecteplase) and postinterventional events.

S. No.	Frequency of tenecteplase application	Additional interventions needed for pleural drainage after tenecteplase	Chest X-ray picture following tenecteplase administration	Concomitant analgesics
1	Four	None	Improved	Paracetamol and naproxen
2	Once	None	Clear	Paracetamol and ibuprofen
3	Once	None	Clear	None
4	Twice	None	Improved	None
5	Twice	None	Clear	Tramadol
6	Twice	Thoracotomy and decortication	No improvement	None
7	Twice	None	Clear	Tramadol
8	Twice	None	Clear	None
9	Twice	None	Clear	Tramadol
10	Twice	None	Clear	None
11	Once	None	Clear	Tramadol
12	Twice	None	Improved	Tramadol
13	Twice	None	Clear	Paracetamol
14	Once	None	Improved	None
15	Four	None	Clear	None

anesthetics, the needle connected to a 20 cc syringe was inserted until the pleural fluid drained freely. Then, the syringe was disconnected, the guide wire was introduced, and after removing the needle, a space was created by blade to insert the dilator to open the tract for the catheter. After dilator removal, a catheter was introduced inside pleural cavity. As soon as the catheter was inside the pleural cavity, the stylet and guide wire were removed; catheter was opened and connected to a drainage box. Suction (ranging from 15 to 20 mmHg) was applied. Thoracic tube insertion was carried out in the traditional way.

Tenecteplase solution was prepared by keeping 3000 IU tenecteplase with 40 cc of 0.9 normal saline mixed 10 cc of 1% of lidocaine. The whole mixture was kept in a 50 mL syringe. The syringe was then connected to a 3-way lock catheter, and the solution was pushed inside the catheter followed by 20 mL normal saline flushing. The catheter was closed for one hour and then drained.

4. Details regarding Tenecteplase Administration and Postadministration Events

All the study participants were administered tenecteplase at 3000 IU. The key details of the intervention and postinterventional events are listed in Table 2. Following tenecteplase, all the participants had complete/near complete drainage of pleural fluid except one who needed additional thoracotomy with decortication for complete resolution. Ten (66.7%) had complete resolution of chest X-ray findings following the drainage after tenecteplase while four (26.7%) showed significant improvement from the baseline. Nearly half (8, 53.3%) required analgesics for pain control following the drainage. The administration of tenecteplase was considered to have failed when there was no improvement in the chest X-ray or absence of any pleural fluid being drained or persistence of fever and/or chest pain. The interval time for evaluation and readministration of tenecteplase was 24 hours.

5. Discussion

We observed that tenecteplase is effective and safe in our patients with complicated parapneumonic effusion. The findings were like the only other report with tenecteplase where the authors have observed an efficacy rate of 92.1% (35/38 patients) and adverse events in only 6.9% (4/38) patients [6]. We observed the treatment failure rate of only one (out of the total 15) patient. Studies have reported around 27% failure rate with chest tube drainage alone [8]. Deoxyribonuclease (DNase) significantly decreases the viscosity of the pus in the pleural fluid and eases the drainage [9]. Intrapleural alteplase with DNase was observed to be successful in 58/61 (93.4%) of patients with bleeding in the pleural fluid requiring blood transfusion encountered in three (4.9%) patients [10]. Thrombolytics alone were observed with significantly lower success rate in large randomized clinical trials [11]. Tenecteplase with DNase is yet to be trialled, and it would be interesting and useful to evaluate the outcomes with this combination. Similarly, tenecteplase was observed to be effective even in our patients with 3 locules as detected by CT scan. Tenecteplase is a long-acting thrombolytic drug thus requiring fewer doses of administration for prolonged effect. We observed that except for two patients (due to partial response), the remaining required only one- or two-times administration. The prolonged duration of action of tenecteplase may be an advantage in patients with pleural effusion associated with inoperable lung cancer. We did not observe any bleeding episodes with tenecteplase despite two patients with the history of cerebrovascular accident. Fibrin-specific thrombolytic has been shown to be effective and safe even when used in patients with thalassemia with baseline anaemia and on anticoagulation therapy [12]. The only side effect observed following intrapleural administration was pain at the local site that was effectively ameliorated in all the patients with analgesics. In fact, nearly half of our patients (8/15) did not require any analgesic as the pain was self-limiting.

6. Conclusion

We observed that intrapleural tenecteplase is effective and safe for facilitating drainage of pleural fluid in parapneumonic effusions. High quality randomized clinical trials with/-without DNase combination are needed for confirming the therapeutic benefit of intrapleural tenecteplase.

Additional Points

Key Messages. (i) Intrapleural thrombolytics are effective in facilitating the drainage of complex pleural effusions. (ii) Previous studies have used streptokinase, urokinase, and alteplase. Only one published study is available encountering tenecteplase. (iii) We observed that tenecteplase is effective and safe in our patients with complicated parapneumonic pleural effusions.

References

[1] S. J. Chapman and R. J. Davies, "Recent advances in parapneumonic effusion and empyema," *Current Opinion in Pulmonary Medicine*, vol. 10, no. 4, pp. 299–304, 2004.

[2] H. E. Davies, R. J. O. Davies, C. W. H. Davies, and on behalf of the BTS Pleural Disease Guideline Group, "Management of pleural infection in adults: British Thoracic Society pleural disease guideline 2010," *Thorax*, vol. 65, Suppl 2, pp. ii41–ii53, 2010.

[3] C. W. Towe, S. R. Carr, J. M. Donahue et al., "Morbidity and 30-day mortality after decortication for parapneumonic empyema and pleural effusion among patients in the Society of Thoracic Surgeons' General Thoracic Surgery Database," *The Journal of Thoracic and Cardiovascular Surgery*, vol. 157, no. 3, pp. 1288–1297.e4, 2019.

[4] A. A. Komissarov, N. Rahman, Y. C. G. Lee et al., "Fibrin turnover and pleural organization: bench to bedside," *American Journal of Physiology. Lung Cellular and Molecular Physiology*, vol. 314, no. 5, pp. L757–L768, 2018.

[5] E. S. Altmann, I. Crossingham, S. Wilson, and H. R. Davies, "Intra-pleural fibrinolytic therapy versus placebo, or a different fibrinolytic agent, in the treatment of adult parapneumonic effusions and empyema," *Cochrane Database of Systematic Reviews*, no. 10, article CD002312, 2019.

[6] A. Refaat, N. Affara, T. Muhsen, and M. Salahuddin, "Intrapleural tenecteplase therapy in treatment of loculated parapneumonic pleural effusions and empyema," *Egyptian Journal of Chest Diseases and Tuberculosis*, vol. 63, no. 4, pp. 913–921, 2014.

[7] S. B. Coutts, E. Berge, B. C. Campbell, K. W. Muir, and M. W. Parsons, "Tenecteplase for the treatment of acute ischemic stroke: a review of completed and ongoing randomized controlled trials," *International Journal of Stroke*, vol. 13, no. 9, pp. 885–892, 2018.

[8] J. M. Porcel, "Chest tube drainage of the pleural space: a concise review for pulmonologists," *Tuberculosis and Respiratory Diseases*, vol. 81, no. 2, pp. 106–115, 2018.

[9] F. Piccolo, N. Popowicz, D. Wong, and Y. C. Lee, "Intrapleural tissue plasminogen activator and deoxyribonuclease therapy for pleural infection," *Journal of Thoracic Disease*, vol. 7, no. 6, pp. 999–1008, 2015.

[10] N. Popowicz, O. Bintcliffe, D. de Fonseka et al., "Dose de-escalation of intrapleural tissue plasminogen activator therapy for pleural infection. The alteplase dose assessment for pleural infection therapy project," *Annals of the American Thoracic Society*, vol. 14, no. 6, pp. 929–936, 2017.

[11] N. A. Maskell, C. W. Davies, A. J. Nunn et al., "U.K. controlled trial of intrapleural streptokinase for pleural infection," *The New England Journal of Medicine*, vol. 352, no. 9, pp. 865–874, 2005.

[12] X. K. Cheong, A. Yu-Lin Ban, and M. F. Abdul Hamid, "Short-course intrapleural alteplase and DNase in complex effusion with bleeding risk," *Respirology Case Reports*, vol. 8, no. 7, article e00648, 2020.

3

Respiratory Involvement in Patients with Neuromuscular Diseases

Athanasios Voulgaris ,[1,2] Maria Antoniadou,[1,3] Michalis Agrafiotis ,[1,3] and Paschalis Steiropoulos [1,2]

[1]*MSc Program in Sleep Medicine, Medical School, Democritus University of Thrace, Alexandroupolis, Greece*
[2]*Department of Pneumonology, Medical School, Democritus University of Thrace, Alexandroupolis, Greece*
[3]*Department of Pneumonology, General Hospital "G. Papanikolaou", Thessaloniki, Greece*

Correspondence should be addressed to Paschalis Steiropoulos; steiropoulos@yahoo.com

Academic Editor: Roberto Walter Dal Negro

Respiratory muscle weakness is a major cause of morbidity and mortality in patients with neuromuscular diseases (NMDs). Respiratory involvement in NMDs can manifest broadly, ranging from milder insufficiency that may affect only sleep initially to severe insufficiency that can be life threatening. Patients with neuromuscular diseases exhibit very often sleep-disordered breathing, which is frequently overlooked until symptoms become more severe leading to irreversible respiratory failure necessitating noninvasive ventilation (NIV) or even tracheostomy. Close monitoring of respiratory function and sleep evaluation is currently the standard of care. Early recognition of sleep disturbances and initiation of NIV can improve the quality of life and prolong survival. This review discusses the respiratory impairment during sleep in patients with NMDs, the diagnostic tools available for early recognition of sleep-disordered breathing and the therapeutic options available for overall respiratory management of patients with NMDs.

1. Introduction

Neuromuscular diseases (NMDs) encompass a diverse group of diseases which may affect the upper motor neurons, lower motor neurons, peripheral nerves, the neuromuscular junction, and muscles. Although this definition may include a large variety of disorders, the term "neuromuscular" is reserved for inherited or acquired diseases predominately manifesting with motor dysfunction. From the pulmonologist's perspective all NMDs present with a common trait: impairment of ventilatory function. This impairment is caused by either compromised airway patency and protective reflexes and/or by reduced respiratory pump efficiency. These pathophysiological events result in sleep-disordered breathing, followed by diurnal hypoventilation at later disease stages. In addition, patients with NMDs are prone to developing various other respiratory complications such as infections, atelectasis, and aspiration syndromes [1, 2]. The introduction of ventilatory support in the early stages of symptomatic sleep hypoventilation, especially in the form of noninvasive ventilation (NIV), as well as various other advances in respiratory care have contributed significantly to the improvement of survival and the quality of life of patients with NMDs [3–6].

NMDs can be hereditary or acquired, slowly or rapidly progressive [7, 8]. Inherited NMDs are not uncommon, with an estimated prevalence exceeding 1 in 3000 among newborns [9]. The prevalence of the majority of NMDs generally ranges between 1 and 10/100000 population; however some disorders are much more common e.g. postpolio syndrome and Charcot-Marie-Tooth disease with a prevalence greater than 10/100000, whereas others are quite rare, e.g. Lambert-Eaton myasthenic syndrome and congenital muscular dystrophies with a prevalence of less than 1/100000 [10]. In a European survey, among patients treated with domiciliary mechanical ventilation, neuromuscular patients were most likely to receive prolonged (>6 years) ventilatory support and to undergo tracheostomy procedures [11].

NMDs cause respiratory disease mainly by causing respiratory muscle dysfunction. Respiratory insufficiency had been the main cause of morbidity and mortality in patients with NMDs until recent respiratory care became available [12, 13]. Respiratory complications and failure will eventually develop in the majority of the patients with NMDs although the age of onset might vary depending on the rate of disease progression. For example, most of the children with spinal muscular atrophy (SMA) type 1 will develop respiratory failure and die before the age of 3 years without adequate respiratory management, while respiratory failure will present later in childhood in only 40% of patients with SMA type 2 [14, 15]. In patients with Duchenne muscular dystrophy (DMD), respiratory failure commonly appears after the loss of ambulation [16]. Conversely, respiratory failure can precede non respiratory muscle weakness, in patients with Pompe's disease and amyotrophic lateral sclerosis [17, 18].

NMDs can also present with various non respiratory manifestations. DMD may cause left ventricular insufficiency and conduction abnormalities [19]. Patients with NMDs may also manifest bony deformities such as chest wall and spine abnormalities. In DMD, scoliosis commonly presents during the second decade of life, after patients become wheelchair-bound, as a result of paravertebral muscle atonia [20]. Conversely, and unless ventilatory support is provided, patients with SMA types 1 and 2 develop bell-shaped chest deformity and pectus excavatum attributed to the preferential involvement of intercostal muscles and the relative sparing of the diaphragm [21]. Patients with myotonic dystrophy commonly exhibit a mild cognitive impairment and a narcolepsy-like clinical phenotype, associated with excessive daytime sleepiness without adequate management for SDB [22, 23].

2. Respiratory Function in Patients with Neuromuscular Diseases

From a practical point of view, the respiratory muscles can be grouped into inspiratory (main and accessory), expiratory, and the upper airway muscles. Dysfunction of these groups can manifest as three different types of failure: (1) respiratory pump failure (inspiratory muscles' dysfunction) (2) upper airway failure, and swallowing dysfunction (upper airway muscles' dysfunction) and (3) cough failure (inspiratory, expiratory, and upper airway muscles dysfunction) [1, 13].

The respiratory pump is responsible for moving the air in and out of the lungs. The respiratory pump fails when it operates against an increased workload or when the respiratory muscles fail to generate enough force. Both of these circumstances predispose to respiratory muscle fatigue, which is defined as the inability to sustain a contractile force against a constant workload [24]. As fatigue increases the patient develops a rapid shallow breathing pattern, which is not fatigue-specific, but rather a reflex response to increased work of breathing [25].

In patients with NMDs the contractile function of the inspiratory and expiratory muscles is impaired. Moreover, chest wall compliance is decreased as a result of scoliosis and stiffening of the thoracic cage tendons and ligaments, while recurrent aspirations, microatelectasis, and pulmonary congestion due to cardiac disease are responsible for a decrease in lung compliance [26]. In addition, the upper airway collapsibility and hypotonia lead to increased resistance to airflow, which also contributes to the increased workload of the failing respiratory pump [27]. Although the initial physiologic response to these events is an increase in respiratory drive, this mechanism is eventually insufficient to maintain alveolar ventilation and hypoventilation finally ensues [28, 29]. Moreover, upper airway muscle failure also accounts for swallowing dysfunction and impaired airway protection, leading to recurrent episodes of aspiration and pneumonia [13].

Normal cough consists of an initial inspiratory phase to reach a lung volume equal to 85–90% of TLC; a compression phase characterized by rapid closure of the glottis for 0.2 seconds with simultaneous contraction of the expiratory muscles to create a pressure greater than 200 cm H_2O; and an expulsion phase characterized by rapid opening of the glottis while the expiratory muscles continue to contract in order to produce an expiratory cough flow greater than 400 L/min [30]. High cough flows are essential for removing secretions and debris and clearing the airways. Therefore, impairment of either the inspiratory, expiratory or glottic muscles in patients with NMDs might compromise effective cough function leading to increased susceptibility to respiratory infections, atelectasis and respiratory failure [1, 31].

3. Respiratory Function during Sleep in Patients with Neuromuscular Diseases

Normal sleep is characterized by a decrease in alveolar ventilation by 1-2 L/min mainly caused by a decrease in tidal volume, while the pattern of breathing becomes shallow and irregular [32]. As a result PCO_2 increases and O_2 decreases by 2–8 mmHg each, while the ventilatory response to hypoxemia and hypercapnia is attenuated [33, 34]. These changes become more pronounced during deep sleep and especially during phasic REM sleep [32]. There are several reasons accounting for these physiologic events, including the reduced lung volume in the supine position, the withdrawal of the wakefulness drive to breathe and the reduced chemosensitivity of respiratory control center [35]. In addition, the tone of the intercostal muscles decreases during sleep [36], while the tone of the diaphragm decreases during NREM but is maintained during REM sleep; as a result, normal ventilation during REM sleep becomes totally dependent on the diaphragmatic function [37]. Finally, the activity of the pharyngeal dilator muscles -particularly of the genioglossus- decreases gradually during sleep resulting in increased upper airway resistance which becomes maximal during REM sleep [38].

These events are more pronounced in patients with NMDs as a result of respiratory and upper airway muscle weakness. The most frequent breathing disorder in NMDs is hypoventilation presenting at first during REM sleep and then occurring at all sleep stages and finally when the patient is awake [39, 40]. Symptoms suggestive of nocturnal hypoventilation are sudden arousals, morning headache, daytime sleepiness, and fatigue [41].

The most common respiratory event during sleep in NMDs is central hypopnea [42–45]. Central hypopneas are most commonly observed during phasic REM sleep, as a result of the decreased tone of the intercostal and accessory muscles combined with inadequate function of the diaphragm [42, 44–46]. Obstructive events are also observed in patients with NMDs, especially in DMD and acid maltase deficiency. In these disorders, sleep disordered breathing follows a bimodal distribution with obstructive events occurring early in the course of the disease while frank hypoventilation prevails at later years [43, 47]. In addition, obstructive events do not appear to be more likely in bulbar ALS patients, although the evidence here is equivocal [48, 49]. Some studies suggest that obstructive events are more likely in patients with a higher body mass index (BMI), in snorers, in those with anatomic abnormalities such as macroglossia, and in those with increased upper airway resistance during REM sleep [42, 43, 50]. Furthermore, Cheyne-Stokes breathing and other central sleep apnea syndromes in association with cardiomyopathy and unstable control of breathing have also been reported [51, 52]. During sleep, patients with NMDs also exhibit hypoxemia which is related to the presence of hypoventilation, apneas and hypopneas, and ventilation-perfusion mismatch due to atelectasis occurring in the supine position [53].

4. Evaluation of Respiratory Function and Cough in Patients with Neuromuscular Diseases

Respiratory assessment in patients with NMDs includes evaluation of respiratory muscle strength, gas exchange, and cough efficiency. Spirometry, arterial blood gas, mouth and nasal pressures are among the most widely used techniques.

In NMDs impairment of respiratory muscle contractile function leads to respiratory pump failure, characterized by decreases in vital capacity (VC), total lung capacity (TLC) and functional residual capacity (FRC) [54]. This reduction in VC is further augmented in the supine position and a drop of greater than 25% is considered 90% sensitive and 79% specific for the diagnosis of diaphragmatic weakness [55]. Interestingly, a decrease in VC can be observed earlier in the course of the disease as compared to TLC, due to the increased residual volume (RV) observed in patients with expiratory muscle weakness [56]. However, although VC is considered a robust index for the respiratory evaluation of patients with NMDs, it can be fairly insensitive in early disease stages. In a study involving patients with various types of NMDs, an inspiratory VC of less than 60% predicted the presence of sleep apnea syndrome and a VC of less than 40% was associated with sleep hypoventilation with a sensitivity of 91% and 94% and a specificity of 89% and 79% respectively; patients with a VC of less than 25% suffered from daytime ventilatory failure [39]. In a cohort involving more than 1000 patients with ALS, forced vital capacity (FVC) less than 75% was associated with a median survival of 2.91 years as opposed to 4.08 years for patients with FVC of greater than 75% [57]. In another study, a supine FVC of less than 80% was 94.6% sensitive in predicting death or tracheostomy within the first year in a group of patients with ALS [58]. In patients with DMD, VC increases until the age of 10–12 years, when it reaches a plateau, followed by a decline which can be as high as 10.7% per year [59]. Loss of ambulation and establishment of scoliosis is associated with an accelerated decline in lung function in DMD patients and a VC of less than 1L predicts a 5-year survival rate of 8% without adequate noninvasive respiratory support [8, 60, 61]. Moreover, an inspiratory VC of less than 1.1 L could reliably identify patients at high risk for severe chest infections in a retrospective study involving children and adolescents with various NMDs [62].

An increased PCO_2 value in arterial blood gas indicates the presence of diurnal respiratory pump failure. In addition, an increased alveolar-arterial difference should point towards a concurrent parenchymal lung disease. Of note, PCO_2 commonly appears reduced at initial disease stages but increases later when respiratory muscle impairment has progressed significantly [63]. Importantly, either diurnal hypercapnia or an increased bicarbonate or base excess (BE) level might indicate coexistent nocturnal hypoventilation. In a study of patients with DMD, values of PCO_2 >45 mmHg and BE > 4 mmol/L predicted nocturnal hypoventilation with a sensitivity of 99% and 55% and a specificity of 75% and 100% respectively [64].

Cough efficiency is assessed by measuring cough flow variables, of which the most important are peak expiratory cough flow (PECF) and cough volume acceleration (CVA). Either a customary handheld peak flow meter, which is used for patients with asthma, or an office spirometer, can be used for cough flow measurements; however it should be noted that significant differences between pneumotachograph- and peak flow meter-based assessments have been reported [65]. Nevertheless, an inefficient cough is characterized by a lower peak inspiratory cough flow, a longer compression phase and a lower PECF [66].

PECF is the highest cough flow obtained after instructing the patient to take a deep breath and cough forcibly. For adults and older children, a PECF of less than 160 L/min is associated with ineffective secretion clearance and tracheostomy decannulation failure [67]. Moreover, a PECF less than 270 L/min is associated with higher risk for acute respiratory failure and higher respiratory morbidity during the course of a trivial respiratory tract infection [68–70]. Most authorities would consider a PECF less than 270 L/min as an indication for commencement of cough augmentation strategies [71, 72].

CVA is derived by dividing PECF by the time required to reach its value (peak expiratory flow rise time, PEFRT). In a prospective study involving stable ALS patients, a CVA of less than 28.9 L/sec^2 was slightly more reliable than PECF in predicting ineffective cough during a respiratory tract infection [69]. In addition, when compared to PECF and PEFRT, CVA was the most reliable predictor of aspiration in patients with ALS [66]. In another study, the strength of cough in patients with ALS correlated with the ability to produce transient cough spikes during a maximal flow-volume maneuver; the absence of these spikes also correlated with increased mortality [73, 74].

Maximum insufflation capacity (MIC) and lung insufflation capacity are also important variables in the assessment of cough function. MIC is defined as the maximum volume of air that can be held in the lungs while the glottis is closed and is obtained by instructing the patient to stack several volumes of air after taking a deep breath. Air stacking can be performed with the use of a volume ventilator or a resuscitation bag with an one way valve, or with the technique of glossopharyngeal breathing [75]. When the glottic function is not intact, the same effect can be obtained via the use of a manual resuscitator with the expiratory port blocked, or a volume ventilator set to deliver volumes close to the subject's inspiratory capacity or a mechanical insufflator-exsufflator device (MI-E); in that instance the term lung insufflation capacity is preferred (LIC) [76]. MIC/LIC can be measured with a simple spirometer and the greater the difference between VC and MIC/LIC, the higher the PECF that will be achieved when the patient coughs from maximum insufflation [72, 76, 77].

Measurements of maximal static mouth pressures are among the most common methods used to assess inspiratory and expiratory muscle strength in daily clinical practice. They are measured via a mouthpiece, which is connected to a manometer. One limitation of the static mouth pressures is that they cannot be measured reliably in patients with facial muscle weakness [78]. Maximum inspiratory pressure (MIP) is the average pressure sustained over 1 sec when the patient takes a deep breath against a blocked mouthpiece from the RV (Mueller maneuver). MIP correlates well with VC in children and adults with various types of NMDs [39, 79–81]. When evaluated in a mixed population of children and adolescents with NMDs, a MIP less than −46 cm H_2O predicted the presence of sleep apnea and a MIP less than −40 cm H_2O was associated with sleep hypoventilation with a sensitivity of 82 and 95% and specificity of 89% and 65%, respectively [39]. Unlike VC, MIP is neither related to the number of chest infections nor the total days of antibiotic therapy during the preceding year [62].

Maximal expiratory pressure (MEP) is the average pressure sustained over 1 sec when the subject blows against a blocked mouthpiece from TLC (Valsava maneuver). A MEP greater than +60 H_2O is required to produce an efficient cough, while a MEP of less than +45 H_2O suggests impaired expiratory muscle function and decreased ability to cough [82]. In a study involving children and adolescents with DMD, MEP correlated with VC, but its rate of decline during the course of the disease was higher as compared to MIP and VC [81]. MEP has also been shown to correlate with the number of infections and the number of days on antibiotic therapy in the preceding year, although the correlation is weaker than for VC and PECF [62].

Nasal pressures are measured via a plug wedged into the nostril and connected to a manometer, while the subject performs a quick sniff, i.e., a sharp voluntary inspiratory maneuver through the nostril (sniff nasal inspiratory pressure, SNIP). This maneuver is performed from FRC and although it might be easier to perform and more suitable for patients with facial muscle weakness, more than 10 attempts are often required before a plateau is reached [78, 83]. SNIP has a strong correlation with PCO_2 in nonbulbar patients with ALS and a SNIP of less than −40 cm H_2O was the most reliable noninvasive predictor of hypercapnic respiratory failure in nonbulbar ALS patients with a sensitivity of 85% and a specificity of 81% [63, 84]. In a prospective study of 98 patients with ALS, a SNIP < −40 cm H_2O was significantly correlated with the severity of nocturnal hypoxemia, while no such association was established for MIP and VC; in the same study, a SNIP < −40 cm H_2O was associated with a median survival of 6 months [85]. In a more recent study of patients with ALS, a SNIP of less than −34 cm H_2O could predict death or tracheostomy within one year with a sensitivity of 75% and a specificity of 72% [86]. Another study evaluated the evolution of MIP, SNIP, and VC in patients with DMD and Becker muscular dystrophy (BMD), between 5 and 20 years old. In patients with DMD, MIP remained stable, while VC and SNIP decreased consistently after an initial increase; however, SNIP showed an earlier decline than VC (at 10.5 years versus 12.5 years, respectively) [87].

5. Evaluation of Sleep-Disordered Breathing in Patients with Neuromuscular Diseases

Polysomnography (PSG) complemented by capnography is the gold standard method for the assessment of sleepdisordered breathing in patients with neuromuscular diseases, and overnight PSG should be applied when available [14, 16, 20, 88]. The American Thoracic Society recommends annual evaluation of sleep disordered breathing in children with DMD, ideally using PSG with simultaneous measurement of CO_2 [16, 20]. However, in younger children with uncertain course of the disease or with rapid clinical deterioration or in patients with recurrent infections, sleep monitoring should be performed more frequently [16, 20, 88]. Nevertheless, and especially in cases where polysomnography is not available, other types of sleep studies such as cardiorespiratory polygraphy or pulse oximetry should be considered although these may not be sensitive enough to detect sleep-disordered breathing in NMDs [88, 89]. Indeed, although a "sagging" oximetry profile is a feature of sleep hypoventilation in patients with NMDs, short or mild episodes or hypoventilation might be missed by overnight pulse oximetry; however, some authorities assert that clinical significant hypoventilation is unlikely in asymptomatic patients who do not desaturate below 93% [88, 90]. Nevertheless, according to several authors, a desaturation to a value <88% (or 90%) for 5 consecutive minutes or a desaturation to a value <90% for 10% (or 30%) of the total recording time might be indicators of sleep hypoventilation in neuromuscular patients [90–93]. The addition of capnography might increase the diagnostic sensitivity of oximetry and the use of oxicapnometry could be considered as a more practical approach for neuromuscular patients when polysomnography is not available [88, 94–96]. According to the American Academy of Sleep Medicine scoring rules, sleep hypoventilation in adults is defined as 1) an increase in PCO_2 (arterial, transcutaneous or end-tidal) to a value >55 mmHg for ≥10 minutes or (2) an increase in PCO_2 by >10 mmHg, to a value >50 mmHg for ≥10 minutes. In children, sleep hypoventilation is scored when PCO_2 exceeds 50 mmHg for >25% of total sleep time [97]. Some authors have employed alternative definitions of sleep hypoventilation, including a peak transcutaneous PCO_2 > 49 mmHg [93] or a mean transcutaneous PCO_2 > 50 mmHg [3, 15]. However, because various definitions are used for sleep hypoventilation [98], levels of CO_2 approaching 50 mmHg during sleep are suggestive of nocturnal hypoventilation and should indicate institution of nocturnal NIV [6, 16, 20, 88]. Apart from hypoventilation, the detection of upper airway obstructive events before or after the initiation of NIV might also be of prognostic significance in certain diseases, e.g. ALS [99, 100]. As a rule, initiation of NIV should not be delayed when abnormal findings on oxicapnography combined with morning signs of nocturnal hypoventilation are detected [88].

6. Respiratory Management of Patients with Neuromuscular Diseases

The aim of respiratory management of patients with NMDs is threefold: ventilatory support, cough augmentation, and lung volume recruitment. Ventilatory support assists the function of the feeble respiratory muscles and stabilizes gas exchange; cough augmentation improves cough flows and supports secretion clearance; and lung volume recruitment aims to avert functional decline as a result of atelectasis and chest wall contractures [76, 101].

Ventilatory support can be provided either via a noninvasive interface (e.g. nasal, oronasal mask or a mouthpiece) or invasively via a tracheostomy. Although, ventilatory support was initially applied in the form of negative pressure ventilation to treat patients with poliomyelitis in the 1950s, it is now most commonly administered in the form of positive pressure ventilation and is the treatment of choice for patients with NMDs and acute or chronic ventilatory failure [5, 6, 88, 91, 102].

The mechanisms which account for the beneficial effect of NIV on respiratory physiology of patients with NMDs remain unclear. Possible mechanisms include the unloading of the respiratory muscles, the resetting of the respiratory center and improvement in lung mechanics [103]. Nickol et al. suggested that the main benefit of NIV in restrictive lung diseases (kyphoscoliosis and neuromuscular diseases) is associated with the resetting of the chemoreceptors to a lower level of PCO_2, probably due to reduced renal retention of bicarbonates [104].

Many authorities suggest that NIV should be started in patients with symptoms of nocturnal hypoventilation (e.g. headache, fatigue, daytime sleepiness) plus abnormal findings in oximetry or capnometry (as discussed above). Other indications include a reduced VC (e.g. <50%), decreased respiratory muscle pressures (e.g. SNIP < 40 cm H_2O or MIP < 65 cm H_2O) or a daytime PCO_2 > 45 mmHg [16, 90–92, 105, 106].

It should be noted that tracheostomy ventilation used to be the standard treatment for patients with prolonged or total ventilator dependence and for those with impaired secretion clearance due to weak cough; however the combination of nasal or mouthpiece ventilation (MPV) with cough augmentation strategies has made this option obsolete for the majority of patients with NMDs, except for those with advanced bulbar disease [107–110].

NIV should be administered early during the course of the disease to treat patients with symptomatic sleep hypoventilation. In a randomized controlled trial, which compared NIV to supportive care in normocapnic patients with neuromuscular and chest wall disease and sleep hypoventilation, patients who did not receive NIV experienced faster deterioration, earlier establishment of daytime hypercapnia and more symptoms [3].

Several studies have suggested that NIV can prolong survival in patients with NMDs. A randomized controlled trial, in patients with ALS comparing NIV to supportive care, noted that NIV offered a survival advantage of 205 days, although this benefit was limited to nonbulbar patients. However, some indices of quality of life improved both in bulbar and nonbulbar patients [111]. In addition, a recent retrospective cohort study also observed an overall survival advantage of 15 months for both bulbar and nonbulbar patients with ALS who received treatment with NIV [112]. Simonds et al. conducted an observational study of 23 patients with DMD and diurnal and nocturnal ventilatory failure, who received NIV via nasal mask, and observed 1½ year survival rates of 73% and 85%, respectively [113]. A retrospective study in the total populations of DMD patients in Denmark reported a decrease in mortality from 4.7% to 2.6% per 100 years between 1977 and 2001, which was attributed to an increase in the use of mechanical ventilation from 0.9% to 43.4% during the same period [114].

Institution of NIV in patients with NMDs also improves daytime symptoms, quality of life and parameters of gas exchange. In a prospective observational study of ALS patients treated with NIV for 1 month, nocturnal oxygen and carbon dioxide improved in both bulbar and nonbulbar patients, while sleep quality and electroencephalographic indices of sleep fragmentation improved only in the nonbulbar subgroup [115]. An improvement in sleep and respiratory outcomes which persisted for 15 months was also noted in a retrospective study of bulbar and nonbulbar ALS patients treated with NIV [116]. In the study by Simonds et al., institution of NIV in patients with DMD was associated with an improvement in arterial blood gas values, which persisted throughout the treatment period, while the quality of life was equivalent to other groups of patients with nonprogressive respiratory disorders also treated with NIV [113]. Similarly, in patients with spinal muscular atrophy, NIV normalized sleep architecture and improved respiratory parameters, as well as symptoms of sleep-disordered breathing [117, 118]. In a study of 20 patients with various NMDs, application of NIV was associated with amelioration of the respiratory disturbance index, oxygen saturation, and transcutaneous PCO_2 as well as indices of daytime sleepiness, as Epworth Sleepiness Scale and Multiple Sleep Latency Test [119].

In the majority of the aforementioned studies [115–119] NIV titration was performed based on sleep oximetric or polysomnographic readings, while relatively low-span bilevel settings (<18 cm H_2O) were used. However, other authors have criticized this strategy as inadequate to effect complete respiratory muscle rest. These experts prefer the term "noninvasive ventilatory support (NVS)" to emphasize the role of this modality in substituting the respiratory muscles in the work of breathing [5, 6]. Their alternative approach does not employ sleep studies (e.g. polysomnography) for NIV initiation and titration. In fact, it consists of initially implementing NVS during sleep based on reduced supine VC and symptoms of sleep hypoventilation (fatigue, morning headaches, somnolence etc) using either tidal volumes at the range of 0.8–1.5 L in the volume-preset mode or high-span drive pressures

(18–25 cm H_2O) in pressure-preset modes with a back-up respiratory rate commonly set to 12–14 breaths/minute; single limb circuits with true exhalation valves and nasal or oronasal or lipcover interfaces are commonly used. NVS is subsequently applied most of the day during wakefulness when the patient develops symptoms of breathlessness most commonly in volume-preset mode with an angled 15 mm mouthpiece used as interface. This set up allows the patient vary the inhaled tidal volume according to his needs and air-stack ad lib. Nasal masks can be alternatively used for patients with weak mouth muscles who are unable to grab the mouthpiece, while pressure-preset modes can be employed for patients who are unable to air-stack (e.g. infants). This approach is complemented by advanced secretion management strategies i.e., air-stacking and mechanical insufflation exsufflation (MI-E) and also incorporates specifically designed protocols to decannulate tracheostomized patients to 24-hour full ventilatory support [5,6]. According to these protocols, an assisted PECF > 160 L/min effected by a combination of MI-E and abdominal thrust is associated with a very high rate of tracheostomy decannulation success [110, 120].

The aim of the NVS strategy is to avert the use of invasive tubes (tracheostomies), improve survival rates and quality of life and reduce the number of hospital admissions [5, 6, 121]. Thus, in a study reporting on postpolio survivors, MPV was used for 1.028 patient-years (or 14.8 years per patient) for a total mortality of 1 per 60.5 patient-years [122]. In addition, a study on DMD patients under treatment with continuous NVS and mechanically assisted coughing plus cardiac interventions, observed a 50% survival rate of 39.6 months for the continuous NVS group versus 18.1 and 28.9 months for historical patients treated with supplemental oxygen or tracheostomy, respectively [61]. Last, in a study reporting on the use of MPV in 42 final stage DMD patients, 51% of the patients were alive at 7 years post implementation and 50% survived to a mean age of 31 [123]. In addition, the application of continuous NVS plus MI-E to children with SMA 1 was associated with improved survival (sometimes surpassing 20 years of age) and better quality of life for both patients and caregivers [124, 125]. Other authors have also reported on patients with ALS without symptoms of airway spasticity who have been using continuous NVS for many years before tracheostomy [6]. Moreover, in a study by Tzeng and Bach which included neuromuscular patients with PECF of less than 270 L/min or at least 1 episode of respiratory decompensation, the combination of NVS with cough augmentation techniques was associated with a significant reduction in total admissions and the duration in hospital stay due to respiratory exacerbations [68].

For neuromuscular patients with weak cough and reduced cough flows, various cough augmentation strategies should be employed. These techniques could assist either the inspiratory or the expulsive cough phase or both. The former consist of various breath-stacking or lung insufflation maneuvers (see above), while the later consist of manual abdomen or thoracic compression maneuvers [75]. Manually assisted cough with or without breath-stacking or lung insufflation maneuvers should be taught in all patients with PECF < 270/L/min. For patients with PECF < 160/L/min, the use of mechanical insufflation-exsufflation (MI-E) which augments both inspiratory and expulsive cough phases, should be considered [92, 105, 106, 126, 127].

Lung volume recruitment employs the same lung insufflation strategies used for cough augmentation and in fact these two strategies complement each other. Lung volume recruitment is based on achieving maximal lung inflation either with the use of air-stacking techniques or with a MI-E device [76, 128]. Standard lung volume recruitment sessions consist of performing 3–5 (or even more) lung inflation maneuvers twice daily [76, 128]. In cohort of 282 patients with various NMDs, lung volume recruitment applied over several years resulted in increased MIC and LIC, despite a decrease in VC, indicating a higher number of recruitable lung units [76]. In a study including 151 patients with DMD, lung volume recruitment delayed the maximal VC decline by at least 5 years compared to previously reported series [129]. In addition, in a retrospective study of 16 individuals with DMD followed over a median of 6 years, the prescription of lung volume recruitment decreased the rate of VC decline from 4.5% predicted/year to 0.5% predicted/year [128]. McKim et al. also reported retrospectively an 89% decrease in VC decline over a period of 78 months follow-up in 22 DMD patients who were prescribed lung volume recruitment sessions [130]. In another retrospective study on a mixed population of 21 patients with NMDs, the regular use of the MI-E device resulted in improvement in VC by 28% during the first year and stabilization during the second year [131].

In the case of acute respiratory failure (ARF) in patients with NMD, NIV, and aggressive secretion management with MI-E should be introduced. Importantly, NIV should be considered in patients with NMDs who present with an acute illness and exhibit tachypnea (respiratory rate >20/min), even if hypercapnia is absent, especially in those with a known VC < 1 L [132, 133]. Adequate hydration should be ensured and the clinician should have a low threshold for administering antibiotics, particularly when there is high probability of an underlying chest infection [134]. The role of NIV combined with MI-E has been investigated in a prospective non-controlled study involving 16 children with NMDs and acute respiratory failure treated in a pediatric intensive care unit [135]. Hypercapnic respiratory failure was present in 15 cases (mean $PaCO_2$ 73.2 mmHg), whereas one had experienced hypoxemic ARF. NIV and MI-E were successfully delivered in 12 cases (75%) with a significant drop in $PaCO_2$ levels (>20 mmHg). Interestingly, all patients, including those who were invasively ventilated after intubation, were discharged from the hospital without the need for tracheostomy [135]. Nevertheless, failure of NIV and secretion management strategies (e.g. in the case of severe upper airway obstruction, cranio-facial abnormalities, or coma) should not delay early initiation of invasive ventilation.

7. Conclusions

Patients with neuromuscular diseases are at high risk for respiratory complications during the course of their disease. Early recognition of respiratory impairment is vital and a multidisciplinary approach should be adopted in order to provide the best optimal treatment. Noninvasive positive pressure ventilation and advanced cough management strategies are currently the standard of care in neuromuscular diseases as they improve survival, sleep, and quality of life.

References

[1] J. O. Benditt, "The neuromuscular respiratory system: physiology, pathophysiology, and a respiratory care approach to patients," *Respiratory Care*, vol. 51, no. 8, pp. 829–837, 2006, Discussion 837-839.

[2] A. K. Simonds, "NIV and neuromuscular disease," *Noninvasive Ventilation*, vol. 41, pp. 224–239, European Respiratory Society, 2008.

[3] S. Ward, M. Chatwin, S. Heather, and A. K. Simonds, "Randomised controlled trial of noninvasive ventilation (NIV) for nocturnal hypoventilation in neuromuscular and chest wall disease patients with daytime normocapnia," *Thorax*, vol. 60, no. 12, pp. 1019–1024, 2005.

[4] L. F. Wolfe, N. C. Joyce, C. M. McDonald, J. O. Benditt, and J. Finder, "Management of pulmonary complications in neuromuscular disease," *Physical Medicine and Rehabilitation Clinics of North America*, vol. 23, no. 4, pp. 829–853, 2012.

[5] J. R. Bach, "Noninvasive positive pressure ventilatory support begins during sleep," *Sleep Medicine Clinics*, vol. 12, no. 4, pp. 607–615, 2017.

[6] J. R. Bach, "Noninvasive respiratory management of patients with neuromuscular disease," *Annals of Rehabilitation Medicine*, vol. 41, no. 4, pp. 519–538, 2017.

[7] C. M. McDonald, "Clinical approach to the diagnostic evaluation of hereditary and acquired neuromuscular diseases," *Physical Medicine and Rehabilitation Clinics of North America*, vol. 23, no. 3, pp. 495–563, 2012.

[8] N. Ambrosino, N. Carpenè, and M. Gherardi, "Chronic respiratory care for neuromuscular diseases in adults," *European Respiratory Journal*, vol. 34, no. 2, pp. 444–451, 2009.

[9] A. E. Emery, "Population frequencies of inherited neuromuscular diseases–a world survey," *Neuromuscular Diseases*, vol. 1, no. 1, pp. 19–29, 1991.

[10] J. C. Deenen, C. G. Horlings, J. J. Verschuuren, and A. L. Verbeek, B. G. Van Engelen, "The epidemiology of neuromuscular diseases: a comprehensive overview of the literature," *Journal of Neuromuscular Diseases*, vol. 2, no. 1, pp. 73–85, 2015.

[11] S. J. Lloyd-Owen, G. C. Donaldson, N. Ambrosino et al., "Patterns of home mechanical ventilation use in Europe: results from the Eurovent survey," *European Respiratory Journal*, vol. 25, no. 6, pp. 1025–1031, 2005.

[12] R. S. Howard, C. M. Wiles, N. P. Hirsch, and G. T. Spencer, "Respiratory involvement in primary muscle disorders: assessment and management," *QJM: An International Journal of Medicine*, vol. 86, no. 3, pp. 175–189, 1993.

[13] C. Perrin, J. N. Unterborn, C. D. Ambrosio, and N. S. Hill, "Pulmonary complications of chronic neuromuscular diseases and their management," *Muscle & Nerve*, vol. 29, no. 1, pp. 5–27, 2004.

[14] C. H. Wang, R. S. Finkel, E. S. Bertini et al., "Consensus statement for standard of care in spinal muscular atrophy," *Journal of Child Neurology*, vol. 22, no. 8, pp. 1027–1049, 2007.

[15] A. K. Simonds, "Chronic hypoventilation and its management," *European Respiratory Review*, vol. 22, no. 129, pp. 325–332, 2013.

[16] J. D. Finder, D. Birnkrant, J. Carl et al., "Respiratory care of the patient with Duchenne muscular dystrophy: ATS consensus statement," *American Journal of Respiratory and Critical Care Medicine*, vol. 170, no. 4, pp. 456–465, 2004.

[17] E. C. Rosenow and A. G. Engel, "Acid maltase deficiency in adults presenting as respiratory failure," *The American Journal of Medicine*, vol. 64, no. 3, pp. 485–491, 1978.

[18] B. Al-Shaikh, W. Kinnear, T. W. Higenbottam, H. S. Smith, J. M. Shneerson, and I. Wilkinson, "Motor neurone disease presenting as respiratory failure," *British Medical Journal (Clinical Research Ed.)*, vol. 292, no. 6531, pp. 1325–1326, 1986.

[19] A. E. H. Emery, "The muscular dystrophies," *Lancet*, vol. 359, no. 9307, pp. 687–695, 2002.

[20] J. D. Finder, "A 2009 perspective on the 2004 American Thoracic Society statement, respiratory care of the patient with Duchenne muscular dystrophy," *Pediatrics*, vol. 123, 4, pp. S239–S241, 2009.

[21] W. D. Arnold, D. Kassar, and J. T. Kissel, "Spinal muscular atrophy: diagnosis and management in a new therapeutic era," *Muscle & Nerve*, vol. 51, no. 2, pp. 157–167, 2015.

[22] A. Modoni, G. Silvestri, M. G. Vita, D. Quaranta, P. A. Tonali, and C. Marra, "Cognitive impairment in myotonic dystrophy type 1 (DM1): a longitudinal follow-up study," *Journal of Neurology*, vol. 255, no. 11, pp. 1737–1742, 2008.

[23] D. Hilton-Jones, "Myotonic dystrophy–forgotten aspects of an often neglected condition," *Current Opinion in Neurology*, vol. 10, no. 5, pp. 399–401, 1997.

[24] C. Roussos and S. Zakynthinos, "Fatigue of the respiratory muscles," *Intensive Care Medicine*, vol. 22, no. 2, pp. 134–155, 1996.

[25] M. J. Tobin, W. Perez, S. M. Guenther et al., "The pattern of breathing during successful and unsuccessful trials of weaning from mechanical ventilation," *American Review of Respiratory Disease*, vol. 134, no. 6, pp. 1111–1118, 1986.

[26] J. O. Benditt, "Management of pulmonary complications in neuromuscular disease," *Physical Medicine and Rehabilitation Clinics of North America*, vol. 9, no. 1, pp. 167–185, 1998.

[27] M. Eikermann, F. M. Vogt, F. Herbstreit et al., "The predisposition to inspiratory upper airway collapse during partial neuromuscular blockade," *American Journal of Respiratory and Critical Care Medicine*, vol. 175, no. 1, pp. 9–15, 2007.

[28] B. Fauroux and S. Khirani, "Neuromuscular disease and respiratory physiology in children: putting lung function into perspective," *Respirology*, vol. 19, no. 6, pp. 782–791, 2014.

[29] L. T. Mulreany, D. J. Weiner, J. M. McDonough, H. B. Panitch, and J. L. Allen, "Noninvasive measurement of the tension-time index in children with neuromuscular disease," *Journal of Applied Physiology*, vol. 95, no. 3, pp. 931–937, 2003.

[30] F. D. McCool and D. E. Leith, "Pathophysiology of cough," *Clinics in Chest Medicine*, vol. 8, no. 2, pp. 189–195, 1987.

[31] J. M. Poponick, I. Jacobs, G. Supinski, and A. F. DiMarco, "Effect of upper respiratory tract infection in patients with

neuromuscular disease," *American Journal of Respiratory and Critical Care Medicine*, vol. 156, no. 2, pp. 659–664, 1997.

[32] G. A. Gould, M. Gugger, J. Molloy, V. Tsara, C. M. Shapiro, and N. J. Douglas, "Breathing pattern and eye movement density during REM sleep in humans," *American Review of Respiratory Disease*, vol. 138, no. 4, pp. 874–877, 1988.

[33] N. J. Douglas, D. P. White, J. V. Weil et al., "Hypoxic ventilatory response decreases during sleep in normal men," *The American Review of Respiratory Disease*, vol. 125, no. 3, pp. 286–289, 1982.

[34] N. J. Douglas, D. P. White, J. V. Weil, C. K. Pickett, and C. W. Zwillich, "Hypercapnic ventilatory response in sleeping adults," *The American Review of Respiratory Disease*, vol. 126, no. 5, pp. 758–762, 1982.

[35] V. Malik, D. Smith, and T. Lee-Chiong, "Respiratory physiology during sleep," *Sleep Medicine Clinics*, vol. 7, no. 3, pp. 497–505, 2012.

[36] D. W. Hudgel and P. Devadatta, "Decrease in functional residual capacity during sleep in normal humans," *Journal of Applied Physiology*, vol. 57, no. 5, pp. 1319–1322, 1984.

[37] E. Tabachnik, N. L. Muller, A. C. Bryan, and H. Levison, "Changes in ventilation and chest wall mechanics during sleep in normal adolescents," *Journal of Applied Physiology*, vol. 51, no. 3, pp. 557–564, 1981.

[38] A. Kay, J. Trinder, and Y. Kim, "Progressive changes in airway resistance during sleep," *Journal of Applied Physiology*, vol. 81, no. 1, pp. 282–292, 1996.

[39] R. Ragette, U. Mellies, C. Schwake, T. Voit, and H. Teschler, "Patterns and predictors of sleep disordered breathing in primary myopathies," *Thorax*, vol. 57, no. 8, pp. 724–728, 2002.

[40] K. Rezania, F. D. Goldenberg, and S. White, "Neuromuscular diseases and acute respiratory failure: diagnosis and management," *Neurologic Clinics*, vol. 30, no. 1, pp. 161–185, 2012.

[41] J. M. Shneerson and A. K. Simonds, "Noninvasive ventilation for chest wall and neuromuscular diseases," *European Respiratory Journal*, vol. 20, no. 2, pp. 480–487, 2002.

[42] F. Barbé, M. A. Quera-Salva, C. McCann et al., "Sleep-related respiratory disturbances in patients with Duchenne muscular dystrophy," *European Respiratory Journal*, vol. 7, no. 8, pp. 1403–1408, 1994.

[43] Y. Khan and J. Z. Heckmatt, "Obstructive apnoeas in Duchenne muscular dystrophy," *Thorax*, vol. 49, no. 2, pp. 157–161, 1994.

[44] P. E. Smith, P. M. Calverley, and R. H. Edwards, "Hypoxemia during sleep in Duchenne muscular dystrophy," *American Review of Respiratory Disease*, vol. 137, no. 4, pp. 884–888, 1988.

[45] F. Cirignotta, S. Mondini, M. Zucconi et al., "Sleep-related breathing impairment in myotonic dystrophy," *Journal of Neurology*, vol. 235, no. 2, pp. 80–85, 1987.

[46] J. E. White, M. J. Drinnan, A. J. Smithson, C. J. Griffiths, and G. J. Gibson, "Respiratory muscle activity and oxygenation during sleep in patients with muscle weakness," *European Respiratory Journal*, vol. 8, no. 5, pp. 807–814, 1995.

[47] U. Mellies, R. Ragette, C. Schwake, M. Baethmann, T. Voit, and H. Teschler, "Sleep-disordered breathing and respiratory failure in acid maltase deficiency," *Neurology*, vol. 57, no. 7, pp. 1290–1295, 2001.

[48] C. Santos, A. Braghiroli, L. Mazzini, R. Pratesi, L. V. Oliveira, and G. Mora, "Sleep-related breathing disorders in amyotrophic lateral sclerosis," *Monaldi Archives for Chest Disease*, vol. 59, no. 2, pp. 160–165, 2003.

[49] K. A. Ferguson, M. J. Strong, D. Ahmad, and C. F. George, "Sleep-disordered breathing in amyotrophic lateral sclerosis," *Chest*, vol. 110, no. 3, pp. 664–669, 1996.

[50] M. Labanowski, W. Schmidt-Nowara, and C. Guilleminault, "Sleep and neuromuscular disease: frequency of sleep-disordered breathing in a neuromuscular disease clinic population," *Neurology*, vol. 47, no. 5, pp. 1173–1180, 1996.

[51] J. Lemay, F. Sériès, M. Sénéchal, B. Maranda, and F. Maltais, "Unusual respiratory manifestations in two young adults with Duchenne muscular dystrophy," *Canadian Respiratory Journal*, vol. 19, no. 1, pp. 37–40, 2012.

[52] A. Sankari, A. T. Bascom, S. Chowdhuri, and M. S. Badr, "Tetraplegia is a risk factor for central sleep apnea," *Journal of Applied Physiology*, vol. 116, no. 3, pp. 345–353, 2014.

[53] S. C. Bourke and G. J. Gibson, "Sleep and breathing in neuromuscular disease," *European Respiratory Journal*, vol. 19, no. 6, pp. 1194–1201, 2002.

[54] F. Laghi and M. J. Tobin, "Disorders of the respiratory muscles," *American Journal of Respiratory and Critical Care Medicine*, vol. 168, no. 1, pp. 10–48, 2003.

[55] C. Fromageot, F. Lofaso, D. Annane et al., "Supine fall in lung volumes in the assessment of diaphragmatic weakness in neuromuscular diseases," *Archives of Physical Medicine and Rehabilitation*, vol. 82, no. 1, pp. 123–128, 2001.

[56] L. S. Aboussouan, "Sleep-disordered breathing in neuromuscular disease," *American Journal of Respiratory and Critical Care Medicine*, vol. 191, no. 9, pp. 979–989, 2015.

[57] A. Czaplinski, A. A. Yen, and S. H. Appel, "Forced vital capacity (FVC) as an indicator of survival and disease progression in an ALS clinic population," *Journal of Neurology, Neurosurgery & Psychiatry*, vol. 77, no. 3, pp. 390–392, 2006.

[58] E. P. Schmidt, D. B. Drachman, C. M. Wiener, L. Clawson, R. Kimball, and N. Lechtzin, "Pulmonary predictors of survival in amyotrophic lateral sclerosis: use in clinical trial design," *Muscle & Nerve*, vol. 33, no. 1, pp. 127–132, 2006.

[59] J. Gayraud, M. Ramonatxo, F. Rivier, V. Humberclaude, B. Petrof, and S. Matecki, "Ventilatory parameters and maximal respiratory pressure changes with age in Duchenne muscular dystrophy patients," *Pediatric Pulmonology*, vol. 45, no. 6, pp. 552–559, 2010.

[60] M. F. Phillips, R. C. Quinlivan, R. H. Edwards, and P. M. Calverley, "Changes in spirometry over time as a prognostic marker in patients with Duchenne muscular dystrophy," *American Journal of Respiratory and Critical Care Medicine*, vol. 164, no. 12, pp. 2191–2194, 2001.

[61] Y. Ishikawa, T. Miura, Y. Ishikawa et al., "Duchenne muscular dystrophy: survival by cardio-respiratory interventions," *Neuromuscular Diseases*, vol. 21, no. 1, pp. 47–51, 2011.

[62] C. Dohna-Schwake, R. Ragette, H. Teschler, T. Voit, and U. Mellies, "Predictors of severe chest infections in pediatric neuromuscular diseases," *Neuromuscular Diseases*, vol. 16, no. 5, pp. 325–328, 2006.

[63] R. A. Lyall, N. Donaldson, M. I. Polkey, P. N. Leigh, and J. Moxham, "Respiratory muscle strength and ventilatory failure in amyotrophic lateral sclerosis," *Brain Journal of Neurology*, vol. 124, no. 10, pp. 2000–2013, 2001.

[64] C. A. Hukins and D. R. Hillman, "Daytime predictors of sleep hypoventilation in Duchenne muscular dystrophy," *American Journal of Respiratory and Critical Care Medicine*, vol. 161, no. 1, pp. 166–170, 2000.

[65] S. T. Kulnik, V. MacBean, S. S. Birring, J. Moxham, G. F. Rafferty, and L. Kalra, "Accuracy of portable devices in measuring peak cough flow," *Physiological Measurement*, vol. 36, no. 2, pp. 243–257, 2015.

[66] E. K. Plowman, S. A. Watts, R. Robison et al., "Voluntary cough airflow differentiates safe versus unsafe swallowing in amyotrophic lateral sclerosis," *Dysphagia*, vol. 31, no. 3, pp. 383–390, 2016.

[67] J. R. Bach and L. R. Saporito, "Criteria for extubation and tracheostomy tube removal for patients with ventilatory failure. A different approach to weaning," *Chest*, vol. 110, no. 6, pp. 1566–1571, 1996.

[68] A. C. Tzeng and J. R. Bach, "Prevention of pulmonary morbidity for patients with neuromuscular disease," *Chest*, vol. 118, no. 5, pp. 1390–1396, 2000.

[69] J. Sancho, E. Servera, J. Díaz, and J. Marín, "Predictors of ineffective cough during a chest infection in patients with stable amyotrophic lateral sclerosis," *American Journal of Respiratory and Critical Care Medicine*, vol. 175, no. 12, pp. 1266–1271, 2007.

[70] J. R. Bach, Y. Ishikawa, and H. Kim, "Prevention of pulmonary morbidity for patients with Duchenne muscular dystrophy," *Chest*, vol. 112, no. 4, pp. 1024–1028, 1997.

[71] L. J. Boitano, "Management of airway clearance in neuromuscular disease," *Respiratory Care*, vol. 51, no. 8, pp. 913–922, 2006.Discussion 922-924

[72] S. W. Kang and J. R. Bach, "Maximum insufflation capacity: vital capacity and cough flows in neuromuscular disease," *American Journal of Physical Medicine & Rehabilitation*, vol. 79, no. 3, pp. 222–227, 2000.

[73] M. I. Polkey, R. A. Lyall, M. Green, P. Nigel Leigh, and J. Moxham, "Expiratory muscle function in amyotrophic lateral sclerosis," *American Journal of Respiratory and Critical Care Medicine*, vol. 158, no. 3, pp. 734–741, 1998.

[74] M. B. Chaudri, C. Liu, R. Hubbard, D. Jefferson, and W. J. Kinnear, "Relationship between supramaximal flow during cough and mortality in motor neurone disease," *European Respiratory Journal*, vol. 19, no. 3, pp. 434–438, 2002.

[75] Y. Ishikawa and J. R. Bach, "Physical medicine respiratory muscle aids to avert respiratory complications of pediatric chest wall and vertebral deformity and muscle dysfunction," *European Journal of Physical and Rehabilitation Medicine*, vol. 46, no. 4, pp. 581–597, 2010.

[76] J. R. Bach, K. Mahajan, B. Lipa, L. Saporito, M. Goncalves, and E. Komaroff, "Lung insufflation capacity in neuromuscular disease," *American Journal of Physical Medicine & Rehabilitation*, vol. 87, no. 9, pp. 720–725, 2008.

[77] S. W. Kang and J. R. Bach, "Maximum insufflation capacity," *Chest*, vol. 118, no. 1, pp. 61–65, 2000.

[78] J. W. Fitting, "Volitional assessment of respiratory muscle strength," *Monaldi Archives for Chest Disease*, vol. 77, no. 1, pp. 19–22, 2012.

[79] U. Mellies, R. Ragette, C. Schwake, H. Boehm, T. Voit, and H. Teschler, "Daytime predictors of sleep disordered breathing in children and adolescents with neuromuscular diseases," *Neuromuscular Diseases*, vol. 13, no. 2, pp. 123–128, 2003.

[80] M. Toussaint, M. Steens, and P. Soudon, "Lung function accurately predicts hypercapnia in patients with Duchenne muscular dystrophy," *Chest*, vol. 131, no. 2, pp. 368–375, 2007.

[81] A. Hahn, J. R. Bach, A. Delaubier, A. Renardel-Irani, C. Guillou, and Y. Rideau, "Clinical implications of maximal respiratory pressure determinations for individuals with Duchenne muscular dystrophy," *Archives of Physical Medicine and Rehabilitation*, vol. 78, no. 1, pp. 1–6, 1997.

[82] R. M. Kravitz, "Airway clearance in Duchenne muscular dystrophy," *Pediatrics*, vol. 123, 4, pp. S231–S235, 2009.

[83] F. Lofaso, F. Nicot, M. Lejaille et al., "Sniff nasal inspiratory pressure: what is the optimal number of sniffs?," *European Respiratory Journal*, vol. 27, no. 5, pp. 980–982, 2006.

[84] M. B. Chaudri, C. Liu, L. Watson, D. Jefferson, and W. J. Kinnear, "Sniff nasal inspiratory pressure as a marker of respiratory function in motor neuron disease," *European Respiratory Journal*, vol. 15, no. 3, pp. 539–542, 2000.

[85] R. K. Morgan, S. McNally, M. Alexander, R. Conroy, O. Hardiman, and R. W. Costello, "Use of Sniff nasal-inspiratory force to predict survival in amyotrophic lateral sclerosis," *American Journal of Respiratory and Critical Care Medicine*, vol. 171, no. 3, pp. 269–274, 2005.

[86] R. Capozzo, V. N. Quaranta, F. Pellegrini et al., "Sniff nasal inspiratory pressure as a prognostic factor of tracheostomy or death in amyotrophic lateral sclerosis," *Journal of Neurology*, vol. 262, no. 3, pp. 593–603, 2015.

[87] V. Nève, J.-M. Cuisset, J.-L. Edmé et al., "Sniff nasal inspiratory pressure in the longitudinal assessment of young Duchenne muscular dystrophy children," *European Respiratory Journal*, vol. 42, no. 3, pp. 671–680, 2013.

[88] J. Hull, R. Aniapravan, E. Chan et al., "British Thoracic Society guideline for respiratory management of children with neuromuscular weakness," *Thorax*, vol. 67, 1pp. i1–i40, 2012.

[89] R. B. Berry, A. Chediak, L. K. Brown et al., "Best clinical practices for the sleep center adjustment of noninvasive positive pressure ventilation (NPPV) in stable chronic alveolar hypoventilation syndromes," *Journal of Clinical Sleep Medicine*, vol. 6, no. 5, pp. 491–509, 2010.

[90] M. Boentert, H. Prigent, K. Várdi et al., "Practical recommendations for diagnosis and management of respiratory muscle weakness in late-onset pompe disease," *International Journal of Molecular Sciences*, vol. 17, no. 10, p. 1735, 2016.

[91] PlumX Metrics, "Clinical indications for noninvasive positive pressure ventilation in chronic respiratory failure due to restrictive lung disease, COPD, and nocturnal hypoventilation—a consensus conference report," *Chest*, vol. 116, no. 2, pp. 521–534, 1999.

[92] V. A. Sansone, C. Gagnon, and Participants of the 207th ENMC Workshop, "207th ENMC Workshop on chronic respiratory insufficiency in myotonic dystrophies: management and implications for research, 27–29 June 2014, Naarden, The Netherlands," *Neuromuscular Diseases*, vol. 25, no. 5, pp. 432–442, 2015.

[93] M. M. Grigg-Damberger, L. K. Wagner, and L. K. Brown, "Sleep hypoventilation in patients with neuromuscular diseases," *Sleep Medicine Clinics*, vol. 7, no. 4, pp. 667–687, 2012.

[94] J. Nardi, H. Prigent, A. Adala et al., "Nocturnal oximetry and transcutaneous carbon dioxide in home-ventilated neuromuscular patients," *Respiratory Care*, vol. 57, no. 9, pp. 1425–1430, 2012.

[95] K. A. Bauman, A. Kurili, S. L. Schmidt, G. M. Rodriguez, A. E. Chiodo, and R. G. Sitrin, "Home-based overnight transcutaneous capnography/pulse oximetry for diagnosing nocturnal hypoventilation associated with neuromuscular diseases," *Archives of Physical Medicine and Rehabilitation*, vol. 94, no. 1, pp. 46–52, 2013.

[96] K. A. Bauman, A. Kurili, H. M. Schotland, G. M. Rodriguez, A. E. Chiodo, and R. G. Sitrin, "Simplified approach to diagnosing sleep-disordered breathing and nocturnal hypercapnia in individuals with spinal cord injury," *Archives of Physical Medicine and Rehabilitation*, vol. 97, no. 3, pp. 363–371, 2016.

[97] R. B. Berry, R. Budhiraja, D. J. Gottlieb et al., "Rules for scoring respiratory events in sleep: update of the 2007 AASM manual for the scoring of sleep and associated events. Deliberations of the sleep apnea definitions task force of the American Academy of Sleep Medicine," *Journal of Clinical Sleep Medicine*, vol. 8, no. 5, pp. 597–619, 2012.

[98] A. Ogna, M.-A. Quera Salva, H. Prigent et al., "Nocturnal hypoventilation in neuromuscular disease: prevalence according to different definitions issued from the literature," *Sleep and Breathing*, vol. 20, no. 2, pp. 575–581, 2016.

[99] M. Georges, V. Attali, J. L. Golmard et al., "Reduced survival in patients with ALS with upper airway obstructive events on noninvasive ventilation," *Journal of Neurology, Neurosurgery & Psychiatry*, vol. 87, no. 10, pp. 1045–1050, 2016.

[100] V. N. Quaranta, P. Carratù, M. F. Damiani et al., "The prognostic role of obstructive sleep apnea at the onset of amyotrophic lateral sclerosis," *Neurodegenerative Diseases*, vol. 17, no. 1, pp. 14–21, 2017.

[101] Y. Molgat-Seon, L. M. Hannan, P. B. Dominelli et al., "Lung volume recruitment acutely increases respiratory system compliance in individuals with severe respiratory muscle weakness," *ERJ Open Research*, vol. 3, no. 1, p. 00135, 2017.

[102] D. R. Hess, "The growing role of noninvasive ventilation in patients requiring prolonged mechanical ventilation," *Respiratory Care*, vol. 57, no. 6, pp. 900–918, 2012, Discussion 918-920.

[103] N. S. Hill, "Noninvasive ventilation. Does it work, for whom, and how?," *American Review of Respiratory Disease*, vol. 147, no. 4, pp. 1050–1055, 1993.

[104] A. H. Nickol, N. Hart, N. S. Hopkinson, J. Moxham, A. Simonds, and M. I. Polkey, "Mechanisms of improvement of respiratory failure in patients with restrictive thoracic disease treated with noninvasive ventilation," *Thorax*, vol. 60, no. 9, pp. 754–760, 2005.

[105] EFNS Task Force on Diagnosis and Management of Amyotrophic Lateral Sclerosis, P. M. Andersen, S. Abrahams et al., "EFNS guidelines on the clinical management of amyotrophic lateral sclerosis (MALS)—revised report of an EFNS task force," *European Journal of Neurology*, vol. 19, no. 3, pp. 360–375, 2012.

[106] D. A. McKim, J. Road, M. Avendano et al., "Home mechanical ventilation: a Canadian Thoracic Society clinical practice guideline," *Canadian Respiratory Journal*, vol. 18, no. 4, pp. 197–215, 2011.

[107] "International consensus conferences in intensive care medicine: noninvasive positive pressure ventilation in acute respiratory failure," *American Journal of Respiratory and Critical Care Medicine*, vol. 163, no. 1, pp. 283–291, 2001.

[108] M. Agrafiotis, K. Nikolaou, D. Siopi, and D. Chloros, "Open-circuit mouthpiece ventilation: indications, evidence and practicalities," *Noninvasive Ventilation in Medicine—Recent Updates*, IntechOpen, 2018.

[109] J. R. Bach, A. S. Alba, and L. R. Saporito, "Intermittent positive pressure ventilation via the mouth as an alternative to tracheostomy for 257 ventilator users," *Chest*, vol. 103, no. 1, pp. 174–182, 1993.

[110] J. R. Bach, M. R. Gonçalves, I. Hamdani, and J. C. Winck, "Extubation of patients with neuromuscular weakness: a new management paradigm," *Chest*, vol. 137, no. 5, pp. 1033–1039, 2010.

[111] S. C. Bourke, M. Tomlinson, T. L. Williams, R. E. Bullock, P. J. Shaw, and G. J. Gibson, "Effects of noninvasive ventilation on survival and quality of life in patients with amyotrophic lateral sclerosis: a randomised controlled trial," *The Lancet Neurology*, vol. 5, no. 2, pp. 140–147, 2006.

[112] D. J. Berlowitz, M. E. Howard, J. F. Fiore et al., "Identifying who will benefit from non-invasive ventilation in amyotrophic lateral sclerosis/motor neurone disease in a clinical cohort," *Journal of Neurology, Neurosurgery & Psychiatry*, vol. 87, no. 3, pp. 280–286, 2016.

[113] A. K. Simonds, F. Muntoni, S. Heather, and S. Fielding, "Impact of nasal ventilation on survival in hypercapnic Duchenne muscular dystrophy," *Thorax*, vol. 53, no. 11, pp. 949–952, 1998.

[114] J. Jeppesen, A. Green, B. F. Steffensen, and J. Rahbek, "The Duchenne muscular dystrophy population in Denmark, 1977–2001: prevalence, incidence and survival in relation to the introduction of ventilator use," *Neuromuscular Diseases*, vol. 13, no. 10, pp. 804–812, 2003.

[115] B. Vrijsen, B. Buyse, C. Belge et al., "Noninvasive ventilation improves sleep in amyotrophic lateral sclerosis: a prospective polysomnographic study," *Journal of Clinical Sleep Medicine*, vol. 11, no. 5, pp. 559–566, 2015.

[116] M. Boentert, I. Brenscheidt, C. Glatz, and P. Young, "Effects of noninvasive ventilation on objective sleep and nocturnal respiration in patients with amyotrophic lateral sclerosis," *Journal of Neurology*, vol. 262, no. 9, pp. 2073–2082, 2015.

[117] U. Mellies, C. Dohna-Schwake, F. Stehling, and T. Voit, "Sleep disordered breathing in spinal muscular atrophy," *Neuromuscular Diseases*, vol. 14, no. 12, pp. 797–803, 2004.

[118] A. Petrone, M. Pavone, M. B. C. Testa, F. Petreschi, E. Bertini, and R. Cutrera, "Noninvasive ventilation in children with spinal muscular atrophy types 1 and 2," *American Journal of Physical Medicine & Rehabilitation*, vol. 86, no. 3, pp. 216–221, 2007.

[119] C. Guilleminault, P. Philip, and A. Robinson, "Sleep and neuromuscular disease: bilevel positive airway pressure by nasal mask as a treatment for sleep disordered breathing in patients with neuromuscular disease," *Journal of Neurology, Neurosurgery & Psychiatry*, vol. 65, no. 2, pp. 225–232, 1998.

[120] J. R. Bach, L. R. Saporito, H. R. Shah, and D. Sinquee, "Decanulation of patients with severe respiratory muscle insufficiency: efficacy of mechanical insufflation-exsufflation," *Journal of Rehabilitation Medicine*, vol. 46, no. 10, pp. 1037–1041, 2014.

[121] J. R. Bach, M. R. Gonçalves, A. Hon et al., "Changing trends in the management of end-stage neuromuscular respiratory muscle failure: recommendations of an international consensus," *American Journal of Physical Medicine & Rehabilitation*, vol. 92, no. 3, pp. 267–277, 2013.

[122] J. R. Bach, A. S. Alba, G. Bohatiuk, L. Saporito, and M. Lee, "Mouth intermittent positive pressure ventilation in the management of postpolio respiratory insufficiency," *Chest*, vol. 91, no. 6, pp. 859–864, 1987.

[123] M. Toussaint, M. Steens, G. Wasteels, and P. Soudon, "Diurnal ventilation via mouthpiece: survival in end-stage Duchenne patients," *European Respiratory Journal*, vol. 28, no. 3, pp. 549–555, 2006.

[124] J. R. Bach, V. Niranjan, and B. Weaver, "Spinal muscular atrophy type 1: a noninvasive respiratory management approach," *Chest*, vol. 117, no. 4, pp. 1100–1105, 2000.

[125] J. R. Bach, "POINT: Is noninvasive ventilation always the most appropriate manner of long-term ventilation for infants with spinal muscular atrophy type 1? yes, almost always," *Chest*, vol. 151, no. 5, pp. 962–965, 2017.

[126] M. Toussaint, M. Chatwin, J. Gonzales, D. J. Berlowitz, and ENMC Respiratory Therapy Consortium, "228th ENMC International Workshop: Airway clearance techniques in neuromuscular diseases Naarden, The Netherlands, 3–5 March, 2017," *Neuromuscular Diseases*, vol. 28, no. 3, pp. 289–298, 2018.

[127] M. Chatwin, M. Toussaint, M. R. Gonçalves et al., "Airway clearance techniques in neuromuscular diseases: a state of the art review," *Respiratory Medicine*, vol. 136, pp. 98–110, 2018.

[128] S. L. Katz, N. Barrowman, A. Monsour, S. Su, L. Hoey, and D. McKim, "Long-term effects of lung volume recruitment on maximal inspiratory capacity and vital capacity in Duchenne muscular dystrophy," *Annals of the American Thoracic Society*, vol. 13, no. 2, pp. 217–222, 2016.

[129] M. Chiou, J. R. Bach, L. Jethani, and M. F. Gallagher, "Active lung volume recruitment to preserve vital capacity in Duchenne muscular dystrophy," *Journal of Rehabilitation Medicine*, vol. 49, no. 1, pp. 49–53, 2017.

[130] D. A. McKim, S. L. Katz, N. Barrowman, A. Ni, and C. LeBlanc, "Lung volume recruitment slows pulmonary function decline in Duchenne muscular dystrophy," *Archives of Physical Medicine and Rehabilitation*, vol. 93, no. 7, pp. 1117–1122, 2012.

[131] F. Stehling, A. Bouikidis, U. Schara, and U. Mellies, "Mechanical insufflation/exsufflation improves vital capacity in neuromuscular diseases," *Chronic Respiratory Disease*, vol. 12, no. 1, pp. 31–35, 2015.

[132] F. Racca, L. Del Sorbo, T. Mongini, A. Vianello, and V. M. Ranieri, "Respiratory management of acute respiratory failure in neuromuscular diseases," *Minerva Anestesiologica*, vol. 76, no. 1, pp. 51–62, 2010.

[133] A. C. Davidson, S. Banham, M. Elliott et al., "BTS/ICS guideline for the ventilatory management of acute hypercapnic respiratory failure in adults," *Thorax*, vol. 71, no. Suppl 2, pp. i1–i35, 2016.

[134] A. K. Simonds, "Ventilator support in children with neuromuscular diseases," *Caring for the Ventilator Dependent Child: A Clinical Guide*, L. M. Sterni and J. L. Carroll, Eds., pp. 283–298, Springer, New York, NY, 2016.

[135] T.-H. Chen, J.-H. Hsu, J.-R. Wu et al., "Combined noninvasive ventilation and mechanical in-exsufflator in the treatment of pediatric acute neuromuscular respiratory failure," *Pediatric Pulmonology*, vol. 49, no. 6, pp. 589–596, 2014.

4

Chronic Pulmonary Silicone Embolism from Breast Augmentation is not a Common Finding in Explanted Lungs

Jarmanjeet Singh,[1] **Hanine Inaty**,[2] **Sanjay Mukhopadhyay**,[3] **and Atul C. Mehta**[2]

[1]*Internal Medicine Residency Program, The Cleveland Clinic Foundation, Cleveland, OH, USA*
[2]*Respiratory Institute, The Cleveland Clinic Foundation, Cleveland, OH, USA*
[3]*Department of Pathology, The Cleveland Clinic Foundation, Cleveland, OH, USA*

Correspondence should be addressed to Atul C. Mehta; mehtaa1@ccf.org

Academic Editor: Roberto Walter Dal Negro

Objective. Acute pulmonary silicone embolism (APSE) related to subcutaneous silicone injections is a well-known entity. Recently, a few cases of pathologically confirmed chronic pulmonary silicone embolism (CPSE) from breast implants have been reported. The prevalence of CPSE in women with breast augmentation is unknown. This study was done to determine the prevalence of CPSE in female lung transplant recipients with a history of breast augmentation and to determine whether breast augmentation plays a role in chronic lung diseases requiring lung transplantation. *Methods.* A retrospective chart review was performed to identify female lung transplant recipients with a history of breast augmentation prior to or at the time of lung transplantation. Ten patients meeting these criteria were identified. The pathologic features of the explanted lungs of these patients were reexamined for CPSE by a board-certified pathologist with expertise in lung transplantation and pulmonary embolism. *Results.* Of 1518 lung transplant recipients at Cleveland Clinic, 578 were females. Of 578 females, 10 (1.73%) had history of breast augmentation. A total of 84 H&E-stained slides from the explanted lungs from 10 cases were examined. No pathologic evidence of chronic silicone embolism was seen in any of the 10 cases. *Conclusions.* CPSE is not associated with pulmonary disease leading to lung transplantation. Breast augmentation is not a significant contributor to pulmonary disease requiring lung transplantation. Further studies are required to ascertain the prevalence of CPSE in the general breast augmentation populace and to define the relationship between breast augmentation and pulmonary disease.

1. Introduction

The concept of breast implantation was introduced in the 18th century by Vincenz Czerny who used a lipoma for breast augmentation [1]. Since then, breast implantation has evolved considerably, and breast implants are composed of an outer elastomer shell of silicone and an inner filler, which can be either silicone gel or saline. Silicone used in breast implants is polydimethylsiloxane (PDMS) and is considered safe [2]. Acute pulmonary silicone embolism (APSE) from cosmetic silicone injections is well known to cause lung disease [3–8]. Recently, cases of chronic pulmonary silicone embolism (CPSE) related to silicone and saline breast implants causing dyspnea and pulmonary infiltrates have been reported [9–13] (Table 1). CPSE is embolization of silicone to the lungs in women with breast implantation but with no history of subcutaneous silicone injection. These cases made us wonder whether CPSE is an underrecognized contributor to chronic pulmonary ailments. This study was done to determine the prevalence of CPSE in female lung transplant recipients with a history of breast augmentation and to determine whether breast augmentation plays a role in chronic lung diseases requiring lung transplantation.

2. Methods

Medical records of the lung transplant population at Cleveland Clinic (July 1990–May 2016) were reviewed retrospectively to identify female lung transplant recipients who had undergone breast implantation prior to the

TABLE 1: Reported cases of chronic pulmonary silicone embolism from the breast implants.

Case	Age/sex	Symptoms	Radiographic finding on CT chest	Type of implant (silicone versus saline)	Histopathology (microscopic and energy-dispersive X-ray analysis, EDX$)
1	41/F	Dyspnea	Diffuse GGO*	Silicone	(i) Clear, nonbirefringent globules characteristic of silicone emboli (ii) EDX not performed
2	45/F	Dyspnea	Diffuse GGO	Saline	(i) Clear, nonbirefringent globules on microscopy (ii) Energy-dispersive X-ray microanalysis (EDX) showed silicone emboli
3	72/F	Dyspnea	Diffuse GGO and reticular opacities	Silicone	(i) Clear, nonbirefringent globules on microscopy (ii) Energy-dispersive X-ray microanalysis (EDX) showed silicone emboli
4	56/F	Chronic illness	Not available	Silicone	(i) Silicone plaques in the lungs on microscopy (ii) Energy-dispersive X-ray microanalysis (EDX) showed silicone emboli
5	59/F	Dyspnea	Diffuse pulmonary infiltrates and consolidations	Double lumen prosthesis (cohesive gel and saline solution)	(i) Translucent vacuolated globular deposits of silicone

*GGO: ground glass opacities; $EDX: energy-dispersive X-ray analysis.

lung transplantation. Data was gathered for the following variables: demographics, current status of patient (alive or deceased), smoking history, type of breast implant (saline or silicone), duration of breast augmentation prior to transplantation, history of implant rupture, unilateral versus bilateral lung transplantation, primary diagnosis leading to lung transplantation, radiologic and pathologic findings, and survival of candidate after transplantation.

2.1. Pathologic Examination. Histopathologic examination of explanted lungs was performed by a fellowship-trained pulmonary pathologist with expertise in pulmonary silicone embolism [10, 14]. Standard protocol including analysis of 3 sections (peripheral, mid, and central) of alveolated lung per lobe was used. Additional sections were taken if areas of special interest were identified on gross examination such as a nodule, cyst, and cavity. These sections were reexamined specifically for evidence of silicone embolization within pulmonary blood vessels.

3. Results

Of 1518 lung transplant recipients, 578 were females. Of these females, 10 (1.73%) had history of breast augmentation; 3 had silicone implants, 1 had saline implant, and, in 6, the type of implant could not be determined. The mean duration of breast implantation prior to lung transplantation was 29.25 years (4/10). 2 females had evidence of implant rupture on gross examination at the time of surgery. 8 were smokers with a mean of 34.4 pack-years and 2 were nonsmokers. Lung transplantation was unilateral in 7 and bilateral in 3. 8 had emphysema and 2 had bronchiectasis on chest CT. Indication for lung transplantation was chronic obstructive pulmonary disease in 7 patients, and cystic fibrosis, ciliary dyskinesia, and alpha-1 antitrypsin deficiency in one patient each. 4 patients were alive at the time of this study, with a mean age of 66.25 years (range: 59–77). The mean age at death was 52.2 years (range: 21–70). A total of 84 hematoxylin-eosin-stained slides from the explanted lungs (range: 3–23 slides per case; mean: 8.4) were examined for evidence of silicone emboli. None of the slides showed pathologic evidence of silicone embolism (Table 2).

4. Discussion

Reported pulmonary complications from silicone breast implants include silicone thorax [15, 16], pleural effusions [17], silicone-related complaints [18–20], siliconosis, autoimmune/inflammatory syndrome induced by adjuvants (ASIA) [21–23], and anaplastic large cell lymphoma [24, 25]. The presumed pathogenesis behind these complications is the inflammatory response elicited by migration of silicone particles into tissues [26]. Silicone particles and silicone-laden macrophages have been demonstrated at distant sites in affected individuals [12, 27, 28].

Prompted by safety concerns, a moratorium was placed on use of silicone breast implants in the United States between 1992 and 2006 [19]. After reapproval from the FDA in 2006, silicone implants regained their popularity. At present, breast implantation is the most common cosmetic surgery

TABLE 2: Radiographic and pathologic findings of the explanted lungs.

Case	Duration of breast implantation before lung transplant (in years)	Radiographic diagnosis before lung transplantation	Number of slides studied	Pathologic diagnosis	Evidence of breast implant rupture at the time of lung transplantation surgery	Silicone emboli in explanted lungs
1	Unknown	Bronchiectasis	9	Bronchiectasis	Not available	Absent
2	Unknown	Emphysema	6	Emphysema	Not available	Absent
3	25	Emphysema	5	Emphysema	Not available	Absent
4	Unknown	Emphysema	6	Emphysema	Not available	Absent
5	Unknown	Emphysema	8	Emphysema	Not available	Absent
6	Unknown	Emphysema	8	Emphysema	Not available	Absent
7	25	Emphysema	3	Emphysema	Intracapsular rupture	Absent
8	Unknown	Bronchiectasis	23	Bronchiectasis	Not available	Absent
9	30	Emphysema	9	Emphysema	Not available	Absent
10	35	Emphysema	7	Emphysema	Focal rupture	Absent

in the United States, with approximately 279,143 cosmetic and 106,338 reconstructive breast implantations performed in 2015 alone [29]. The recent discovery of CPSE related to breast implants has rekindled the controversy regarding the safety of breast augmentation.

Since both cosmetic silicone injections and breast implants contain PDMS, acute pulmonary silicone embolism from silicone injections can help us in understanding the disease spectrum of CPSE due to molecular similarity. Clinicopathological findings in APSE include congestion, pneumonitis, diffuse alveolar damage causing adult respiratory distress syndrome (ARDS), and death [3–8]. Schmid et al. showed that acute silicone embolism can have the same critical presentation as fat embolism with a mean Schonfeld score of 9 [8]. Therefore, CPSE also carries the potential of causing grave complications like acute respiratory failure and death. Fortunately, the reported cases of CPSE have presented as a chronic form of lung disease mimicking interstitial lung disease (ILD) [9–13].

In our study, we did not see any evidence of pulmonary silicone embolism from breast implants in the explanted lungs of the lung transplant recipients. Due to small sample size of 10 patients, we cannot entirely exclude the occurrence of CPSE in the studied population but the data is strongly convincing towards lack of association. Moreover, only 10 females (1.73%) had history of breast implantation among a total of 578 female lung transplant recipients, suggesting no significant association between the two. This lack of association does underline the rarity of CPSE.

To our knowledge, this is the first original study that has attempted to identify CPSE in women with breast implants by pathologic analysis of the explanted lungs. We acknowledge that female lung transplant recipients with breast augmentation constitute an extremely small fraction of the general population that undergoes breast augmentation. The absence of CPSE in this small sample should not be generalizable to regular breast implant recipients in general. However, the absence of CPSE in this large female lung transplant population at our hospital shows its rarity and insignificance in lung transplantation epidemiology. Nevertheless, pulmonologists should be aware of this rare but potentially grave complication and should consider CPSE in the differential of pulmonary pathology in patients with breast implants. Larger studies are required to ascertain the extent to which CPSE might cause occult or symptomatic lung disease not necessarily requiring lung transplantation in general breast implant population.

5. Summary/Conclusion

Our study did not show any evidence of CPSE in female lung transplant recipients who had undergone breast augmentation prior to lung transplantation. We conclude that breast augmentation is not a significant contributor to pulmonary diseases requiring lung transplantation. Based upon reported cases, CPSE can cause significant pulmonary morbidity. Further studies are required to determine the prevalence of CPSE in the general breast implant population and to define the relationship between breast augmentation, CPSE, and pulmonary diseases.

Disclosure

An abstract/poster from this study has been presented at (1) Fleischner Society (*Atul C. Mehta*, "Chronic Pulmonary Silicon Embolism from Breast Augmentation Is Not a Common Finding in Explanted Lungs"), 48th Annual Meeting of the Fleischner Society, Beverly, MA, June 15-16, 2017; (2) American Thoracic Society (*Jarmanjeet Singh, Hanine Inaty, Sanjay Mukhopadhyay,* and *Atul C. Mehta*, "Chronic Pulmonary Silicon Embolism from Breast Augmentation Is Not a Common Finding in Explanted Lungs"), American Journal of Respiratory and Critical Care Medicine 2017, 195:A3584. All the authors approve of this version to be final and ready for publication. All the authors are in agreement to be accountable for all aspects of the work ensuring that questions related to the accuracy or integrity of any part of the work are appropriately investigated and resolved.

Authors' Contributions

Jarmanjeet Singh, M.B.B.S., M.D., prepared research protocol, carried out data collection, and wrote the manuscript. Hanine Inaty, M.D., carried out data collection and took part in manuscript writing. Sanjay Mukhopadhyay, M.D., prepared research protocol, performed pathological specimen testing (board-certified pathologist), and took part in manuscript writing. Atul C. Mehta, M.B.B.S., F.C.C.P., and F.A.C.P., prepared research protocol, carried out data collection, took part in manuscript writing, and provided guidance and supervision.

References

[1] M. C. Champaneria, W. W. Wong, M. E. Hill, and S. C. Gupta, "The evolution of breast reconstruction: A historical perspective," *World Journal of Surgery*, vol. 36, no. 4, pp. 730–742, 2012.

[2] D. C. C. França, A. L. de Castro, A. M. P. Soubhia, S. M. H. C. Á. de Aguiar, and M. C. Goiato, "Evaluation of the biocompatibility of silicone gel implants - histomorphometric study," *Acta Informatica Medica*, vol. 21, no. 2, pp. 93–97, 2013.

[3] K. Y. Chung, S. H. Kim, I. H. Kwon et al., "Clinicopathologic review of pulmonary silicone embolism with special emphasis on the resultant histologic diversity in the lung—a review of five cases," *Yonsei Medical Journal*, vol. 43, no. 2, pp. 152–159, 2002.

[4] K. Lyapichev, F. M. Chinea, J. Poveda, J. Pereda, P. A. Bejarano, and M. T. Garcia-Buitrago, "Pulmonary empty spaces: silicone embolism—a decade of increased incidence and its histological diagnosis," *Case Reports in Pathology*, vol. 2016, Article ID 3741291, pp. 1–5, 2016.

[5] C. S. Restrepo, M. Artunduaga, J. A. Carrillo et al., "Silicone pulmonary embolism: report of 10 cases and review of the literature," *Journal of Computer Assisted Tomography*, vol. 33, no. 2, pp. 233–237, 2009.

[6] J. Chastre, P. Brun, and P. Soler, "Acute and latent pneumonitis after subcutaneous injections of silicone intranssexual men," *The American Review of Respiratory Disease*, vol. 135, no. 1, pp. 236–240, 1987.

[7] P. Gopie, S. Sakhamuri, A. Sharma, S. Solomon, and S. Teelucksingh, "Acute pneumonitis secondary to subcutaneous silicone injection," *Journal of General Internal Medicine*, vol. 4, pp. 477–479, 2011.

[8] A. Schmid, A. Tzur, L. Leshko, and B. P. Krieger, "Silicone embolism syndrome: a case report, review of the literature, and comparison with fat embolism syndrome," *CHEST*, vol. 127, no. 6, pp. 2276–2281, 2005.

[9] P. P. Gopinath, A. Ali, F. Van Tornout, A. Kamath, M. Crawford, and A. G. Nicholson, "Chronic silicone embolism syndrome due to PIP breast implant leakage - a new entity?" *Histopathology*, vol. 66, no. 6, pp. 904–906, 2015.

[10] A. Arora, H. Inaty, S. Mukhopadhyay, M. Abu-Hijleh, and A. C. Mehta, "Chronic pulmonary silicone embolism related to saline breast implants," *Annals of the American Thoracic Society*, vol. 13, no. 1, pp. 139–141, 2016.

[11] M. C. Bois, X. Hu, A. C. Roden, E. S. Yi, J. H. Ryu, and M. P. Alexander, "Increasing pulmonary infiltrates in a 72-year-old woman with metastatic breast cancer," *CHEST*, vol. 146, no. 6, pp. e208–e211, 2014.

[12] R. M. Kappel, L. L. Boer, and H. Dijkman, "Gel bleed and rupture of silicone breast implants investigated by light-, electron microscopy and energy dispersive X-ray analysis of internal organs and nervous tissue," *Clinical Medical Reviews and Case Reports*, vol. 3, no. 6, article 087, 2016.

[13] S. Paredes Vila, F. J. Gonzalez Barcala, J. Suarez Antelo, M. Moldes Rodriguez, I. Abdulkader Nallib, and L. Valdes Cuadrado, "Pneumonitis caused by silicone gel following breast implant rupture," *Irish Journal of Medical Science*, vol. 179, no. 1, pp. 141–145, 2010.

[14] S. Mukhopadhyay, *Non-Neoplastic Pulmonary Pathology: An Algorithmic Approach to Histologic Findings in the Lung*, Cambridge University Press, Cambridge, UK, 2016.

[15] R. L. Levine, T. C. Allen, J. Cartwright Jr., and P. T. Cagle, "Silicone thorax due to a ruptured breast implant," *CHEST*, vol. 127, no. 5, pp. 1854–1857, 2005.

[16] J. B. Sykes and P. A. Rosella, "Intrathoracic migration of a silicone breast implant 5 months after video-assisted thoracoscopic surgery," *Journal of Computer Assisted Tomography*, vol. 36, no. 3, pp. 306-307, 2012.

[17] I. H. Shaik, B. Gandrapu, F. Gonzalez-Ibarra, D. Flores, J. Matta, and A. K. Syed, "Silicone Breast Implants: A Rare Cause of Pleural Effusion," *Case Reports in Pulmonology*, vol. 2015, pp. 1–3, 2015.

[18] A. E. Brawer, "Bones, groans, and silicone.," *Lupus*, vol. 21, no. 11, pp. 1155–1157, 2012.

[19] A. K. Brawer, "Chronology of systemic disease development in 300 symptomatic recipients of silicone gel-filled breast implants," *ournal of Clean Technology, Environmental Toxicology and Occupational Medicine*, vol. 5, pp. 223–233, 1996.

[20] A. E. Brawer, "Silicon and matrix macromolecules: New research opportunities for old diseases from analysis of potential mechanisms of breast implant toxicity," *Medical Hypotheses*, vol. 51, no. 1, pp. 27–35, 1998.

[21] Y. Shoenfeld and N. Agmon-Levin, "'ASIA'—autoimmune/inflammatory syndrome induced by adjuvants," *Journal of Autoimmunity*, vol. 36, no. 1, pp. 4–8, 2011.

[22] M. J. L. Colaris, M. de Boer, R. R. van der Hulst, and J. W. Cohen Tervaert, "Two hundreds cases of ASIA syndrome following silicone implants: a comparative study of 30 years and a review of current literature," *Immunologic Research*, vol. 65, no. 1, pp. 120–128, 2017.

[23] C. Perricone, S. Colafrancesco, R. D. Mazor, A. Soriano, N. Agmon-Levin, and Y. Shoenfeld, "Autoimmune/inflammatory syndrome induced by adjuvants (ASIA) 2013: Unveiling the pathogenic, clinical and diagnostic aspects," *Journal of Autoimmunity*, vol. 47, pp. 1–16, 2013.

[24] O. Moling, A. Piccin, M. Tauber et al., "Intravascular large B-cell lymphoma associated with silicone breast implant, HLA-DRB1∗11:01, and HLA-DQB1∗03:01 manifesting as macrophage activation syndrome and with severe neurological symptoms: A

case report," *Journal of Medical Case Reports*, vol. 10, no. 1, article 254, 2016.

[25] G. Ramos-Gallardo, J. Cuenca-Pardo, E. Rodríguez-Olivares et al., "Breast implant and anaplastic large cell lymphoma meta-analysis," *Journal of Investigative Surgery*, vol. 30, no. 1, pp. 56–65, 2016.

[26] N. Kossovsky and C. J. Freiman, "Silicone breast implant pathology. Clinical data and immunologic consequences," *Archives of Pathology & Laboratory Medicine*, vol. 118, no. 7, pp. 686–693, 1994.

[27] W. H. Beekman, R. Feitz, P. J. Van Diest, and J. J. Hage, "Migration of silicone through the fibrous capsules of mammary prostheses," *Annals of Plastic Surgery*, vol. 38, no. 5, pp. 441–445, 1997.

[28] W. Greene, D. Raso, L. Walsh, R. Harley, and R. Silver, "Electron probe microanalysis of silicon and the role of the macrophage in proximal (Capsule) and distant sites in augmentation mammaplasty patients," *Plastic and Reconstructive Surgery*, vol. 95, no. 3, pp. 513–519, 1995.

[29] American Society of Plastic Surgeons, "Complete plastic surgery statistics report 2015," https://www.plasticsurgery.org/news/plastic-surgery-statistics.

5

Successful Use of Hyperbaric Oxygen as Adjunctive Therapy for a Nonhealing Venous Ulcer in a Patient with Systemic Sclerosis and Pulmonary Arterial Hypertension

Isaac Biney,[1] Tina Dudney,[1] Mitchell Goldman,[2] Lee Carder,[2] and Elise Schriver[1]

[1]*Department of Medicine, Division of Pulmonary Disease and Critical Care Medicine, University of Tennessee Graduate School of Medicine, Knoxville, TN, USA*
[2]*Department of Surgery, University of Tennessee Graduate School of Medicine, Knoxville, TN, USA*

Correspondence should be addressed to Isaac Biney; isaacbiney@yahoo.co.uk

Academic Editor: Takeshi Terashima

Skin ulcers are a common complication of systemic sclerosis (SSc) that can significantly impact the quality of life. There have been recent reports on the use of hyperbaric oxygen therapy (HBO_2T) in the management of nonhealing systemic sclerosis skin ulcers. The effect of HBO_2T on pulmonary arterial hypertension (PAH), another common and potentially life-threatening complication of SSc, is unclear with literature on the subject lacking. We present the case of a 65-year-old female with limited SSc complicated by severe PAH and a nonhealing left lower extremity venous ulcer. HBO_2T was successfully used as an adjunct in her management resulting in complete resolution of the venous ulcer and improved quality of life without any adverse effects on her pulmonary arterial hypertension.

1. Introduction

Systemic sclerosis (SSc) is a chronic connective tissue disease with multiorgan involvement characterized by diffuse microangiopathy and the deposition of collagen into the skin and internal organs leading to progressive fibrosis. It is a subtype of a heterogeneous group of autoimmune diseases referred to as scleroderma and can be subcategorized by the degree of skin and internal organ fibrosis into limited SSc and diffuse SSc [1]. Skin ulcers are recorded in up to 50% of patients with SSc, and pathogenic mechanisms include microvascular damage and vasospasm [2]. Vascular impairment may also cause nonhealing of ulcers arising due to other mechanisms. These ulcers can be very painful and can cause a significant decline in a patient's quality of life. Management of these ulcers can be very challenging, and therapeutic guidelines remain controversial [2].

Hyperbaric oxygen therapy (HBO_2T) involves the administration of 100% oxygen in a closed chamber pressurized to greater than 1 atmosphere absolute (ATA). Its use in ischemic and nonhealing wounds has been documented since the mid-20th century, and there are well-established indications [3]. Its benefits for these indications have been attributed to antihypoxic, antimicrobial, antiedema, anti-inflammatory, and angiogenetic effects [4]. Recently, there have been several case reports of successful use of HBO_2T in nonhealing ulcers, involving both the digits and extremities, in patients with SSc [4–6].

One relatively common and harmful complication of SSc is pulmonary arterial hypertension (PAH). Prevalence rates up to 19% have been reported in the literature and it is stated as the leading cause of death in this population [7–12]. There have been concerns raised by experts about the safety of HBO_2T in patients with significant PAH. In a recent study looking at HBO_2T-treated ulcers in SSc subjects, patients with moderate to severe pulmonary hypertension were excluded [13]. There is currently no literature evaluating effects of HBO_2T in patients with PAH.

We report a case of successful use of HBO_2T as adjunctive therapy for the treatment of a nonhealing venous ulcer in a patient with limited SSc complicated by PAH.

2. Case Presentation

A 65-year-old female was diagnosed with limited systemic sclerosis 11 years previously after presenting with Raynaud's phenomenon complicated by digital necrosis resulting in amputation of the tip of her left third finger and interstitial lung disease. Her SSc had been managed with various disease-modifying agents, but each had to be discontinued due to intolerance. She was maintained on chronic low-dose prednisone. Her first encounter with our facility was when she presented to vascular surgery with chronic venous insufficiency and a nonhealing venous ulcer on the medial aspect of her left lower leg which had developed in October 2016. At the time, her functional status had declined from being fully functional to being confined to a wheelchair or a walker due to the discomfort from her leg ulcer and exertional dyspnea. She had debridement of the wound and radiofrequency ablation of her left saphenous vein and developed hypotension following the procedure requiring ICU admission. During workup for the hypotension, she had an echocardiogram which showed a left ventricular ejection fraction (LVEF) of 30-35%, a severely dilated right ventricle (RV) with moderately reduced function as measured by a tricuspid annular plane systolic excursion (TAPSE) of 1.1 cm and an estimated right ventricular systolic pressure of 66 mmHg. A noncontrast CT scan of her chest showed mild interstitial lung disease. She subsequently had a right heart catheterization which showed a pulmonary artery pressure of 91/37 mmHg with a mean of 55, a transpulmonary gradient of 47 mmHg, a pulmonary capillary wedge pressure of 8 mmHg, and a pulmonary vascular resistance of 18.1 Woods units. Her cardiac output was 2.6 L/min and cardiac index was 1.8 L/min/m^2. She had a normal ventilation perfusion scan. She was diagnosed with PAH with a World Health Organization (WHO) functional class of IV. A repeat echocardiogram prior to the initiation PAH therapy showed a LVEF of 55-60%. The patient refused parenteral prostanoids. She was treated with sildenafil and macitentan and inhaled treprostinil with improvement of her WHO functional class to class III.

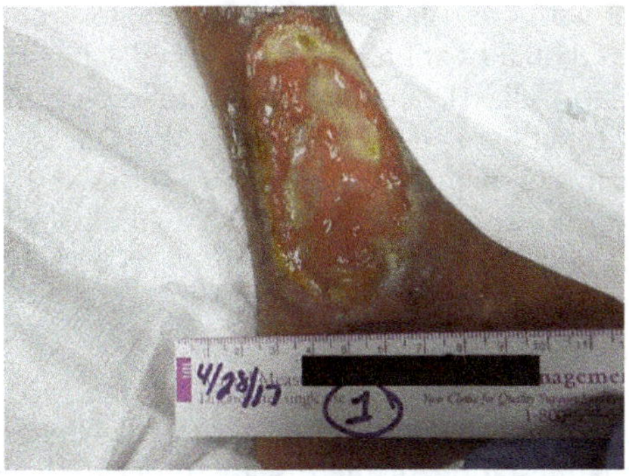

FIGURE 1: Left lower extremity venous ulcer at the time of initial presentation to the wound care center.

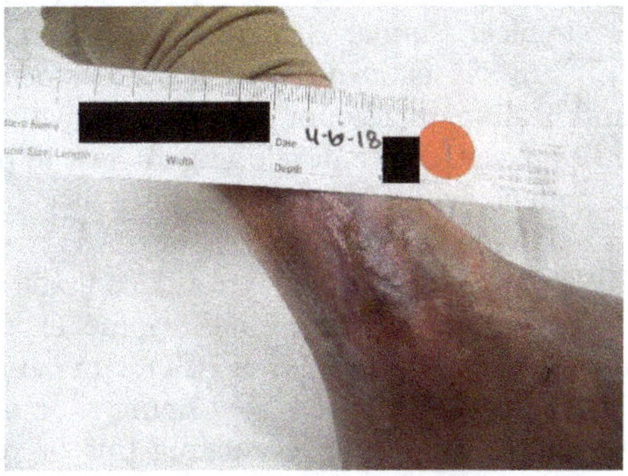

FIGURE 2: Left lower extremity demonstrating complete resolution of venous ulcer after a year of treatment.

She began treatment of her left lower extremity wound at our wound care center in April 2017. At her initial evaluation, her wound measured 10 cm long, 5.3 cm wide, and 0.3 cm deep with an area of 41.626 cm^2 and a volume of 12.488 cm^3. It was described as a full-thickness wound without exposed structures, with well-defined borders, a large amount of serosanguineous exudate and with medium amount of granulation tissue (Figure 1). Initial treatment was with nonadherent Silvercel as the primary dressing and Kerlix with ABD pad applied as the secondary dressing. After 2 months, the primary dressing was changed to the bioengineered skin substitute Apligraf and Mepitel One. Three months later, it was switched to Adaptic. The maximum reduction in wound area achieved with these modalities was 78.1% reduction after 7 months of treatment. The patient was thought to have exhausted her options at this point. After a thorough search of the literature, consulting with the patient's pulmonologist and cardiologist, and detailed discussion with the patient outlining the potential risks involved and possible benefits, a joint decision was made to attempt HBO_2T which started in November 2017. Her most recent echocardiogram had been obtained 4 months prior, and it showed an LVEF of 61%, grade 1 diastolic dysfunction, a moderately dilated RV with mildly reduced function, TAPSE 1.6 cm, and an estimated RVSP of 72 mmHg. The patient received 30 treatments between 11/13/2017 and 12/19/2017 in a monoplace chamber at 2 ATA with 90 minutes of oxygen with no air breaks. Duration of each treatment ranged from 106 to 110 minutes. No immediate adverse events were noted during any of the treatment sessions, and she did not experience any worsening of her exercise tolerance. After completion of HBO_2T, wound care continued with Apligraf, Adaptic, and Xeroform. Complete wound closure was achieved by April 2018 (Figure 2). She had 3 wound debridements during her treatment at the wound care center, 2 while receiving HBO_2T. At follow-up, her functional status has improved to WHO class II, echocardiogram showed a LVEF of 65-70%, mild left atrial enlargement, grade II diastolic dysfunction, mild right atrial enlargement, and a mildly to moderately dilated right ventricle with normal function measured by a TAPSE of 1.9 cm. She had started exercising on a stationary bicycle and worked 5-7 hours per day. Prior to HBO_2T, significant nocturnal wound pain interfered with her sleep. After wound closure, her pain resolved and quality of life vastly improved. The patient continues to do well. At her most recent follow-up in October 2019, her functional status remains at WHO class II, serum brain natriuretic peptide level was 45 pg/mL, and her echocardiogram showed a normal-sized RV with normal function and an RVSP of 33.9 mmHg.

3. Discussion

Ulcers related to SSc (SSc-SU) have been known to be a challenging manifestation of the disease, often difficult to heal and recurrent. Their management has improved over the last decade with a multidisciplinary approach involving the combined use of systemic and advanced local treatments but has still been described as suboptimal [2]. Though our patient had a venous ulcer, similar challenges can be encountered in a patient with SSc as the disease has been associated with poor wound healing on account of the vasculopathy.

There has recently been developing interest in the use of HBO_2T in patients with SSc with intractable ulcers with several published case reports demonstrating its success. In our patient, HBO_2T was successfully used as an adjunct for treatment of her nonhealing ulcer [4–6]. Some experts have expressed concerns about the use of HBO_2T in patients with PAH. Whether this is a generalized opinion or not, there have been no human studies evaluating this or reports of adverse events of HBO_2T when used in patients with PAH. A recent study found that patients with SSc complicated by skin ulcers were more likely to have increased pulmonary arterial pressures [2]. Most studies looking at ulcers in systemic sclerosis have focused on digital ulcers with very little attention to nonhealing lower extremity ulcers [14]. Development of PAH and right ventricular dysfunction are likely to add to the challenge of managing such ulcers. In a study evaluating lower extremity ulcers in patients with SSc, 10 out of 249 patients had active nondigital leg ulcers. Of these, one patient had PAH and venous insufficiency and was among the 3 patients who had a nonhealing ulcer [14]. It is reasonable to deduce that patients with PAH will form a significant proportion of patients with SSc-SU who get to the point of being considered for HBO_2T if indeed HBO_2T becomes a standard adjunctive therapy in intractable SSc-SU.

There is scant literature evaluating the effect of HBO_2T on the pulmonary circulation in humans. Pulmonary oxygen toxicity manifesting as an acute exudative phase and subacute proliferative phase occurs with increasing fraction of inspired oxygen and partial pressure of oxygen. However, current applications of HBO_2T have not been shown to cause pulmonary symptoms or clinically significant pulmonary function defects [15]. Weaver et al. reported pulmonary artery catheter data in 10 normal subjects exposed to 40 minutes of hyperbaric air followed by 40 minutes of HBO_2T. Pulmonary vascular resistance (PVR) decreased by up to 48% during HBO_2T with reduction in pulmonary artery pressure (PAP) by up to 19%. Measurements returned to baseline after removal of hyperbaric conditions [16]. Long-term effects are unknown. In a study evaluating the effect of hyperoxia on the pulmonary circulation in rats, pulmonary vascular remodeling with altered hemodynamics including an increase in PVR and PAP was observed after continuous exposure to hyperoxia for 7 days at normobaric pressure [17]. Jacobson et al. demonstrated the development of pulmonary hypertension in rabbits after hyperbaric exposure to 100% oxygen for 1 hour with evidence to suggest that this was due to increased synthesis of thromboxane [18]. Armstrong et al. evaluated the safety of HBO_2T in SSc patients. Two patients were said to have not received HBO_2T on account of moderate to severe pulmonary hypertension, the underlying reason for this was not discussed. There have been case reports associating HBO_2T with pulmonary edema in patients with left-sided heart failure [19, 20]. Possible mechanisms attributed to this finding include increased peripheral vasoconstriction leading to increased cardiac afterload, increased oxidative myocardial stress, decreased left ventricular (LV) compliance by oxygen radical-mediated reduction in nitric oxide right and left ventricular imbalance, and increased pulmonary capillary permeability. A study of the effect of HBO_2T on cardiac performance in anesthetized dogs showed increased systemic vascular resistance but no change in PVR, and the data suggested that HBO_2T may act by a differential effect on the autonomic innervation of the right and left ventricles [21].

Our successful use of HBO_2T as adjunctive therapy in our patient suggests that it may be safe to use in patients with PAH, but further research is needed to fully evaluate this as the risk benefit is unknown. With increasing interest in HBO_2T use in SSc-SU and with the high prevalence of PAH in this population, it will be important to not automatically exclude patients who could benefit from a potentially life-changing therapy.

References

[1] C. Ferreli, G. Gasparini, A. Parodi, E. Cozzani, F. Rongioletti, and L. Atzori, "Cutaneous manifestations of scleroderma and scleroderma-like disorders: a comprehensive review," *Clinical Reviews in Allergy & Immunology*, vol. 53, no. 3, pp. 306–336, 2017.

[2] D. Giuggioli, A. Manfredi, F. Lumetti, M. Colaci, and C. Ferri, "Scleroderma skin ulcers definition, classification and treatment strategies our experience and review of the literature," *Autoimmunity Reviews*, vol. 17, no. 2, pp. 155–164, 2018.

[3] G. Lam, R. Fontaine, F. L. Ross, and E. S. Chiu, "Hyperbaric oxygen therapy: exploring the clinical evidence," *Advances in Skin & Wound Care*, vol. 30, no. 4, pp. 181–190, 2017.

[4] B. Mirasoglu, B. S. Bagli, and S. Aktas, "Hyperbaric oxygen therapy for chronic ulcers in systemic sclerosis - case series," *International Journal of Dermatology*, vol. 56, no. 6, pp. 636–640, 2017.

[5] Y. M. Markus, M. J. Bell, and A. W. Evans, "Ischemic scleroderma wounds successfully treated with hyperbaric oxygen therapy," *The Journal of Rheumatology*, vol. 33, no. 8, pp. 1694–1696, 2006.

[6] E. Poirier, H. Wind, and N. Cordel, "Efficacy of hyperbaric oxygen therapy in the treatment of ischemic toe ulcer in a patient presenting systemic sclerosis," *Annales de dermatologie et de venereologie*, vol. 144, no. 1, pp. 55–59, 2017.

[7] G. Lefèvre, L. Dauchet, E. Hachulla et al., "Survival and prognostic factors in systemic sclerosis-associated pulmonary hypertension: a systematic review and meta-analysis," *Arthritis and Rheumatism*, vol. 65, no. 9, pp. 2412–2423, 2013.

[8] V. D. Steen and T. A. Medsger, "Changes in causes of death in systemic sclerosis, 1972-2002," *Annals of the Rheumatic Diseases*, vol. 66, no. 7, pp. 940–944, 2007.

[9] J. G. Coghlan, C. P. Denton, E. Grünig et al., "Evidence-based detection of pulmonary arterial hypertension in systemic sclerosis: the DETECT study," *Annals of the Rheumatic Diseases*, vol. 73, no. 7, pp. 1340–1349, 2014.

[10] C. Muangchan, Canadian Scleroderma Research Group, M. Baron, and J. Pope, "The 15% rule in scleroderma: the frequency of severe organ complications in systemic sclerosis. A systematic review," *The Journal of Rheumatology*, vol. 40, no. 9, pp. 1545–1556, 2013.

[11] L. Schachna, F. M. Wigley, B. Chang, B. White, R. A. Wise, and A. C. Gelber, "Age and risk of pulmonary arterial hypertension in scleroderma," *Chest*, vol. 124, no. 6, pp. 2098–2104, 2003.

[12] K. Morrisroe, the Australian Scleroderma Interest Group (ASIG), M. Huq et al., "Risk factors for development of pulmonary arterial hypertension in Australian systemic sclerosis patients: results from a large multicenter cohort study," *BMC Pulmonary Medicine*, vol. 16, no. 1, p. 134, 2016.

[13] S. Armstrong, A. W. Evans, Z. Ahmad, and S. R. Johnson, "Safety and effectiveness of hyperbaric oxygen therapy for systemic sclerosis ulcers," 2016, https://acrabstracts.org/abstract/safety-and-effectiveness-of-hyperbaric-oxygen-therapy-for-systemic-sclerosis-ulcers/.

[14] V. K. Shanmugam, P. Price, C. E. Attinger, and V. D. Steen, "Lower extremity ulcers in systemic sclerosis: features and response to therapy," *International Journal of Rheumatology*, vol. 2010, Article ID 747946, 8 pages, 2010.

[15] M. Heyboer III, D. Sharma, W. Santiago, and N. McCulloch, "Hyperbaric oxygen therapy: side effects defined and quantified," *Advances in Wound Care*, vol. 6, no. 6, pp. 210–224, 2017.

[16] L. K. Weaver, S. Howe, G. L. Snow, and K. Deru, "Arterial and pulmonary arterial hemodynamics and oxygen delivery/extraction in normal humans exposed to hyperbaric air and oxygen," *Journal of Applied Physiology*, vol. 107, no. 1, pp. 336–345, 2009.

[17] R. Jones, W. M. Zapol, and L. Reid, "Pulmonary artery remodeling and pulmonary hypertension after exposure to hyperoxia for 7 days. A morphometric and hemodynamic study," *The American Journal of Pathology*, vol. 117, no. 2, pp. 273–285, 1984.

[18] J. M. Jacobson, J. R. Michael, R. A. Meyers, M. B. Bradley, A. M. Sciuto, and G. H. Gurtner, "Hyperbaric oxygen toxicity: role of thromboxane," *Journal of Applied Physiology*, vol. 72, no. 2, pp. 416–422, 1992.

[19] L. K. Weaver and S. Churchill, "Pulmonary edema associated with hyperbaric oxygen therapy," *Chest*, vol. 120, no. 4, pp. 1407–1409, 2001.

[20] C. Obiagwu, V. Paul, S. Chadha, G. Hollander, and J. Shani, "Acute pulmonary edema secondary to hyperbaric oxygen therapy," *Oxford Medical Case Reports*, vol. 2015, no. 2, pp. 183-184, 2015.

[21] F. L. Abel, J. E. McNamee, D. L. Cone, D. Clarke, and J. Tao, "Effects of hyperbaric oxygen on ventricular performance, pulmonary blood volume, and systemic and pulmonary vascular resistance," *Undersea & Hyperbaric Medicine*, vol. 27, no. 2, pp. 67–73, 2000.

6

One Lung Soldier: A Ventilation Conundrum in a Postpneumonectomy Syndrome Complicated by Acute Respiratory Syndrome

Jaskaran K. Purewal,[1] **N. F. N. Sakul**,[1] **Nikhita R. Balabbigari**,[1] **Alberto Nenninger**,[1] **and Nisha Kotecha**[2]

[1]*Department of Medicine, Overlook Medical Center, Summit, NJ 07901, USA*
[2]*Department of Pulmonary Critical Care, Overlook Medical Center, Summit, NJ 07901, USA*

Correspondence should be addressed to Jaskaran K. Purewal; jaskaran.purewal@gmail.com

Academic Editor: Tun-Chieh Chen

Postpneumonectomy syndrome involves mediastinal shift causing dynamic airway obstruction via compression of the main bronchus and distal trachea. A few case reports describe the development of ARDS in patients with postpneumonectomy syndrome. Reeb et al. (2017) describe the mortality of postpneumonectomy ARDS anywhere from 33% to 88%. One may encounter difficulty in intubation and ventilation as parameters based on ideal body weight may not apply. Prone positioning ventilation and ECMO have been successfully used in isolated cases. We present such a case and highlight challenges in management. A 70-year-old male Vietnam veteran with remote history of right pneumonectomy thirty years prior presented with fever, cough, and dyspnea. Physical exam was significant for T 36.3°C, BP 162/73, heart rate 145 BPM, RR 22 breaths/minute, ht. 1.72 m, and wt. 78 kg, with transmitted right lung sounds and rhonchi on the left. Labs showed WBC 23.92/nL and procalcitonin 0.84 ng/mL. CXR showed left infiltrate and opacification of right hemithorax with right mediastinal shift. EKG showed atrial fibrillation. He was started on broad spectrum antibiotics for pneumonia, but deteriorated, and was intubated for respiratory distress from ARDS. Vasopressors were initiated for shock. Given the history of pneumonectomy, he was initially ventilated with lower tidal volumes (320 mL). However, incremental changes were made to tidal volumes, and ETT was repositioned several times for hypoxia. Epoprostenol and cisatracurium were also initiated. Positional changes would lead to sudden desaturation; hence, prone positioning ventilation was not done. He was not considered for ECMO due to his pneumonectomy status. Unfortunately, his condition worsened progressively and he expired. The guidelines for ARDS are well established. However, postpneumonectomy patients are unique as seen in our patient. It is unclear whether an endobronchial tube advanced into the left bronchus could have helped difficult airway management resulting from suspected postpneumonectomy syndrome as suggested by CXR. Higher tidal volumes were also unsuccessful in alleviating hypoxia and led to persistently elevated plateau pressures and driving pressures as high as 23, which was inconsistent with our goal of lung protective ventilation. Few case reports describe the successful use of prone positioning ventilation or ECMO in postpneumonectomy patients with ARDS. Although not well studied, low tidal volumes supported with ECMO may have been a favorable strategy for our patient.

1. Introduction

The postpneumonectomy state is a unique entity with associated anatomical and physiological challenges. One such challenge is the postpneumonectomy syndrome, more commonly seen in patients with right pneumonectomies, which involves dynamic airway obstruction resulting from compression of the main bronchus and distal trachea by the vertebral column or aorta due to the rotation and right mediastinal shift. These patients pose particularly difficult challenges in ventilation due to the increased respiratory dead space and decreased venous return and are prone to shunting and development of pulmonary edema [1]. The management of ARDS in these patients is not well established but usually is conservative and often involves mechanical ventilation once it becomes necessary. Due to the unique anatomy and physiology, one may encounter difficulty in endotracheal tube positioning and selecting ventilation parameters. Studies regarding ventilator management in ARDS excluded patients with pneumonectomy. The usual lung protective ventilation parameters dependent on ideal body weight may not apply to patients with a single lung. But at the same time, the attempt to lower the tidal volume further may be impossible due to difficulty in oxygenation of such patients. Prone positioning ventilation and extracorporeal membrane oxygenation (ECMO) have been successfully used in isolated similar cases but have been generally reserved for postsurgical pneumonectomy patients who develop ARDS. In a small retrospective study by Reeb et al., the use of VV-ECMO in postpneumonectomy ARDS patients was studied and subsequently showed improved hospital survival [2]. We present a patient with remote history of pneumonectomy now admitted with ARDS and highlight unique challenges associated with its management.

2. Case Presentation

A 70-year-old male with hypertension and remote history of carcinoid tumor requiring right pneumonectomy thirty years prior presented with one week of generalized malaise, fever, nonproductive cough, and worsening dyspnea on exertion. He was in his usual state of health until one week prior to his presentation; overall, he was very healthy with good functional status with slightly decreased stamina. Initial physical exam was significant for temperature 36.3°C, BP 162/73, irregular heart rate 145 beats/minute, respiratory rate 22 breaths/minute, height 1.72 m, and weight 78 kg. He was a thin male with transmitted lung sounds on the right and significant rhonchi on the left. The remainder of the physical exam was otherwise within normal limits. Initial lab results showed leukocytosis (WBC 23.92/nL), positive procalcitonin (0.84 ng/mL), negative Legionella and S. pneumoniae urine antigen, negative respiratory viral panel, and mild respiratory alkalosis on ABG (7.49/39/69/24.6). EKG showed atrial fibrillation with rapid ventricular response. Initial CXR showed left-sided infiltrate with pleural effusion as well as complete opacification of the right hemithorax with right mediastinal shift (Figure 1). Overall, there was concern for severe sepsis due to multilobar community-acquired pneumonia. He was subsequently started on ceftriaxone and azithromycin and placed on high-flow nasal cannula. He was also started on a continuous infusion of diltiazem and received full-dose enoxaparin for anticoagulation in the setting of uncontrolled atrial fibrillation. He quickly converted to normal sinus rhythm within a few hours and was started on oral diltiazem. However, within four hours of hospital admission, his respiratory status quickly deteriorated and a rapid response was called for hypoxia and increased work of breathing. Oxygen requirements on high-flow nasal cannula had increased significantly, and while he was able to speak in full sentences, he was clearly anxious, air hungry, and using accessory muscles to breathe. ECHO showed normal left ventricular function with an ejection fraction of 55% and a sclerotic aortic valve without stenosis but was not significant for any cardiac shunt, such as patent foramen ovale. Repeat ABG showed worsening hypoxia with a $PaO_2:FiO_2$ ratio of 71 mmHg. Repeat CXR showed worsening of the left-sided infiltrate (Figure 2). Further imaging with CT chest or even a bronchoscopy was needed to further qualify the worsening infiltrate as well as possible obstruction from postpneumonectomy syndrome; however, the patient was never hemodynamically stable for this. He required transfer to the intensive care unit and intubation for significant respiratory distress, with concern for developing ARDS and septic shock. Antibiotic coverage was broadened to vancomycin, piperacillin-tazobactam, and azithromycin; stress dose steroids and vasopressors were also initiated. Given the history of pneumonectomy, he was initially ventilated with low tidal volumes (320 mL). While the goal was to maintain lung protective ventilation, incremental changes were made to

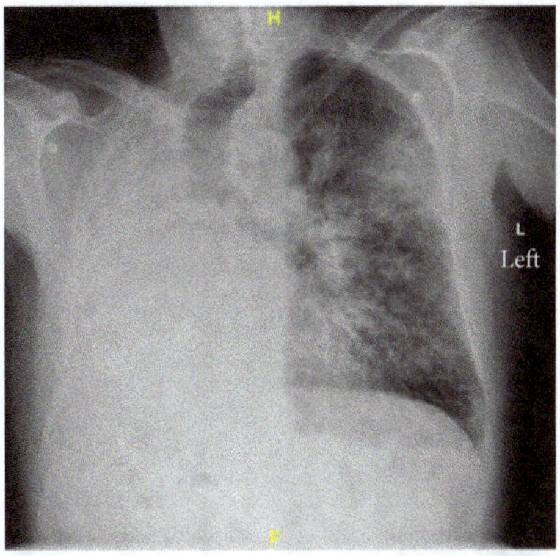

Figure 1: Initial chest X-ray showing complete opacification of the right hemithorax from pneumonectomy. Right mediastinal shift present. Diffuse infiltrates noted in the left lung.

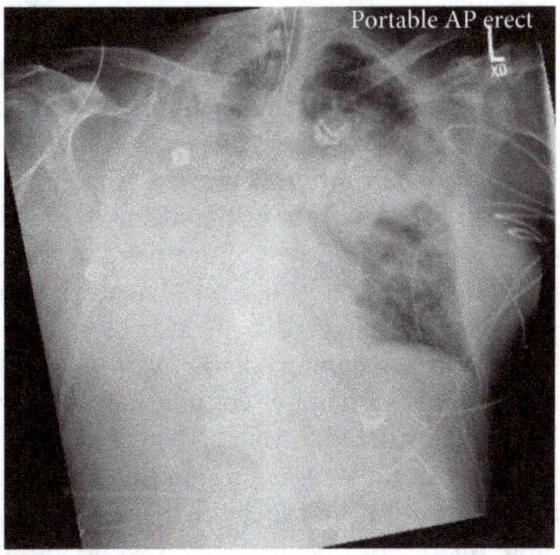

Figure 2: Repeat chest X-ray done one day after admission. Patient noted to have worsening hypoxia and increased work of breathing and was subsequently intubated. Chest X-ray significant for worsening of the left-sided superior perihilar infiltrate.

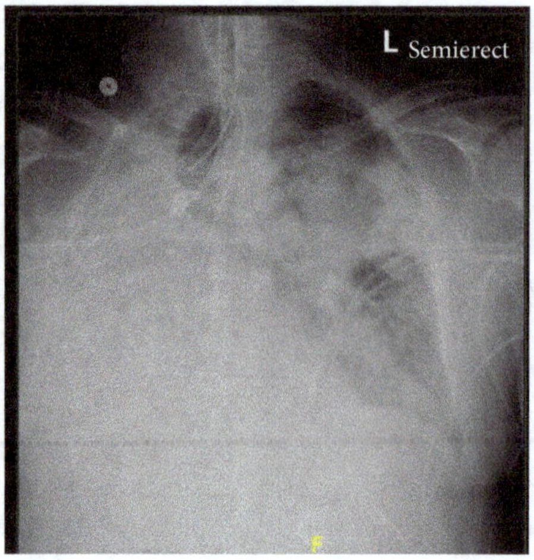

FIGURE 3: Chest X-ray done after advancement of the endotracheal tube, shown in the image to be projected toward the right side of the trachea. Persistent airspace disease noted in the left upper lobe.

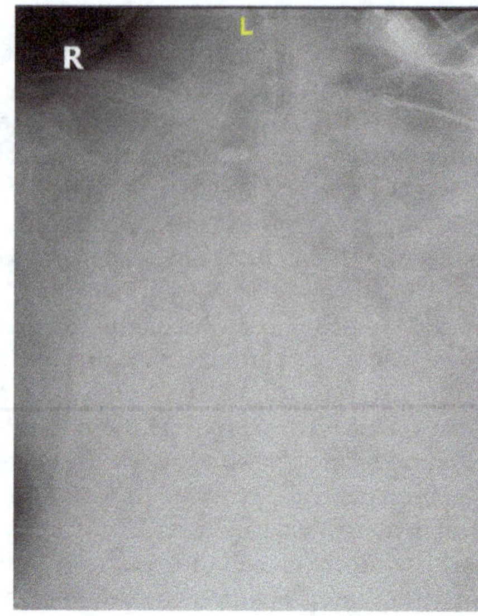

FIGURE 4: Chest X-ray showing significant worsening of the L-sided infiltrate, leading to complete opacification of the left lung.

his tidal volume to maintain oxygenation but were not effective. Throughout his ICU course, oxygenation and ventilation proved to be difficult. In addition, his endotracheal tube was repositioned several times leading to temporary improvements in oxygenation (Figure 3). Epoprostenol and neuromuscular blockade were initiated for oxygenation and ventilator synchrony; however, they were only beneficial temporarily. Furthermore, peak and plateau pressures were consistently elevated, suggestive of an obstructive component, possibly from worsening edema from ARDS exacerbating his underlying postpneumonectomy state. While proning ventilation was considered, it was not done as even minimal changes in his position lead to sudden hemodynamic instability with desaturation and tachycardia. Furthermore, due to his remote history of pneumonectomy and clinical severity, he was not considered a good candidate for ECMO. Unfortunately, due to his progressively worsening clinical condition, which was also verified by the worsening chest X-ray (Figure 4), he was transitioned to comfort care measures and expired.

3. Discussion

ARDS is a well-recognized clinical entity in an ICU setting, and its management involves treatment of the underlying etiology as well as ventilation management. Several guidelines and studies have been conducted to direct treatment and escalation of care to prone ventilation and ECMO. However, postpneumonectomy patients have particular anatomical and physiological changes that pose challenges in their management of ARDS as seen in our patient.

Pneumonectomies are indicated for numerous reasons including removal of malignancy or in a trauma setting. While uncommon, postpneumonectomy syndrome can occur within weeks or even years after removal of the lung. It is more commonly seen after right pneumonectomy, possibly due to the more severe anatomical changes. The postpneumonectomy syndrome results in airway obstruction due to rotation and mediastinal shift towards the pneumonectomy site. This results in eventual herniation and overinflation of the remaining lung and leads to central airway compression [3]. Patients will often present with stridor, worsening dyspnea, or recurrent pulmonary infections as a result. This was clearly seen in our patient. Imaging findings clearly described with relation to postpneumonectomy syndrome were clearly also illustrated in our patient's initial admitting chest X-ray (Figure 1). While he was asymptomatic from the clear anatomical changes noted on his imaging, infection and subsequent edema may have exacerbated his underlying postpneumonectomy state. In a study done in 2008, surgical correction of the syndrome with prostheses led to improved flow rates, decreased FVC, and correction of the hyperinflation, as well as an improved FEV1/FVC ratio. However, more than the changes noted on PFTs, patients experienced significant improvement in their symptoms [3]. It is clear that this syndrome causes airway compression, and thus, airway management may be difficult. Besides the difficulty in intubation from mechanical obstruction, the associated hypercapnia, hypoxia, increased respiratory dead space, and overall decreased venous return can contribute to ventilation problems, as was seen in our patient [1]. Initial airway management was difficult due to poor placement of the ETT (Figures 2 and 3). While a CT chest would have been ideal to visualize the extent this played in his ventilation problems, it was not feasible. A similar case was described in 2015, in which a patient underwent a left-sided pneumonectomy for a persistent mycobacterial infection and three months later became symptomatic. CT imaging in this patient showed significant obstruction of the bronchus intermedius and right lower bronchus. The case report also describes difficulty in oxygenating the patient, and eventually, the patient's endotracheal tube was then temporarily replaced with an endobronchial tube until surgery was viable. The authors additionally describe considering the use of an endobronchial stent but mention uncertainty in its efficacy or long-term risks [4]. In the anesthesia literature, mediastinal masses often create airway obstruction, which are managed with the use of endobronchial tubes [5]. Whether a single lumen endobronchial tube advanced up to the left bronchus could have been used to decompress the airway and overcome this obstruction to provide better ventilation remains unclear. Another potential concern was a possible platypnea-orthodeoxia syndrome caused by interatrial shunting after pneumonectomy [6]. However, this was highly unlikely as no intracardiac shunt was noted on ECHO, and furthermore, our patient was not symptomatic from this condition prior to presentation, even in the setting of his pneumonectomy done thirty years ago.

Since the PROSEVA trial in 2013, early initiation of proning in patients with severe ARDS had an associated mortality benefit [7]. However, there is limited literature regarding postpneumonectomy patients affected with ARDS and the subsequent effect of proning. While prone ventilation was not an option for our patient due to hemodynamic instability, case reports have demonstrated significant improvement in similar patients [8, 9]. Furthermore, it is uncertain whether typical ventilation strategies used in ARDS management may be as effective due to a combination of the underlying pathophysiology of postpneumonectomy syndrome and ARDS. Initial ventilator settings were to maintain low tidal volumes and were adjusted based on the patient's pneumonectomy status; we still had difficulty maintaining adequate oxygenation despite adjustments and increases to the tidal volume. These increments in tidal volume led to persistently elevated plateau pressures > 30 and driving pressures as high as 23, which oppose the goal of lung protective ventilation. Low tidal volumes when supported with ECMO may have been a favorable strategy for our patient and allowed us to ventilate with a lower plateau and driving pressures. A small study done by Reeb et al. showed that the use of VV-ECMO in postpneumonectomy ARDS patients decreased the mortality from 80 to 50%. ECMO had allowed for greater lung protective strategies, decreased tidal volumes, adequate gas exchange, and overall better recovery of lung tissue [2]. ECMO was not considered in our patient but may have been beneficial and may have allowed for the use of improved lung protective strategies. While it is difficult in this particular set of patients, greater study is needed regarding ARDS management in postpneumonectomy patients.

4. Conclusion

Few case reports describe improved mortality with prone ventilation as well as ECMO in postpneumonectomy ARDS, which in hindsight may have been beneficial for our patient given the difficulties we had in managing our patient's ventilation. While this has not been well studied due to the unique nature of these disease states, it is important to keep in mind as a possibility for management in postpneumonectomy patients. Our case highlights how better guidelines with regard to treatment concerning single lung ventilation and a possible postpneumonectomy syndrome may have been life changing in his scenario.

Abbreviations

ECMO:	Extracorporeal membrane oxygenation
ARDS:	Acute respiratory distress syndrome
CXR:	Chest X-ray
EKG:	Electrocardiogram
ABG:	Arterial blood gas
WBC:	White blood cell
FEV1:	Forced expiratory volume
FVC:	Forced vital capacity
PFTs:	Pulmonary function tests
ETT:	Endotracheal tube
VV-ECMO:	Venovenous extracorporeal membrane oxygenation.

Additional Points

Key Points. Postpneumonectomy syndrome is a rare entity that leads to mechanical airway obstruction due to mediastinal shift, which can contribute to difficult airway management. The use of prone ventilation and ECMO have been used in isolated cases of postpneumonectomy ARDS, but their utility and subsequent effects are not well understood. Further study is needed on ventilation in patients with pneumonectomies.

References

[1] M. Sharifpour and E. A. Bittner, "Postpneumonectomy syndrome," *Anesthesiology*, vol. 121, no. 6, p. 1334, 2014.

[2] J. Reeb, A. Olland, J. Pottecher et al., "Extracorporeal membrane oxygenation for acute respiratory distress syndrome after pneumonectomy," *The Annals of Thoracic Surgery*, vol. 103, no. 3, pp. 881–889, 2017.

[3] K. R. Shen, J. C. Wain, C. D. Wright, H. C. Grillo, and D. J. Mathisen, "Postpneumonectomy syndrome: surgical management and long-term results," *The Journal of Thoracic and Cardiovascular Surgery*, vol. 135, no. 6, pp. 1210–1219.e6, 2008.

[4] T. Karasaki and M. Tanaka, "Life-threatening postpneumonectomy syndrome complicated with right aortic arch after left pneumonectomy," *Case Reports in Surgery*, vol. 2015, Article ID 768067, 4 pages, 2015.

[5] B. Harte, M. Jaklitsch, S. McKenna, and S. Body, "Use of a modified single-lumen endobronchial tube in severe tracheobronchial compression," *Anesthesiology*, vol. 96, no. 2, pp. 510-511, 2002.

[6] T. Komatsu and D. Bethune, "Platypnea orthodeoxia syndrome and bronchopleural fistula following right pneumonectomy: the first case of double misfortune following pneumonectomy," *International Journal of Surgery Case Reports*, vol. 2, no. 4, pp. 47-48, 2011.

[7] C. Guérin, J. Reignier, J. Richard et al., "Prone positioning in severe acute respiratory distress syndrome," *The New England Journal of Medicine*, vol. 368, no. 23, pp. 2159–2168, 2013.

[8] S. Tatineni, S. Sasikumar, and V. Shanbhag, "Prone position for management of refractory hypoxaemia in a patient with single lung," *Indian Journal Of Respiratory Care*, vol. 1, no. 1, pp. 69–71, 2012.

[9] R. Cornejo, C. Romero, D. Goñi et al., "Ventilación en posición prono prolongada como alternativa en el tratamiento del síndrome de distrés respiratorio agudo grave posneumonectomía: caso clínico," *Revista Médica de Chile*, vol. 137, no. 10, 2009.

7

A Retrospective Study of Ultrasound Characteristics and Macroscopic Findings in Confirmed Malignant Pleural Effusion

Nevenka Piskac Zivkovic,[1] Igor Cikara,[1,2] Nina Petra Novak,[1] Boris Brkljacic,[1,3] and Neven Tudoric[1,3]

[1] *University Hospital Dubrava, Zagreb, Croatia*
[2] *Faculty of Medicine Osijek, University Josip Juraj Strossmayer Osijek, Croatia*
[3] *School of Medicine, University of Zagreb, Zagreb, Croatia*

Correspondence should be addressed to Nevenka Piskac Zivkovic; npiskac@kbd.hr

Academic Editor: Roberto Walter Dal Negro

Background. A definitive diagnosis of malignant pleural effusion (MPE) is reached by cytological or histological assessment, but thorough analysis of the ultrasound features of the effusion as well as pleural thickening or nodularity can also be of significant diagnostic help. *Objective.* To assess the relationship of specific ultrasound characterisctics and macroscopic features of confirmed malignant pleural effusion, thus increasing the diagnostic potential of thoracic ultrasound. *Methods.* The findings of thoracic ultrasonography performed prior to initial thoracentesis in 104 patients with subsequently confirmed malignant pleural effusion were analyzed with regard to the macroscopic features of the pleural effusion. *Results.* Distribution in terms of frequency of hemorrhagic/sanguinolent (n=64) in relation to nonhemorrhagic transparent/opaque (n=40) MPE, regardless of their ultrasound characteristics, did not yield a statistically significant correlation (p=0.159). Conversely, the frequency distribution of hemorrhagic pleural effusions (n=8) in relation to nonhemorrhagic effusions (n=1), in the group of septated MPE, showed a statistically significant difference (p<0.001). The least number of patients (0.96%) had a complex septated MPE combined with the macroscopic appearance of a serous/transparent nonhemorrhagic effusion, which suggests that this combination is a sporadic occurrence and may have a diagnostic significance for this patient group. *Conclusion.* The incidence of specific combinations of the ultrasound characteristics and macroscopic appearance of MPEs showed different frequency distributions, which may improve the diagnostic value of thoracic ultrasound in this patient population.

1. Introduction

Pleural effusion is a common manifestation of various malignancies, suggesting advanced disease and a poor prognosis. Approximately 30% of malignant pleural effusions originate from lung carcinoma and result in survival rates of 8-10 months [1]. Detection of pleural effusion often leads to prompt implementation of standardized diagnostic procedures with thoracocentesis as the initial step.

Thoracic ultrasound (TUS) is an important, often initial, diagnostic method for the detection and localization of pleural effusion, as well as for the safe performance of further invasive diagnostic procedures. Since it enables real-time visualization, TUS significantly increases diagnostic accuracy, considerably diminishing the number of potential complications. A detailed thoracic ultrasound examination incorporates the analysis of sonographic features of the effusion, the visceral and parietal pleura, and the visible lung parenchyma. Although the definitive diagnosis of malignant effusion is made from a cytological or histological assessment, a thorough analysis of the ultrasound findings has significant diagnostic value.

According to Yang et al. [2], pleural effusion is classified as anechoic, complex septated, complex nonseptated, or homogeneously echogenic. The echogenicity of the pleural effusion is assessed by comparing it with the echogenicity of the liver (hypoechoic, isoechoic, and hyperechoic), while the reference value for anechogenicity is the echogenicity of bile in the gallbladder. The terms "complex" or "heterogeneous" are used to denote findings of echogenic zones within an anechoic effusion. Fibrinous septation is a relatively common finding in pleural effusion and varies in intensity, ranging from a few separated, often floating, fibrin strands to dense reticular structures with a honeycomb appearance [3–5]. Fibrinous septation is the consequence of an increased amount of proteins in the effusion, therefore being a common finding in exudates, including tuberculous, pleural empyema, hematothorax, and parapneumonic effusions [6, 7].

According to Yang et al. [2] transudate pleural effusion is always anechoic, whereas exudates, both malignant and nonmalignant, may be anechoic or echogenic. The authors reported findings of anechoic pleural effusion in 27% of nonmalignant and 40% of malignant pleural effusions, a similar distribution of various types of echogenic effusions. Conversely, Bugalho et al. [7] found only 5% of anechoic malignant effusions, which is in line with the results of others [6, 8]. In most cases, the malignant effusion presented features of complex nonseptated effusion [2].

The potential cause for the lower incidence of fibrinous septation in malignant effusion has been analyzed at the molecular level. It was proposed to be the consequence of increased fibrinolytic activity in malignant effusion resulting from a higher level of tissue plasminogen activator (tPA). In contrast, tuberculous exudates were characterized by an increased level of the inhibitor type-1 of tissue plasminogen activator (PAI -1) and tumor necrosis factor alpha (TNF-alpha) [9, 10]. The fibrinous septation was also reported to be a consequence of repeated thoracocenteses and pleurodesis, where increased levels of inflammatory cytokines (TNF-alpha, IL-1, IL-5, IL-6, and IL-8) were found [11, 12].

Malignant pleural effusion has biochemical features of exudate and only rarely presents as transudate [13, 14]. Macroscopically, malignant pleural effusions can be serous, sanguinolent, or hemorrhagic. Cytological analysis reveals predominance of lymphocytes, macrophages, and mesothelial cells, whereas there are usually less than 25% of polymorphonuclears and between 8 and 12% of eosinophils [15] found.

A complete chest sonography includes an estimate of pleural thickness, possible detection of pleural nodes, and an examination of the adjacent lung parenchyma (presence of the air bronchogram or possible pulmonary consolidation). TUS also enables measurement of the thickness of the diaphragm, as well as the possible detection of liver metastases. Although the finding of the thickened visceral, parietal, and diaphragmal pleura is common in malignant effusions, if it is less than 1 cm, it does not have specific diagnostic relevance [7, 8]. On the contrary, pleural thickening greater than 1 cm, along with the finding of pleural nodes, is very indicative. Bugalho et al. [7] reported these findings in 79% of malignant and only 9% of nonmalignant pleural effusions. The presence of air bronchogram is more common in nonmalignant effusions.

As proof of malignant etiology, cytological analysis of the pleural effusion sampled at initial thoracocentesis has a sensitivity of 62%. The repeated procedures increase the sensitivity up to 72% (49-91%) [16]. This indicates that for a large number of patients further diagnostic evaluation is necessary. Targeted TUS-guided pleural biopsy increases the number of successfully diagnosed malignant effusions with sensitivity of almost 90% [17–19]. However, in the case of some pleural effusions collected in patients with lung carcinoma, the presence of malignant cells or pleural involvement cannot be detected. Such cases are classified as paramalignant pleural effusions resulting from diverse causes, including atelectasis, pulmonary embolism, hypoalbuminemia, chylothorax, radiotherapy, and chemotherapy [20].

The objective of our study was to assess the relationship of specific ultrasound characterisctics and macroscopic features of confirmed malignant pleural effusion, thus increasing the diagnostic potential of thoracic ultrasound.

2. Materials and Methods

This retrospective, single-center study was conducted at the Division of Pulmonology of the University Hospital Dubrava in Zagreb, Croatia, during a 4-year period (January 2014–June 2018). It has been approved by the institutional Ethics Committee.

2.1. Subjects. The studied subjects were selected among patients referred for thoracic ultrasonography because of suspected pleural effusion at the standard chest X-ray. In the studied group of patients, the malignant etiology of effusion was subsequently established using regular diagnostic procedures. This means that, in case of repeatedly negative cytoanalysis of effusion, ultrasound- or CT-guided pleural needle biopsy was performed. A few patients underwent video-assisted thoracoscopy (VATS) with biopsy of the pleura and/or lung parenchyma. All collected samples were analyzed at the Department of Cytology and Pathology in the same institution. Patients with contraindications for thoracentesis and those who did not give their consent to participate in the study were excluded.

2.2. Ultrasonography. The procedure was performed using the Aloka 7 Utrasound System (Aloka, Japan). A 2-5 MHz convex probe was used for the analysis of the pleural effusion, visceral pleura, and lung parenchyma, whereas the parietal pleura and thoracic wall were examined with the use of a linear 5-10 MHz probe. The examination was conducted with the patient placed in the sitting position, by a pulmonologist experienced in the use of TUS (15Y). The thoracic cavity was systematically examined by moving the probe from dorsal to ventral along the intercostal spaces from the diaphragm to the lung apices.

Based on the ultrasound features, the pleural effusions were classified as anechoic, homogeneously echogenic, complex septated, or complex nonseptated. Furthermore, the appearance and thickness of the parietal, visceral, and diaphragmal pleura were analyzed, as well as the available lung parenchyma and the thoracic wall structures. After ultrasonography, ultrasound-guided pleural puncture was performed in accordance with the British Thoracic Society (BTS) guidelines [20]. The gross features of the obtained samples (transparent clear to pale yellow, pale yellow with cloudy appearance, opaque, sanguinolent, and hemorrhagic) were recorded, before the samples were referred

Table 1: Primary origin and type of malignant disease in patients with malignant pleural effusion.

Site and type of tumor	Patients (N)
Lung adenocarcinoma	34
Small cell lung carcinoma	5
Non-small cell lung carcinoma	4
Pleural mesothelioma	6
Gastric adenocarcinoma	9
Colon adenocarcinoma	16
Invasive ductal breast cancer	14
Ovarian carcinoma	4
Endometrial carcinoma	2
Thymic carcinoma	1
Papillary carcinoma of the urinary bladder	1
Melanoma	2
Non-Hodgkin lymphoma	5
Acute myeloid leukemia	1

for further biochemical, microbiological, and cytologocal assessment.

2.3. Statistical Analysis. The collected data were entered into the Excel spreadsheet (MS Office 2007) and the cumulative frequency for the ultrasound features and gross findings of the malignant pleural effusions was calculated. Statistical analysis of the frequency table was done by Chi-square test, using the SAS Studio 3.5 statistical software package (SAS Institute Inc., Cary, NC, USA). $P<0.05$ was considered statistically significant.

3. Results

In the above-mentioned 4-year period, 104 patients (55 females, 49 males, mean age 69 years) with confirmed MPE were recorded by means of retrospective analysis. The malignant nature of the effusion was confirmed by the finding of malignant cells in pleural effusion samples from 72 (69%) patients, in transthoracic pleural biopsy samples from 26 (25%) patients, and in samples obtained by surgical pleural biopsy during VATS from 6 (6%) patients. In 97 patients the pleural effusion was a result of solid tumor metastasis, while 7 patients had a dissemination of hematologic disease. In the majority of the cases, the primary sites of the tumors were the lungs (41%), organs of the gastrointestinal tract (24%), and the breasts (13%). Table 1 lists the primary sites as well as the types of tumors and hematologic diseases diagnosed in the patients with MPEs.

Based on the ultrasound features, 95 (91.35%) patients had a nonseptated pleural effusion (in 11 patients the pleural effusion was classified as anechoic, in 16 patients as homogeneously echogenic, and in 68 patients as complex nonseptated), and 9 (8.65%) patients were found to have a septated pleural effusion. Table 2 lists the ultrasound characteristics of the MPEs as well as their gross features. Figure 1 shows the typical ultrasound finding of fibrinous septations in a complex septated pleural effusion, and in Figure 2 a complex nonseptated pleural effusion can be seen.

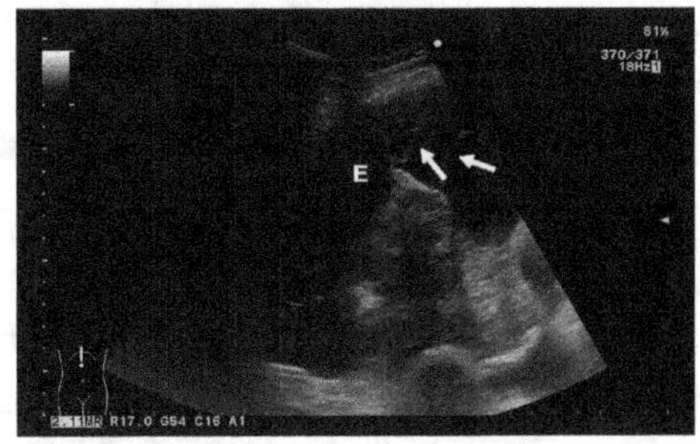

Figure 1: Typical ultrasonographic image of malignant pleural effusion with fibrinous septation. Fibrin strands within a pleural effusion can be seen (white arrows); E = pleural effusion.

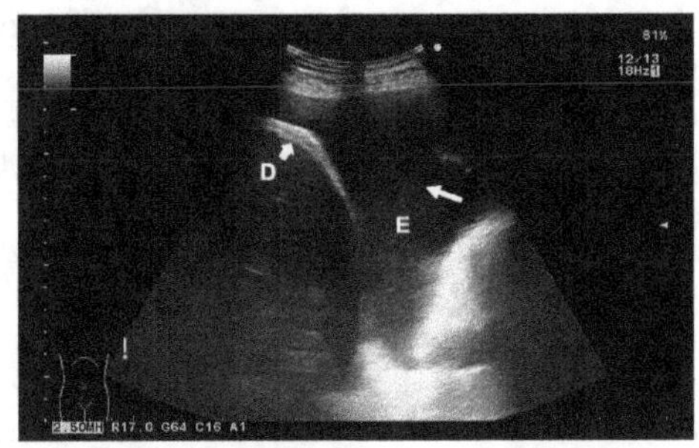

Figure 2: Typical ultrasonographic image of complex nonseptated malignant pleural effusion. Heterogeneously hyperechoic spots inside effusion (right white arrow) without fibrinous septations can be seen. D = diaphragm (left bold white arrow); E = pleural effusion.

According to the macroscopic characteristics, in 64 patients (62%) pleural effusion was sanguinolent/hemorrhagic, in 15 patients (14%) transparent and clear, while in the remaining 25 patients (24%) the effusion was pale yellow with cloudy appearance or opaque. The frequency distribution of the hemorrhagic/sanguinolent (n=64) in comparison with the nonhemorrhagic transparent or cloudy/opaque MPEs (n=40), regardless of their ultrasound characteristics, did not yield a statistically significant correlation (p=0.159).

The frequency distribution of the septated (n=8) in relation to the nonseptated pleural effusions (n=56) within the group of hemorrhagic effusions showed a statistically significant difference (p=0.0001).

In view of the specific ultrasound findings, special attention was given to the analysis of pleural effusions with fibrinous septations. Out of the 9 patients with MPEs with fibrinous septations, 3 had metastasis originating from lung tumors, in 2 cases the primary malignancies were adenocarcinomas of the lung, and there was one case of small cell lung carcinoma. Out of the remaining 6 complex septated pleural effusions, three were caused by the propagation of solid extrathoracic tumors (gastric carcinoma, melanoma, and papillary urinary bladder carcinoma), and 3 were the result of malignant hematologic disease dissemination (non-Hodgkin lymphoma and acute myelogenous leukemia). In 8

TABLE 2: Ultrasound features and macroscopic appearance of malignant pleural effusions.

Ultrasound characteristic					Macroscopic finding					
					Sanguinolent/ hemorrhagic		Serous transparent		Serous opaque	
	n	%	n	%	n	%	n	%	n	%
Complex septated	9	8.65	9	8.65	8	88.89	1	11.11	0	0.00
Homogeneously echogenic	16	15.39								
Anechoic	11	10.58	95	91.35	56	58.95	14	14.74	25	26.31
Complex non-septated	68	65.38								
Total	104	100.00	104	100.00						

patients from this group the pleural effusion was sanguinolent or hemorrhagic, and only one patient (non-Hodgkin lymphoma) had a transparent serous pleural effusion. The frequency distribution of hemorrhagic pleural effusions (n=8) as compared to nonhemorrhagic effusions (n=1), within the group of MPEs with fibrinous septations, showed a statistically significant difference (p<0.0001). From the data listed in Table 2 it can be concluded that the combination of a macroscopically nonhemorrhagic pleural effusion and fibrinous septations was a sporadic occurrence in the MPE group, found only in one of the 104 patients.

Pleural nodularity was established in 53 patient samples, 75% of which were macroscopically hemorrhagic/sanguinolent. Pleural thickening (>10 mm) was confirmed in 45 patients, 64% of which had gross features of hemorrhagic/sanguinolent pleural effusion.

The majority of the analyzed pleural effusions were lymphocytic (>50% lymphocytes). The number of polymorphonuclears was lower than 25%, and the amount of eosinophils was less than 12%. In 3 (3%) patients the malignant pleural effusion had transudate characteristics.

4. Discussion

This is the first study to compare the macroscopic characteristics with the ultrasound findings in MPE. Consistent with the results of other authors [21, 22], distribution analysis of the macroscopic findings in MPE, regardless of the ultrasound features, did not yield a statistically significant difference (p=0.159). Yang et al. [2] were the first to describe the ultrasound characteristics of MPE, whereas Qureshi et al. [8] repoted that malignancies had been diagnosed by TUS in 26/33 patients. Out of 7 false-negative results, the CT findings were negative in 6 (86%) patients. The authors concluded that ultrasound findings of pleural nodularity accompanied by a thickening of the parietal costal pleura by >10 mm and the diaphragmatic pleura by >7 mm represented a significant predictor of a malignant etiology of the pleural effusion, with a procedure sensitivity of 73% and a specificity of 100%. It has to be emphasized that pleural nodularity was confrmed in specific pleural effusions as well [7]. Due to that fact, the finding of pleural nodularity is not considered pathognomonic for MPE, especially in regions where tuberculosis is common, although it still remains a significant predictor of malignancy in undiagnosed pleural effusion (sensitivity 78.8%, specificity 91.0%). In our patient cohort pleural nodularity was established in 51% of the cases. In 75% of these patients the effusion was hemorrhagic or sanguinolent. Consistent with that, a >10 mm thickening of the parietal pleura was confirmed in 43% of the patients, out of which 56% had a hemorrhagic or sanguinolent effusion. Furthermore, the literature describes two more ultrasound findings, i.e., the invasion of thoracic wall structures and the presence of liver metastasis, which suggest a malignant etiology of the pleural effusion with a high sensitivity and specificity [7, 23]. These ultrasound criteria are present in a smaller number of MPE patents. Negative cytological findings combined with ultrasound criteria which suggest a malignant etiology of the pleural effusion require a further diagnostic workup and obtaining samples for pathohistological analysis.

Two further ultrasound characteristics with a higher incidence in MPE in relation to nonmalignant pleural effusion (NMPE) are the absence of air bronchograms in the peripheral lung infiltrate (p=0.001) and the absence of fibrinous septations in the pleural effusion (p=0.006) [7]. The cited parameters display a high sensitivity, but low specificity. The absence of air bronchograms has a sensitivity of 92.4% and a specificity of 31.3% [7]. False-negative findings are most often due to malignant obstructive pneumonia. Fibrinous sepations are a relatively rare finding in MPE, reported by various authors at an incidence of 4-7.5% [6–8]. TUS is a very reliable method for the assessment of septations in pleural effusion, with a sensitivity of 92.4% [7]. However, due to its low specificity (25%), the analysis of fibrinous septations has a limited diagnostic value. The possibility of errors in the ultrasound evaluation of fibrinous septations in the effusion needs to be taken into account. This applies to the findings of floating visceral pleura of an atelectatic lung lobe (Figure 3) and pleural adhesions (Figure 4), which are common in effusions with transudate features that have been present for a longer period of time. They are usually supradiaphragmatic, with cytological features of reactively changed, macrophage-transformed mesothelial cells [24].

Taking into account the results of studies conducted so far, and with the aim of improving the effectiveness of TUS in MPE patients, macroscopic findings of pleural effusion were analyzed retrospectively within the context of their ultrasound characteristics. Upon statistical analysis and the correlation of frequency distributions of specific combinations of macroscopic appearance and ultrasound characteristics of MPEs, significant results were obtained. The frequency distribution of hemorrhagic/sanguinolent (n=64) in relation to nonhemorrhagic transparent/opaque (n=40) malignant pleural effusions, regardless of their ultrasound

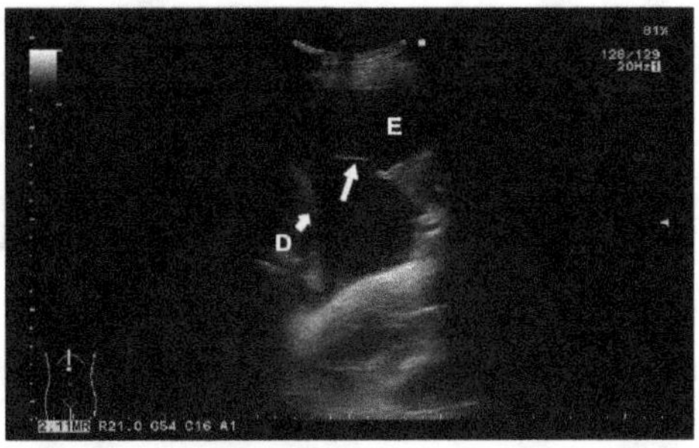

FIGURE 3: Floating visceral pleura due to atelectasis of the lung lobe (right white arrow). D = diaphragm (left bold white arrow); E = pleural effusion.

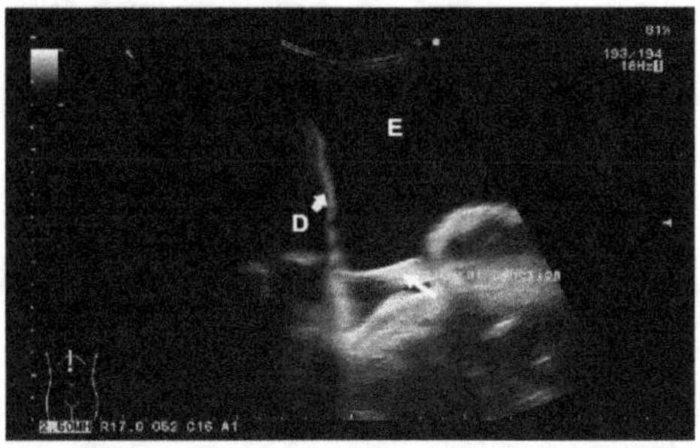

FIGURE 4: Pleural adhesions. Pleural adhesions (right white arrow) with sharp contours, hyperechoic, connecting the diaphragmatic pleura and parenchyma of the collapsed lung. D = diaphragm (left bold white arrow); E = pleural effusion.

characteristics, did not yield a statistically significant correlation (p=0.159). In contrast, the frequency distribution of hemorrhagic (n=8) as compared to nonhemorrhagic pleural effusions (n=1), within the group of malignant pleural effusions with fibrinous septations, showed a statistically significant difference (p<0.0001). The least number of patients (0.96%) had a complex septated MPE combined with the macroscopic appearance of a serous/transparent nonhemorrhagic effusion, which suggests that this combination is a sporadic occurrence and may have a diagnostic significance for this patient group.

The authors are aware of the study limitations, particularly in view of the fact that it was a retrospective investigation which did not include patients with nonmalignant pleural effusion. We believe that prospective study, which would also include patients with nonmalignant pleural effusion, would help in better evaluation of diagnostic value of thorasis ultrasound in the assessment of malignant etiology in undiagnosed pleural effusions.

References

[1] V. B. Antony, R. Loddenkemper, P. Astoul et al., "Management of malignant pleural effusions," *European Respiratory Journal*, vol. 18, no. 2, pp. 402–419, 2001.

[2] P.-C. Yang, K.-T. Luh, D.-B. Chang, H.-D. Wu, C.-J. Yu, and S.-H. Kuo, "Value of sonography in determining the nature of pleural effusion: Analysis of 320 cases," *American Journal of Roentgenology*, vol. 159, no. 1, pp. 29–33, 1992.

[3] J. Reuß, "Sonographic imaging of the pleura: Nearly 30 years experience," *European Journal of Ultrasound*, vol. 3, no. 2, pp. 125–139, 1996.

[4] K. Wernecke, "Ultrasound study of the pleura," *European Radiology*, vol. 10, no. 10, pp. 1515–1523, 2000.

[5] C. Görg, I. Restrepo, and W. B. Schwerk, "Sonography of malignant pleural effusion," *European Radiology*, vol. 7, no. 8, pp. 1195–1198, 1997.

[6] H.-J. Chen, W.-H. Hsu, C.-Y. Tu et al., "Sonographic septation in lymphocyte-rich exudative pleural effusions: A useful diagnostic predictor for tuberculosis," *Journal of Ultrasound in Medicine*, vol. 25, no. 7, pp. 857–863, 2006.

[7] A. Bugalho, D. Ferreira, S. S. Dias et al., "The diagnostic value of transthoracic ultrasonographic features in predicting malignancy in undiagnosed pleural effusions: A prospective observational study," *Respiration*, vol. 87, no. 4, pp. 270–278, 2014.

[8] N. R. Qureshi, N. M. Rahman, and F. V. Gleeson, "Thoracic ultrasound in the diagnosis of malignant pleural effusion," *Thorax*, vol. 64, no. 2, pp. 139–143, 2009.

[9] C. C. Hua, L. C. Chang, Y. C. Chen, and S. C. Chang, "Proinflammatory cytokines and fibrinolytic enzymes in tuberculous and malignant pleural effusions," *CHEST*, vol. 116, no. 5, pp. 1292–1296, 1999.

[10] F. Philip-Joet, M.-C. Alessi, C. Philip-Joet et al., "Fibrinolytic and inflammatory processes in pleural effusions," *European Respiratory Journal*, vol. 8, no. 8, pp. 1352–1356, 1995.

[11] C. S. Grove and Y. C. G. Lee, "Vascular endothelial growth factor: the key mediator in pleural effusion formation," *Current Opinion in Pulmonary Medicine*, vol. 8, no. 4, pp. 294–301, 2002.

[12] C. Chung, C. Yeh, J. Sheu, Y. Chen, and S. Chang, "Repeated thoracenteses affect proinflammatory cytokines, vascular endothelial growth factor, and fibrinolytic activity in pleural transudates," *The American Journal of the Medical Sciences*, vol. 334, no. 6, pp. 452–457, 2007.

[13] M. Ashchi, J. Golish, P. Eng, and P. O'Donovan, "Transudative malignant pleural effusions: Prevalence and mechanisms," *Southern Medical Journal*, vol. 91, no. 1, pp. 23–26, 1998.

[14] Z. Assi, J. L. Caruso, J. Herndon, and E. F. Patz Jr., "Cytologically proved malignant pleural effusions: Distribution of transudates and exudates," *CHEST*, vol. 113, no. 5, pp. 1302–1304, 1998.

[15] R. W. Light, Y. S. Erozan, and W. C. Ball, "Cells in Pleural Fluid: Their Value in Differential Diagnosis," *JAMA Internal Medicine*, vol. 132, no. 6, pp. 854–860, 1973.

[16] M. P. Rivera, A. C. Mehta, and M. M. Wahidi, "Establishing the diagnosis of lung cancer: diagnosis and management of lung cancer, 3rd ed: American college of chest physicians evidence-based clinical practice guidelines," *CHEST*, vol. 143, no. 5, pp. e142S–e165S, 2013.

[17] I. Psallidas, I. Kalomenidis, J. M. Porcel, B. W. Robinson, and G. T. Stathopoulos, "Malignant pleural effusion: From bench to bedside," *European Respiratory Review*, vol. 25, no. 140, pp. 189–198, 2016.

[18] R. Loddenkemper, "Thoracoscopy - state of the art," *European Respiratory Journal*, vol. 11, pp. 213–221, 1998.

[19] C. F. N. Koegelenberg, E. M. Irusen, F. Von Groote-Bidlingmaier, J. W. Bruwer, E. M. A. Batubara, and A. H. Diacon, "The utility of ultrasound-guided thoracentesis and pleural biopsy in undiagnosed pleural exudates," *Thorax*, vol. 70, no. 10, pp. 995–997, 2015.

[20] C. Hooper, Y. C. G. Lee, and N. Maskell, "Investigation of a unilateral pleural effusion in adults: British Thoracic Society

pleural disease guideline 2010," *Thorax*, vol. 65, supplement 2, pp. ii4–ii17, 2010.

[21] V. Villena, A. López-Encuentra, R. García-Luján, J. Echave-Sustaeta, and C. J. Á. Martínez, "Clinical implications of appearance of pleural fluid at thoracentesis," *CHEST*, vol. 125, no. 1, pp. 156–159, 2004.

[22] R. W. Light, "Useful tests on the pleural fluid in the management of patients with pleural effusions," *Current Opinion in Pulmonary Medicine*, vol. 5, no. 4, pp. 245–249, 1999.

[23] V. Bandi, W. Lunn, A. Ernst, R. Eberhardt, H. Hoffmann, and F. J. F. Herth, "Ultrasound vs CT in detecting chest wall invasion by tumor: A prospective study," *CHEST*, vol. 133, no. 4, pp. 881–886, 2008.

[24] A. Churg, T. V. Colby, P. Cagle et al., "The separation of benign and malignant mesothelial proliferations," *The American Journal of Surgical Pathology*, vol. 24, no. 9, pp. 1183–1200, 2000.

8

Diagnostic Yield of Combined Pulmonary Cryobiopsies and Electromagnetic Navigation in Small Pulmonary Nodules

Olivier Taton[1], **Benjamin Bondue**[1], **Pierre Alain Gevenois**[2]
Myriam Remmelink[3] **and Dimitri Leduc**[1]

[1]*Department of Pneumology, Hôpital Erasme, Université Libre de Bruxelles, 808 Route de Lennik, 1070 Brussels, Belgium*
[2]*Department of Radiology, Hôpital Erasme, Université Libre de Bruxelles, 808 Route de Lennik, 1070 Brussels, Belgium*
[3]*Department of Pathology, Hôpital Erasme, Université Libre de Bruxelles, 808 Route de Lennik, 1070 Brussels, Belgium*

Correspondence should be addressed to Olivier Taton; olivier.taton@erasme.ulb.ac.be

Olivier Taton and Benjamin Bondue contributed equally to this work.

Academic Editor: Nicole S. L. Goh

Background. An increasing number of pulmonary nodules of unknown nature are detected as a result of screening by CT in high lung cancer risk patients. *Objectives.* The purposes of this study were to assess the diagnostic yield of electromagnetic navigation bronchoscopy (ENB) combined with transbronchial lung cryobiopsy (TBLC) and to compare it with standard transbronchial biopsy (TBB) in pulmonary nodules of less than 2 cm in diameter. *Methods.* We prospectively included 32 patients (18 men and 14 women, mean age 68 ± 9 years) with nodules of less than 2 cm in diameter and no metastasis at ^{18}FDG PET-CT. The nodule position was determined by ENB, radial endobronchial ultrasonography miniprobe, and fluoroscopy. Eight samples were obtained, six by TBB and two by TBLC. *Results.* Nodule diameter averaged 16 ± 3 mm. Twenty-five nodules were malignant and 18 were surgically resected. Surgery was avoided in four patients as the biopsies revealed a benign disease. The samples obtained by TBLC were five times larger than those by TBB. The diagnostic yields of TBLC and TBB were 69% and 38%, respectively (p=0.017). Adverse events consisted in 15 mild or moderate bleedings and one pneumothorax. *Conclusions.* In the setting of peripheral pulmonary lesions of less than 20 mm in diameter, ENB-combined TBLC is feasible and safe, provides larger samples, and has higher diagnostic yield than TBB.

1. Introduction

Since the report of decreased lung cancer mortality associated with screening trials in subjects at high lung cancer risk [1], the number of chest CT scans performed for the detection of lung cancer increased dramatically. As a consequence, an increasing number of solid and nonsolid (ground glass) nodules of unknown etiology are detected [2]. The challenge for the physician is to determine safely and accurately the pathological nature of these nodules.

It is acknowledged that flexible bronchoscopy under fluoroscopic guidance has a diagnostic yield lower than 30% for nodules less than 2 cm in diameter as compared to higher than 60% in those larger than 2 cm in diameter [3]. Interestingly, Eberhardt et al. [4] reported that the diagnostic yield of bronchoscopy could be improved up to 88% by combining electromagnetic navigation bronchoscopy (ENB) with endobronchial ultrasonography (EBUS) in order to guide transbronchial biopsy (TBB). However, their study group included patients with a wide range of nodule sizes with only 23 patients with nodules smaller than 2 cm in diameter.

On the other hand, the size of tissue samples obtained with standard forceps usually limits the diagnostic yield in small nodules especially in the era of immunohistochemical and molecular testing required for lung cancer targeted therapies [5]. Transbronchial lung cryobiopsy (TBLC) is an emerging technique that allows tissue samples larger than those obtained with standard TBB in the setting of interstitial lung diseases [6, 7] and has been shown to be feasible under

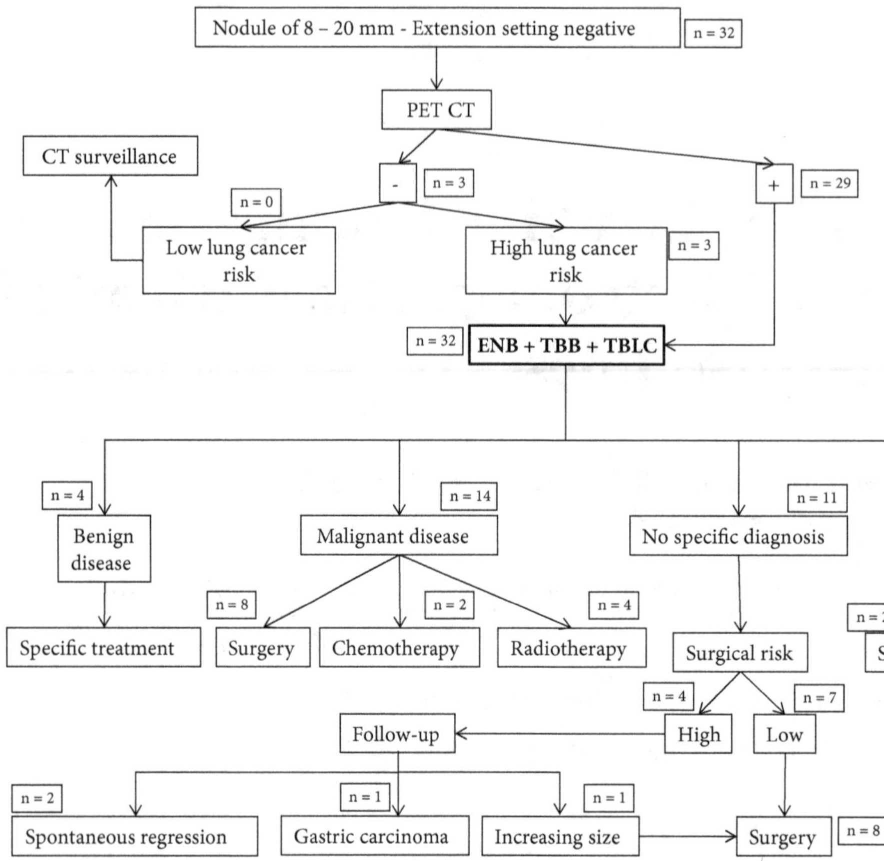

FIGURE 1: Flowchart summarizing the management of patients with pulmonary nodules from 8 to 20 mm in diameter without locoregional or distant metastasis with the frequencies in each category. Benign diseases consisted in tuberculosis in three patients, sarcoidosis in one patient, and cryptogenic organizing pneumonia in one patient. Abbreviations: ENB = electromagnetic navigation bronchoscopy; EBUS = endobronchial ultrasonography; TBB = transbronchial biopsy; TBLC = transbronchial lung cryobiopsy.

EBUS guidance in the setting of pulmonary nodules [8, 9]. We thus hypothesized that TBLC could perform better than TBB in the workup of nodules smaller than 2 cm in diameter. The purpose of this prospective study was therefore to compare the diagnostic yield of TBLC and TBB, both guided by an EBUS miniprobe combined with ENB, in this particular setting.

2. Materials and Methods

2.1. Study Design and Patients. This study protocol was approved by our institutional ethics committee and written informed consent was obtained from all patients.

From December 2016 to March 2018, 32 consecutive patients (18 men and 14 women, mean age (± standard deviation, SD) 68 ± 9 years) were prospectively enrolled. Twelve patients were current smokers and 17 patients were ex-smokers. On average, the smokers had smoked 37 ± 23 pack-years. All patients underwent chest CT scan the day before bronchoscopy. The location and the size of each nodule were recorded. Patients with pulmonary solid or nonsolid nodules were considered for inclusion in our study group if they fulfilled the following criteria: age over 18 years; a CT-detected solid or nonsolid nodule with a diameter ranging from 8 to 20 mm without any evidence of locoregional or distant metastasis; no endobronchial abnormality; platelets count higher than 80,000/mm^3; systolic pulmonary arterial pressure lower than 45 mmHg at transthoracic ultrasonography; no coagulation tests abnormality; no severe respiratory dysfunction defined as FEV_1 < 1L, FVC < 50% predicted, or DLCO < 25% predicted; and no contraindication to general anesthesia or bronchoscopy. Metabolic activity of lung nodules was assessed by a ^{18}FDG PET-CT scan. In absence of ^{18}FDG uptake, patients at high lung cancer risk (age of 55 to 74 years, more than 30 pack-years of smoking history, growing lung lesion, or neoplasm history) were also included. Figure 1 summarizes the management of these patients.

2.2. Tissue Sampling. General anesthesia and muscles paralysis were obtained with remifentanil (Ultiva®, Aspen Pharma, Dublin, Ireland), propofol (Propolipid®, Fresenius Kabi, Hesse, Germany), and rocuronium (Esmeron®, MSD, Kenilworth, NJ). After insertion of a rigid bronchoscope, a guide sheath (Edge™ Firm Tip, endobronchial procedure kit, 180° catheter, Covidien, MA, USA) was first inserted through a flexible bronchoscope (BF-1TH190, Olympus, Tokyo, Japan) in the segmental bronchus close to the target nodule with the previously described ENB technique (superDimension/Bronchus, Herzliya, Israel) [10]. The ENB was considered successful if the distance from the sensor probe to the target center was less than 10 mm according to Becker et al. [10]. The average fiducial target registration error, which is the discrepancy between the virtual and real bronchoscopy, was not assessed in this study. A radial EBUS miniprobe (UM-S20-17S, 20 MHz, Olympus, Tokyo, Japan) was then inserted in the guide sheath in order to check its position close to the target nodule. Finally, the position holding of the catheter was checked at regular time intervals by fluoroscopy.

Six samples were obtained through the bronchial wall (i.e., TBB) with a standard pair of forceps (FB-233D, 3 Fr, Olympus, Tokyo, Japan), the position holding of the catheter having been checked by ENB after the three first samples. All the material was then removed in order to place a Fogarty balloon into the segmental bronchus, which was inflated prophylactically after each cryobiopsy for controlling possible bleeding following TBLC. The ENB procedure was performed again. A first TBLC sample was obtained through a flexible cryoprobe of 115 cm in length and 1.9 mm in diameter (ERBE, Medizintechnik GmbH, Tubingen, Germany) inserted into the guide sheath. Once in position, the probe was cooled for 7 to 8 seconds; then the guide sheath, the cryoprobe, and the bronchoscope were together removed out of the airway and the frozen specimen was thawed first in saline at room temperature and afterwards transferred to formalin for fixation [6]. A second TBLC sample was obtained if no significant complication was observed. ENB technique and fluoroscopy were performed before each TBLC in order to position again the guide sheath. Adverse events occurring during and after completion of the procedure were recorded.

Among possible complications, bleeding was scored as follows: score 0, when no bleeding occurred; score 1, when bleeding stopped within five minutes either spontaneously or by inflation of the Fogarty balloon; score 2, when bleeding was prolonged for more than five minutes or needed cold saline instillation; and score 3, when bleeding required embolization, selective bronchial intubation, transfusion, or admission in the intensive care unit or resulted in prolonged hospital stay or patient's death [6].

All samples were analyzed by a pathologist (blind for review) with more than 25 years of experience in lung pathology. If the diagnosis based on TBB and TBLC samples was uncertain or inconsistent with the clinical presentation, operable patients were referred for surgical resection and nonoperable patients were followed up by CT six months thereafter. Depending on histological analyses, microbiological analyses (i.e., specific staining and culture) were requested if needed. Pathological analysis of the surgical specimen and CT follow-up were considered as the independent methods of reference for establishing the final diagnosis.

2.3. Statistics. Continuous data were expressed using means ± SD. Categorical data were expressed as percentages. The diagnostic yield of each technique is the ratio of correctly diagnosed cases to the total number of patients expressed in percentage. Comparisons between groups were performed using the chi-square or Fisher's exact test when appropriate. A two-tailed p value of less than 0.05 was considered as statistically significant. Statistical analysis was performed using SAS (SAS Institute, Cary, NC).

Table 1: Patients characteristics.

Patients characteristics at inclusion in the study	
Male gender (%)	56 (18/32)
Age (yrs)	68 ± 9
Current smoker (%)	37 (12/32)
Previous smoker (%)	53 (17/32)
Pack-year	37 ± 23
Body height (cm)	169 ± 8
Body weight (kg)	73 ± 15
FEV_1 (ml)	1851 ± 716
FEV_1 (% predicted)	71.5 ± 20.1
DLCO (% predicted)	58.8 ± 19.2
PAPs (mmHg)	30 ± 5
Lesion size (mm)	16 ± 3
Lobar distribution of nodules at initial CT scan	
Right upper lobe	8
Middle lobe	1
Right lower lobe	8
Left upper lobe	7
Left lower lobe	8
Malignancy at the end of follow-up	
Lung adenocarcinoma	20
Squamous cell cancer	2
Small cell lung cancer	2
Metastatic carcinoma	1

Note: data are presented as frequencies or means ± SD. Abbreviations: FEV_1 = forced expiration volume in 1 second; DLCO = carbon monoxide diffusing capacity; PAPs = systolic pressure of pulmonary artery.

3. Results

3.1. Patients and Nodules Characteristics. Patients and nodules characteristics are summarized in Table 1. The mean diameter of the target nodules was 16 ± 3 mm. All patients but one presented one single nodule. One patient presented four nodules. In that particular patient, the largest nodule (16 mm in diameter) was selected for biopsy. All nodules were solid but one was nonsolid. Fifteen, sixteen, and one patient, respectively, had the nodule in their upper, lower, or middle lobe. Eleven patients presented a bronchus sign at CT [11]. Figure 2 showed 4 representative patients in our study group.

Fifteen patients were operable at the time of inclusion according to the ERS guidelines [12] but preferred to have first the endoscopic evaluation before a surgical procedure. At the end of this study, eleven among these 15 operable patients had surgery that revealed a malignant disease and surgery was avoided in four patients as the endoscopic procedures could yield the diagnosis of a benign disease.

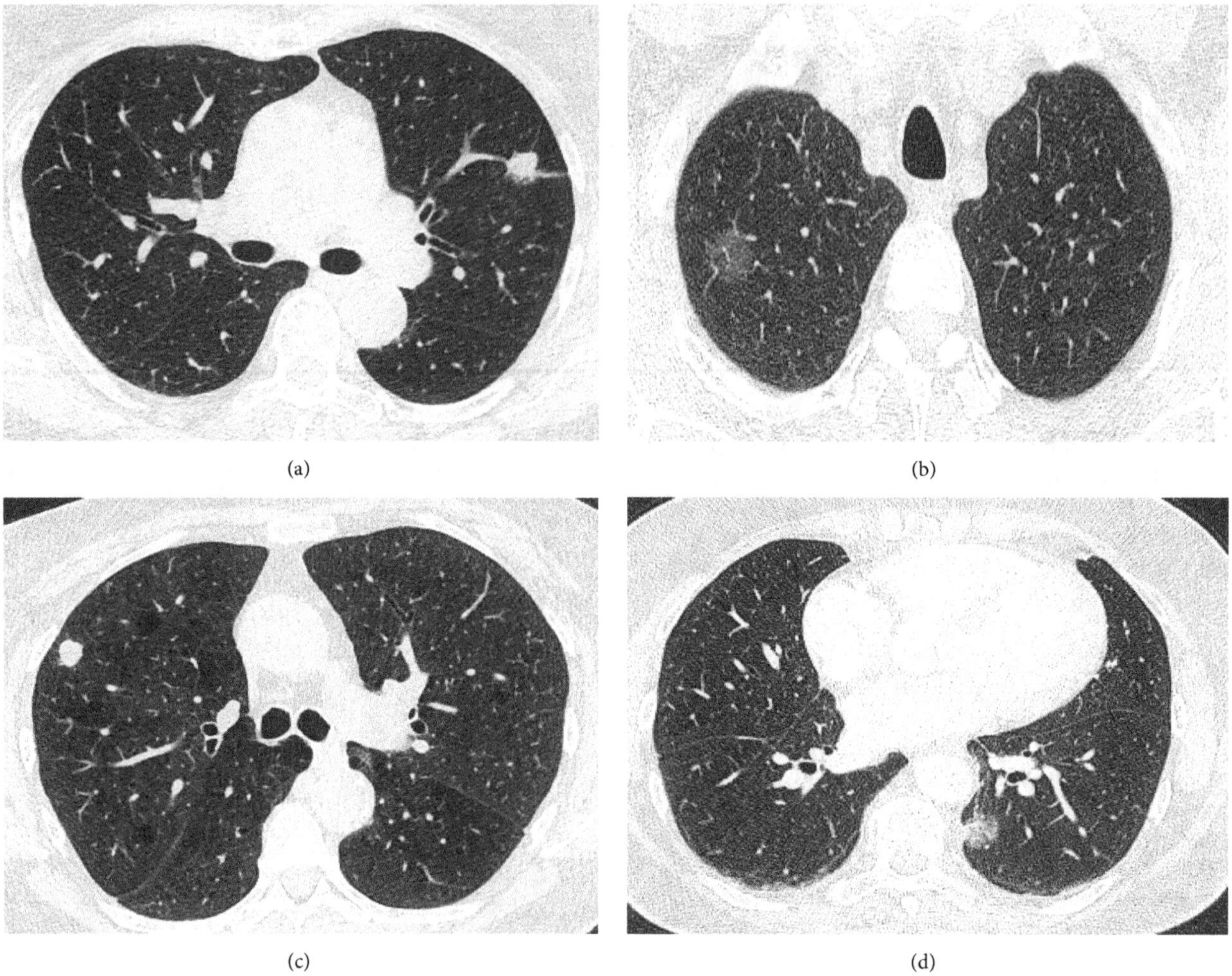

FIGURE 2: CT scans in four representative patients. Panel (a) presents a solid nodule of 16 mm in diameter in the left upper lobe in a 75-year-old woman. The final diagnosis was tuberculosis. Panel (b) presents a nonsolid nodule of 20 mm in diameter in the right upper lobe in a 57-year-old man. The final diagnosis was lung adenocarcinoma. Panel (c) presents a solid nodule of 11 mm in diameter in the right upper lobe in a 72-year-old woman. The final diagnosis was small cell lung carcinoma. Panel (d) presents a nonsolid nodule of 14 mm in diameter in the left lower lobe in a 67-year-old woman. The final diagnosis was lung adenocarcinoma.

3.2. Final Diagnosis. Malignancy was diagnosed in 25 patients. Among these 25 patients, 20 presented a lung adenocarcinoma, two a squamous cell cancer, two a small cell lung cancer, and one a metastasis of a gastric carcinoma. The diagnosis was confirmed by surgery in 18 patients and by TBLC/TBB in six patients. In one patient, a gastric carcinoma was diagnosed by gastric biopsy during the follow-up and the pulmonary nodule was assumed to be a lung metastasis from the gastric carcinoma. Other diagnoses included tuberculosis in three patients, nonspecific inflammation with spontaneous regression in two patients, cryptogenic organizing pneumonia in one patient, and sarcoidosis in one patient.

3.3. Technical Results. In three patients, we were unable to reach the target with the ENB. As a consequence, the method was successful in 29 patients. Among these 29 patients, the nodule was visualized at fluoroscopy in eight patients and at EBUS miniprobe in 19 patients.

3.4. Comparison between TBLC and TBB. The mean diameters of the samples, respectively, obtained by TBLC and TBB were 5.3 mm ± 0.7 and 1.1 mm ± 0.6 ($p< 0.001$) (Table 2).

Among the 29 patients in whom both TBLC and TBB could be obtained, their overall diagnostic yield was 69% (20/29) and 38% (11/29), respectively (p=0.017). Considering the three patients in whom the target nodule could not be reached with ENB, the diagnostic yield was 63% (20/32) and 34% (11/32), respectively (p=0.024).

Among the 29 patients in whom both TBLC and TBB could be obtained, the sensitivity and specificity of TBLC for the diagnosis of a malignant nodule were, respectively, 61% and 100% as compared to 35% and 100% for TBB (p=0.008 and p>0.999, respectively). The corresponding positive and negative predictive values of TBLC were, respectively, 100% and 40% as compared to 100% and 29% for TBB (p>0.999 and p=0.277, respectively).

The lobar location of the nodule, the bronchus sign, the nodule size, the malignant vs. benign disease, or the

TABLE 2: Comparison between TBB and TBLC in 29 patients in whom both TBLC and TBB were obtained.

	TBB	TBLC	*p* value
Sample size (mm)	1.1 ± 0.6	5.3 ± 0.7	<0.001
Diagnostic yield *	38 % (11/29)	69 % (20/29)	0.017
Sensitivity	35%	61%	0.008
Specificity	100%	100%	>0.999
Positive PV	100%	100%	>0.999
Negative PV	29%	40%	0.277
Bleeding			
Grade 1	7%	38%	0.005
Grade 2	0%	14%	0.043
Grade 3	0%	0%	>0.999

Note: abbreviations: TBB = transbronchial biopsy; TBLC = transbronchial lung cryobiopsy; PV = predictive value. *: diagnosis was obtained by TBLC alone in 9 patients and by both TBB and TBLC in 11 patients.

TABLE 3: Comparison between diagnosis accuracy by TBB and that by TBLC.

	< 15 mm	≥ 15 mm	*p*
TBB	5/11 (45 %)	6/18 (33 %)	0,540
TBLC	6/11 (54 %)	14/18 (78 %)	0,230
	Lower lobes	Other lobes	
TBB	6/15 (40 %)	5/14 (36 %)	0,820
TBLC	10/15 (67 %)	10/14 (71 %)	0,791
	Malignant disease	Benign disease	
TBB	8/23 (35 %)	3/6 (50 %)	0,555
TBLC	14/23 (61 %)	4/6 (67 %)	0,73
	EBUS +	EBUS -	
TBB	7/19 (37 %)	4/10 (40 %)	0,876
TBLC	13/19 (68 %)	7/10 (70 %)	0,934
	Bronchus sign +	Bronchus sign -	
TBB	3/11 (27 %)	8/18 (44 %)	0,329
TBLC	8/11 (73 %)	12/18 (67 %)	0,816

Note: abbreviations: TBB = transbronchial biopsy; TBLC = transbronchial lung cryobiopsy; EBUS = endobronchial ultrasonography; EBUS + = nodule visualization by EBUS miniprobe. EBUS - = no nodule visualization by EBUS miniprobe. Bronchus sign + = presence of a bronchus sign. Bronchus sign - = absence of bronchus sign.

technique used (nodule visualization or not with EBUS miniprobe) for visualizing the nodule in addition to ENB had no statically significant impact on the diagnostic performance (*p* ranging from 0.073 to 0.934) (Table 3).

We have also calculated the number needed to be tested (by endoscopic procedure) to diagnose benign disease and we obtained the number of 8. It means that we have to perform 8 endoscopic procedures to diagnose one benign disease and to avoid an inadequate treatment such as surgical resection or stereotactic ablative radiotherapy.

3.5. Adverse Events. Bleeding was graded 1 and 2 in, respectively, eleven and four patients. Pneumothorax needing pleural drainage for three days was observed in one patient. No other adverse event was observed and no mortality was recorded.

4. Discussion

This study shows that, in the workup of pulmonary nodules smaller than 2 cm in diameter, TBLC performs better than TBB and is safe with no or minimal associated adverse events.

We used TBLC in order to obtain as large as possible tissue samples and we combined it with fluoroscopy, EBUS miniprobe, and ENB in order to accurately reach the target nodules. With this strategy, the overall diagnostic yield of TBLC reaches 63%, a figure in line with results reported by Wang et al. in their meta-analysis also focused on lesions smaller than 20 mm in diameter (60.9% with a 95% confidence interval ranging from 54.0 to 67.7%) [13].

As compared to TBB, TBLC provides larger tissue samples and has also the theoretical advantage of reaching nodules adjacent to bronchus segments between successive divisions that are inaccessible by TBB as it requires that the pair of forceps faces the target nodule. The difference of diagnostic yields between TBLC and TBB—respectively, around 70% and 40%—confirms these advantages. As previously reported [7], the samples obtained by TBLC are indeed approximately five times larger than those by TBB. This larger size could probably explain that the diagnostic yield and sensitivity of TBLC are higher than those of TBB in lung nodules. However, the sensitivity and the negative predictive value remain low with prevalence of malignancy approximating 80% in our study group, very close to that reported by Gex et al. (76.5% with a 95% confidence interval ranging from 70.2% to 81.2%) in their systematic review [14].

TBLC associated with ENB could be the best option in the diagnosis of nodules smaller than 20 mm in diameter. CT-guided transthoracic needle biopsy is an alternative to assess peripheral lesions but is associated with a higher complication rate than endoscopy [15], especially in lesions smaller than 30 mm in diameter, in which the rate of pneumothorax reaches 32.3% [16]. In our study group, the rate of bleeding and pneumothorax was particularly low, rising the interest of TBLC associated with ENB in the particular setting of small-size nodules. Indeed, we observed lower bleeding—with no severe bleeding—and pneumothorax rates than in the setting of interstitial lung disease [17]. The only patient who required chest tube drainage had a nodule adjacent to the pleura, suggesting avoidance of cryobiopsy in this particular location.

In order to improve the accuracy of lesion targeting, new guidance techniques have been developed. However, despite the use of three complementary localization techniques (fluoroscopy, EBUS miniprobe, and ENB), the diagnostic yield of TBB in our study was much lower than 65% and 67% reported in two recent systematic reviews [10, 13]. Our low diagnostic yield could be explained, at least in part, by the recruitment in our tertiary hospital of more challenging cases, including small targets, a very low frequency of the CT bronchus sign, a sign considered as a key variable conditioning ENB yield with an odd's ratio averaging 7.6 [11], and a low proportion of nodules visualized with the EBUS miniprobe, such visualization being also associated with an increased yield [4].

Whereas surgical resection is the currently recommended treatment in operable patients with lung nodule, high lung cancer risk, and no metastasis [18], 15 of our patients preferred to have first an endoscopic evaluation. Among them, four patients presented a benign disease and surgery could thus be avoided. In five other patients, malignancy was proved by an endoscopic procedure and they were operated on. The six remaining patients had no specific diagnosis after endoscopic procedure and were also operated on with a subsequent diagnosis of lung cancer in all of them. The actual benefit of endoscopic procedures appears thus lower in operable patients than in nonoperable ones but could nevertheless be an option in selected patients and could be discussed with them. On the other hand for nonoperable patients, stereotactic ablative radiotherapy has proven efficacy in the control of early stage cancer with few adverse events [19]. Considering this locoregional treatment and systemic treatment currently available, in nonoperable patients or in patients with intermediate lung cancer risk (for example, nongrowing or PET-negative nodules), cryobiopsy could be considered in order to propose specific treatments. We could also speculate that combining endoscopic approaches (ENB, EBUS miniprobe, and fluoroscopy), TBLC, and rapid on-site pathological examination followed by surgery would be an interesting future option to investigate.

Our study has two important limitations. First, the small number of included patients precludes definite conclusions on the appropriateness of TBLC in small lung nodules. Second, this is a monocentric study limiting the impact of procedural variability. Our results should therefore encourage further randomized and multicentric studies with a standardized approach of the nodules of less than 20 mm in diameter.

In conclusion, in the setting of peripheral pulmonary lesions of less than 20 mm in diameter, ENB-combined TBLC is feasible and safe, provides larger tissue samples, and has higher diagnostic yield than TBB. This approach could be proposed in nonoperable or low/intermediate lung cancer risk patients.

Abbreviations

DLCO: Diffusing capacity for carbon monoxide
EBUS: Endobronchial ultrasonography
ENB: Electromagnetic navigation bronchoscopy
FEV_1: Forced expiration volume in one second
FVC: Forced vital capacity
TBB: Transbronchial biopsy
TBLC: Transbronchial lung cryobiopsy.

Disclosure

The authors participate in endoscopic workshops with ERBE and Medtronic.

Authors' Contributions

Olivier Taton and Benjamin Bondue contributed equally to the realization of this work.

Acknowledgments

This work was supported by the Erasme Fund for Medical Research.

References

[1] D. R. Aberle, A. M. Adams, and C. D. Berg, "Reduced lung-cancer mortality with low-dose computed tomographic screening," *The New England Journal of Medicine*, vol. 365, no. 5, pp. 395–409, 2011.

[2] M. K. Gould, T. Tang, I.-L. A. Liu et al., "Recent trends in the identification of incidental pulmonary nodules," *American Journal of Respiratory and Critical Care Medicine*, vol. 192, no. 10, pp. 1208–1214, 2015.

[3] G. Schreiber and D. C. McCrory, "Performance characteristics

of different modalities for diagnosis of suspected lung cancer: Summary of published evidence," *CHEST*, vol. 123, no. 1, 2003.

[4] R. Eberhardt, D. Anantham, A. Ernst, D. Feller-Kopman, and F. Herth, "Multimodality bronchoscopic diagnosis of peripheral lung lesions: A randomized controlled trial," *American Journal of Respiratory and Critical Care Medicine*, vol. 176, no. 1, pp. 36–41, 2007.

[5] W. D. Travis, E. Brambilla, M. Noguchi et al., "Diagnosis of lung cancer in small biopsies and cytology: Implications of the 2011 International Association for the Study of Lung Cancer/American Thoracic Society/European respiratory society classification," *Archives of Pathology & Laboratory Medicine*, vol. 137, no. 5, pp. 668–684, 2013.

[6] B. Bondue, T. Pieters, P. Alexander et al., "Role of transbronchial lung cryobiopsies in diffuse parenchymal lung diseases: Interest of a sequential approach," *Pulmonary Medicine*, vol. 2017, 2017.

[7] V. Pajares, C. Puzo, D. Castillo et al., "Diagnostic yield of transbronchial cryobiopsy in interstitial lung disease: a randomized trial," *Respirology*, vol. 19, no. 6, pp. 900–906, 2014.

[8] M. Schuhmann, K. Bostanci, A. Bugalho et al., "Endobronchial ultrasound-guided cryobiopsies in peripheral pulmonary lesions: a feasibility study," *European Respiratory Society*, vol. 43, no. 1, pp. 233–239, 2014.

[9] S. Herath and E. Yap, "Novel hybrid cryo-radial method: an emerging alternative to CT-guided biopsy in suspected lung cancer. A prospective case series and description of technique," *Respirology Case Reports*, vol. 6, no. 2, p. e00287, 2018.

[10] H. D. Becher, F. Herth, A. Ernst, and Y. Schwarz, "Bronchoscopic biopsy of peripheral lung lesions under electromagnetic guidance: A pilot study," *Journal of Bronchology & Interventional Pulmonology*, vol. 12, no. 1, pp. 9–13, 2005.

[11] L. M. Seijo, J. P. de Torres, M. D. Lozano et al., "Diagnostic yield of electromagnetic navigation bronchoscopy is highly dependent on the presence of a bronchus sign on CT imaging: results from a prospective study," *CHEST*, vol. 138, no. 6, pp. 1316–1321, 2010.

[12] A. Brunelli, A. Charloux, C. T. Bolliger et al., "ERS/ESTS clinical guidelines on fitness for radical therapy in lung cancer patients (surgery and chemo-radiotherapy)," *European Respiratory Journal*, vol. 34, no. 1, pp. 17–41, 2009.

[13] J. S. Wang Memoli, P. J. Nietert, and G. A. Silvestri, "Meta-analysis of guided bronchoscopy for the evaluation of the pulmonary nodule," *CHEST*, vol. 142, no. 2, pp. 385–393, 2012.

[14] G. Gex, J. A. Pralong, C. Combescure, L. Seijo, T. Rochat, and P. M. Soccal, "Diagnostic yield and safety of electromagnetic navigation bronchoscopy for lung nodules: a systematic review and meta-analysis," *Respiration*, vol. 87, no. 2, pp. 165–176, 2014.

[15] R. S. Wiener, L. M. Schwartz, S. Woloshin, and H. Gilbert Welch, "Population-based risk for complications after transthoracic needle lung biopsy of a pulmonary nodule: an analysis of discharge records," *Annals of Internal Medicine*, vol. 155, no. 3, pp. 137–144, 2011.

[16] F. F. Görgülü, F. Y. Öksüzler, S. A. Arslan, M. Arslan, İ. E. Özsoy, and O. Görgülü, "Computed tomography-guided transthoracic biopsy: Factors influencing diagnostic and complication rates," *Journal of International Medical Research*, vol. 45, no. 2, pp. 808–815, 2017.

[17] K. A. Johannson, V. S. Marcoux, P. E. Ronksley, and C. J. Ryerson, "Diagnostic yield and complications of transbronchial lung cryobiopsy for interstitial lung disease: A systematic review and metaanalysis," *Annals of the American Thoracic Society*, vol. 13, no. 10, pp. 1828–1838, 2016.

[18] G. A. Silvestri, A. V. Gonzalez, M. A. Jantz et al., "Methods for staging non-small cell lung cancer: diagnosis and management of lung cancer, 3rd ed: American college of chest physicians evidence-based clinical practice guidelines," *CHEST*, vol. 143, no. 5, pp. e211–e250, 2013.

[19] J. A. Klapper, S. A. Hittinger, and C. E. Denlinger, "Alternatives to lobectomy for high-risk patients with early-stage non-small cell lung cancer," *The Annals of Thoracic Surgery*, vol. 103, no. 4, pp. 1330–1339, 2017.

9

Saddle Pulmonary Embolus Caught in Transit across a Patent Foramen Ovale

Aram Barbaryan,[1] Stefania Bailuc,[1] Travis Abicht,[2] Sergey Barsamyan,[3] Yonatan Gizaw,[1] and Aibek E. Mirrakhimov[4]

[1] *Division of General, Geriatric & Hospital Medicine, University of Kansas Health System, Kansas City, KS, USA*
[2] *Department of Cardiothoracic Surgery, University of Kansas Health System, Kansas City, KS, USA*
[3] *Department of Cardiology, John Radcliffe Hospital, Oxford University Hospitals NHS Trust, Oxford, UK*
[4] *Division of Pulmonary and Critical Care Medicine, University of New Mexico, Albuquerque, USA*

Correspondence should be addressed to Aram Barbaryan; abarbaryan@kumc.edu

Academic Editor: John Murchison

Impending paradoxical embolism (IPE) also described in the literature as thrombus straddling a patent foramen ovale (PFO) or paradoxical embolus in transit is a rare condition when thrombus (originating mostly in deep veins of lower extremities) embolized to the heart gets caught in PFO or in atrial septal defect without systemic embolization. We present a case of a 39-year-old female on oral contraceptive pills who presented to the emergency department with chief complaint of dyspnea and chest pain. She was found to have saddle pulmonary embolus (PE) extending through PFO to left atrium and into the left ventricle. Patient underwent emergent open pulmonary embolectomy, removal of right and left atrial thrombi, and closure of patent foramen ovale. She tolerated the surgery well and was discharged home on chronic anticoagulation therapy.

1. Introduction

Impending paradoxical embolism (IPE) also described in the literature as thrombus straddling a patent foramen ovale (PFO) or paradoxical embolus in transit is a rare condition when thrombus (originating mostly in deep veins of lower extremities) embolized to the heart gets caught in PFO or in atrial septal defect without systemic embolization. In 1877, Cohnheim documented the first cadaveric diagnosis of an IPE [1]. More than century later in 1985 Nellessen first described IPE using echocardiography [2]. The prevalence of PFO in adult population is 27% [3]. Normally because of left to right pressure gradient there is shunt between left and right atrium. However, in the setting pulmonary artery pressure elevation often occurs with massive and large PE that gradient reverses and the clot can migrate through PFO to left atrium causing paradoxical systemic embolization, or a clot that is larger than PFO can be trapped in PFO causing IPE [4]. We present a case of a 39-year-old female who was found to have IPE. She subsequently underwent surgical thrombectomy with excellent outcome.

2. Case Presentation

A 39-year-old female with history of asthma, obesity, and menorrhagia presented to the hospital with one-week history of exertional shortness of breath. In addition to dyspnea, she reported right lower extremity swelling and pain, which started 4 days prior to this presentation. The patient denied chest pain, palpitations, recent weight loss, known history of personal or family history of blood clots, history of miscarriages, and recent travel. Her only medication was oral contraceptive pill for menorrhagia.

She was hypoxic requiring 2 liters of supplemental oxygen via nasal cannula to maintain oxygen saturation >90%, with respiratory rate 18 breaths per minute. She was mildly tachycardic with a heart rate of 108 bpm and blood pressure was 144/90, and the temperature was 36.6°C. The physical examination was significant for morbid obesity and right lower extremity swelling without sings of phlegmasia cerulea dolens. Troponin I level was normal, BNP was elevated at 704 pg/ml (reference 0-100 pg/ml), 12 lead ECG showed sinus rhythm 95 bpm with $S_1Q_3T_3$ pattern (Figure 1): Chest

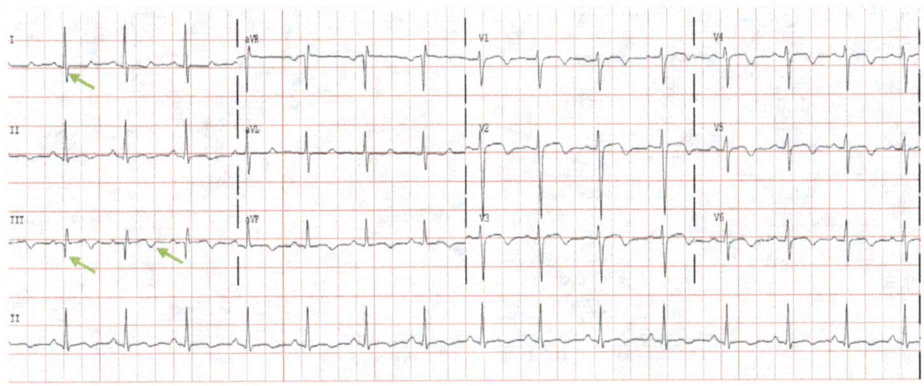

FIGURE 1: 12 lead ECG on admission showing sinus rhythm 95 bpm with $S_1Q_3T_3$ pattern (prominent S wave in lead I, Q wave and inverted T wave in lead III, green arrows).

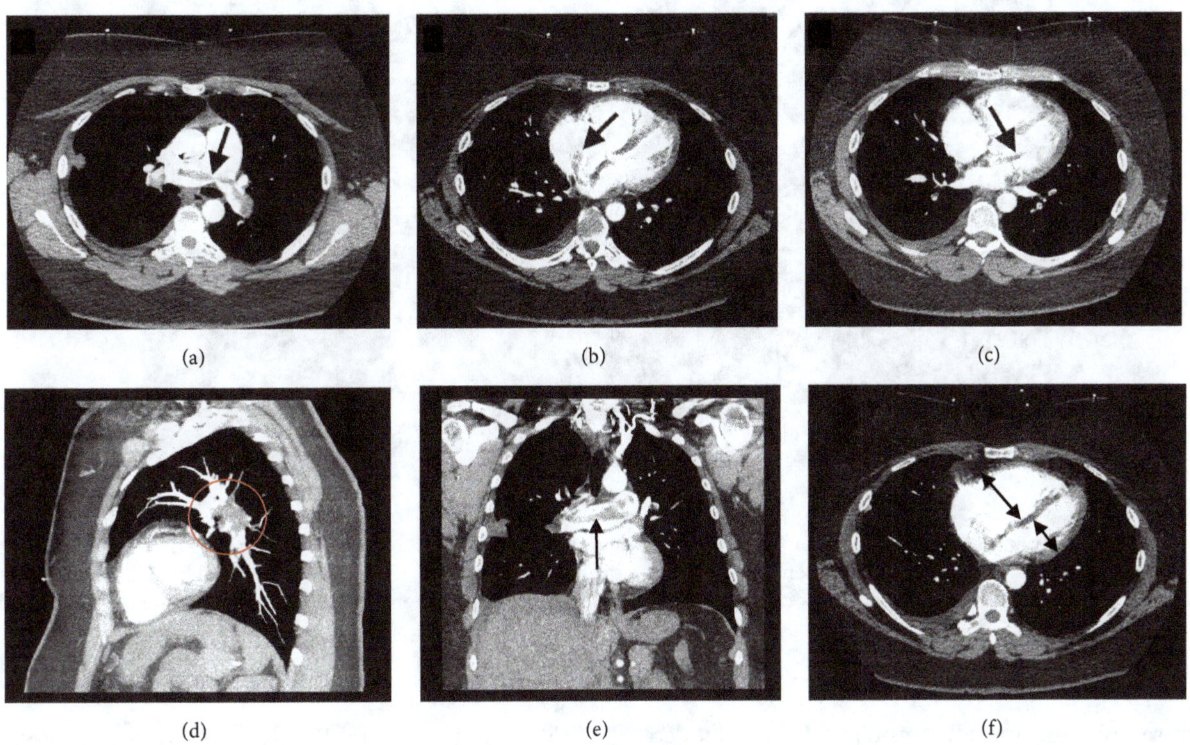

FIGURE 2: CTPA showing saddle PE (a), intracardiac thrombus extending from RA to LA through PFO (b) and further prolapsing into the left ventricle through mitral valve leaflets (c): all axial reconstruction. The same clot in sagittal view ((d), inside the red circle) and coronal view (e). RV enlargement relative to LV compressing the LV in characteristic "D shaped" pattern ((f), double arrows) all consistent with RV strain.

X-ray was unremarkable. Wells' score was 7.5 (3 points for clinical signs and symptoms of deep vein thrombosis, 3 points of PE being the most likely diagnosis, and 1.5 points for heart rate > 100 bpm) rendering high chance of PE; therefore, CT pulmonary angiogram (CTPA) was performed (Figure 2). It demonstrated saddle type pulmonary embolus with extension into multiple segmental and subsegmental branches in the bilateral upper and bilateral lower lobes along with right ventricular (RV) strain (RV end-diastolic diameter was increased with RV to left ventricular (LV) diameter ratio >1) and mild dilatation of main pulmonary artery (35mm, normal is < 29 mm) [5–7]. CTPA also showed a linear band of low density extending within the left atrium and into the left ventricle most compatible with thrombus.

The patient was started on unfractionated heparin infusion. Transthoracic echocardiogram (TTE) was performed to further assess the intracardiac clot burden, the RV strain and to identify right-to-left shunt. TTE (Figure 3) showed a large mobile mass straddling the interatrial septum with elements in both atria, extending to and past the mitral valve and prolapsing into the left ventricle during diastole. This was highly suggestive of a communication between the atria consistent with large patent foramen ovale or atrial septal defect. Moderately dilated RV (RV/LV diameter ratio

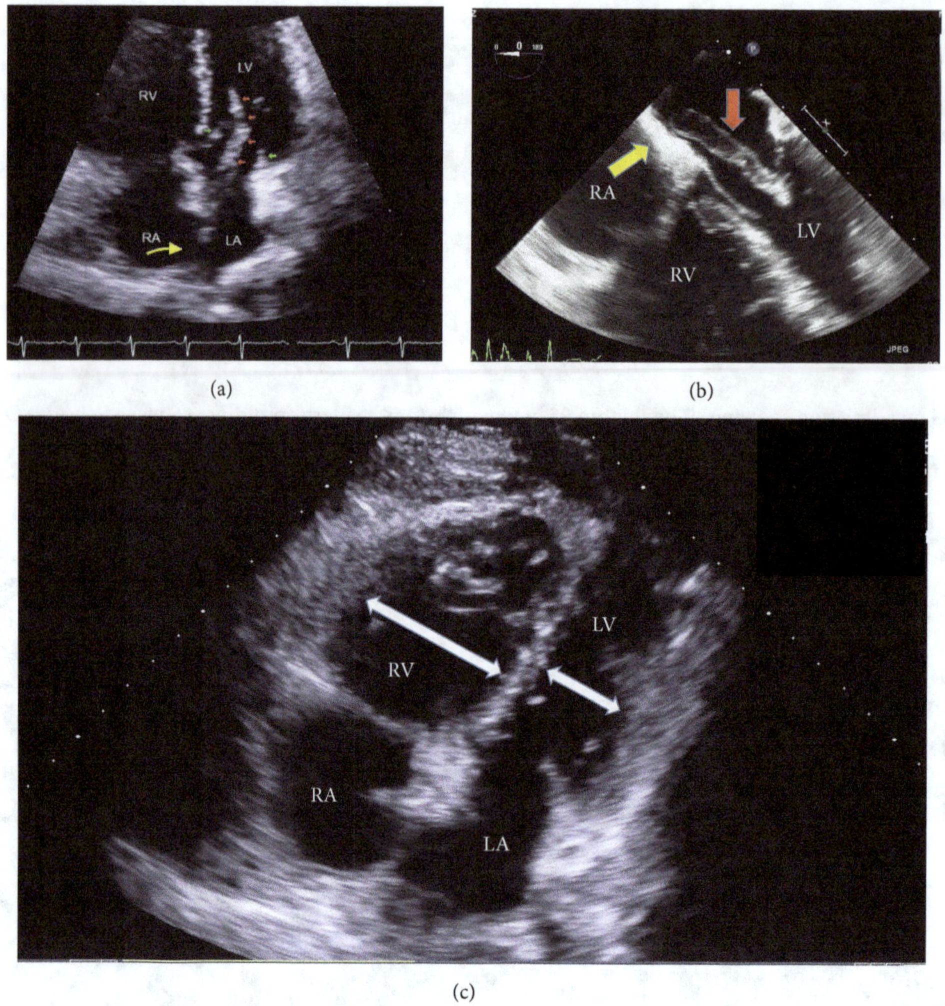

FIGURE 3: Echocardiography: (a) TTE apical four-chamber view demonstrating elongated LA thrombus (red arrows) prolapsing through PFO and LA into the LV during the diastole. Green arrows depict mitral valve leaflets. (b) The same clot is clearly visualized on TEE attached to interatrial septum. Yellow arrow depicts the location of PFO. (c) TTE subcostal view enlarged right heart chambers exceeding their left counterparts in size.

>1) with severely impaired RV systolic function, moderate RA dilation, moderate to severe tricuspid regurgitation, pulmonary artery systolic pressure of 73 mmHg and systolic flattening of the interventricular septum were also noted. All these findings were consistent with RV strain caused by PE. Lower extremity venous doppler ultrasound showed unstable occlusive extensive thrombus within the right femoral vein extending through the right popliteal vein.

Because of large clot burden as well as impending paradoxical embolization, the patient underwent emergent open pulmonary embolectomy, removal of right and left atrial thrombi, and PFO closure (Figure 4). Intraoperative transesophageal echocardiogram (TEE) confirmed the TTE findings (Figure 3): because of the presence of an unstable extensive lower extremity venous thrombus an inferior vena cava filter was also placed. The patient tolerated the surgery well and was discharged from the hospital on oral anticoagulation with warfarin. Six month later during her follow-up visit repeat TTE demonstrated improvement in RV dilation, TV regurgitation, and PA pressure (PA systolic pressure was reduced to 26 mmHg).

3. Discussion

According to the International Cooperative Pulmonary Embolism Registry of 1,135 patients with PE, 42 (4%) were found to have right heart thrombus [8]. According to European Society of Cardiology 2014 guidelines on the diagnosis and management of acute pulmonary embolism, this patient is classified as having intermediate high-risk PE because of presence of RV dysfunction signs on imaging and elevated cardiac biomarkers. Intermediate risk PE patients have 30-day mortality of 3.2 - 24.5% [9–11]. Meanwhile, the presence of right heart thrombus in the setting of PE is associated with increased mortality (27-45%) with majority of fatal events occurring in the first 24 hours [8, 12]. The presence of PFO in patient with PE is an independent predictor of death, systemic embolization, and complicated hospital course [13].

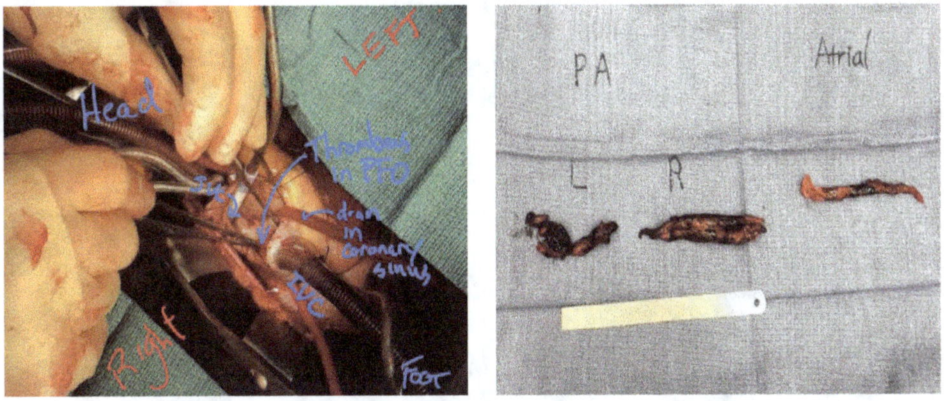

FIGURE 4: Photographs from surgical thrombectomy. Saddle pulmonary embolus was extracted from the pulmonary artery. The embolus that extended to all visualized segments of the branch pulmonary arteries was removed as well. The thrombus that was straddling the PFO was also removed en bloc. The PFO was surgically closed.

Because of the complexity and heterogeneity of this patient population, the management options are individualized and no guidelines exist underlying the most cost-effective diagnostic and treatment strategies due to rarity.

Treatment can be surgical (thromboembolectomy), catheter-based (without or without thrombolysis), or conservative (systemic anticoagulation or thrombolysis). In their systematic literature review (1985-2008) that included 174 patients with IPE, Meyers et al. showed 18% mortality with cardiogenic shock and stroke among the most common causes of death. Surgical thromboembolectomy demonstrated significant decrease in composite of mortality and systemic embolization compared with anticoagulation or thrombolysis [14]. According to another systematic review surgery was associated with the lowest risk of embolization while thrombolytic therapy had the highest mortality compared with thromboembolectomy or heparin [15]. The abovementioned findings were confirmed in the most recent literature review by Seo WW et al. that included 194 patients with thrombus trapped in PFO. In this review, surgical thrombectomy was associated with statistically significant decrease in mortality and systemic embolization compared with anticoagulation and thrombolysis. Interestingly, systemic thrombolysis was associated with higher mortality and posttreatment embolization compared with surgery and anticoagulation especially in patients without hemodynamic compromise and cardiac arrest [16].

In large PE without cardiac arrest catheter directed thrombolysis (CDT) has been shown to provide similar clinical results as systemic thrombolysis but with less hemorrhagic risks because of much lower dose of thrombolytic agents (1/3 of the dose used in systemic thrombolysis) [17, 18]. However, in a patient with thrombus straddling the PFO performing CDT might disrupt the clot in RA [19]. Ultrasound-accelerated CDT (UACDT) that delivers uniform radial US energy on top of continuous small doses of thrombolytic is another approach without major bleeding complications, but it is not without risks of clot fragmentation in this patient population [20]. Percutaneous mechanical thrombectomy via clot aspiration, fragmentation, or rheolysis through high pressure saline has a success rate of up to 80% with low bleeding complications. However, in the process of clot aspiration the fragmented pieces of clot might cause systemic embolization through PFO [9]. The discussed treatment options are summarized in Figure 5 [21].

The specific treatment strategy should take into consideration individual parameters such as patient's age, hemodynamic stability, comorbidities, and bleeding risk. In general, surgical thromboembolectomy with PFO closure is favored over anticoagulation and thrombolysis, and thrombolysis is favored in hemodynamically unstable patients with contraindications to surgery [14, 15]. 2011 American Heart Association guidelines recommend echocardiographic screening for PFO in patients with massive or submassive PE (class IIb, level of evidence C). They also give class IIb, level of evidence C recommendation in favor of surgical thromboembolectomy in IPE [22].

4. Conclusions

Since IPE has high mortality, echocardiographic screening for PFO should be recommended in patient with massive or submassive PE. Common diseases can have rare deadly presentations. Diagnosis is easy and can significantly change the treatment strategy and improve mortality. Coordination of care and multidisciplinary team approach is important for the favorable outcome in these cases. Some medical centers employ a so-called Pulmonary Embolism Response Team (PERT), consisting of experts in cardiology, vascular surgery, pulmonary and critical care medicine, cardiac surgery, hematology, and emergency medicine [23]. Priority should be given to surgical thromboembolectomy since it has less systemic embolization compared with thrombolytic therapy and anticoagulation and it has been proven to decrease mortality.

Abbreviations

APRN: Advanced practice registered nurse
IPE: Impending paradoxical embolism

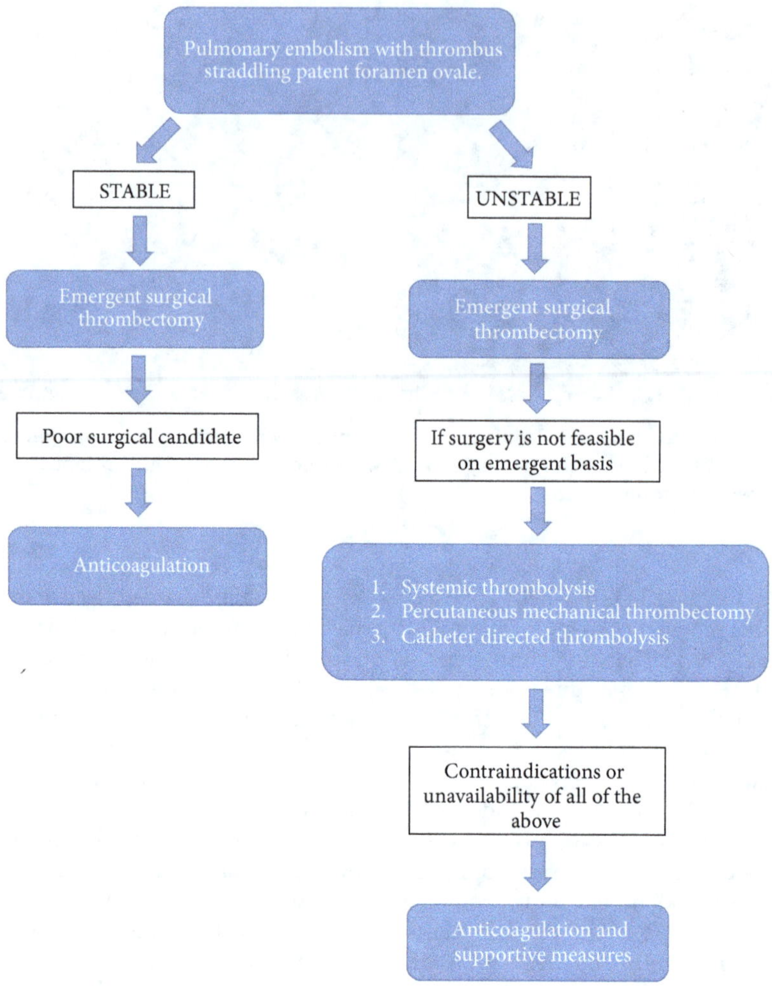

FIGURE 5

LV: Left ventricle, left ventricular
PE: Pulmonary embolus, pulmonary embolism
PERT: Pulmonary Embolism Response Team
PFO: Patent foramen ovale
RV: Right ventricle, right ventricular
TEE: Transesophageal echocardiogram
TTE: Transthoracic echocardiogram.

Acknowledgments

We thank Katherine Lysaught APRN for her assistance in obtaining intraoperative images and pictures presented in this case report.

References

[1] I. Cohnheim, J. Thrombose, and Embolie, *Vorlesungen iiber Allgemeine Pathologic*, vol. 1, article no. 134, Hirschwald, Berlin, Germany, 1877.

[2] U. Nellessen, W. G. Daniel, G. Matheis, H. Oelert, K. Depping, and P. R. Lichtlen, "Impending paradoxical embolism from atrial thrombus: correct diagnosis by transesophageal echocardiography and prevention by surgery," *Journal of the American College of Cardiology*, vol. 5, no. 4, pp. 1002–1004, 1985.

[3] P. T. Hagen, D. G. Scholz, and W. D. Edwards, "Incidence and size of patent foramen ovale during the first 10 decades of life: an autopsy study of 965 normal hearts," *Mayo Clinic Proceedings*, vol. 59, no. 1, pp. 17–20, 1984.

[4] F. P. Chan and T. R. Jones, "Images in clinical medicine. Paradoxical embolus.," *The New England Journal of Medicine*, vol. 345, no. 11, p. 803, 2001.

[5] Q. A. Truong, J. M. Massaro, I. S. Rogers et al., "Reference values for normal pulmonary artery dimensions by noncontrast cardiac computed tomography the framingham heart study," *Circulation: Cardiovascular Imaging*, vol. 5, no. 1, pp. 147–154, 2012.

[6] K. K. Kumamaru, A. R. Hunsaker, N. Wake et al., "The variability in prognostic values of right ventricular-to-left ventricular diameter ratios derived from different measurement methods on computed tomography pulmonary angiography: A patient outcome study," *Journal of Thoracic Imaging*, vol. 27, no. 5, pp. 331–336, 2012.

[7] D. K. Kang, C. Thilo, U. J. Schoepf et al., "CT signs of right ventricular dysfunction: Prognostic role in acute pulmonary embolism," *JACC: Cardiovascular Imaging*, vol. 4, no. 8, pp. 841–849, 2011.

[8] A. Torbicki, N. Galié, A. Covezzoli, E. Rossi, M. De Rosa, and S. Z. Goldhaber, "Right heart thrombi in pulmonary embolism: results from the international cooperative pulmonary embolism registry," *Journal of the American College of Cardiology*, vol. 41, no. 12, pp. 2245–2251, 2003.

[9] S. V. Konstantinides, A. Torbicki, G. Agnelli et al., "Task Force for the Diagnosis and Management of Acute Pulmonary Embolism of the European Society of Cardiology (ESC).. 2014 ESC guidelines on the diagnosis and management of acute pulmonary embolism," *European Heart Journal*, vol. 35, no. 43, pp. 3033–3069, 2014.

[10] D. Aujesky, D. S. Obrosky, R. A. Stone et al., "Derivation and validation of a prognostic model for pulmonary embolism," *American Journal of Respiratory and Critical Care Medicine*, vol. 172, no. 8, pp. 1041–1046, 2005.

[11] D. Jiménez, D. Aujesky, L. Moores et al., "Simplification of the pulmonary embolism severity index for prognostication in patients with acute symptomatic pulmonary embolism," *JAMA Internal Medicine*, vol. 170, no. 15, pp. 1383–1389, 2010.

[12] P. S. Rose, N. M. Punjabi, and D. B. Pearse, "Treatment of right heart thromboemboli," *CHEST*, vol. 121, no. 3, pp. 806–814, 2002.

[13] S. Konstantinides, A. Geibel, W. Kasper, M. Olschewski, L. Blümel, and H. Just, "Patent foramen ovale is an important predictor of adverse outcome in patients with major pulmonary embolism," *Circulation*, vol. 97, no. 19, pp. 1946–1951, 1998.

[14] P. O. Myers, H. Bounameaux, A. Panos, R. Lerch, and A. Kalangos, "Impending paradoxical embolism: systematic review of prognostic factors and treatment," *CHEST*, vol. 137, no. 1, pp. 164–170, 2010.

[15] E. Fauveaua, A. Cohen, N. Bonnet, K. Gacem, and H. Lardoux, "Surgical or medical treatment for thrombus straddling the patent foramen ovale: Impending paradoxical embolism? Report of four clinical cases and literature review," *Archives of Cardiovascular Diseases*, vol. 101, no. 10, pp. 637–644, 2008.

[16] W.-W. Seo, S. E. Kim, M.-S. Park et al., "Systematic review of treatment for trapped thrombus in patent foramen ovale," *Korean Circulation Journal*, vol. 47, no. 5, pp. 776–785, 2017.

[17] W. T. Kuo, M. K. Gould, J. D. Louie, J. K. Rosenberg, D. Y. Sze, and L. V. Hofmann, "Catheter-directed therapy for the treatment of massive pulmonary embolism: systematic review and meta-analysis of modern techniques," *Journal of Vascular and Interventional Radiology*, vol. 20, no. 11, pp. 1431–1440, 2009.

[18] W. T. Kuo, A. Banerjee, P. S. Kim et al., "Pulmonary embolism response to fragmentation, embolectomy, and catheter thrombolysis (PERFECT): Initial results from a prospective multicenter registry," *CHEST*, vol. 148, no. 3, pp. 667–673, 2015.

[19] C. Kabrhel, J. S. Rempell, L. L. Avery, D. M. Dudzinski, and I. Weinberg, "Case 29-2014: A 60-year-old woman with syncope," *The New England Journal of Medicine*, vol. 371, no. 12, pp. 1143–1150, 2014.

[20] M. Dumantepe, I. Uyar, B. Teymen, O. Ugur, and Y. Enc, "Improvements in pulmonary artery pressure and right ventricular function after ultrasound-accelerated catheter-directed thrombolysis for the treatment of pulmonary embolism," *Journal of Cardiac Surgery*, vol. 29, no. 4, pp. 455–463, 2014.

[21] K. Nakamura, G. A. Alba, J. A. Scheske et al., "A 57-year-old man with insidious dyspnea and nonpleuritic chest and back pain," *CHEST*, vol. 150, no. 2, pp. e41–e47, 2016.

[22] M. R. Jaff, M. S. McMurtry, S. L. Archer et al., "Management of massive and submassive pulmonary embolism, iliofemoral deep vein thrombosis, and chronic thromboembolic pulmonary hypertension: a scientific statement from the american heart association," *Circulation*, vol. 123, no. 16, pp. 1788–1830, 2011.

[23] D. M. Dudzinski and G. Piazza, "Multidisciplinary pulmonary embolism response teams," *Circulation*, vol. 133, no. 1, pp. 98–103, 2016.

10

A Case of Acute Life-Threatening Pulmonary Hemorrhage from Synthetic Cannabinoid Abuse

Muhammad Imtiaz,[1] Biplab Saha,[2] Uzma Sana Ullah,[3] and Aditi Saha[4]

[1]*Division of Pulmonary and Critical Care Medicine, Conemaugh Memorial Medical Center, Johnstown, Pennsylvania, USA*
[2]*Division of Pulmonary and Critical Care Medicine, Albany Medical Center, Albany, New York, USA*
[3]*Department of Medicine, Conemaugh Memorial Medical Center, Johnstown, Pennsylvania, USA*
[4]*Department of Medicine, Saint Barnabas Medical Center, Livingston, New Jersey, USA*

Correspondence should be addressed to Biplab Saha; spanophiliac@yahoo.com

Academic Editor: Luis Borderías

We report a case of alveolar hemorrhage secondary to inhalation of synthetic cannabinoid. The patient developed hemoptysis and respiratory failure 48 hours after the episode. Alveolar hemorrhage from synthetic cannabinoid use is a rare entity that has been reported only thrice previously. The unique feature of this case was that the initial urine and blood toxicology screens were negative for cannabinoids and the diagnosis was confirmed via detection of serum metabolites of a synthetic cannabinoid.

1. Background

Use of synthetic cannabinoid (SC) is on the rise. Numerous new compounds with minimal chemical modification and similar biologic activity have been designed over the years. Many of these SC compounds are now considered schedule 1 controlled substances. Most of the SC abused in the United States are produced overseas and are often available to the consumers over the internet or sold as "fake marijuana" at head shops. A prompt diagnosis of SC toxicity requires high index of suspicion in the right clinical setting as well as an appropriate work-up. Diffuse alveolar hemorrhage (DAH) is a life-threatening condition that predominantly stems from infectious, inflammatory, coagulopathy, and cardiac etiology [1]. DAH secondary to inhalational toxin exposure has also been reported [2, 3]. We report a case of DAH after SC use in a 27-year-old man. A unique aspect of this case was that a urine drug screen for tetrahydrocannabinol (THC) was negative and the diagnosis was confirmed by the presence of the serum metabolite of a SC, UR-144.

2. Case Presentation

A 27-year-old man with history of polysubstance abuse was witnessed to inhale "K2," a synthetic cannabinoid. Over the next hour, he became unresponsive and was brought to an emergency room where he was found to be hypoxemic. There was no evidence of traumatic injury. He was intubated and admitted to the intensive care unit (ICU).

He had no other significant past medical history. Physical examination revealed an intubated and sedated patient; temperature was 97.1 °F, blood pressure was 144/84 mmHg, pulse was 98 beats/min, and oxygen saturation was 100% on FiO_2 0.5; and bilateral coarse crackles were audible on chest auscultation.

Laboratory evaluation revealed WBC 10,900/dL, hemoglobin 12.6 g/dL, hematocrit 39.8 %, platelets 191,000/dL, sodium 140 meq/L, potassium 3.7 meq/L, chloride 102 meq/L, bicarbonate 19 mmol/L, BUN 13 mg/dL, creatinine 1.2 mg/dL, and creatine kinase 1,952 IU/L. Computed tomography (CT) of the brain showed no acute intracranial pathology. His initial arterial blood gas (ABG) values were pH 7.28, pCO_2 58 mmHg, and pO_2 125 mmHg on 50% oxygen. Chest radiography revealed alveolar opacities in the right upper lobe (Figure 1(a)).

The patient was started on broad-spectrum antibiotics. A urine and blood toxicology screen was positive for benzodiazepines (which he received after intubation) and negative for amphetamines, barbiturates, cocaine, opiates, phencyclidine,

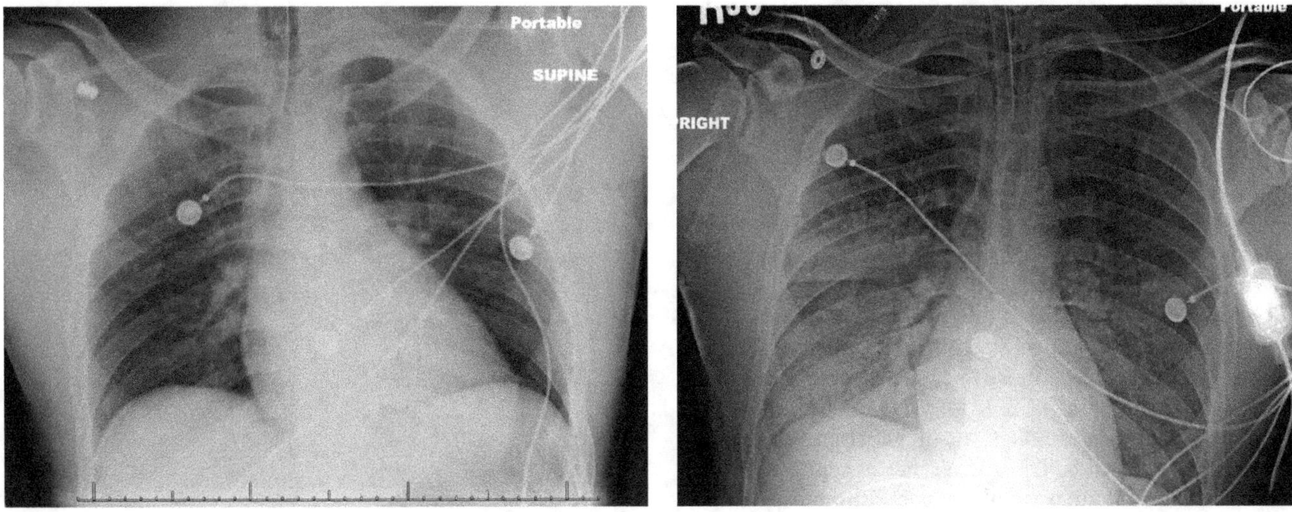

(a) Chest radiograph on admission, showing equivocal opacities at the right lung base

(b) Chest radiograph 36 hours after admission, showing diffuse lung opacities

FIGURE 1

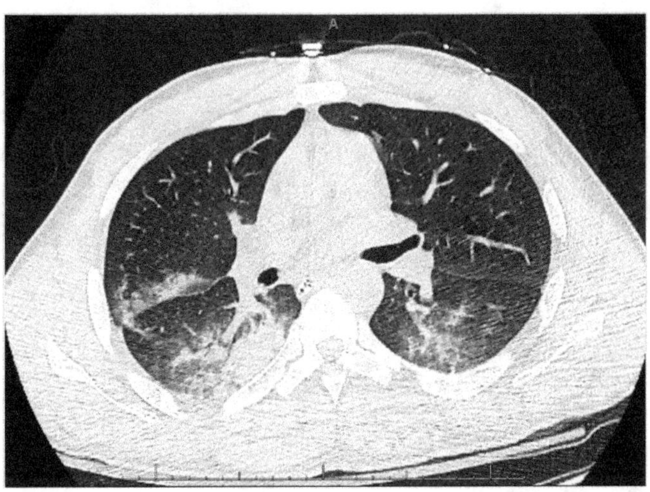

FIGURE 2: Computerized tomography (CT) of the chest 36 hours after admission, showing bilateral parenchymal opacities.

methadone, and cannabinoids. On the second day, frank blood was noted on suction from the endotracheal tube. His gas exchange worsened requiring a FiO_2 1.0 to maintain adequate oxygenation. A blood gas showed profound hypoxemia with a pO_2 110 mmHg. A chest radiograph revealed worsening bilateral alveolar infiltrates (Figure 1(b)). A CT of the chest revealed patchy ground glass opacities and diffuse lung consolidation (Figure 2). Bronchoscopy was performed and showed oozing of blood from all right lung airways and the left lower lobe bronchus. Sequential bronchoalveolar lavage (BAL) confirmed diffuse alveolar hemorrhage by demonstrating increasingly bloody return. Hemosiderin laden macrophages were seen in BAL fluid on microscopy. Measurements of serum anti-nuclear antibody, anti-neutrophil cytoplasmic antibody, and anti-glomerular basement membrane antibody were negative. Urine analysis was negative for hematuria. BAL was negative for an infectious etiology. An echocardiogram was normal. There was no evidence of coagulopathy. UR- 144 N (4/5-hydroxypentyl), a metabolite of UR-144, was identified in the patient's blood by qualitative enzyme-linked immunosorbent assay (ELISA).

The patient was empirically treated with high-dose steroid for 3 days, followed by prednisone 40 mg/day that was tapered to 10 mg/day over 4 days and then discontinued. Over the 48 hours after corticosteroid administration, his oxygenation improved significantly. A chest radiograph performed 96 hours after admission showed complete resolution of the alveolar opacities. The patient was successfully extubated and transferred out of ICU. He was discharged 10 days after admission, neurologically and functionally intact.

3. Discussion

We have presented a patient with alveolar hemorrhage from inhalation of UR-144, a SC. SC abuse is becoming more frequent [4]. Most users are young and have a history of marijuana or polysubstance abuse [5]. There are very few reports documenting potential life-threatening respiratory conditions developing after SC inhalation, including diffuse alveolar hemorrhage and respiratory failure in otherwise healthy individuals. In previous cases [4, 6, 7] as well as ours, no other identifiable etiology for alveolar hemorrhage was found, suggesting that SC was the cause. In all these cases, alveolar hemorrhage developed within 24-48 hours after SC inhalation, suggesting a temporal relationship.

Synthetic cannabinoids interact with CB_1 and CB_2 receptors and are more potent than their natural counterpart, tetrahydrocannabinol (THC) [8]. The exact mechanism by which these compounds cause alveolar hemorrhage is currently unknown. The most likely explanation is direct injury to the alveolocapillary membrane following inhalation. What was uniquely important in our patient's case was that the initial urine drug screen for cannabinoids was negative, and yet a serum metabolite of UR-144, UR-144 N (4/5-hydroxypentyl), was identified. Therefore, a negative urine drug screen for THC does not exclude the possibility of SC toxicity and a dedicated urine or serum study is necessary [8, 9].

We believe that the diagnosis of synthetic cannabinoid-induced respiratory failure can be established by the acute onset of hemoptysis and respiratory failure that is delayed 24-48 hours after inhalation of the drug, provided that alternative conditions including infection, coagulopathy, malignancy, autoimmune, or connective tissue diseases have been excluded. The presence of UR-144 metabolite in serum solidifies the diagnosis, although the diagnosis can be usually made on clinical grounds. Treatment remains supportive. The use of corticosteroids may be of benefit, although presently this remains conjectural.

4. Conclusion

DAH from synthetic cannabinoid use is rare. Clinicians need to be aware of the time delay between synthetic cannabinoid inhalation and the onset of respiratory failure. A negative cannabinoid urine screen does not exclude the diagnosis and a serum and urine metabolite screening is necessary to identify the culprit compound.

References

[1] M. S. Park, "Diffuse alveolar hemorrhage," *Tuberculosis and Respiratory Diseases*, vol. 74, no. 4, pp. 151–162, 2013.

[2] P. Kelchen, F. Jamous, and M. K. Huntington, "Diffuse alveolar haemorrhage associated with aerosol propellant use," *BMJ Case Reports*, vol. 2013, Article ID bcr2013200022, 2013.

[3] R. J. Murray, R. J. Albin, W. Mergner, and G. J. Criner, "Diffuse alveolar hemorrhage temporally related to cocaine smoking," *CHEST*, vol. 93, no. 2, pp. 427–429, 1988.

[4] M. Adelman, M. Thorp, and R. Smith, "Diffuse alveolar hemorrhage due to K2 inhalation," *CHEST*, vol. 150, no. 4, p. 1248A, 2016.

[5] M. S. Castaneto, D. A. Gorelick, N. A. Desrosiers, R. L. Hartman, S. Pirard, and M. A. Huestis, "Synthetic cannabinoids: epidemiology, pharmacodynamics, and clinical implications," *Drug and Alcohol Dependence*, vol. 144, pp. 12–41, 2014.

[6] S. Alhadi, A. Tiwari, R. Vohra, R. Gerona, J. Acharya, and K. Bilello, "High times, low sats: diffuse pulmonary infiltrates associated with chronic synthetic cannabinoid use," *Journal of Medical Toxicology*, vol. 9, no. 2, pp. 199–206, 2013.

[7] A. Loschner, A. Cihla, F. Jalali, and S. Ghamande, "Diffuse alveolar hemorrhage: add "greenhouse effect" to the growing list," *CHEST*, vol. 140, no. 4, p. 149A, 2011.

[8] J. L. Wiley, J. A. Marusich, and J. W. Huffman, "Moving around the molecule: Relationship between chemical structure and in vivo activity of synthetic cannabinoids," *Life Sciences*, vol. 97, no. 1, pp. 55–63, 2014.

[9] A. J. Barnes, E. Spinelli, S. Young, T. M. Martin, K. L. Kleete, and M. A. Huestis, "Validation of an ELISA synthetic cannabinoids urine assay," *Therapeutic Drug Monitoring*, vol. 37, no. 5, pp. 661–669, 2015.

11

A Case of Vaping TCH Oil Leading to Vaping Associated Pulmonary Injury: Our Approach to its Diagnosis, Management and Recommendations

Anshika Singh, Qiuxue Tan, Nicole M. Saccone, and David H. Lindner

NCH Healthcare System, Naples, FL 34102, USA

Correspondence should be addressed to Anshika Singh; anshika.singh@nchmd.org

Academic Editor: Samer Al-Saad

Vaping's popularity has grown exponentially since its introduction to the US market in 2003. Its use has sky-rocketed since the unveiling of the vaping pods in 2017 which may account for the advent of the vaping related illnesses we are now seeing. Substances such as nicotine solution, tetrahydrocannabinol (THC) oil, cannabidiol (CBD) oil, and butane hash oil (BHC) packaged in cartridges available in various flavors and concentrations are aerosolized by the heating of metal coils in the e-cigarette/vaping devices. Cases from all over the country have recently been coming to light in which vaping has led to severe acute pulmonary disease or vaping-associated-pulmonary-injury (VAPI). A vast majority of the presenting patients in the reported cases have required hospitalization and intensive care, needing supplemental oxygen and even endotracheal intubation and mechanical ventilation. 98% of patients present with respiratory symptoms (dyspnea, hypoxia, chest pain, cough, hemoptysis), 81% of patients have gastrointestinal symptoms (nausea, vomiting, diarrhea, and abdominal pain), and 100% of patients have constitutional symptoms such as fever, chills, and fatigue/malaise on presentation. Although based on history and clinical presentation it is reasonable to have a high suspicion for VAPI, diagnostic workup to rule out alternative underlying causes such as infection, malignancy, or autoimmune process should be performed before establishing the diagnosis. Computed Tomography (CT) scans of the chest have predominantly shown ground-glass opacity in the lungs, often with areas of lobular or subpleural sparing. Although lung biopsies have been performed on a relatively low number of cases, lung injury patterns so far have shown acute fibrinous pneumonitis, diffuse alveolar hemorrhage, or organizing pneumonia, usually bronchiolocentric, and accompanied by bronchiolitis. Treatment plans that have led to clinical improvement in the reported cases center around high-dose systemic steroids, although there are a lack of data regarding the best regimen and the absolute need for corticosteroids. The role of antibiotics appears to be limited once infection has definitively been ruled out. We present the case of a young male who vaped THC oil and developed severe acute pulmonary injury requiring mechanical ventilation and showed a remarkable response to high dose steroid therapy with improvement in clinical symptoms and resolution of diffuse ground glass opacity on repeat HRCT scan.

1. Introduction

An electronic cigarette or "e-cigarette" is a battery-powered device that vaporizes (hence the term "vaping") a liquid solution in order to simulate smoking without burning the tobacco. Since its introduction in the market in 2003, its use and popularity has grown exponentially. When activated, usually by pressing a button, the metal coil in the device heats and vaporizes the liquid nicotine, emitting steam which is orally inhaled. Water vapor mixed with chemical byproducts are then exhaled. Apart from nicotine, other substances such as tetrahydrocannabinol (THC), cannabidiol (CBD), and butane hash oil (BHC) can also be inhaled using an e-cigarette device. There is an increasing concern surrounding the practice of vaping as well as an existing knowledge gap regarding vaping-induced-pulmonary-injury (VAPI), its precise mechanism of pathogenesis, and the best course of management in VAPI cases. Our case aims to contribute to this growing literature to help others further understand this relatively new syndrome.

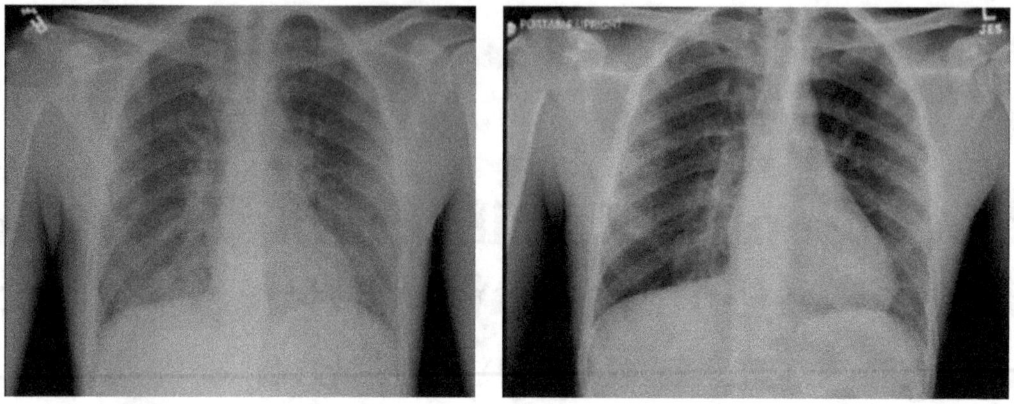

(a) (b)

FIGURE 1: (a) Portable chest X-ray done in the ER on presentation showing bibasilar infiltrates and interstitial prominence. (b) Portable chest X-ray on hospital day 4 prior to discharge with improvement in aeration of the lungs, especially the right lung medially and left lingula. There continues to be minimal interstitial infiltrates present.

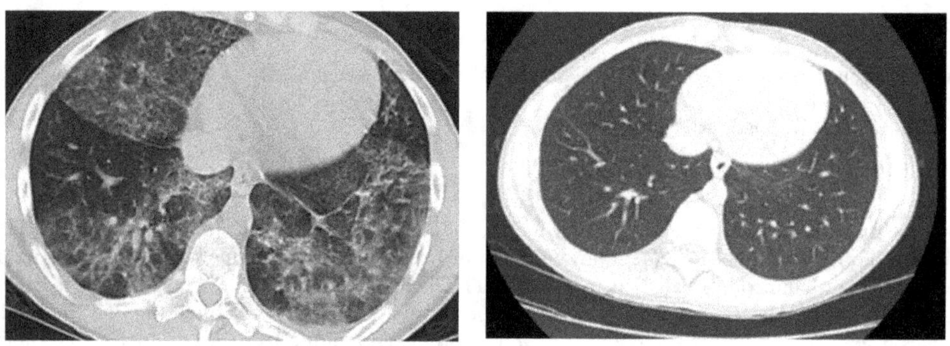

(a) (b)

FIGURE 2: (a) CT scan of the chest without contrast done prior to steroids demonstrating bilateral, multilobar diffuse interstitial and mixed infiltrates evident as "honey combing" and "ground glass" appearance, with well-defined fissure line showing that the infiltrate do no cross between lobes. (b) HRCT scan of the chest post steroid therapy showing resolution of the previously evident diffuse opacity. The scans are 5 weeks apart.

2. Case Presentation

A twenty-year-old male with no significant past medical history presented to our ER with fever, nonbloody vomiting of gastric content, and epigastric abdominal pain. Symptoms began four days prior to this presentation along with worsening dyspnea, a nonproductive cough, and one episode of submassive hemoptysis. He was recently seen one day prior at an urgent care center, during which a 2-view chest X-ray showed left perihilar and right basilar interstitial prominence. At that time, he was assessed to have community-acquired pneumonia and sent home on 250 mg of oral Azithromycin. Despite taking azithromycin for one day, his dyspnea worsened and he began to cough up yellow-brown sputum. He denied any previous similar symptoms and denied previous hospital admission for pneumonia. He denied any recent sick contacts or recent travel. Family history and past surgical history was negative. Social history was significant for marijuana use and occasional drinking with friends. He informed us that he has been vaping THC oil cartridges for 3-4 years. He denied smoking cigarettes or vaping nicotine.

At rest, his respiratory rate was 22/min, heart rate 118/min, blood pressure 135/75 mmHg, temperature 39.3°C, and oxygen saturation 94% on room air. Basic labs were significant for mild leukocytosis of 11.6TH/UL with a neutrophil predominance (92%) and no eosinophils, procalcitonin 0.39, ESR 69, CRP 32, and cannabinoid in urine drug screen. A complete metabolic panel was within normal limits. Blood cultures and respiratory viral PCR were negative. A portable chest X-ray in the ER on this admission showed interval increasing bibasilar infiltrates and persistent left perihilar interstitial prominence (Figure 1), as compared to that from the day prior. Therefore, due to his presenting symptoms, he went for a CT chest which showed bilateral diffuse interstitial and mixed infiltrates in his lungs (Figure 2(a)). Given his acute presentation and suspicion for impending respiratory failure, he was admitted to the critical care unit. Intravenous 125 mg of methylprednisolone was subsequently given, and he was continued on community-acquired pneumonia empiric treatment with ceftriaxone and azithromycin.

However, chest X-rays on the patient's first and second day in the hospital showed no interval improvement of bibasilar

Table 1: Infectious and autoimmune labs tested.

Significant lab	Patient's lab results	Lab reference range
IGE	1900 IU/ml	0–100 IU/ml
IGG	666 mg/dl	700–1600 mg/dl
IGM	143 mg/dl	40–230 mg/dl
IGA	180 mg/dl	70–400 mg/dl
CRP	26.2 mg/dl	<0.3 mg/dl
ESR	69 mm/hr	0–10 mm/hr
Procalcitonin	0.30 ng/ml	<0.05 ng/ml
Lactate dehydrogenase	234 IU/L	87–241 IU/ml
Urine cannabinoids	Positive	Threshold 50 ng/ml
ANA screen	Negative	—
Scl-70	<1.0 AI	—
C3	125 mg/dl	90–180 mg/dl
C4	26.6 mg/dl	10–40 mg/dl
RA	<10 IU/dl	=<15 IU/dl
Cyclic citrullinated peptide	16	Weak positive: 20–39
ANCA	Negative p-anca, c-anca, atypical anca	—
Cryoglobulins	None detected	—
Glom basement Membrane IGG	<1.0 AI	—
AFB culture and smear	Negative	—
Fungus culture and smear	Negative	—
Legionella culture	Negative	—
Pneumocystis smear	Negative	—
Lower respiratory culture	Negative	—
S. pneumoniae Antigen urine	Negative	—
Urine culture	Negative	—
Influenza A/B antigen	Negative	—
RP panel	Negative	—
HIV Ab/Ag, 4th gen	Nonreactive	—

infiltrates, and neither did the patient demonstrate any clinical improvement. All the tests ordered to detect infectious and rheumatological causes came back within normal limits (Table 1). Due to the episode of submassive hemoptysis and negative workups thus far, he underwent flexible bronchoscopy on hospital day 2. No biopsies were taken. The serial aliquots did not get bloody, ruling out diffuse alveolar hemorrhage (DAH). Bronchoscopy cultures sent included lower respiratory culture, AFB culture, fungal cultures, viral culture, influenza A/B and CMV, legionella pneumophila PCR, and pneumocystis smear, all of which returned negative. Cytology was negative for malignancy. Flow cytometry results reported lymphocytes: 3%, monocytes: 0%, granulocytes: 95%, CD45 Dim: 0.3%, CD45 Neg: 0.2%. Due to high suspicion for vaping pneumonitis, the patient was given another 120 mg of IV methylprednisolone on hospital day 2.

On hospital day 3, he became increasingly dyspneic, requiring 50 L oxygen via heated high flow nasal cannula. The patient was given another four doses of methylprednisolone 40 mg on this day. On hospital day 4, the patient's dyspnea improved. The chest X-ray taken this day showed improvement in aeration of the lungs, especially the medial right lung and left lingula, along with continued minimal interstitial infiltrates. Antibiotics were discontinued, and he was given another 80 mg of intravenous methylprednisolone prior to hospital discharge on hospital day 4. He was discharged to his home on nine days of tapering prednisone starting at 60 mg daily.

Five weeks after his hospital admission, the patient presented to our pulmonary clinic for a follow-up. He reported feeling "90% back to normal" and said he has been able to help his uncle move some furniture without feeling exhausted or short of breath in doing so. He had felt short of breath with a mild dry cough for the first few days post-hospital discharge; however, he reported that these symptoms have greatly improved. His oxygen saturation was 98% on room air with a respiratory rate of 18/min at rest. His physical exam with respiratory focus was benign. High-resolution chest CT on this day did not convey any findings of acute or active pulmonary parenchymal disease (Figure 2(b)). The previously described bilateral ground-glass opacity and patchy infiltrates encompassing five lobes were no longer present or visible. A pulmonary function test was normal, with no evidence of airway disease.

3. Discussion

There is an increasing prevalence of cannabis use in e-cigarettes among the US youth. A study that examined data from about 20,000 middle and high school students regarding the use of e-cigarette devices with a substance other than nicotine reported cannabis use in e-cigarettes by 8.9% of all students and 30.6% of those who ever used e-cigarettes [1]. It is not uncommon for e-cigarette users to view vaping as the healthier alternative to smoking traditional cigarettes. However, in the medical community, there is a growing concern regarding the adverse health implications of vaping, as cases of vaping induced pulmonary injury (VAPI) as seen in our twenty-year-old male patient are being increasingly reported in recent years. So far, about 200 cases have come to light in which pulmonary pathologies such as acute hypersensitivity pneumonitis, lipoid pneumonia, chemical pneumonitis, acute eosinophilic pneumonia, and diffuse alveolar hemorrhage can temporally be related to patients' use of vaping devices. As per the Center for Disease Control and Prevention surveillance case definition, our patient is a "Confirmed" case [2].

The proposed reason explaining why vaping THC oil damages the lung tissue is largely debated and may be the direct impact of cannabinoid vapors or the inflammation from the flavoring and diluting additives in the cartridges. There are growing reports of illegal contamination of TCH cartridges with vitamin-E acetate oil as a diluting agent. Vitamin-E oil, which is otherwise harmless on topical application, is known to cause severe inflammatory reaction in the pulmonary parenchyma when inhaled [3, 4]. Another incriminated agent is diacetyl or 2,3-butanedione, which is a commonly used flavoring agent in the food industry and is now being used as a flavoring agent in vape cartridges to impart a pleasant buttery flavor to the inhaled vapors. The FDA has listed Diacetyl as safe for gastrointestinal consumption, but no regulation exists regarding its use in inhaled tobacco or e-cigarette solutions. Currently, the FDA has not identified any compound present in the cartridges to be the cause of the severe pulmonary injury, although they are working it in collaboration with the CDC while further investigations are in progress. Another potential contributor to pulmonary cytotoxicity is the transfer of metal ions from the heated alloy coils of the devices into the vaping solution and subsequently into the inhaled aerosols [5, 6].

A large case series with a cluster of 53 cases of severe pulmonary disease associated with vaping, reported to the Wisconsin Department of Health Services and the Illinois Department of Public Health, described 98% of patients as having respiratory symptoms (dyspnea, hypoxia, chest pain, cough, and hemoptysis), 81% of patients as having gastrointestinal symptoms (nausea, vomiting, diarrhea and abdominal pain), and 100% of patients as having constitutional symptoms like fever, chills, and fatigue/malaise on presentation. Possibly due to the symptom profile resembling community-acquired pneumonia, patients often end up receiving empiric antibiotics in the ER without much improvement in their condition [7]. Our patient was also prescribed oral azithromycin by the urgent care center to which he had first presented. His condition deteriorated and required him to seek medical attention again after two days. We therefore strongly recommend keeping VAPI high in the differentials, especially in presenting patients who are young and lack any major past medical history that would cause such acute respiratory symptoms. The role of good history-taking skills to guide healthcare practitioners towards this diagnosis cannot be stressed enough. We suggest making it common practice to ask patients if they "vape" instead of limiting the social history to the traditionally-asked question, "do you smoke?" As per a health advisory issued by Pennsylvania Department of Health, information regarding the vaping device used, the substance and the source of the substance, the pattern of vaping, and the timing of use relative to symptom onset must be obtained [8]. A vast majority of the presenting patients in the reported cases have required hospitalization to intensive care, needing supplemental oxygen, and even endotracheal intubation and mechanical ventilation. Two reported cases have also resulted in death due to severe respiratory failure, reemphasizing the need to strongly discourage vaping, regardless of whether it is recreational or an off-label tool to help one quit smoking [7]. Other sources have also reported up to 20–30 deaths in the past year attributable to VAPI [3].

Although based on history and clinical presentation it is reasonable to have a high suspicion for VAPI, a diagnostic workup to rule out infection, malignancy, or autoimmune processes as the underlying cause should be performed before establishing the diagnosis. CT chest scans on several reported cases of VAPI have predominantly shown ground-glass opacity, often with areas of lobular or subpleural sparing. Cases of vaping-associated acute lipoid pneumonia may additionally demonstrate nodular tree-in-bud opacities [7]. Subpleural sparing on chest CT has been noted in some but not all cases and was not present in our case [8]. Despite having mild and nonspecific changes on X-ray, our patient's CT scan showed much more severe interstitial disease and inflammatory changes. Therefore, it would be reasonable to consider obtaining a CT scan of the chest for patients with high suspicion for vaping pneumonitis, regardless of benign-looking chest X-rays. At present, there is no definite guideline established regarding performing bronchoscopy and lung biopsy in either "confirmed" or "probable" cases, but they can be a useful tool to differentiate between various histopathological patterns of VAPI, in addition to ruling out infection, malignancy, and rheumatologic causes of the patients' symptoms as well as excluding diffuse alveolar hemorrhage (DAH). Since this is a newly recognized condition, there are insufficient data regarding the most specific histopathological findings that can be deemed diagnostic of VAPI. A review of lung biopsies from 17 patients with VAPI has shown lung injury patterns ranging from acute fibrinous pneumonitis, diffuse alveolar hemorrhage, or organizing pneumonia, usually bronchiolocentric and accompanied by bronchiolitis [9]. In our patient, a lung biopsy was not obtained; however, negative serial aliquots during bronchoscopy excluded DAH and a cytology report of BAL specimen, which was grossly dark and turbid, showed pulmonary macrophages, neutrophils, and proteinaceous debris, along with pigment-laden histiocytes indicative of a degree of alveolar hemorrhage. No obvious malignant cells or viral inclusions were seen. Flow Differential (%) and Population Analysis reported lymphocytes: 3%, monocytes: 0%, granulocytes: 95%, CD45 Dim: 0.3%, CD45 Neg: 0.2%. His CD4/CD8 ratio of the BAL specimen was 1.38, indicating possible hypersensitivity pneumonitis due to the vaping. Negative antibodies testing for systemic sclerosis, granulomatosis with polyangiitis, SLE, RA factor, AntiCCP, and cryoglobulins helped us rule out the autoimmune conditions from our differentials. We did initially entertain the idea of ANCA negative vasculitis in our patient, however, in absence of renal, upper respiratory tract and cutaneous manifestations it eventually was low on our differentials. We suggest it would be valuable to do BAL with cytology and microbiologic studies and reserve a lung biopsy for specific cases when a better understanding of VAPI's pathogenesis is needed or the possibility of another diagnosis remains. Besides gaining insight about the pattern of pulmonary injury and the extent of damage, it would also help identify other histopathological features that probably have not been recognized or associated with VAPI yet. On our search of the literature, it was interesting to note that there is a knowledge gap regarding correlation between the substance vaped (THC oil vs. butane hash oil vs. various flavored nicotine solutions) and the type of acute lung injury the substance causes.

Treatment plans that have led to clinical improvement in the reported cases center around respiratory support and high-dose systemic steroids, although there is a lack of data regarding the best regimen and the absolute need for corticosteroids. The role of antibiotics appears to be limited once infection has definitively been ruled out. Many centers tend to empirically cover for community-acquired pneumonia. However, clinical improvement has largely been noted, mostly after administering high-dose steroids [7]. Our patient received 120 mg of intravenous methylprednisolone on day 2, day 3, and day 4, followed by 80 mg on day 5 of his hospital stay with the goal of slowly weaning him to oral steroids upon discharge. Again, due to the emerging nature of this syndrome, the total duration of steroid therapy necessary to ensure complete recovery is indeterminate, although tapering the oral dose over 4–6 weeks with repeat lung scans and outpatient follow-up so far appears to be a reasonable course of action. It is still too early to comment on the superiority of one treatment approach over another. High resolution CT (HRCT) scan of the chest in our patient, performed after 5 weeks of initiating steroid therapy, showed complete resolution of the ground-glass opacity and patchy infiltrates in both the right and left lung. A pulmonary function test after the steroid therapy was normal with no evidence of airway disease. Although clinically our patient was back to his baseline, we would like to endorse the importance of regular pulmonary follow-up for these patients in order to watch out for possible long-term complications of vaping THC oil. We did not come across any study looking into the long-term pulmonary outcomes of VAPI following clinical resolution.

4. Conclusions

In summary, our case adds to the growing body of literature on VAPI, for which suspicion should be high in patients who use e-cigarettes and present with acute respiratory symptoms. It also goes on to highlight that high dose steroid therapy can be lifesaving. Bilateral ground-glass opacity in the lungs on CT; negative blood, sputum, and BAL culture for infection; and negative rheumatological markers in such a setting are highly suggestive of this diagnosis. The decision to do flexible bronchoscopy with biopsy and BAL specimen cytology should be tailored on a case-by-case basis, but doing so would expand our knowledge of this newly-emerging syndrome.

References

[1] K. F. Trivers, E. Phillips, A. S. Gentzke, M. A. Tynan, and L. J. Neff, "Prevalence of cannabis use in electronic cigarettes among US youth," *JAMA Pediatrics*, vol. 172, no. 11, pp. 1097–1099, 2018.

[2] J. G. Schier, J. G. Meiman, J. Layden et al., "Severe pulmonary disease associated with electronic-cigarette–product use—interim guidance," *Morbidity and Mortality Weekly Report*, vol. 68, no. 36, pp. 787–790, 2019.

[3] Vitamin E Acetate Products Investigated in THC Oil Deaths, 2019, https://vaping360.com/vape-news/84181/vitamin-e-acetate-products-investigated-in-thc-oil-deaths/.

[4] Vape Pen Lung Disease, 2019, https://www.leafly.com/news/health/vape-pen-lung-disease-vitamin-e-oil-explained.

[5] G. Kaur, T. Muthumalage, and I. Rahman, "Mechanisms of toxicity and biomarkers of flavoring and flavor enhancing chemicals in emerging tobacco and nontobacco products," *Toxicology Letters*, vol. 288, pp. 143–155, 2018.

[6] P. Olmedo, W. Goessler, S. Tanda et al., "Metal concentrations in e-cigarette liquid and aerosol samples: the contribution of metallic coils," *Environmental Health Perspectives*, vol. 126, p. 2, 2018.

[7] J. E. Layden, I. Ghinai, I. Pray et al., "Pulmonary illness related to e-cigarette use in illinois and wisconsin—preliminary report," *New England Journal of Medicine*, 2019.

[8] Pennsylvania Department of Health, "2019—PAHAN—454–08-16-ADV severe acute pulmonary disease associated with vaping," 2019, https://www.health.pa.gov/topics/Documents/HAN/2019-PAHAN--454-08-16-ADV-Vaping.pdf.

[9] Y. M. Butt, M. L. Smith, H. D. Tazelaar et al., "Pathology of vaping-associated lung injury," *New England Journal of Medicine*, vol. 381, no. 18, pp. 1780–1781, 2019.

12

Pulmonary Langerhans Cell Histiocytosis Presenting as a Solitary Pulmonary Nodule on a Lung Cancer Screening CT

Hassan Baig,[1] **Sushilkumar Sonavane**,[2] **Ian Makey**,[3] **Jorge Mallea**,[1] **and Andras Khoor**[4]

[1]*Department of Pulmonary and Critical Care Medicine, Mayo Clinic Florida, 4500 San Pablo Road, Jacksonville, FL 32224, USA*
[2]*Department of Diagnostic Radiology, Mayo Clinic Florida, 4500 San Pablo Road, Jacksonville, FL 32224, USA*
[3]*Department of Thoracic Surgery, Mayo Clinic Florida, 4500 San Pablo Road, Jacksonville, FL 32224, USA*
[4]*Department of Anatomic and Clinical Pathology, Mayo Clinic Florida, 4500 San Pablo Road, Jacksonville, FL 32224, USA*

Correspondence should be addressed to Hassan Baig; baig.hassan@mayo.edu

Academic Editor: Inger F. Oey

Pulmonary Langerhans cell histiocytosis (PLCH) is a rare inflammatory condition that mostly affects lungs in smokers. On imaging, it usually presents as multiple, upper lobe predominant, solid, and cavitary nodules, but presentation as solitary pulmonary nodule (SPN) is rare. We describe a case of SPN seen on low-dose lung cancer screening CT (LDCT) that was FDG avid on PET/CT. Given concern for malignancy, lobectomy was planned if intraoperative frozen section was consistent with malignancy. Lobectomy was performed based on frozen section; however, on formal pathology review, the nodule was ultimately found to be PLCH. This case illustrates an atypical presentation of PLCH as a solitary nodule. Furthermore, it helps demonstrate how rare etiologies (like PLCH) may be more frequently encountered and should be considered in the differential diagnosis for solitary lung nodules, especially in the era of lung cancer screening.

1. Background

The evaluation of a solitary pulmonary nodule (SPN) involves appropriate risk stratification for malignancy and weighing potential harms of interventions, especially in the current era of computed tomography (CT) screening for lung cancer. The etiology of lung nodules seen in lung cancer screening programs is predominantly benign [1] such as from infection, inflammation, or granulomatous disease [2]. Pulmonary Langerhans cell histiocytosis (PLCH) is a rare inflammatory condition that mostly affects lungs in smokers [3]. On imaging, it can be seen as multiple, upper lobe predominant, solid, and cavitary nodules, but presentation as a solitary pulmonary nodule is rare. We describe a case of a SPN seen on low-dose lung cancer screening CT (LDCT) that was suspicious on positron emission tomography (PET) scan and was ultimately found to be PLCH on surgical pathology. This case presented a diagnostic dilemma, as intraoperative frozen sections were suggestive of malignancy.

2. Case Presentation

A 63-year-old female patient, current smoker with a 15 pack-year history, presented to the pulmonary clinic for evaluation and management of a single lung nodule detected on LDCT at another facility. The LDCT chest demonstrated a left upper lobe, 11 mm nodule with spiculated borders. Other imaging features included upper lobe predominant centrilobular emphysema, a few, tiny, calcified nodules, presumably old granulomas, and two small, thin-walled parenchymal cysts (Figure 1). She had already completed a whole body PET/CT scan as recommended. The PET/CT scan displayed (18)F-fluorodeoxyglucose (FDG) avidity of the nodule with a standardized uptake value (SUV) of 4.2 (Figure 2) and no abnormal uptake elsewhere in the body. Her symptoms included occasional nonproductive cough. She denied significant shortness of breath, fever, chills, night sweats, weight loss, or hemoptysis.

Given the patient's age, smoking status, and imaging characteristics, the concern for lung cancer was high. After

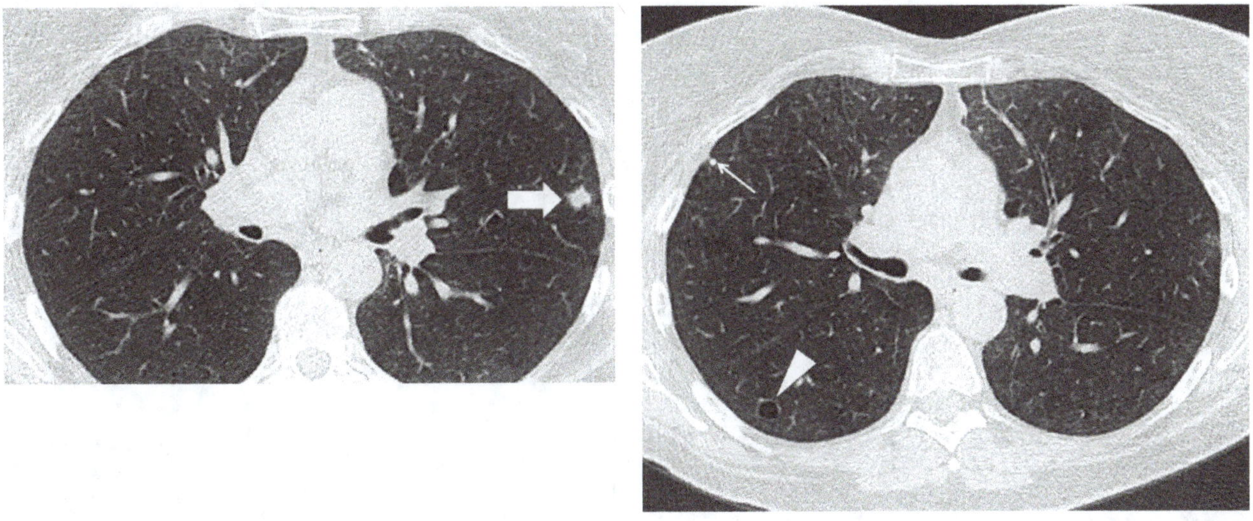

(a) (b)

FIGURE 1: (a, b) Axial chest CT images show an irregular shape, 1.1 cm, left upper lobe nodule with spiculated margins (block arrow), and a thin-walled parenchymal cyst in right lower lobe (arrowhead). Please note mild centrilobular, paraseptal emphysema, and a tiny, calcified right upper lobe nodule (thin arrow).

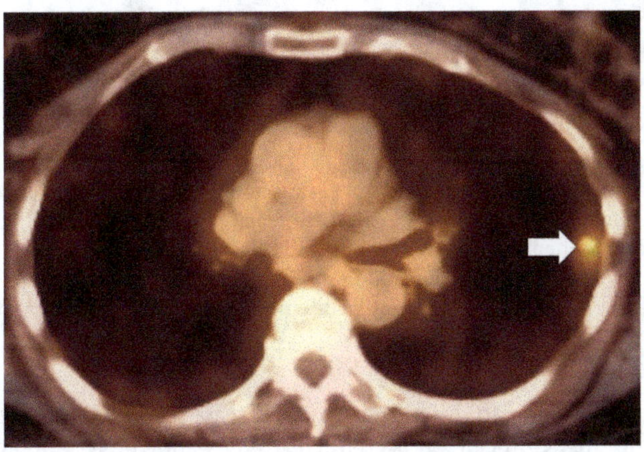

FIGURE 2: Axial, fused FDG PET–CT image shows increased FDG uptake in the left upper lobe nodule with SUV of 4.2 (arrow).

evaluation by the thoracic surgery team and presentation at a multidisciplinary conference, it was decided to proceed with diagnostic wedge resection and subsequent left upper lobectomy if indicated. During the procedure, frozen section analysis of the wedge resection showed a 10 mm nodule with atypical alveolar type II cell proliferation. Adenocarcinoma with lepidic features was suspected, and the left upper lobectomy was completed. The patient was discharged without complications.

Sections of the formalin-fixed paraffin-embedded nodule revealed alveolar septal expansion with numerous eosinophils, alveolar macrophage accumulation (desquamative interstitial pneumonia-like reaction), and focal organizing pneumonia (Figure 3). The alveolar type II cell proliferation, which had appeared atypical in the previous frozen sections, now looked reactive in nature. The histologic findings were consistent with pulmonary Langerhans cell histiocytosis. Immunohistochemical studies exhibited clusters of S100, CD1a, and langerin-positive Langerhans cells within the lesion, confirming the diagnosis.

In the outpatient setting, the patient was advised smoking cessation as the most important intervention to prevent disease progression. Regular follow-up every 3-6 months initially was advised with pulmonary function tests and chest CT to assess for further lung parenchymal involvement in the form of worsening nodular or cystic disease and the development of fibrosis.

3. Discussion

Lung nodules are commonly detected incidentally on chest radiographs, routine chest CT, or LDCT for lung cancer screening. The overall chance of the nodule being cancerous, even among high-risk patients, tends to be low [1]. Certain imaging features such as nodule size and spiculated margins can raise the suspicion for malignancy. PET/CT scan provides useful information for lung cancer diagnosis and staging but can have a false-positive rate of 25% and even up to 40% in areas with endemic infections such as fungal or tuberculous [4]. In our case, the patient's smoking status, nodule size of 11 mm, and high FDG avidity on PET/CT scan led to further surgical diagnostic evaluation. Of note, the calculated lung cancer risk based on a validated tool (Brock University cancer prediction equation) was 31% [1], and 80% was accounting for the PET/CT data (based on Herder prediction model) [5], conferring a moderate to high malignant risk. Due to a possibility of a nonnegligible false-negative result, CT-guided biopsy might not have been sufficient to confidently rule out malignancy. Nondiagnostic biopsies in lesions less than 3 centimeters have been reported in up to 36% of cases [6]. This and other aspects of the different diagnostic interventions were discussed with patient. She actively participated in the shared decision-making process,

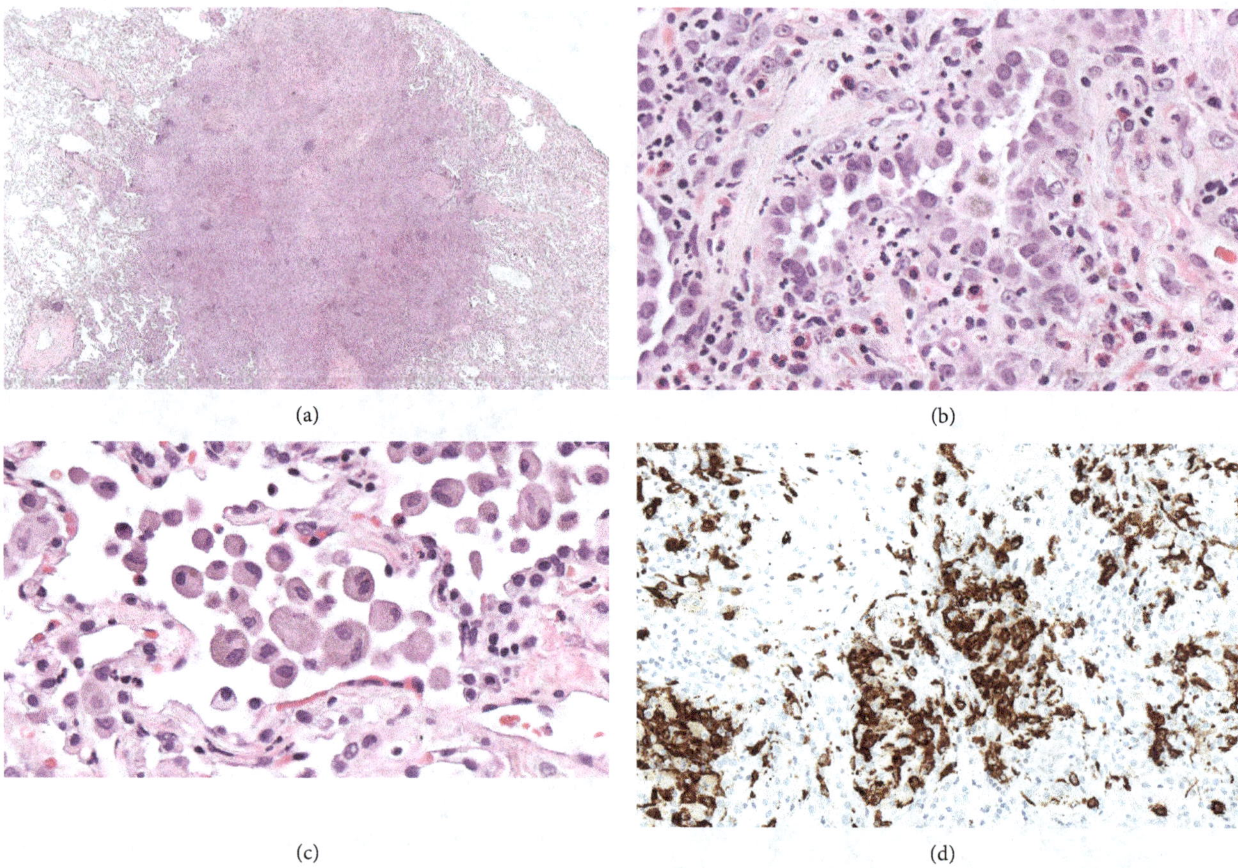

Figure 3: Histologic features of the pulmonary nodule. (a) Low magnification image shows a solid appearing nodule with indistinct edges (hematoxylin-eosin stain, original magnification 8x). (b) A high magnification view exhibits marked reactive alveolar type II cell hyperplasia. The alveolar septa are expanded and contain scattered eosinophils (hematoxylin-eosin stain, original magnification 400x). (c) Another high magnification view shows alveolar macrophage accumulation at the edge of the nodule (hematoxylin-eosin stain, original magnification 400x). (d) Immunohistochemistry for langerin reveals clusters of Langerhans cells within the nodule (original magnification 400x).

highlighting the importance of such a process when ordering and discussing the results of screening CTs.

After formal pathology review, the diagnosis of pulmonary Langerhans cell histiocytosis was made. The initial diagnostic wedge resection demonstrated a nodule with significant atypical type II alveolar cell proliferation. This raised the suspicion of adenocarcinoma; however, on formal pathology review after lobectomy, it was not the case. Small lung adenocarcinoma diagnosis can pose challenges on frozen section because alveolar cell atypia and artifacts can simulate malignancy. Frozen section analysis can have an error rate up to 6% [7]. Furthermore, a sublobar resection instead of lobectomy could have been considered. Based on the only randomized controlled trial, limited resections are associated with higher local recurrent rates, lower overall survival, and equivalent perioperative morbidity as compared to lobectomy [8]. However, increasing evidence from observational studies has demonstrated similar outcomes including recurrence rates and overall survival in those patients intentionally chosen to undergo sublobar resection (as opposed to necessity due to underlying comorbidities) [9]. Further, randomized trials are underway, and until then, the standard of care in a low-surgical-risk patient remains lobectomy.

PLCH is an interstitial lung disease closely linked to smoking. Clinically, it is characterized by shortness of breath and cough with minimal crackles on lung auscultation [3]. On imaging, the upper and mid lung zones show greater involvement compared to lower lung zones. Small, stellate, or irregular-shape centrilobular nodules are present, some of which can show faint central lucencies. The nodules are usually solid density and can also have surrounding ground glass density [10]. In advanced stage of the disease, the cysts become larger, irregular, or bizarre shaped [11]. Histologically, the disease is characterized by peribronchiolar nodules, containing a mix of smoker's macrophages, eosinophils, and Langerhans cells along with varying degrees of fibrosis. Langerhans cells can be identified by their pale blue nucleus with nucleolar infoldings and with special stains including S100, CD1a, and langerin [12].

Management of PLCH typically involves smoking cessation with clinical and imaging follow-up as necessary. If the disease progresses, steroids and even chemotherapy can be considered [13]. Lung transplantation is reserved for severe, intractable cases [14].

The unique aspect of this case is that PLCH presenting as a solitary pulmonary nodule is extremely rare. Only a handful of cases have been described that presented similarly as a SPN concerning for malignancy and were resected [15-17]. On follow-up imaging ranging from 2 up to 24 years, no significant sequelae had been noted in these reported cases. Furthermore, in the era of low-dose CT scans for lung cancer screening, nodules requiring further diagnostic workup are likely to become more prevalent and will require careful consideration of all etiologies, including those less commonly encountered.

References

[1] A. McWilliams, M. C. Tammemagi, J. R. Mayo et al., "Probability of cancer in pulmonary nodules detected on first screening CT," *The New England Journal of Medicine*, vol. 369, no. 10, pp. 910–919, 2013.

[2] D. Ost, A. M. Fein, and S. H. Feinsilver, "Clinical practice. The solitary pulmonary nodule," *The New England Journal of Medicine*, vol. 348, no. 25, pp. 2535–2542, 2003.

[3] J. H. Ryu, T. V. Colby, T. E. Hartman, and R. Vassallo, "Smoking-related interstitial lung diseases: a concise review," *The European Respiratory Journal*, vol. 17, no. 1, pp. 122–132, 2001.

[4] S. A. Deppen, J. D. Blume, C. D. Kensinger et al., "Accuracy of FDG-PET to diagnose lung cancer in areas with infectious lung disease: a meta-analysis," *Journal of the American Medical Association*, vol. 312, no. 12, pp. 1227–1236, 2014.

[5] G. J. Herder, H. van Tinteren, R. P. Golding et al., "Clinical Prediction Model To Characterize Pulmonary Nodules: Validation and Added Value of," *Chest*, vol. 128, no. 4, pp. 2490–2496, 2005.

[6] R. C. Larscheid, P. E. Thorpe, and W. J. Scott, "Percutaneous transthoracic needle aspiration biopsy: a comprehensive review of its current role in the diagnosis and treatment of lung tumors," *Chest*, vol. 114, no. 3, pp. 704–709, 1998.

[7] R. Gupta, R. McKenna Jr., and A. M. Marchevsky, "Lessons learned from mistakes and deferrals in the frozen section diagnosis of bronchioloalveolar carcinoma and well-differentiated pulmonary adenocarcinoma: an evidence-based pathology approach," *American Journal of Clinical Pathology*, vol. 130, no. 1, pp. 11–20, 2008.

[8] R. J. Ginsberg and L. V. Rubinstein, "Randomized trial of lobectomy versus limited resection for T1 N0 non-small cell lung cancer. Lung Cancer Study Group," *The Annals of Thoracic Surgery*, vol. 60, no. 3, pp. 615–623, 1995.

[9] C. Cao, D. Chandrakumar, S. Gupta, T. D. Yan, and D. H. Tian, "Could less be more?-a systematic review and meta-analysis of sublobar resections versus lobectomy for non-small cell lung cancer according to patient selection," *Lung Cancer*, vol. 89, no. 2, pp. 121–132, 2015.

[10] Y. Zhou, Y. Li, L. Fan, and S. Liu, "A solitary pulmonary ground-glass nodule in adult systemic Langerhans' cell histiocytosis," *International Journal of Clinical and Experimental Pathology*, vol. 8, no. 10, pp. 13561–13564, 2015.

[11] L. Hagmeyer and W. Randerath, "Smoking-related interstitial lung disease," *Deutsches Ärzteblatt International*, vol. 112, no. 4, pp. 43–50, 2015.

[12] A. C. Roden and E. S. Yi, "Pulmonary Langerhans cell histiocytosis: an update from the pathologists' perspective," *Archives of Pathology & Laboratory Medicine*, vol. 140, no. 3, pp. 230–240, 2016.

[13] N. Schönfeld, W. Frank, S. Wenig et al., "Clinical and radiologic features, lung function and therapeutic results in pulmonary histiocytosis X," *Respiration*, vol. 60, no. 1, pp. 38–44, 2004.

[14] G. Dauriat, H. Mal, G. Thabut et al., "Lung transplantation for pulmonary Langerhans' cell histiocytosis: a multicenter analysis," *Transplantation*, vol. 81, no. 5, pp. 746–750, 2006.

[15] A. Khoor, J. L. Myers, H. D. Tazelaar, and S. J. Swensen, "Pulmonary Langerhans cell histiocytosis presenting as a solitary nodule," *Mayo Clinic Proceedings*, vol. 76, no. 2, pp. 209–211, 2001.

[16] C. J. Fichtenbaum, G. M. Kleinman, and R. G. Haddad, "Eosinophilic granuloma of the lung presenting as a solitary pulmonary nodule," *Thorax*, vol. 45, no. 11, pp. 905-906, 1990.

[17] G. P. M. ten Velde, F. B. J. M. Thunnissen, J. M. A. van Engelshoven, and E. F. M. Wouters, "A solitary pulmonary nodule due to eosinophilic granuloma," *The European Respiratory Journal*, vol. 7, no. 8, pp. 1539-1540, 1994.

13

Recurrent Pneumothorax with CPAP Therapy for Obstructive Sleep Apnea

Kartikeya Rajdev,[1] Pretty Sara Idiculla,[2] Shubham Sharma,[3] Susanna G. Von Essen,[1] Peter J. Murphy,[1] and Sabin Bista[1]

[1]*Department of Internal Medicine, Division of Pulmonary, Critical Care & Sleep Medicine, University of Nebraska Medical Center, 42nd and Emile St., Omaha, Nebraska 68198-7400, USA*
[2]*Sree Gokulam Medical College & Research Foundation, Kerala, India*
[3]*University College of Medical Sciences & GTB Hospital, New Delhi, India*

Correspondence should be addressed to Kartikeya Rajdev; kartikeyarajdev@gmail.com

Academic Editor: Antonio Corrado

Pulmonary barotrauma such as pneumothorax (PTX) is a known complication of invasive mechanical ventilation. However, it is uncommonly reported with the use of noninvasive positive pressure ventilation (NPPV) and CPAP (continuous positive airway pressure) therapy. We present a case of a 66-year-old female who presented with chronic dyspnea on exertion secondary to right-sided diaphragmatic hernia. The patient also underwent a home sleep study which suggested obstructive sleep apnea (OSA) for which she was initiated on CPAP. She then underwent surgical repair of her right diaphragmatic hernia. The patient developed pneumothorax three times over the course of the following several months, once on the right side and twice on the left side. The patient's incidences of PTX had a temporal association with the CPAP initiation. Her CPAP therapy was discontinued permanently after the third occurrence of PTX. With this case report, we highlight the risk of barotrauma with the use of CPAP for OSA. There are very few reported cases of PTX in association with NPPV therapy for OSA. The lung-protective ventilation strategies and limiting the positive airway pressures can help reduce the risk of pulmonary barotrauma with CPAP.

1. Introduction

Positive pressure ventilation can be applied invasively and through noninvasive methods. Noninvasive positive pressure ventilation (NPPV) is the method of employing mechanical ventilation without endotracheal intubation, thereby eliminating the complications of invasive mechanical ventilation. It utilizes a tight-fitting nasal or facemask to deliver pressurized gas that increases the transpulmonary pressure and subsequently inflates the lungs. The process is followed by exhalation, which results from lung recoiling and expiratory muscle efforts. Continuous positive airway pressure (CPAP) is a mode where positive pressure is applied and maintained throughout the respiratory cycle to keep the upper airways patent and to increase mean airway pressure to improve oxygenation. CPAP is not strictly a ventilation method, but a broad definition of NPPV could include CPAP. CPAP is commonly utilized for the management of patients with obstructive sleep apnea (OSA). Pneumothorax (PTX) is a known complication of invasive mechanical ventilation; however, it is less common with the use of NPPV and occurrence in patients with OSA is rare. We illustrate a case of a 66-year-old female who developed recurrent PTX with CPAP therapy for OSA.

2. Case Report

A 66-year-old Hispanic female, with a past medical history of hypertension and morbid obesity (BMI-40), presented to the emergency department (ED) with complaints of right flank pain of two-day duration. She also complained of dyspnea on exertion (MMRC-2) and daytime fatigue for the past 2

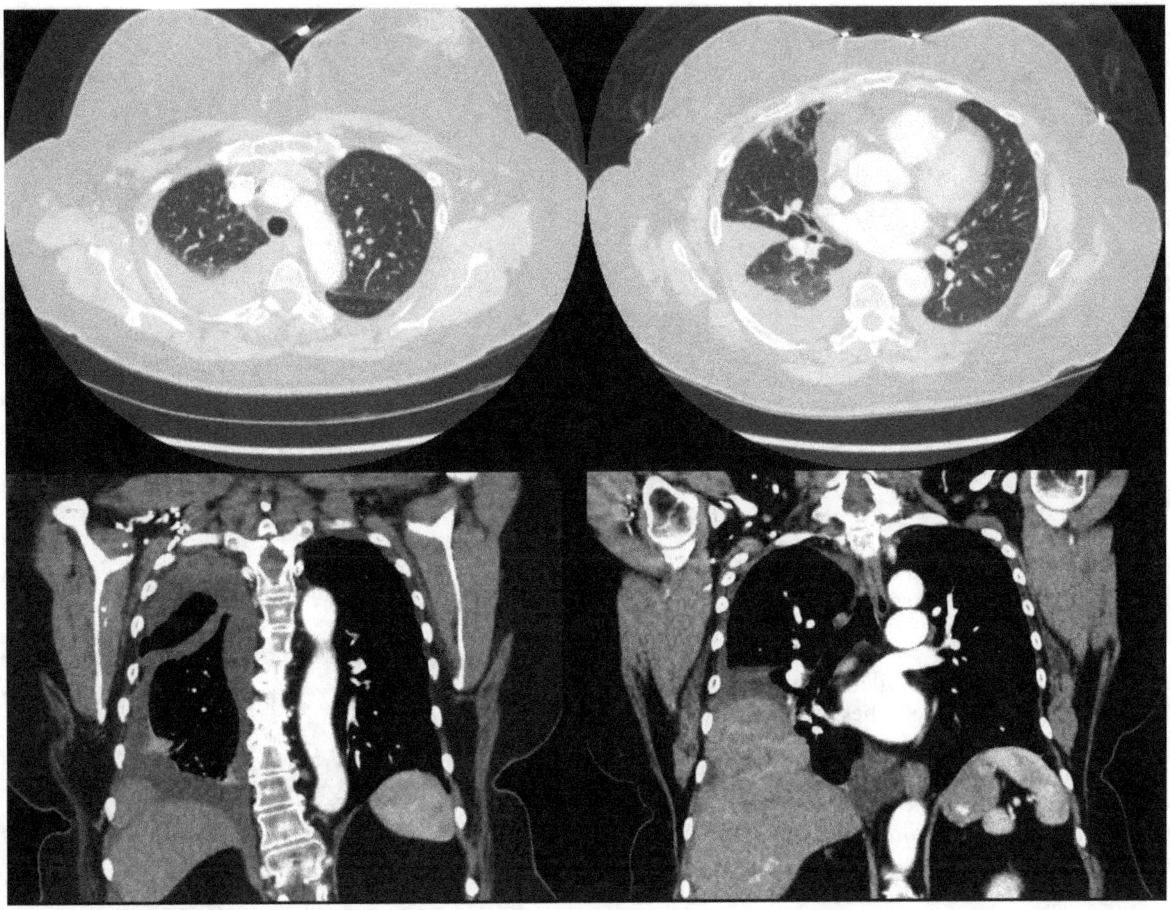

Figure 1: CT chest and abdomen showing right-sided pleural effusion and right lateral diaphragmatic hernia.

years. She denied any fever, cough, chest pain, nausea, or vomiting or any other symptoms. She underwent a computed tomography (CT) scan of her chest and abdomen which revealed moderate right-sided pleural effusion and a small loculated pleural effusion on the left. There were also right pleural space masses displaying associated hepatic vasculature which suggested a lateral diaphragmatic hernia containing liver (Figure 1). Thoracentesis was performed on the right side which demonstrated an exudative pleural effusion. The fluid cytology showed reactive mesothelial cells and negative for malignancy. The pleural fluid bacterial, fungal, and AFB cultures and adenosine deaminase were negative. The patient was offered surgical repair of her right-sided diaphragmatic hernia as her shortness of breath (SOB) was affecting her daily activities and exercise tolerance. Around that time, the patient also underwent a home sleep apnea test (HST) which showed mild OSA with a apnea-hypopnea index (AHI) of 13.0 per hour for a total recording time of 10 h. CPAP therapy was recommended because of potential under calling of the severity and hypoxemia that was noted out of proportion to the severity of sleep apnea. She was started on auto-CPAP with the pressure range of 4-20 cm H_2O with ResMed Airsense 10 Auto device and nasal mask.

One month later, she underwent right diaphragmatic hernia repair through muscle-sparing thoracotomy and a wedge biopsy of the right lower lobe of the lung. Surgical biopsy showed nonspecific chronic inflammation, mild fibrosis, and intra-alveolar hemorrhage. The etiology of her pleural disease was unclear. Her postoperative period was uneventful, and a follow-up chest X-ray (CXR) demonstrated small, bilateral, residual pleural effusions with adjacent atelectasis. She was discharged home in a stable condition and resumed CPAP one week later.

Five weeks after her surgery, she was seen in the clinic where she described feeling mild right-sided pleuritic chest pain and cough for one-day duration. CXR revealed a moderate right apicolateral PTX, measuring about 1.7 cm and small stable bilateral pleural effusions (Figure 2). She was managed conservatively and advised to come to the ED if her symptoms worsen. Her CPAP was temporarily discontinued. Two weeks later, she was seen in the clinic and got a CXR which showed complete resolution of the PTX. At this point, she was advised to resume her CPAP use. Her CPAP compliance report after her surgery until she developed PTX was reviewed and showed a 95th percentile pressure of 14.8 cm of water and median pressure of 10.6 cm of water. The 95th percentile air leak was mildly increased at 29.7 L/min (considering <24 L/min as acceptable). The residual AHI was 0.8. The patient continued to use her CPAP every night and reported improvement in her daytime fatigue and morning headaches with the use of CPAP.

Around 6 months after her first episode of PTX, she presented to the ED with complaints of sudden onset of SOB and left-sided chest pain. CXR showed a large left pneumothorax

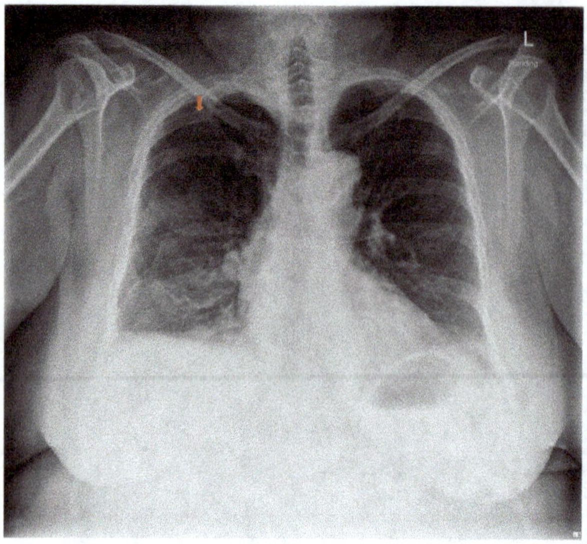

FIGURE 2: Chest X-ray showing moderate right-sided apicolateral pneumothorax (depicted by red arrow).

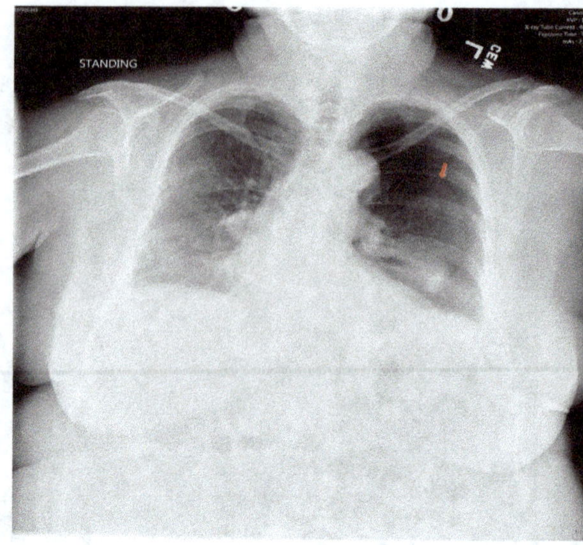

FIGURE 3: Chest X-ray showing large left-sided pneumothorax and lung collapse (depicted by red arrow).

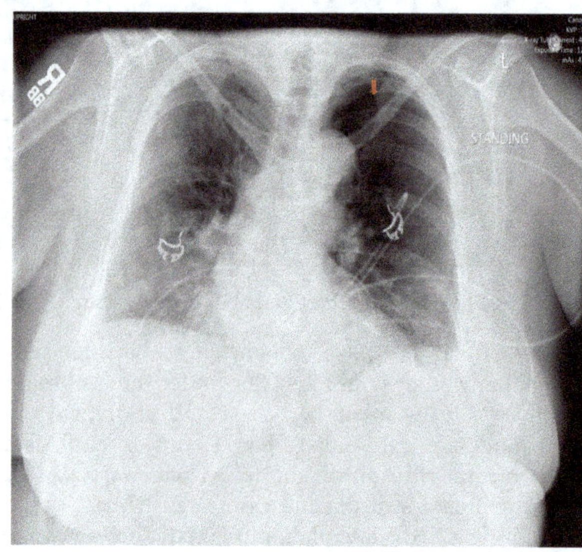

FIGURE 4: Chest X-ray showing large left-sided pneumothorax (depicted by red arrow).

and lung collapse, with small bilateral pleural effusions (Figure 3). A 12 French pigtailed chest tube was placed on the left side. CT scan of the chest showed tiny residual left PTX and small bilateral layering pleural effusions with bilateral atelectatic changes. Her chest tube was removed after two days. She was discharged home and advised to discontinue the CPAP use. Two weeks later, she was seen in the clinic where she reported resolution of her symptoms, and CXR did not show any PTX. At this point, her CPAP was resumed with the same pressure settings. Her CPAP compliance report for the few months prior to her second episode of PTX showed a 95th percentile pressure of 16.8 cm of water and median pressure of 11.8 cm of water. The 95th percentile air leak was borderline increased at 25.9 L/min. The residual AHI was 1.1. The patient's OSA was being managed by her pulmonologist and not by a sleep specialist.

Around twelve days after resuming CPAP, she presented to the ED with sudden onset of SOB. Chest imaging again revealed a moderate to large PTX on the left for which a chest tube was placed (Figure 4). The chest tube was removed after two days, and she was discharged home in a stable condition. Due to the recurrent PTX with a strong temporal association with the resumption of CPAP, it was decided to discontinue the CPAP permanently. The patient was initiated on nocturnal oxygen for nocturnal hypoxemia. The patient is currently doing well with no recurrence of PTX for the last one year.

3. Discussion

NPPV is a noninvasive ventilation that uses some form of an interface to ventilate the lungs. These interfaces include nasal pillow masks that fit into the nostrils, nasal masks that cover the nose, oral masks that fit into the mouth, oronasal or full-face masks that fit into both the nose and mouth, and helmet masks that cover the entire face [1]. CPAP and BPAP (bilevel positive airway pressure) are the two most commonly used types of NPPV. CPAP provides continuous pressure during the entire breathing cycle [2]. BPAP delivers preset inspiratory and expiratory pressures at alternating levels. The pressure delivered in BPAP is higher during inspiration and lower during expiration [3]. NPPV is used in the management of many clinical conditions that cause respiratory failure such as chronic obstructive pulmonary disease (COPD), asthma, thoracic wall deformity, neuromuscular diseases, obesity hypoventilation syndrome, OSA, pneumonia, pulmonary edema, and acute respiratory distress syndrome (ARDS) [4]. When applied at optimal levels to selected patients, NPPV is generally safe and well-tolerated. The side effects are usually minor, and severe complications occur very rarely. Interface-related complications include discomfort, skin rash, nasal bridge sores, nasal obstruction, claustrophobia, increased dead space, aspiration, hypersalivation, salivary retention, pressure sores, and dental problems. These

TABLE 1: Characteristics of patients who developed pneumothorax with NPPV therapy for OSA.

Case	Age (years)	Sex	NPPV indication	Underlying lung pathology	NPPV type	NPPV pressure settings
Current case—Rajdev et al.	66	F	Obstructive sleep apnea	Right-sided pleural effusion and diaphragmatic hernia	CPAP with nasal mask	(i) Auto-CPAP pressure-4-20 cm H_2O
Langner et al. [6]	68	NA	Obstructive sleep apnea	None	CPAP	(i) Initial therapy pressure-9 cm H_2O (ii) Pressure later increased-13 cm H_2O
Herrejón Silvestre et al. [8]	67	M	Obstructive sleep apnea	Pan acinar emphysema	BPAP with nasal mask	(i) Inspiratory pressure-10 cm H_2O (ii) Expiratory pressure-5 cm H_2O
Mao et al. [20]	64	M	Obstructive sleep apnea	None	PAP (ASV)	(i) Pressure support-5-10 cm H_2O (ii) EPAP-15 cm H_2O
Chicote Álvarez et al. [21]	72	NA	Obstructive sleep apnea	NA	CPAP	(i) NA

ASV: adaptive support ventilation; BPAP: bilevel positive airway pressure; CPAP continuous positive airway pressure; EPAP: expiratory positive airway pressure; F: female; H_2O: water; M: male; NA: not available; NPPV: noninvasive positive pressure ventilation; OSA: obstructive sleep apnea.

are usually corrected by mask adjustment or changing the type of mask. The pressure-related complications include discomfort, ear/sinus pain, gastric insufflation, and flow-related side effects which are nasal/oral congestion, nasal/oral dryness, runny nose, nosebleed, and eye irritation. The major complications of NPPV are rare and include aspiration, mucus plugging, hypoxemia, hypotension, and barotrauma [5].

PTX is a potentially fatal complication in patients who undergo mechanical ventilation and has been reported more commonly with invasive mechanical ventilation. Pulmonary barotrauma can occur in mechanically ventilated patients as a result of a sustained increase in regional transmural pressure that causes overdistension and subsequent rupture of the alveoli. This causes air leak into the perivascular adventitia causing interstitial emphysema. Air can also dissect along the perivascular sheaths and the cervical fascial planes leading pneumomediastinum and subcutaneous emphysema, respectively. If the tension is not released, the high pressure can eventually cause rupture of the mediastinal pleura, resulting in PTX [6].

Though described mainly with invasive mechanical ventilation, the same mechanism may apply for NPPV. The application of high noninvasive positive pressures can be detrimental as it leads to high airway pressures and subsequent alveolar overdistension [7]. Due to the scarcity of literature, the exact incidence of PTX in patients who undergo NPPV is not known. It has been reported in patients who received NPPV for hypoxemia, OSA, acute respiratory failure, and chronic respiratory failure. The presence of an underlying lung condition was noted in most of the reported cases such as COPD [8–11]; cystic fibrosis [12]; Duchenne muscular dystrophy [13, 14] and chronic nonprogressive myopathy [15], pneumonia [10, 16, 17], asthma [18], and interstitial lung disease [10]; and COVID-19 [19]. The onset of PTX varied from occurring within hours of initiation to years after the initiation of NPPV therapy. After an extensive review of literature, we found only 4 other cases of PTX occurring with the use of NPPV for OSA [6, 8, 20, 21]. The characteristics of these patients with OSA and the NPPV settings, including our patient, are summarized in Table 1 and Table 2.

Imaging with chest radiograph or CT scan should be performed for patients on NPPV who present with sudden onset of dyspnea and chest pain, to evaluate for PTX. Large, symptomatic PTX requires drainage with the help of a chest tube. Choo-Kang et al. treated their case of recurrent PTX from NPPV with chemical pleurodesis using doxycycline initially followed by open pleurodesis, when the former failed [15]. The application of lung-protective strategies during mechanical ventilation can help reduce the risk of lung parenchymal injury and PTX. The protective settings for NPPV include maintaining low P_{pl} (<30 cm H_2O), low tidal volume, and sound use of PEEP (positive end-expiratory pressure) to balance the distending end-inspiratory pressures as well as meet the required target of arterial oxygen pressure [7]. Since underlying lung pathologies can increase the risk of barotrauma, they should be treated appropriately. In cases that occur while on the volume-limited device, switching to a pressure-limited device is suggested especially if the PTX is slow to resolve or recur [13, 22]. This is probably because pressure-limited ventilation limits the peak airway pressure, thereby decreasing the risk of barotrauma [13].

As described above, PTX is an uncommonly reported but serious complication with the use of NPPV, and cases of PTX with NPPV use for OSA are extremely limited. In this case report, we present a case of recurrent pneumothorax secondary to CPAP therapy for OSA, with a strong temporal association with the initiation of CPAP. There has not been a consensus on the best treatment modality for mild OSA due to limited evidence base, and many physicians would offer CPAP to patients with mild OSA. The American Academy of Sleep Medicine (AASM) recommends offering positive airway pressure therapy to all patients who have been diagnosed with OSA [23, 24]. They defined OSA as either a respiratory disturbance index (RDI) ≥ 15 events per hour with or without symptoms or an obstructive RDI between 5 and 14 events per hour that is accompanied by any of the following: fatigue, nonrestorative sleep, sleepiness, or insomnia symptoms; habitual snoring and/or breathing interruptions; waking up with gasping, breath-holding, or

Table 2: Features of PTX in the affected patients.

Case	First PTX onset after NPPV	PTX frequency	Intervention for PTX
Current case—Rajdev et al.	2 months	Three times	Chest tube
Langner et al. [6]	Years	Once	Chest tube
Herrejón Silvestre et al. [8]	Within hours	Once	Chest tube
Mao et al. [20]	NA	Twice	Chest tube
Chicote Álvarez et al. [21]	NA	Once	Chest tube

NA: not available; NPPV: noninvasive positive pressure ventilation; PTX: pneumothorax.

choking; and hypertension, cognitive dysfunction, mood disorder, coronary artery disease, congestive heart failure, stroke, type 2 diabetes, or atrial fibrillation [25]. The obstructive RDI is defined as the number of obstructive apneas, obstructive hypopneas, and respiratory effort related arousals (RERAs) per hour of sleep. A recent randomized clinical trial by Wimms et al. found an improvement in the quality of life in patients with mild OSA treated with CPAP [26]. That being said, we believe that our patient's severity of OSA on the HST was underestimated as the total recording time was 10 h, whereas the usual sleep duration as reported by the patient and the average CPAP use on the compliance report was around 7-8 h. This is because the HST measures RDI over a total recording time, unlike in-laboratory study which uses total sleep time. The literature supports that the treatment provided by sleep and nonsleep specialists resulted in a similar quality of life, symptom scores, and adherence [27]. However, with this article, we would like to highlight that the involvement of a sleep specialist in patients with a complicated course of OSA treatment may be useful. A high air leak can lead to the generation of high CPAP pressures. Therefore, air leak should be addressed, especially in patients who are mouth breathers and are on a nasal mask. An in-laboratory titration study can be pursued to determine the optimal positive pressure level required to normalize the AHI (<5) in order to help limit the positive pressures. Nocturnal oxygen therapy for OSA significantly improves oxygen saturation and intermittent hypoxia in patients with OSA [28]. However, with the current evidence, it is difficult to recommend oxygen therapy over CPAP for the treatment of patients who are unable to tolerate CPAP therapy. Oxygen therapy has been shown to prolong the duration of apnea and hypopnea events, perhaps as a result of suppressing hypoxic respiratory drive which can potentially worsen acidosis [28]. It also does not address the upper airway obstruction that is central to the pathophysiology of OSA. Oral appliances like mandibular advancement devices, weight loss, positional therapy, and upper airway surgical options are some of the alternatives that can be utilized in patients who are not able to tolerate positive airway pressure therapy.

In conclusion, health-care providers should be aware of pneumothorax as a potential complication from the use of NPPV for OSA and limiting the positive airway pressures or use of alternative therapy when feasible might help decrease the risk of such complications. A timely referral to a sleep specialist may be warranted in managing CPAP-related complication while treating OSA.

Consent

An informed consent was obtained from the patient for publication of this case report and any accompanying images.

Authors' Contributions

All authors have been involved in the preparation of this manuscript. All authors have read and approved the manuscript.

References

[1] A. Bachour, H. Avellan-Hietanen, T. Palotie, and P. Virkkula, "Practical aspects of interface application in CPAP treatment," *Canadian Respiratory Journal*, vol. 2019, Article ID 7215258, 8 pages, 2019.

[2] J. A. Katz and J. D. Marks, "Inspiratory work with and without continuous positive airway pressure in patients with acute respiratory failure," *Anesthesiology*, vol. 63, no. 6, pp. 598–607, 1985.

[3] B. Kraynek, "What are the clinical indications for noninvasive positive pressure ventilation?," *The Hospitalist*, vol. 2011, no. 12, 2011.

[4] S. Mehta and N. S. Hill, "Noninvasive ventilation," *American Journal of Respiratory and Critical Care Medicine*, vol. 163, no. 2, pp. 540–577, 2001.

[5] P. C. Gay, "Complications of noninvasive ventilation in acute care," *Respiratory Care*, vol. 54, no. 2, pp. 246–258, 2009.

[6] S. Langner, M. Kolditz, J. Kleymann et al., "Großer Pneumothorax unter CPAP-Therapie beim Schlafapnoepatienten ohne vorbekannte Lungen- und Thoraxerkrankungen – ein Fallbericht [Large pneumothorax in a sleep apnea patient with CPAP without previously known lung and thoracic diseases - a case report]," *Pneumologie (Stuttgart, Germany)*, vol. 74, no. 4, pp. 217–221, 2020.

[7] N. R. MacIntyre, "Physiologic effects of noninvasive ventilation," *Respiratory Care*, vol. 64, no. 6, pp. 617–628, 2019.

[8] A. Herrejón Silvestre, I. Inchaurraga Alvarez, and M. Marín González, "Neumotórax espontáneo asociado al uso de BiPAP nocturno con mascarilla nasal," *Archivos de Bronconeumologia*, vol. 34, no. 10, p. 512, 1998.

[9] R. Raghavan, A. K. Ellis, W. Wobeser, K. B. Sutherland, and D. E. O'Donnell, "Hemopneumothorax in a COPD patient treated with noninvasive positive pressure ventilation: the risk of attendant anticoagulation," *Canadian Respiratory Journal*, vol. 11, Article ID 971743, 4 pages, 2004.

[10] K. Fukushima, K. Marut, C. Kiyofuji, and M. Sugimoto, "Evaluation of the incidence of pneumothorax and background of

patients with pneumothorax during noninvasive positive pressure ventilation," *Nihon Kokyuki Gakkai Zasshi*, vol. 46, no. 11, pp. 870–874, 2008.

[11] D. J. McCracken, E. O. Bedawi, M. Hassan, D. Stavroulias, and N. M. Rahman, "Secondary pneumothorax in end-stage lung disease complicated by noninvasive ventilation and a persistent air leak," *Breathe (Sheffield, England)*, vol. 14, no. 4, pp. e119–e122, 2018.

[12] C. S. Haworth, M. E. Dodd, M. Atkins, A. A. Woodcock, and A. K. Webb, "Pneumothorax in adults with cystic fibrosis dependent on nasal intermittent positive pressure ventilation (NIPPV): a management dilemma," *Thorax*, vol. 55, no. 7, pp. 620–622, 2000.

[13] A. Vianello, G. Arcaro, F. Gallan, C. Ori, and M. Bevilacqua, "Pneumothorax associated with long-term non-invasive positive pressure ventilation in Duchenne muscular dystrophy," *Neuromuscular Disorders*, vol. 14, no. 6, pp. 353–355, 2004.

[14] H. E. Cho, J. Byun, W. A. Choi, M. Kim, K. Y. Kim, and S.-W. Kang, "Analysis of pneumothorax in non-invasive ventilator users with Duchenne muscular dystrophy," *Chest*, 2020.

[15] L. R. Choo-Kang, F. O. Ogunlesi, S. A. McGrath-Morrow, T. O. Crawford, and C. L. Marcus, "Recurrent pneumothoraces associated with nocturnal noninvasive ventilation in a patient with muscular dystrophy," *Pediatric Pulmonology*, vol. 34, no. 1, pp. 73–78, 2002.

[16] M. Carron, G. Gagliardi, F. Michielan, U. Freo, and C. Ori, "Occurrence of pneumothorax during noninvasive positive pressure ventilation through a helmet," *Journal of Clinical Anesthesia*, vol. 19, no. 8, pp. 632–635, 2007.

[17] G. J. Sheehan, L. J. Miedzinski, and D. G. Schroeder, "Pneumothorax complicating BiPAP therapy for Pneumocystis carinii pneumonia," *Chest*, vol. 103, no. 4, p. 1310, 1993.

[18] A. R. Medford and J. C. T. Pepperell, "Pneumothorax following non-invasive ventilation for acute asthma," *Journal of the Royal College of Physicians of Edinburgh*, vol. 36, no. 1, pp. 29–31, 2006.

[19] A. Gidaro, F. Samartin, A. M. Brambilla et al., "Occurrence of pneumothorax and pneumomediastinum in Covid-19 patients during non-invasive ventilation with continuous positive airway pressure," *medRxiv*, 2020.

[20] J. T. Mao, A. Bernabei, N. Cutrufello, and J. D. Kern, "Spontaneous pneumothorax caused by excessive positive airway pressure therapy for obstructive sleep apnea," in *D36. Pleural Disease: Case Reports II*, no. article A6682, 2018American Thoracic Society, 2018.

[21] E. Chicote Álvarez, M. Arlabán Carpintero, and A. González-Castro, "Edema pulmonar ex vacuo tras drenaje de neumotórax," *Medicina Intensiva*, vol. 42, no. 9, pp. e24–e25, 2018.

[22] A. K. Simonds, "Pneumothorax: an important complication of non-invasive ventilation in neuromuscular disease," *Neuromuscular Disorders*, vol. 14, no. 6, pp. 351-352, 2004.

[23] L. J. Epstein, D. Kristo, P. J. Strollo Jr., and Adult Obstructive Sleep Apnea Task Force of the American Academy of Sleep Medicine, "Clinical guideline for the evaluation, management and long-term care of obstructive sleep apnea in adults," *Journal of Clinical Sleep Medicine*, vol. 5, no. 3, pp. 263–276, 2009.

[24] R. B. Berry, R. Budhiraja, D. J. Gottlieb et al., "Rules for scoring respiratory events in sleep: update of the 2007 AASM Manual for the Scoring of Sleep and Associated Events. Deliberations of the Sleep Apnea Definitions Task Force of the American Academy of Sleep Medicine," *Journal of Clinical Sleep Medicine*, vol. 8, no. 5, pp. 597 619, 2012.

[25] American Academy of Sleep Medicine, *International Classification of Sleep Disorders*, American Academy of Sleep Medicine, Darien, IL, 3rd edition, 2014.

[26] A. J. Wimms, J. L. Kelly, C. D. Turnbull et al., "Continuous positive airway pressure versus standard care for the treatment of people with mild obstructive sleep apnoea (MERGE): a multicentre, randomised controlled trial," *Respiratory medicine*, vol. 8, no. 4, pp. 349–358, 2020.

[27] K. M. Kunisaki, N. Greer, W. Khalil et al., "Provider types and outcomes in obstructive sleep apnea case finding and treatment," *Annals of Internal Medicine*, vol. 168, no. 3, pp. 195–202, 2018.

[28] V. Mehta, T. S. Vasu, B. Phillips, and F. Chung, "Obstructive sleep apnea and oxygen therapy: a systematic review of the literature and meta-analysis," *Journal of Clinical Sleep Medicine*, vol. 9, no. 3, pp. 271–279, 2013.

14

Effectiveness of Clinical Decision Tools in Predicting Pulmonary Embolism

Michael A. Simon[1] **Christopher Tan,**[1] **Patrick Hilden,**[2] **Lyle Gesner,**[1] **and Barry Julius**[1]

[1]*Department of Radiology, RWJBH–Saint Barnabas Medical Center, Livingston, New Jersey, USA*
[2]*Department of Biostatistics, RWJBH–Saint Barnabas Medical Center, Livingston, New Jersey, USA*

Correspondence should be addressed to Michael A. Simon; michaelsimonmd@gmail.com

Academic Editor: Yongchun Shen

Objective. The Wells criteria and revised Geneva score are two commonly used clinical decision tools (CDTs) developed to assist physicians in determining when computed tomographic angiograms (CTAs) should be performed to evaluate the high index of suspicion for pulmonary embolism (PE). Studies have shown varied accuracy in these CDTs in identifying PE, and we sought to determine their accuracy within our patient population. *Methods.* Patients admitted to the Emergency Department (ED) who received a CTA for suspected PE from 2019 Jun 1 to 2019 Aug 31 were identified. Two CDTSs, the Wells criteria and revised Geneva score, were calculated based on data available prior to CTA and using the common D-Dimer cutoff of >500 μg/L. We determined the association between confirmed PE and CDT values and determined the association between the D-Dimer result and PE. *Results.* 392 CTAs were identified with 48 (12.1%) positive PE cases. The Wells criteria and revised Geneva score were significantly associated with PE but failed to identify 12.5% and 70.4% of positive PE cases, respectively. Within our cohort, a D-Dimer cutoff of >300 μg/L was significantly associated with PE and captured 95.2% of PE cases. *Conclusions.* Both CDTs were significantly associated with PE but failed to identify PE in a significant number of cases, particularly the revised Geneva score. Alternative D-Dimer cutoffs may provide better accuracy in identifying PE cases.

1. Introduction

Approximately 180,000 people die each year from pulmonary embolism [1]. Chest computed tomographic angiograms (CTA) are frequently used in the Emergency Department (ED) setting to rule out PE [1]. To guide physicians in managing patients with suspected PE and determine the appropriateness of a CTA, two well-known clinical decision tools (CDTs), the Wells criteria and the revised Geneva score, have been developed [2, 3]. The Wells criteria and the revised Geneva score both stratify patients into risk groups based on clinical characteristics and combine these risk groups with the results of a D-Dimer test in order to determine a patient's likelihood of PE and subsequent need for a CTA (Tables 1 and 2).

The Wells criteria have two accepted methods for calculating PE risk and guidance for a CTA, the two-tiered and three-tiered models [2, 4]. The criteria for assigning points based on signs/symptoms remain the same between these models; the stratification of patients into their risk category for PE differs, which in turn changes the recommended action. The three-tiered model separates the patients into low, medium, and high risk which represents patients who scored 0-1, 2-6, and ≥7 points, respectively. According to this model, patients with a high risk score should receive a CTA while those who fall under low or intermediate risk should receive either a standard D-Dimer using the ELISA method or a high sensitivity D-Dimer test using fluorescent immunoarrays. If the D-Dimer is positive, these patients should receive a CTA, whereas the two-tiered model states that patients with scores ≤ 4 are considered PE unlikely and should receive a high sensitivity D-Dimer test. If positive, a CTA should be performed. Patients with scores > 4 are considered PE likely and should subsequently undergo a CTA [2, 4].

Although these clinical decision tools are available to guide physicians on whether or not a CTA is warranted,

Table 1: Wells criteria.

Variable	Score
Clinical signs and symptoms of DVT	3
PE is #1 diagnosis or equally likely	3
Heart rate > 100	1.5
Immobilization[a] or surgery[b]	1.5
Prior, objectively diagnosed PE or DVT	1.5
Hemoptysis	1
Malignancy[c]	1

[a]At least three days; [b]in previous four weeks; [c]treatment within 6 months or palliative care.

Table 2: Revised Geneva score.

Variable	Score
Age > 65	1
Prior DVT or PE	3
Surgery[a] or lower limb fracture in past month	2
Active malignant condition[b]	2
Unilateral lower limb pain	3
Hemoptysis	2
Heart rate	
<75	0
75-94	3
≥95	5
Pain on lower limb palpation and unilateral edema	4

[a]Under general anesthesia; [b]solid or hematologic malignant condition currently active or considered cured <1 year.

many continue to rely on personal experience with several studies highlighting that CDTs are underutilized [1, 5]. The underutilization of CDTs has been attributed to the experience of the treating physician, a lack of trust in CDTs, and concerns about the impact of false-negative findings [6]. However, studies have shown that most clinicians make errors in diagnosis when faced with complex cases, with up to 35% of these mistakes resulting in morbidity [6, 7].

While CTA remains the gold standard for PE evaluation, CTAs put patients at additional risks for malignancy due to high radiation dose targeted to the chest and renal failure due to the usage of iodine contrast. Additionally, given the finite availability of CT time in the emergency setting, CTA should only be utilized when necessary [8–10].

2. Methods

Institutional IRB approval with a waiver for informed consent was obtained for this retrospective study. A chart review was performed between June 1st through August 31st, 2019 (three months immediately prior to the IRB approval and represented approximately 400 cases) and identified CTAs ordered for patients located in the ED with concern for PE. Review of the medical records did not reveal any documented Wells criteria or revised Geneva score by the ED physicians. Therefore, clinical data, i.e., variables for the respective scoring systems, were extracted from the electronic medical record with subsequent calculation of the Wells criteria and revised Geneva score. Only data available to the ordering physician at the time of the patient's CTA was included in the score calculation.

We utilized the two-tiered model of the Wells criteria, which uses a cutoff of ≤4 and >4. This was done to minimize the subjective aspect of the Wells criteria. When calculating the Wells criterion score, the criterion "PE likely or more likely than an alternative diagnosis" was considered positive only if explicit concern was documented in the ED note. When calculating the revised Geneva score, the first recorded heart rate on presentation was used. In line with previous studies, we combined the intermediate- and high-risk groups together and used the cutoff of ≤3 to effectively rule out PE, thus separating the revised Geneva score into two groups with low or intermediate/high risk, separated by their need for further testing [11, 12].

Clinical findings of deep vein thrombosis (DVT) were considered positive based on a physical exam and if ultrasound of the lower extremity demonstrated a DVT. In addition, a high sensitivity D-Dimer value of greater than 500 μg/L was considered positive [13].

An analysis based on the respective CDT algorithms utilizing both the CDT and D-Dimer values was performed. Each CDT was separated based on whether a CTA would have been indicated based on the results of the CDT. The association between PE, patient, and treatment characteristics, and each CDT was assessed using the Wilcoxon rank-sum test for continuous variables and the chi-squared or Fisher's exact test for categorical variables as appropriate. ROC analyses were used to determine the benefit of other potential cutoffs for D-Dimer testing within our population. All analyses were completed in R (version 3.6.2).

3. Results

A total of 392 cases (ED admits) were identified among 376 unique patients; 48 (12.1%) of cases were found to have PE on CTA. 266 (67.9%) of cases were female, and the median (range) age of the study population was 55 (17–97) years. The median Wells score was 1 (0–9) with thirty-eight cases (9.7%) having a score greater than 4. The median revised Geneva score was 4 (0, 12) with 224 (57.1%) of cases having a revised Geneva score greater than 3. D-Dimer values were available for 155 cases (39.5%) with 61 (39.4%) being >500 μg/L.

When analyzing our data according to the accepted algorithms of the Wells criteria and revised Geneva score, both the Wells criteria and revised Geneva score were significantly associated with PE ($p < 0.001$ and $p = 0.033$, respectively) (Table 3). Among patients positive for PE, the Wells criteria appropriately guided the physician in 88% of cases to order a CTA (true positive), while among patients negative for PE, 41% were guided to CTA (false positive). Within the revised Geneva score, only 30% of patients with PE received a CTA correctly while 12% of negative PE patients received a CTA.

Table 3: Wells criteria, revised Geneva score, and D-Dimer association with CTA. Median (range), N (%).

Variable	CTA result Positive	Negative	p value
Wells criteria	1.5 (0.0, 9.0)	0.0 (0.0, 7.5)	<0.001
Wells criteria (D-Dimer cutoff 500)			<0.001
CTA	28 (87.5)	63 (41.2)	
No CTA	4 (12.5)	90 (58.8)	
Missing	16	191	
Revised Geneva score	5.5 (0.0, 12.0)	4.0 (0.0, 12.0)	0.02
Revised Geneva score (D-Dimer cutoff 500)			0.033
CTA	8 (29.6)	25 (12.0)	
No CTA	19 (70.4)	183 (88.0)	
Missing	21	136	
D-Dimer	1066.0 (273.0, 15180.0)	394.0 (150.0, 8653.0)	<0.001
D-Dimer			0.046
≤300	1 (4.8)	32 (25.8)	
>300	20 (95.2)	92 (74.2)	
Missing	27	220	

Among the subset of 155 cases with a D-Dimer, we identified a value of >300 μg/L as being significantly associated with PE ($p = 0.021$) and accurately captured 20/21 (95.2%) positive PE cases among this subset (Tables 4 and 3). As for the 206 patients that did not have a D-Dimer performed and had Wells criteria < 4, there were sixteen cases positive for PE, resulting in a positivity rate of 7.7%. In comparison, our analyzed cohort which had D-Dimers available but Wells criteria < 4, the positivity rate was 10.1%. This difference in positivity rate is suggestive that analyzing by gestalt alone is creating overuse.

Table 4: Demographics, Wells criteria, revised Geneva score, and D-Dimer median (range), N (%).

Variable	Summary
Gender	
Male	126 (32.1)
Female	266 (67.9)
Age at CTA	55 (17, 97)
CTA	
Negative	344 (87.8)
Positive	48 (12.2)
Wells criteria	1 (0, 9)
Revised Geneva score	4 (0, 12)
Wells criteria (D-Dimer cutoff 500)	
CTA	91 (49.2)
No CTA	94 (50.8)
Missing	207
Revised Geneva score (D-Dimer cutoff 500)	
CTA	33 (14.0)
No CTA	202 (86.0)
Missing	157
D-Dimer	421 (150, 15180)
≤300	33 (22.8)
>300	112 (77.2)
Missing	247

Cases were considered missing when the data was not complete, i.e., no D-Dimer.

4. Discussion

When the Wells criterion algorithm was followed utilizing the accepted cutoff of 500 μg/L, the Wells criteria were significantly associated with CTA result accurately directing 28/32 PE cases to subsequent CTA. Although the Wells criteria were significantly associated with CTA, 12.5% of patients would have been missed suggesting that this scoring method and cutoff may not be ideal for our patient population. In addition, the Wells criteria are heavily weighted towards physician evaluation of the patient and are thereby a more subjective scoring system. This could lead to an increased amount of CTAs ordered based on physician experience. The revised Geneva score did not provide a clinically viable alternative scoring system, with 19/27 PE cases not directed to CTA. Similar results have been reported which found the revised Geneva score to be less robust than the Wells score in predicting PE [11, 14].

Our findings reiterate results that have been seen in other studies which describe a modest 10% positive rate of CTAs for PE while using a CDT. This suggests not only a general overuse of CTAs but an inadequacy of our current CDTs [6, 15]. The failure of the current CDTs to predict a positive test could be due to the tools being built on specific patient populations which do not extrapolate to other groups. Therefore, prior to use, a CDT may need to be evaluated for the specific population to ensure its validity.

This has been done in other institutions such as Allegheny General Hospital in Pittsburgh, Pennsylvania, where a study suggested that, although a value of 500 μg/L is accepted as the D-Dimer cutoff, different values could provide for better care. For instance, raising the threshold to 850 μg/L kept the sensitivity at 100% while increasing specificity to 51% in their population [16]. Further analysis of our data revealed that a value of >300 μg/L was significantly associated with positive CTA. Using this cutoff value as opposed to 500 μg/L greatly increases our sensitivity while slightly decreasing the specificity, missing only one positive PE case (4.7% of cases). This new cutoff value in combination with the Wells criteria could potentially reduce the amount of CTAs performed while maintaining an acceptable level of sensitivity. Our data also suggested that the use of D-Dimer alone may be able to predict CTA outcome just as well as a combination of D-Dimer and a CDT.

CTAs are not benign tests. Carcinogenic risks from radiation delivered during imaging studies are often debated. The variability of radiation dose from CT scans and the uncertain effect of the carcinogenic risk from low dose radiation (0-100 mSv) further confound the matter [17]. However, analysis of atomic bomb survivors (long and accurate follow-up) suggests that there is an increased risk of malignancy with radiation doses between 5 and 100 mSv [17]. Further, studies have shown that there is a higher risk of breast cancer 10 years following two CT chest exams than in a female who did not receive any CT exams during the same period [18]. Alterations to the scoring systems, especially for our predominantly female population, to better stratify patients must be determined.

5. Conclusion

Although CDTs may be useful, our data has exposed concerns in the applicability of the Wells and revised Geneva scores within our population. The data we collected suggests that the revised Geneva score is not applicable to our patient population. The Wells criteria, although associated with PE, missed 12.5% of positive cases. This would suggest that further analysis of the Wells criteria is warranted in our patient population. Identifying a better D-Dimer cutoff could be beneficial in reducing scans. Association of D-Dimer alone in comparison to D-Dimer with the Wells criteria is also warranted based on our findings. Based on this, we are currently performing a prospective study to identify an ideal cutoff for D-Dimer in our patient population. The overall low positive rate of CTA with the use of CDTs suggests the need for further refinement of these tests [6, 15].

Furthermore, comparing the lower positivity rates of the low-risk, non-D-Dimer-performed cohort (7.7%) with the low-risk, D-Dimer-performed cohort (10.1%), it is suggested that determining the need for a low-risk patient to undergo a CTA using gestalt instead of using a D-Dimer is less accurate and contributes to overuse.

6. Limitations

This is a retrospective study at a single institution with a limited sample size. Additionally, a misclassification bias may be present in our analysis as the ED physicians did not document the Wells criteria or revised Geneva in the patient's charts. Therefore, assumptions were made when calculating the Wells criteria, such as only adding three points if the concern for PE was expressly documented. This method could have artificially lowered the Wells criteria for multiple patients placing them in a category where a CTA was not needed. Both clinical decision tools rely on D-Dimer testing in conjunction with the scoring system. More than 230 patients from our cohort did not have a D-Dimer performed. Of these patients, 27 had a positive CTA. The lack of D-Dimer testing prevented our team from fully evaluating the usefulness of the scoring systems for evaluation of PE. Our prospective study will include a D-Dimer sample from all patients.

Additional Points

Take Home Points. (1) Our data suggests that the revised Geneva score fails to capture a significant proportion of patients with pulmonary embolism. (2) The Wells criteria were significantly associated with pulmonary embolism when using a D-Dimer cutoff of 500 μg/L; however, the scoring criteria still missed 13% of cases. (3) A D-Dimer cutoff of ≥300 accurately captured 20/21 positive cases (95% sensitivity and 25% specificity), suggesting that the D-Dimer itself may be an adequate screening tool for PE. Further investigation of D-Dimer alone or in conjunction with the Wells criteria is warranted.

Authors' Contributions

All authors substantially contributed to the conception, writing, and revision of the manuscript. In addition, they all are accountable for the manuscript's content. The authors declare that they had full access to all of the data in this study, and the authors take complete responsibility for the integrity of the data and the accuracy of the data analysis.

References

[1] N. Hsu and G. W. Soo Hoo, "Underuse of clinical decision rules and d-dimer in suspected pulmonary embolism: a nationwide survey of the Veterans Administration Healthcare System," *Journal of the American College of Radiology*, 2019.

[2] P. S. Wells, D. R. Anderson, M. Rodger et al., "Excluding pulmonary embolism at the bedside without diagnostic imaging: management of patients with suspected pulmonary embolism presenting to the emergency department by using a simple clinical model and d-dimer," *Annals of Internal Medicine*, vol. 135, no. 2, pp. 98–107, 2001.

[3] G. le Gal, M. Righini, P. M. Roy et al., "Prediction of pulmonary embolism in the emergency department: the revised Geneva score," *Annals of Internal Medicine*, vol. 144, no. 3, pp. 165–171, 2006.

[4] S. J. Wolf, T. R. McCubbin, K. M. Feldhaus, J. P. Faragher, and D. M. Adcock, "Prospective validation of Wells criteria in the evaluation of patients with suspected pulmonary embolism," *Annals of Emergency Medicine*, vol. 44, no. 5, pp. 503–510, 2004.

[5] E. Simon, I. M. Miake-Lye, S. W. Smith et al., "An evaluation of guideline-discordant ordering behavior for CT pulmonary angiography in the emergency department," *Journal of the American College of Radiology*, vol. 16, no. 8, pp. 1064–1072, 2019.

[6] M. M. Costantino, G. Randall, M. Gosselin, M. Brandt, K. Spinning, and C. D. Vegas, "CT angiography in the evaluation of acute pulmonary embolus," *AJR. American Journal of Roentgenology*, vol. 191, no. 2, pp. 471–474, 2008.

[7] C. Cook, "Is clinical gestalt good enough?," *The Journal of Manual & Manipulative Therapy*, vol. 17, no. 1, pp. 6-7, 2013.

[8] R. Smith-Bindman, J. Lipson, R. Marcus, K. P. Kim, M. Mahesh, R. Gould et al., "Radiation dose associated with common computed tomography examinations and the associated lifetime attributable risk of cancer," *Archives of Internal Medicine*, vol. 169, no. 22, pp. 2078–2086, 2009.

[9] E. C. Lin, "Radiation risk from medical imaging," *Mayo Clinic Proceedings*, vol. 85, no. 12, pp. 1142–1146, 2010.

[10] K. H. Shah, B. H. Slovis, D. Runde, B. Godbout, D. H. Newman, and J. Lee, "Radiation exposure among patients with the highest CT scan utilization in the emergency department," *Emergency Radiology*, vol. 20, no. 6, pp. 485–491, 2013.

[11] D. J. Guo, C. Zhao, Y. D. Zou, X. H. Huang, J. M. Hu, and L. Guo, "Values of the Wells and revised Geneva scores combined with D-dimer in diagnosing elderly pulmonary embolism patients," *Chinese Medical Journal*, vol. 128, no. 8, pp. 1052–1057, 2015.

[12] A. Torbicki, A. Perrier, S. Konstantinides et al., "Guidelines on the diagnosis and management of acute pulmonary embolism," *European Heart Journal*, vol. 29, no. 18, pp. 2276–2315, 2008.

[13] M. Righini, J. van Es, P. L. den Exter et al., "Age-adjusted D-dimer cutoff levels to rule out pulmonary embolism: the ADJUST-PE study," *Journal of the American Medical Association*, vol. 311, no. 11, pp. 1117–1124, 2014.

[14] J. H. Shen, H. L. Chen, J. R. Chen, J. L. Xing, P. Gu, and B. F. Zhu, "Comparison of the Wells score with the revised Geneva score for assessing suspected pulmonary embolism: a systematic review and meta-analysis," *Journal of Thrombosis and Thrombolysis*, vol. 41, no. 3, pp. 482–492, 2016.

[15] J. A. Kline, D. M. Courtney, D. M. Beam, M. C. King, and M. Steuerwald, "Incidence and predictors of repeated computed tomographic pulmonary angiography in emergency department patients," *Annals of Emergency Medicine*, vol. 54, no. 1, pp. 41–48, 2009.

[16] S. Alhassan, E. Bihler, K. Patel, S. Lavudi, M. Young, and M. Balaan, "Assessment of the current D-dimer cutoff point in pulmonary embolism workup at a single institution: retrospective study," *Journal of Postgraduate Medicine*, vol. 64, no. 3, pp. 150–154, 2018.

[17] J. M. Albert, "Radiation risk from CT: implications for cancer screening," *AJR. American Journal of Roentgenology*, vol. 201, no. 1, pp. W81–W87, 2013.

[18] G. M. D. Merry, C. Lee, E. Johnson, and R. Smith-Bindman, *Breast cancer risks from medical imaging including computed tomography (CT) and nuclear medicine among females enrolled in a large integrated health care system*, Radiological Society of North America 2012 Scientific assembly and annual meeting, 2012.

15

Assessment of Respiratory Symptoms and Pulmonary Function Status among Workers of Flour Mills in Addis Ababa, Ethiopia

Dessalegn Demeke [1] **and Diresibachew W. Haile** [2]

[1] *Bahir Dar University College of Medicine and Health Sciences, Department of Physiology, Bahir Dar, Ethiopia*
[2] *Addis Ababa University College of Medicine and Health Sciences, Department of Physiology, Addis Ababa, Ethiopia*

Correspondence should be addressed to Dessalegn Demeke; dessalegnd@bdu.edu.et

Academic Editor: Charlie Strange

Background. Flour dust in the respiratory tract affects lung function. Flour dust is a heterogeneous organic substance which can have a tendency to cause respiratory ailments. There is growing consensus on the deleterious effects of flour dust on respiratory symptoms and lung performance of flour mill workers. *Methods.* The study design was comparative cross-sectional. A total of 54 flour mill workers who work for more than eight-hour shift per day and 54 control subjects matched for sex, age, weight, height, and area of residence were enrolled. Anthropometric measurement was done. Lung function was measured by using a digital portable spirometer (Spiro Pro) based on the ATS guidelines. FVC, FEV_1, FEV_1/FVC, PEFR, and $FEF_{25}\%_{-75}\%$ were measured. Productive cough, dry cough, wheeze, and breathlessness were evaluated using BMRC questionnaire guidelines, administered through face-to-face interview. *Result.* This study showed statistically significant reduction in the mean values of pulmonary function tests in flour mill workers as compared to their matched controls. Reduction of pulmonary function indices in study subjects was significant for FVC (4.25±0.93 vs. 5.30±0.71, $p<0.001$), FEV_1 (3.46±0.86 vs. 4.50±0.72, $p<0.001$), PEFR (5.43±2.43 vs. 7.87±2.53, $p<0.001$), and $FEF_{25}\%_{-75}\%$, (3.87±1.61 vs. 4.60±1.60, $p<0.05$), but not significant for FEV_1/FVC (81.93±12.74 vs. 83.40±12.50, $p>0.05$). Flour mill workers developed 27.7% of restrictive type and 11.1% of obstructive type of lung disorders. Percentage prevalence of respiratory symptoms was evaluated as dry cough (27.7% vs. 9.3%), productive cough (11.1% vs. 5.6%), wheeze (14.8% vs. 3.8%), and breathlessness (16.6% vs.7.4%) in flour mill workers and controls, respectively. *Conclusion.* Based on the results of the present study, occupational exposure to flour dust could cause respiratory dysfunction, thereby reducing lung efficiency.

1. Background

Industrialization has been established to optimally fulfill various human needs. Over the course of time, some industries exert hazardous effect on the health of human beings [1]. Those hazard effects do have significant variations in occupational health and safety performance between countries and economic sectors. Occupational hazards and the health problems associated with occupational health and safety follow different approaches like environmental assessment, biological monitoring, medical surveillance, and epidemiological approaches to identify health problems [2].

Occupational lung diseases are a broad group of diagnosis caused by the inhalation of dusts and chemicals. As a result, improper control of these substances can result in a severe threat to site workers because most of the workers are unaware of this hazardous effect on health [3]. According to NIOSH, atmospheric pollutants, like particulates, are capable of producing adverse effects under some condition(s) of exposure and dose through time [4]. Airborne dusts are particular concern to health, as they are to be associated with occupational lung diseases [5] and exposure to flour dust occurs across a range of food industries including grain mills, flour mills, and bakeries [6, 7].

Flour dust is a heterogeneous substance with respiratory sensitizing properties and long-term exposure to it may cause acute or chronic respiratory disease [8]. Several studies showed that prevalence of sensitization for wheat allergens and fungal a-amylase and OAD is high among workers exposed to flour dust [9]. This can have a tendency to cause respiratory ailments [10]. Poor ventilation is a basic problem in flour mills [11] that have continuous exposure of workers. There are more than 250 million work-related accidents every year [2, 6]. Agriculture, basic food processing, and extractive industries are very widespread and can lead to dust exposure. In many countries, several studies investigated pulmonary function and respiratory symptoms in occupational workers worldwide [11–13]. In Ethiopia, there was no documented data related to the effect of flour dust on pulmonary function among flour mill workers.

The study aims to investigate the effect of flour dust on the pulmonary function by analyzing the pulmonary function tests that will estimate the effectiveness of the lung. This study is therefore undertaken to assess the respiratory symptoms and pulmonary function problems related to flour mill workers. It will also encourage communication between various concerned groups and organizations and foster an improved understanding of the potential problems of flour dust in the country.

2. Methods

2.1. Study Designs. Comparative cross-sectional study design was employed to assess respiratory symptoms and pulmonary function parameters in workers of flour mills. The study was conducted in Lideta subcity, Addis Ababa, Ethiopia, from August to September 2016. Addis Ababa encompasses 10 subcities and 116 woredas. It is located at altitude of 2,400 meters above sea level. Based on the data from Lideta subcity trade and development bureau and urban agriculture corporation, ten of 116 woredas are located in Lideta subcity containing a total of 76 flour mills during a time of data collection.

2.2. Sampling Methods. The source populations were all flour mill workers in Addis Ababa city, Ethiopia. The study population were all flour mill workers and controls in Lideta subcity in the age range between 18 and 43 years.

Study group: it consisted of flour mill workers in Lideta subcity in the age range between 18 and 43 years. All subjects were male as there were no female workers in the flour mill industry in the selected sites during the study period.

Control group: non-flour mill workers in Lideta subcity anthropometrically matched to study group were selected as control group.

Double proportion formula was used for the determination of sample size. The proportions of the sample size were calculated from previous study on association of flour dust on PFTs and prevalence of respiratory symptoms of chronic cough for flour mill workers and control groups (37% vs. 13%, respectively) [14]. Then, the following assumption was used: confidence level 95% (1.96), 80% power of test, correction formula was applied then after considering nonresponse rate of 10%, and the final sample size was one hundred and eight.

2.3. Eligibility Criteria

2.3.1. Inclusion Criteria. Millers who were available in the workplace between the age range of 18 and 64 years and working in the flour mill for more than one year were included.

2.3.2. Exclusion Criteria. Subjects with gross clinical abnormalities of the vertebral column, thoracic cage, neuromuscular diseases, known cases of gross anemia, diabetes mellitus, pulmonary tuberculosis, hypertension, drug addicts, known cardio pulmonary disease, cigarette smokers, tobacco and khat chewers, bakery workers, and those who underwent vigorous exercise or abdominal or chest surgery were excluded from the study.

2.4. Sampling Technique. The sample consisted of all flour mill workers in the mill and matched non-flour mill workers in Addis Ababa, Lideta subcity. Lideta subcity was selected randomly by lottery method of the ten subcities. Lideta subcity contains 10 woredas and 76 flour mills. Among 10 woredas 4 woredas were selected by random sampling. There are 30 flour mills in the 4 woredas and 24 flour mills in the 4 woredas were selected for this study until sample size was saturated. Non-flour mill workers in Lideta subcity matched for age, sex, height, and weight to flour mill workers were selected as controls. Flour mill workers and controls age was 18-64 years selected by convenient sampling technique. Selected flour mill workers and controls fulfilling eligibility criteria were interviewed and anthropometry was measured and finally spirometry was done.

Each participant was informed about the objective of the study and the benefit associated with the study immediately before sample collection. Millers who volunteered to participate in the study have answered questions in the questionnaire, which were relevant to their sociodemographic information. A structured questionnaire was prepared in English and translated into Amharic language and was retranslated back to English by a linguist to ensure consistency. Training was given to the data collectors regarding the objectives of the study and ways of administering the questionnaire by the principal investigator. The prepared questionnaire was pretested prior to the actual data collection on seven (7) informants that were not included in the main survey.

2.4.1. Anthropometric Measurements. Height and weight of the study participants were measured. The height was measured without shoes by the use of a meter rule and approximated to the nearest one cm. Weight was also measured using weighing scale (nearest to one kg), with light clothing and without phones or any encumbrance that could alter their appropriate weight. Body mass index (BMI) was calculated through this formula: weight/squared height (kg/m^2)

2.4.2. Spirometric Measurement. Digital pocket-sized Spiro Pro (JEAGER, Germany) was used to measure pulmonary function indices. Spirometric tests in both exposed and control subjects were done based on ATS guideline. Before every test, the mouthpiece was disinfected in standard solution and then attached to the spirometer. Subjects were told to put the nosepiece on the nose to prevent air blowout. Then, they were also instructed to breathe in fully until their lung filled maximally. Precaution was taken to avoid leakage

TABLE 1: Sociodemographic information of flour mill workers and controls.

Variables	Descriptions	Flour mill workers (n=54)	Control Group(n=54)	P -value
Age range(in years)	18-23	(n=20)37.03%	(n=13) 20.04%	
	24-28	(n=15) 27.7%	(n=20) 37.03%	0.591
	29-33	(n=7) 12.9%	(n=12) 22.2%	
	34-38	(n=6) 11.1%	(n=7)12.9%	
	39-43	(n=6)11.1%	(n=2) 3.7%	
Educational status	Illiterate	(n= 9) 16.6%	0(0)	
	Can write and read	(n= 19) 35.1%	(n=4) 7.4%	
	Grade 8 complete	(n= 15) 27.7%	(n=1) 1.8%	<0.01
	Grade 10 complete	(n= 8)14.8%	(n=15) 27.7%	
	Grade 12 complete	(n= 1) 1.8%	(n= 18) 33.3%	
	Diploma	0(0)	(n= 6)11.1%	
	1st degree	(n=2) 3.7%	(n=10)18.5%	
Marital status	Single	(n=37) 68.5%	(n= 35) 64.8%	
	Married	(n= 14) 25.9%	(n= 17) 31.4%	0.868
	Divorced	(n=3) 5.5%	(n=2) 3.7%	

from mouth pieces. The subjects expire forcefully and as fast and complete as possible until there is no more air left to expel. Spirometric measurements were performed in sitting position and at a fixed time of the day at room temperature (20-25°C), to minimize diurnal variations. The measurements were done in three trials, and one of the three trials, which was the best, was taken and interpreted. Prior to the actual tests, calibration with one-liter syringe and familiarization steps were done.

2.4.3. Data Analysis. Data was edited, coded, entered, and analyzed by SPSS version 20. Independent sample t-test was used for the comparison of the actual value mean respiratory score of flour mill workers and controls. Bivariate analyses were computed to test whether there was association between FVC, FEV_1, FEV_1/FVC, PEFR, and $FEF_{25}\%_{-75}\%$ and duration of exposure. Binary logistic regression and odds ratio were used to analyze and estimate the prevalence of respiratory symptoms. Variables having P value <0.05 are considered as statistically significant.

2.4.4. Ethical Consideration. The study was carried out after ethical clearance and approval was obtained from research committee of the Department of Physiology, Addis Ababa University. The study participants were briefed about the objective and procedures of the study. Thereafter, both verbal and written informed consents were obtained from those volunteers and were selected for the study. Confidentiality of information was maintained by excluding personal identifiers.

3. Results

3.1. Sociodemographic Characteristics. All workers included in the study were males. The age of the flour mill workers ranged between 18 and 43 years with a mean of 27.37±6.71 years while the age of the comparison group ranged between 18 and 43 years with a mean of 28.00±5.33 years (Table 1).

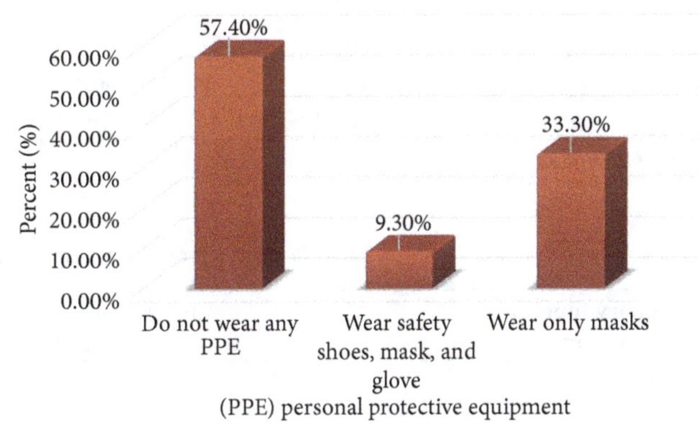

FIGURE 1: Bar chart indicating the use of personal protective equipment.

3.2. Use of Personal Protective Equipment. Personal protective devices used by the workers were investigated in the study area. Among workers, 57.4% (n= 31) do not wear any equipment, 9.3% (n=5) wear safety shoes, masks, and gloves, and 33.3% (n=18) wear only masks (Figure 1). We observed that there is no sufficient personal protective device in the workplace and the workers do not wear the equipment timely even if the material is available. Among the study subjects, 92% of the informants agreed with the idea that all flour mill workers should wear personal protective devices.

3.3. Anthropometric Measurements. Anthropometric parameters of the study subjects in terms of demographic variables demonstrate the comparison between the flour mill workers and their matched control subjects. There were no significant differences between the means of anthropometric parameters: in terms of age, weight, height, and BMI between the groups. The statistical comparison of the matching variables (age, height, weight, and BMI) shows no difference between the two groups (Table 2).

TABLE 2: The anthropometric measurements for flour mill workers and control groups by independent sample t-test.

Parameters	Exposed group(n=54) Mean ±SD	Non exposed group (n=54) Mean ±SD	P-value
Age (years)	27.37±6.71	28.00±5.33	0.591
Weight (kg)	59.72±7.76	61.91±6.39	0.113
Height (meter)	1.66±0.07	1.68±0.05	0.388
BMI (kg/m^2)	21.42±2.25	21.95±1.82	0.185

TABLE 3: Respiratory symptoms of exposed and nonexposed subjects including OR and 95% CI.

Respiratory symptoms		Prevalence % (n=54)	OR	P-value	95% CI Lower	95% CI upper
Dry Cough	case	27.7%(n=15)				
	Control	9.3%(n=5)	3.58	.027*	1.16	11.65
Productive cough	case	11.1%(n=6)				
	Control	5.6%(n=3)	1.76	.467	0.39	7.98
Wheeze	case	14.8% (n=8)				
	Control	3.7%(n=2)	4.25	.084	0.83	21.88
Breathlessness	case	16.6 %(n=9)				
	Control	7.4%(n=4)	2.80	.115	0.78	10.09

Symbol. OR = odd ratio and CI = confidence intervals.

TABLE 4: Percentage predicted lung function tests of exposed and control groups.

Pulmonary function test Parameters	Groups(case n=54 and control n=54)	Mean ±SD	p-value
FVC(L)	Case	88.59±19.05	0.000**
	Control	107.98±14.05	
FEV_1 (L)	Case	87.80±20.47	0.000**
	Control	108.93±16.98	
FEV_1/FVC	Case	98.56±15.99	0.271
	Control	102.01±16.35	
PEFR(L/s)	Case	59.76±25.37	0.000**
	Control	83.00±27.32	
$FEF_{25}\%_{-75}\%$ (L/s)	Case	88.83±35.08	0.001*
	Control	115.09±31.34	

3.4. Respiratory Symptoms. The percentage prevalence of dry cough, productive cough, wheeze, and breathlessness was 27.7%, 11.1%, 14.8%, and 16.6% for exposed informants, respectively, and 9.3%, 5.6%, 3.7%, and 7.4% for control subjects, respectively (Table 3). These values were higher among exposed workers as compared to control groups and the difference was statistically significant for dry cough ($p<0.05$).

Binary logistic regression was used to compare the respiratory symptoms and measure the strength of the association. The odds of dry cough in flour mill workers exposed to flour dust association were found to be statistically significant ($p<0.05$).

3.5. Pulmonary Function Tests. Percentage predicted values of exposed and control groups were indicated (Table 4). There was statistically more significant reduction in the percentage predicted of the exposed group than in healthy control group. Percentage predicted values of control group have largest score when compared to that of the exposed group. The difference was statistically significant ($p<0.05$). However, for FEV_1/FVC difference is not significant ($p>0.05$).

The independent sample t-test (Table 5) for equality of means between two independent groups showed that there is a significant reduction in pulmonary function values of exposed group compared to that in the control ($p<0.05$). The comparison of the mean spirometric indices of flour

TABLE 5: The comparison of the actual value mean spirometric indices of exposed and nonexposed groups by independent sample t-test.

PFTs Parameters	Flour mill workers n=54 and controls n=54)	Mean ±SD	p-value
FVC(L)	Flour mill workers	*4.25±0.93*	p<0.001
	Control	*5.30±0.71*	
FEV_1 (L)	Flour mill workers	*3.46±0.86*	p<0.001
	Control	*4.50±0.72*	
FEV_1%	Flour mill workers	*81.93±12.74*	*p>0.05*
	Control	*83.40±12.50,*	
PEFR(L/s)	Flour mill workers	*5.43±2.43*	*p<0.001*
	Control	*7.87±2.53*	
$FEF_{25}\%_{-75}\%$ (L/s)	Flour mill workers	3.87±1.61	p<0.05
	Control	4.60±1.60	

TABLE 6: Pearson correlation coefficient results between pulmonary function parameters and duration of exposure.

Variables	"r" –value	P-value
FVC	-0.417	0.000**
FEV_1	-0.359	0.000**
FEV_1/FVC	0.060	0.535
PEFR	-0.236	0.014*
$FEF_{25}\%_{-75}\%$	-0.156	0.123

mill and controls groups (mean ±SD) indicates FVC, FEV_1, and PEFR are highly significant (P<0.001) and $FEF_{25}\%_{-75}\%$ are significant (P<0.01). The forced expiratory flow rate at the middle fifty percent ($FEF_{25}\%_{-75}\%$) of the exposed group was lower (3.87L/s) than that of the controls (4.60 L/s). This reduction in flow rate was statistically significant (P <0.01). The PEFR in flour mill workers of the exposed group was lower (5.43 L/s) than that of the controls (7.87 L/s); this reduction was statistically significant (P<0.001).

There was slight reduction in pulmonary function indices (FVC, FEV_1, and FEV1/FVC, PEFR and $FEF_{25}\%_{-75}\%$) as the duration of exposure increases. Both pulmonary function indices and duration of exposure move in opposite direction. Based on their service years (1-12 years) duration of exposure and pulmonary function parameters relationship were determined. Bivariate correlation result showed negative correlation between FVC and duration of exposure which was found to be statistically significant (r= -.417, p <0.001). Pearson's correlation coefficient was used to quantify the degree of linear relationship between pulmonary function indices (FVC, FEV_1, FEV_1/FVC, PEFR, and $FEF_{25}\%_{-75}\%$) and duration of exposure (Table 6).

3.6. Pulmonary Function Status. Flour mill workers were suffering from both obstructive and restrictive disorder. Based on PFTs interpretation results indicate reduction in the pulmonary function efficiency among the flour mill workers. Airflow obstruction which reduces dynamic airway collapse makes expiration difficult. FEV_1/FVC ratio <0.7 and FEV_1 value <80% percentage predicted are considered as obstructive pattern. Restrictive defect needs large amount of elastic work to inflate the lung, which makes inspiration difficult. FEV_1 /FVC ratio >0. 7 and FVC value <80% of percentage predicted are restrictive pattern.

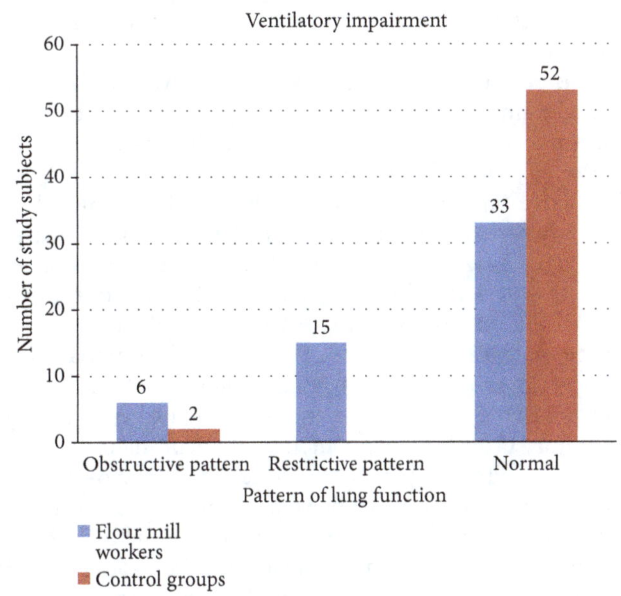

FIGURE 2: Bar chart showing the number of obstructive, restrictive, and normal patterns of lung function in controls and flour mill workers.

Among 54 flour mill workers (n=15), 27.7% developed restrictive and (n=6) 11.1% developed obstructive type of lung disorder. The rest of the study subjects 61.1% (n=33) had normal pulmonary function. Two subjects (3.7%) in the control group developed obstructive type of lung disorder and the rest of the subjects had normal pulmonary function status (Figure 2).

4. Discussion

The present study revealed the prevalence of respiratory symptoms of dry cough (27.7% vs. 9.3%), productive cough (11.1% vs. 5.6%), wheeze (14.8% vs. 3.7%), and breathlessness (16.6% vs. 7.4%) in flour mill workers and controls, respectively. In this study, the higher prevalence of respiratory symptoms in flour mill workers may be due to prolonged exposure of flour dust, unhygienic conditions, and poorly ventilated workplaces of the study areas as compared to the controls. A study by Wagh and his colleagues on the influence of flour dust on flour mill workers compared to the nonexposed controls found that flour mill workers had three times shortness of breath and developed four times frequent coughing compared to controls [11]

Similar findings were reported in Egypt [7] on the effects of exposure to flour dust on respiratory symptoms and lung function of bakery workers. The study showed that flour mill workers had cough, wheezing, and shortness of breath. Another study in Khartoum (Sudan) also showed that daily work related respiratory symptoms were significantly increased in cases compared to controls [5]. Study conducted in India showed the prevalence of respiratory symptoms and disorders among rice mill workers developing phlegm, dyspnea, chest tightness, and cough due to organic dust exposure [15].

The present study investigated the prevalence and the type of pulmonary impairment observed among the flour mill workers. We found 27.7% (n=15) of the workers develop restrictive type of lung disorder while 11.1% (n=6) develop obstructive type of lung disease. On the other hand, there were only two control subjects (3.7%) that showed an obstructive type of lung disorder. Hence, the prevalence of obstructive and restrictive lung diseases was higher in exposed group than in control group. The plausible explanation for the increased prevalence of restrictive lung impairment in exposed group is mainly due to flour dust that reacts with lymphoid and connective tissue in the terminal and respiratory bronchioles and interstitial inflammatory cells.

The results of spirometry done by [16] showed that both controls and mill workers develop lung abnormality. Flour mill workers had five times lung function abnormalities compared to the controls. Similar study showed that workers exposed to flour dust have developed chronic bronchial irritation, which is responsible for the restrictive plus obstructive type of diseases. A study conduct by [17] showed that ventilatory impairments of lung function of flour mill workers were pure restriction and mixed type. Similarly, a study by [11] found that prevalence of ventilatory impairment showed airflow obstruction and restrictive defect were much higher in cases than in controls. This means our study revealed that all lung volumes and flow rates, i.e., FVC, FEV_1, FEV_1 /FVC, $FEF_{25}\%_{-75}\%$, and PEFR, showed statistically significant reductions in the mean values in the flour mill workers as compared to their matched controls.

The findings of the present study were in line with others [17] who reported a decrease in PEFR and association between duration of exposure and pulmonary function change. The longer summative time of exposure to flour dust was associated with reduced spirometric values compared to the controls [18]. Highly significant decrement in PEFR in flour mill workers may suggest the involvement and impairment of the larger airways. This may be due to irritative effect of flour dust causing hypertrophy of mucosal cells with increased secretion of mucous, a cause of obstruction to the exhaled air. PEFR is persistently low and represents collapsing of large airways.

A study by [19] also observed a significant decline in the lung function parameters that include FVC and FEV_1, in workers exposed to flour dust compared to the control group, suggesting that flour dust persistently affects the pulmonary function parameters. The present study is also consistent with another investigation that showed flour dust can adversely affect FVC, FEV_1, and FEV_1/FVC [20]. We found significant negative correlation for FVC, FEV_1, PEFR, and $FEF_{25}\%_{-75}\%$ and duration of flour dust exposure. This is in line with other findings that long-term exposure to flour dust decreased FVC, FEV_1, PEFR, and $FEF_{25}\%_{-75}\%$ values [13, 17, 21]. Reduction in $FEF_{25}\%_{-75}\%$ value in exposed workers may be due to the obstructive pattern of the medium and smaller airways in the flour mill workers.

Similar studies conducted in Nigeria [8] showed that flour millers recorded significantly lower mean lung functions compared with control subjects with an increased risk of developing abnormalities of lung functions and there is an association on the overall mean pulmonary function to the duration of exposure of the flour mill workers.

We found that majority of the workers do not wear any equipment, some workers wear safety shoe, masks, and gloves, and 33.3% wear only masks. Another similar study found that some workers used a mask [16].

5. Limitations of the Study

This study failed to estimate the concentration of organic flour dust in the working area and was unable to determine subclinical cardiopulmonary and other systemic diseases that may affect the result of the study in both cases and controls.

6. Conclusions

Percentage prevalence of respiratory symptoms was higher among exposed workers as compared to control groups and the difference was more vivid for dry cough. Flour mill workers showed significantly reduced values in the pulmonary function tests (FVC, FEV_1, FEV_1 /FVC, PEFR, and $FEF_{25}\%_{-75}\%$) and lung efficiency due to excessive exposure to fine organic flour dust as compared to the controls. There is an inverse relationship between duration of exposure and respiratory function which means that when the duration of exposure increases, there is a deterioration of pulmonary function indices. Flour mill workers develop both restrictive and obstructive types of lung disorder. Personal protective devices were not available at workplaces and the workers usually do not wear the materials.

Acronyms and Abbreviations

ATS:	American Thoracic Society
BMRC:	British Medical Research Council Questionnaire
BMI:	Body mass index
FVC:	Forced vital capacity
FEV_1:	Forced expiratory volume in one second
FEV_1/FVC:	Percentage of the FVC
$FEF_{25}\%_{-75}\%$:	Forced expiratory flow rate at the middle part of FVC

NIOSH: National Institute of Occupational Safety and Health
OAD: Occupational asthma disease
PPE: Personal protective equipment
PFTs: Pulmonary function tests
PEFR: Peak expiratory flow rate
SPSS: Statistical Package for Social Science.

Authors' Contributions

Dessalegn Demeke designed the study, conducted field work, analyzed data, interpreted findings, and wrote the manuscript. Dr.Diresibachew W. Haile supervised the development of proposal, data analysis, manuscript writing, and procedure of spirometric measurement. All authors read the manuscript and agreed to its content.

Acknowledgments

We kindly thank the flour mill workers and data collectors heartfully.

References

[1] Y. Tanko, Y. Olakunle, A. Jimoh, A. Mohammed, A. Goji, and K. Musa, "Effects of wood dust on cardiopulmonary functions and anthropometric parameters of carpenters and non-carpenters in Sabon Gari local government Area, Kaduna State, Nigeria," *Asian journal of medical sciences*, vol. 3, no. 1, pp. 43–46, 2011.

[2] B. O. Alli, *Fundamental principles of occupational health and safety*, 2001.

[3] E. C. Guard, *Occupational Safety and Health Guidance Manual for Hazardous Waste Site Activities*, National Institute for Occupational Safety and Health, 1985.

[4] D. I. Bernstein, M. Chan-yeung, J.-L. Malo, and I. L. Bernstein, *Asthma in the workplace*, CRC Press, 2006.

[5] A. H. Ahmed, I. E. Bilal, and T. H. Merghani, "Effects of exposure to flour dust on respiretory symptoms and lung function of bakery workers: a case control study," *Sudanese Journal of public health*, no. 4, pp. 210–213, 2009.

[6] World health Organization, *Hazard Prevention And Control in The Work Environment, Airborne Dust*, World health Organization, 1999.

[7] H. A. Mohammadien, M. T. Hussein, and R. T. El-Sokkary, "Effects of exposure to flour dust on respiratory symptoms and pulmonary function of mill workers," *Egyptian Journal of Chest Diseases and Tuberculosis*, vol. 62, no. 4, pp. 745–753, 2013.

[8] K. T. Ijadunola, G. E. Erhabor, A. A. Onayade, M. Y. Ijadunola, A. O. Fatusi, and M. C. Asuzu, "Pulmonary functions of wheat flour mill workers and controls in Ibadan, Nigeria," *American Journal of Industrial Medicine*, vol. 48, no. 4, pp. 308–317, 2005.

[9] T. Meijster, E. Tielemans, N. D. Pater, and D. Heederik, "Modelling exposure in flour processing sectors in The Netherlands: A baseline measurement in the context of an intervention program," *Annals of Occupational Hygiene*, vol. 51, no. 3, pp. 293–304, 2007.

[10] D. J. Ross, H. L. Keynes, and J. C. McDonald, "SWORD '96: Surveillance of work-related and occupational respiratory disease in the UK," *Occupational Medicine* , vol. 47, no. 6, pp. 377–381, 1997.

[11] N. D. Wagh, B. G. Pachpande, V. S. Patel, S. B. Attarde, and S. T. Ingle, "The influence of workplace environment on lung function of flour mill workers in Jalgaon urban center," *Journal of Occupational Health*, vol. 48, no. 5, pp. 396–401, 2006.

[12] R. W. Melse, N. W. M. Ogink, and W. H. Rulkens, "Overview of European and Netherlands' regulations on airborne emissions from intensive livestock production with a focus on the application of air scrubbers," *Biosystems Engineering*, vol. 104, no. 3, pp. 289–298, 2009.

[13] M. B. Hosseinabadi, J. Krozhdeh, N. Khanjani, A. Zamani, M. Ranjbar, and M. Mohammadian, "Relationship between lung function and Flour dust in Flour factory workers," *Journal of Community Health Research*, vol. 2, no. 2, pp. 138–146, 2013.

[14] A. Taytard, J. F. Tessier, J. Vergeret et al., "Respiratory function in flour-mill workers," *European Journal of Epidemiology*, vol. 4, no. 1, pp. 104–109, 1988.

[15] T. Ghosh, S. Gangopadhyay, and B. Das, "Prevalence of respiratory symptoms and disorders among rice mill workers in India," *Environmental Health and Preventive Medicine*, vol. 19, no. 3, pp. 226–233, 2014.

[16] C. Melo, S. Konda, T. Shah, and Y. Padwale, "Lung function abnormalities in flour mill workers using spirometry," *International Journal of Medical Science and Public Health*, vol. 5, no. 4, p. 743, 2016.

[17] Y. Nayak, Y. Kacha, H. Mehta, C. Shah, A. Vegad, and M. Varu, "Effects of flour dust on computerized spirometric parameters in flour mill workers," *International Journal of Basic and Applied Physiology*, vol. 2, no. 1, pp. 208–212, 2013.

[18] S. P. Zodpey and R. R. Tiwari, "Peak expiratory flow rate in flour mill workers," *Indian Journal of Physiology and Pharmacology*, vol. 42, no. 4, pp. 521–526, 1998.

[19] M. A. A. El Karim, M. O. G. El Rab, A. A. Omer, and Y. A. A. El Haimi, "Respiratory and allergic disorders in workers exposed to grain and flour dusts," *Archives of Environmental & Occupational Health*, vol. 41, no. 5, pp. 297–301, 1986.

[20] S. A. Meo, "Dose responses of years of exposure on lung functions in flour mill workers," *Journal of Occupational Health*, vol. 46, no. 3, pp. 187–191, 2004.

[21] S. A. Meo and A. M. Al-Drees, "Lung function among non-smoking wheat flour mill workers," *International Journal of Occupational Medicine and Environmental Health*, vol. 18, no. 3, pp. 259–264, 2005.

A Machine Learning Approach to the Interpretation of Cardiopulmonary Exercise Tests: Development and Validation

Or Inbar,[1] Omri Inbar,[2] Ronen Reuveny,[3] Michael J. Segel,[3,4] Hayit Greenspan,[1] and Mickey Scheinowitz[1]

[1]*Department of Biomedical Engineering, Tel-Aviv University, Israel*
[2]*The Edmond and Lily Safra Children's Hospital, Sheba Medical Center, Tel Hashomer, Israel*
[3]*Pulmonary Institute, Sheba Medical Center Tel-Hashomer, Israel*
[4]*Sackler School of Medicine, Tel-Aviv University, Tel-Aviv, Israel*

Correspondence should be addressed to Omri Inbar; inbar@wincol.ac.il

Academic Editor: Yongchun Shen

Objective. At present, there is no consensus on the best strategy for interpreting the cardiopulmonary exercise test's (CPET) results. This study is aimed at assessing the potential of using computer-aided algorithms to evaluate CPET data for identifying chronic heart failure (CHF) and chronic obstructive pulmonary disease (COPD). *Methods.* Data from 234 CPET files from the Pulmonary Institute, at Sheba Medical Center, and the Givat-Washington College, both in Israel, were selected for this study. The selected CPET files included patients with confirmed primary CHF ($n = 73$), COPD ($n = 75$), and healthy subjects ($n = 86$). Of the 234 CPETs, 150 (50 in each group) tests were used for the support vector machine (SVM) learning stage, and the remaining 84 tests were used for the model validation. The performance of the SVM interpretive module was assessed by comparing its interpretation output with the conventional clinical diagnosis using distribution analysis. *Results.* The disease classification results show that the overall predictive power of the proposed interpretive model ranged from 96% to 100%, indicating very high predictive power. Furthermore, the sensitivity, specificity, and overall precision of the proposed interpretive module were 99%, 99%, and 99%, respectively. *Conclusions.* The proposed new computer-aided CPET interpretive module was found to be highly sensitive and specific in classifying patients with CHF or COPD, or healthy. Comparable modules may well be applied to additional and larger populations (pathologies and exercise limitations), thereby making this tool powerful and clinically applicable.

1. Introduction

In the last three decades, clinical exercise testing, in general, and cardiopulmonary exercise testing, in particular, have emerged as an increasingly important tool for patient evaluation in clinical medicine due to a growing awareness of the limitations of traditional resting cardiopulmonary measurements [1]. As noted in the American Heart Association (AHA) Scientific Statement of 2010 [2] "CPET provides a wide array of unique and clinically useful incremental information that heretofore has been poorly understood and underutilized by the practicing clinician." Other authors [3] have pointed out that the data generated from CPET are one of the most challenging sets of results to interpret. They also claim that the resources available to help physicians in the interpretation of CPET results are limited. They state that "...although the American Thoracic Society (ATS)/American College of Chest Physicians (ACCP) statement [4] is comprehensive, it must be approached with "zeal" in order not to be overwhelmed" [3].

Almost all published CPET interpretive strategies are performed manually following expert-based guidelines [4–8]. These interpretation strategies, including flow charts and tables, are cumbersome, complicated, time-consuming, force dichotomous decision making, and partly subjective. They require extensive knowledge and understanding of the meaning and implications of the many CPET variables. As such, potential exists for inconsistent and sometimes inaccurate interpretation of CPET results [9, 10]. This may be at the core of why such a valued and noninvasive procedure (CPET) is underused [2, 11].

At present, there is no consensus on any reported interpretation strategy for CPET test results [4, 10]. In a recent study, Chacey et al. [12] carried out a retrospective review of 77 randomly chosen CPET files to determine the presence of inconsistencies in CPET interpretation from the guidelines issued by ATS/ACCP [4]. They reported that 78% of interpreted CPET studies contained at least one inconsistency. Furthermore, except for Schmid et al. [10], none of the available algorithms were clinically validated [4, 10, 13].

The present study is aimed at assessing the potential of using computer-aided algorithms to evaluate CPET data to identify individuals suffering from chronic heart failure (CHF) or chronic obstructive pulmonary disease (COPD) or are healthy.

In trying to achieve the above goal, we have used classification modules using machine learning algorithms (MLA) such as the support vector machine (SVM). MLAs are increasingly being used in clinical research [14, 15]. Their modeling flexibility makes them valuable tools, especially to describe complex relationships between the outcome and the predictors. Furthermore, in contrast to the standard statistical methods, they do not make any parametric assumptions, which may be potentially advantageous in small studies where the assumptions of classical methods often do not hold. SVM models are used for combining biomarkers through machine learning algorithms in which numerous variables are integrated by a computer program that is first taught to associate one specific clinical value with a combination of dataset [16]. The learned algorithm is then applied to new datasets. It is a model-free method that provides efficient solutions to classification problems without any assumptions regarding the distribution and interdependency of the data. Therefore, it is well suited to be used in studies encompassing multiple factors with minor effects, limited sample sizes, and limited knowledge of underlying biological relationships among attributes [17, 18]. Unsupervised clustering and supervised categorization schemes employed by the SVM facilitate the analysis of large amounts of high-dimensional feature vectors (entailing, in this case, a large set of patient descriptors) [19]. Using clustering techniques enables the automated definition of homogeneous subgroups within the data. In supervised SVM classification, one can learn to model a particular category of patients or discriminate between pathologies and their severity [20].

We hypothesized that a supervised computerized learning algorithm, when given appropriate data from CPET studies, would achieve an acceptable agreement for a major or primary diagnosis with the diagnosis made by conventional manual interpretation.

2. Methods

2.1. Participants. This study used 234 retrospective CPET files (177 men and 57 women), of which 148 were previously diagnosed as having either primary illness, CHF ($n = 73$) or COPD ($n = 75$), or were considered healthy ($n = 86$). The CHF and the COPD patients ($n = 148$) were clinically diagnosed and treated in the cardiology or the pulmonary departments at the Sheba Medical Center in Ramat-Gan. It should be pointed out that some of the studied patients presented with the coexistence of CHF and COPD, and their final group assignment was based on the most prominent clinical findings and symptoms (primary or secondary). The CPET files of the healthy participants were obtained through the CPET database at the exercise physiology laboratory of the Givat-Washington College in Israel. The equipment and all tests' protocols were the same in the two laboratories. The primary criteria for inclusion in the study cohort were valid and confirmed diagnosis of either CHF, COPD, or healthy, technically sound CPET, technically good pulmonary function Test (PFT), maximal effort or symptom-limited CPET tests (respiratory exchange ratio (RER) ≥ 1.00; test duration ≥ 6 min) and age ≥ 25 years old). Healthy normal subjects were older than 25 years, have no history of chronic diseases, have normal cardiorespiratory fitness, and are otherwise in good health. Senior cardiologists and pulmonologists made all clinical diagnoses. The conventional clinical diagnoses of the CHF and COPD patients were made according to the ATS and the American Heart Association (AHA) respective guidelines [21–23] and included some or all of the following procedures; for COPD: spirometry, bronchodilator reversibility, blood tests, chest X-ray or CT scan, sputum examination, and electrocardiogram (ECG) and for CHF: blood tests, chest X-ray, ECG, echocardiogram, stress test, cardiac CT scan, MRI, and, coronary angiogram. CPETs were not included in the conventional clinical diagnostic procedures.

This study was conducted following the amended Declaration of Helsinki. The Institutional Review Board (IRB) of the Sheba Medical Center approved the protocol (No. 1730-14-SMC). Informed consent was not required due to the observational and retrospective nature of the study design.

A flow chart of the study design is shown in Figure 1.

2.2. The Cardiopulmonary Exercise Test (CPET). Before performing the CPET, all study participants completed a pulmonary function test, according to the ATS guidelines [23]. The participants were seated on a cycle ergometer (Ergoselect 1200, Germany). Following a 3 min rest period and 3 min of unloaded pedaling, an incremental symptom-limited maximal exercise test was performed. Expired O_2 and CO_2 gases and the airflow rate were measured breath-by-breath through a facemask connected to a metabolic cart (all from COSMED, Italy). Gas analyzers (O_2 and CO_2) were calibrated before each test. The airflow sensor was calibrated daily. The exercise protocols were designed to ensure that subjects reached volitional exhaustion within 8-12 minutes of incremental exercise. Work rate increments ranged from 5 to 25 watts.min-1.

Before entering the CPET data into the selected SVM learning and the respective validation processes, maximal and submaximal values of each CPET file were obtained using conventional algorithms embedded in the metabolic cart (COSMED, Italy).

Then, the relations of those measured values to their corresponding normal (predicted) values were calculated (% of

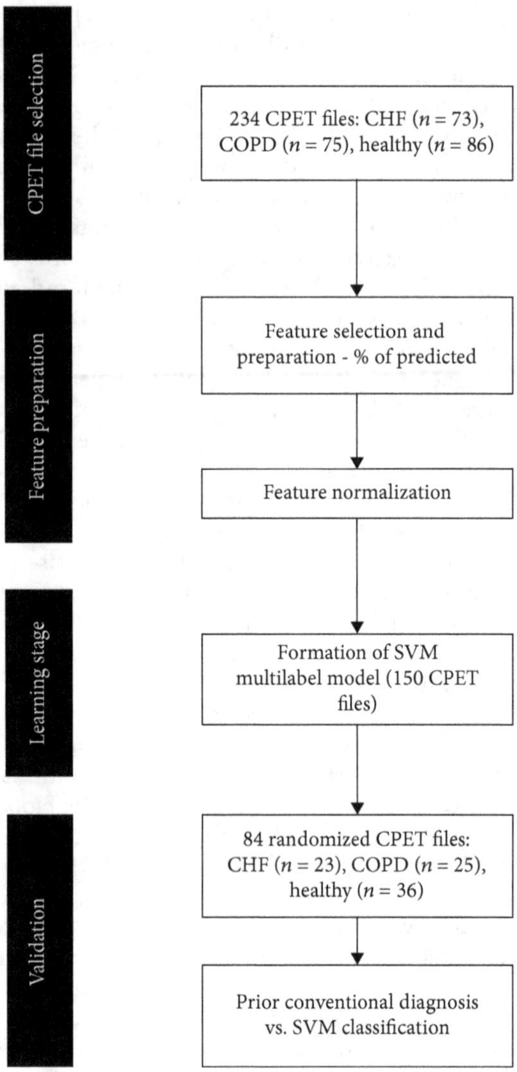

FIGURE 1: Schema of the study's design.

predicted). The predicted normal values were based on Inbar et al. [24] and Wasserman et al. [6] CPET's reference values. The use of % predicted values as input data for the SVM assured unbiased comparisons of the various physiological attributes (peak and submaximal) among wide-ranging test protocols, ergometers, and populations of varied physical, physiological, and pathological characteristics.

2.3. Normalizing Ranges of % of Predicted Values (80%-100%). During CPET, assorted physiological variables are measured with their widely spread respective normal peak values [6, 24]. Table s-1 in the supplementary materials presents an example of normal peak values of a COPD patient and a healthy one, both at age 62 years, and their respective % of predicted ranges and the resulting limits of their % predicted values for two selected CPET attributes (HR and VE). As shown in table s-1, there are widespread spans in the % of predicted values among the displayed CPET attributes (see table s-1, column 7). As shown, one could have a significantly lower than predicted normal peak HR (i.e., 114 beats/min—see column 2), resulting in a 71% of the predicted normal (predicted normal range is 96%-104%; see table s-1, column 7). Simultaneously, a normal healthy peak VE value of 40 L/min will also result in 71% of predicted normal (see table s-1, Column 2) while the predicted normal range is 71%-129% - see table s-1, column 7).

Such cases could hamper the SVM's learning phase and hinder the optimal SVM classification performance [25].

To overcome the above problem and standardize the ranges of the CPET predicted normal limits, we rescaled the original boundaries of all expected normal ranges into equal limits of 80% and 100% of predicted normal (commonly used in medical sciences). It was done by applying a linear regression equation for each CPET variable using three points: the *lower* limit of the predicted normal range was set as 80% of normal, the *average* of the predicted normal range was set as 90% of the normal, and the *upper limit* of the predicted normal range was set as 100% of the normal.

Feature scaling is mapping the feature values of a dataset into the same range and is crucial for machine learning algorithms such as the SVM [25]. Training an SVM classifier includes deciding on a boundary between classes. This boundary is known to have the maximum distance from the nearest point on each data class and differs for nonscaled and scaled cases. Also, the linear scaling of the input data in our study was done to avoid attributes with greater numeric ranges that could dominate those with smaller numeric ranges [25].

Table s-2 in the Supplementary Materials presents comparisons between nonnormalized and normalized CPET values (% predicted) as the input features for the multilabel SVM interpretive model design (from here on will be designated as % of predicted). Table s-2 demonstrates the advantage of using normalized rather than nonnormalized CPET values as input features for the SVM model design.

Following the feature preparation, the SVM learning stage was employed. To explore the high-dimensional space of CPET parameters towards creating the novel rule, discovery correlations, and criteria for disease characterization, we used a linear SVM (multiclass) machine learning tool. The evaluation of the SVM classification results was based upon the SVM probability estimates.

We used SVM procedures to identify (classify) three distinct populations: two highly prevalent chronic diseases, CHF and COPD, and healthy normal subjects (Healthy).

2.4. The SVM Algorithms. SVM is a supervised machine learning technique that is widely used in pattern recognition and classification problems. It includes a set of supervised learning methods developed in the 1990s [17, 20] and is used to solve classification and regression problems. SVM is one of the most popular techniques for supervised classification [26], built on the structural risk minimization (SRM) induction principle, and has found success in a variety of applications [27]. However, the success of many applications using the SVM critically depends on the initial manual choice of features. As indicated above and since this study deals with populations with varied pathophysiological responses during an incremental exercise challenge (due to gender differences,

Table 1: Outcomes (probability estimates (%)) of the SVM multilabel crossvalidation procedure of the learning stage.

Conventional clinical diagnosis	Model cross-validation		SVM classification (%)		
	Sample's splits	No. of iterations	CHF	COPD	Healthy
CHF			**96 ± 5**	3 ± 4	2 ± 2
COPD	Leave-one-out	150	3 ± 6	**95 ± 7**	1 ± 2
Healthy			2 ± 2	2 ± 2	**96 ± 4**
CHF			**95 ± 4**	3 ± 3	2 ± 2
COPD	80% (training) 20% (validation)	300	6 ± 11	**93 ± 11**	1 ± 1
Healthy			1 ± 1	2 ± 2	**97 ± 3**
CHF			**95 ± 4**	3 ± 2	2 ± 2
COPD	70% (training) 30% (validation)	675	6 ± 11	**93 ± 11**	2 ± 2
Healthy			2 ± 2	2 ± 2	**96 ± 4**
CHF			**93 ± 5**	4 ± 3	3 ± 3
COPD	50% (training) 50% (validation)	1875	6 ± 9	**92 ± 9**	2 ± 2
Healthy			3 ± 3	3 ± 3	**94 ± 5**

Data presented as mean ± SD. CHF: chronic heart failure; COPD: chronic obstructive pulmonary disease; Healthy: healthy normal participants; SVM: support vector machine, SD: standard deviation. Bold numbers denote mean ± SD (%) probability estimates of the respective group.

age, weight, height, and physical condition), we used maximal and submaximal CPET values related to respective/relevant normal CPET values (% of predicted values) for the SVM input data (see further elaboration on this issue above).

The SVM model implementations in this study were executed using the Library for Support Vector Machines (LIBSVM) toolbox in MATLAB R2013b [28].

2.5. The SVM Learning Stage. For the SVM learning stage, 150 retrospectively diagnosed individuals with CHF ($N = 50$) and COPD ($N = 50$), as well as healthy participants ($N = 50$) were randomly selected. Patients with varying degrees of disease severity (mild, moderate, and severe) and varying fitness levels (healthy) were included in this stage.

For this stage, we used the Library for Support Vector Machines (LIBSVM) linear multilabel classifier as a learning tool [28, 29] for the three study groups (CHF, COPD, and healthy patients). The SVM multilabel classification model was created based on the input of all CPET parameters (% of predicted).

2.6. The SVM Model Cross-Validation. To evaluate the consistency of the estimates from the newly created SVM model, 4-fold cross-validation procedures were performed on the learning dataset. In each cross-validation stage, the learning dataset was split into the training and validation datasets. This cross-validation process was repeated numerous times (iterations) (see Table 1), allowing each subset to serve once as the test dataset.

2.7. Validation of the Classification Stage. For this stage, the remaining 84 CPET files were added: 23 patients with CHF, 25 with COPD, and 36 healthy participants. Patients with varying degrees of disease severity (mild, moderate, and severe) and varying fitness levels (healthy) were included in this stage. The SVM disease classification (CHF, COPD, or healthy) was based on the SVM probability estimation [30]. A given disease was classified concurring with its highest SVM probability estimate. The SVM classification outcomes (probability estimation) were then compared with the prior official clinical diagnosis.

As indicated above, the validation group included several patients with coexisting respiratory/cardiac illnesses (and in some cases other, more minor diseases). Such a cohort provided more representative patients' samples and consequently a more sensitive assessment of the actual diagnostic accuracy of this algorithm.

2.8. Statistical Analyses. Discrete values (participants' physical characteristics and CPET peak and submaximal values) were calculated and are presented as means ± standard deviation (SD). Comparisons among groups were performed by one-way analysis of variance (ANOVA) (see s-Table 3 and s-Table 4).

The result of the SVM disease classification for each CPET test was compared with its corresponding original clinical diagnosis and considered true positive (TP), false positive (FP), true negative (TN), or false negative (FN). Sensitivity, specificity, accuracy, and overall precision were calculated based on the following formulas:

$$\text{Sensitivity} = \frac{TP}{TP + FN}, \tag{1}$$

$$\text{Sensitivity} = \frac{TN}{TN + FP} \tag{2}$$

$$\text{Accuracy} = \frac{(TP + TN)}{TP + FP + FN + TN}, \tag{3}$$

$$\text{Precision} = \frac{TP}{TP + FP}. \tag{4}$$

Table 2: Physical characteristics of the study participants.

Study stage	Variable	CHF	COPD	Healthy
Learning stage $N = 150$ (113 M, 37 F)	Age (yr)	52.2 ± 13.3	64.4 ± 10.2	45.7 ± 9.3
	Height (cm)	172.3 ± 6.2	169.0 ± 6.7	173.0 ± 4.5
	Weight (kg)	79.4 ± 11.7	70.7 ± 13.3	76.6 ± 5.6
Validation stage $N = 84$ (64 M, 20 F)	Age (yr)	53.7 ± 13.6	66.8 ± 7.6	37.8 ± 13.8
	Height (cm)	172.2 ± 6.9	166.5 ± 6.3	168.9 ± 9.1
	Weight (kg)	81.2 ± 14.9	74.7 ± 14.4	65.1 ± 14.1

Data are presented as mean ± SD. CHF: chronic heart failure; COPD: chronic obstructive pulmonary disease; Healthy: healthy normal participants; M: males; F: females.

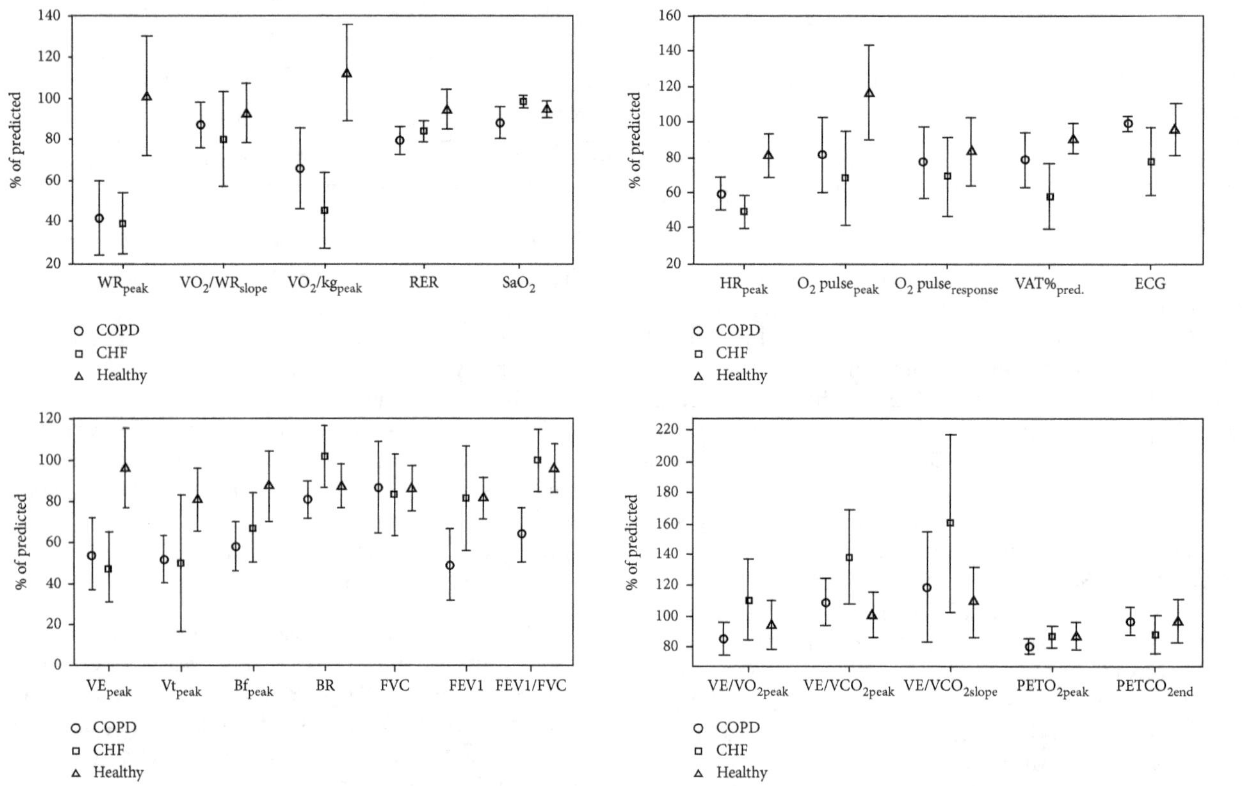

Figure 2: The distribution of CPET results (normalized % of predicted) of all CPET variables of the three study groups (mean ± SD)—validation stage.

TP, FP, TN, and FN represent the number of true positives, false positives, true negatives, and false negatives. A p value of ≤ 0.05 was considered statistically significant.

3. Results

3.1. Participants. The physical characteristics of all study participants (197 males and 37 females) of both the learning and the validation stages, by groups, are summarized in Table 2.

3.2. CPET Results. CPET results, both in absolute and relative (normalized % of predicted) values of all participants by stages (learning and validation) are presented in s-Table 3 and s-Table 4. Focusing on s-Table 4 in the supplementary materials (validation stage), significant differences were observed between the CPET values (normalized % of predicted) of the two patients' groups (CHF and COPD) in half of the CPET attributes (peak VO_2/kg, peak HR, ECG, VAT, peak SaO_2, peak BR, peak VE/VO_2, peak VE/VCO_2, VE/VCO_2 slope, FEV1, and FEV1/FVC) (for respective abbreviations see denotes of s-Table 3). CPET variables differed significantly among the three studied groups (see Table 4 in the supplementary materials and Figure 2 in the text). Therefore, one may argue that, with multiple variables showing significant differences among the three studied groups, it should not be too difficult and time-consuming to discriminate between the three groups, even manually. Nevertheless, when closely examining Figure 2, it is apparent that there is a substantial overlap in the individual data points

Table 3: Summary of the individual probability estimates (%) of the SVM disease classification model.

Conventional clinical diagnosis	Patients' group	SVM probability estimation (%)			
		Mean	SD	Min	Max
CHF	CHF	**92.4**	**10.4**	**57.0**	**100.0**
	COPD	4.2	6.1	0.0	27.0
	Healthy	3.3	5.7	0.0	19.0
COPD	CHF	10.6	13.2	0.0	47.0
	COPD	**79.6**	**16.9**	**45.0**	**100.0**
	Healthy	8.7	13.1	0.0	46.0
Healthy	CHF	5.6	7.8	0.0	36.0
	COPD	8.5	11.7	0.0	43.0
	Healthy	**85.4**	**17.1**	**43.0**	**100.0**

CHF: chronic heart failure; COPD: chronic obstructive pulmonary disease; Healthy: healthy normal participants; SVM: support vector machine; SD: standard deviation; Min: minimum; Max: maximum. Bold numbers denote average probability estimates of the respective group.

in most of the variables measured in the three studied groups. Such overlap could, at least partially, explain the complexity and inconsistency of interpreting individual CPET results. It should be accentuated that the presented dichotomized diagnoses (CHF, COPD, and healthy), reflects, in those demonstrated coexisting pathologies, the primary pathology only (highest probability estimates (%)).

3.3. The Cross-Validation. Table 1 summarizes the results of the cross-validation processes estimating how accurate the SVM-created predictive multilabel model will perform in practice.

In this stage (learning), repeated random subsampling and leave-one-out cross-validation procedures were carried out on the training dataset. Repeated random subsampling cross-validation is a method that splits the dataset into training and validation data. In the present study, we used three splits of cross-validation. The first splits included 80% of the sample files for the model training and 20% of the sample files for the model validation. In the second and third splits, we used 70% for training and 30% for validation and 50% for training, and 50% for validation. Leave-one-out is a particular case of repeated random sub-sampling cross-validation where the validation dataset is 1. The results show a significant separation (very high SVM probability estimates) between the three study populations and a very high similarity within each group (low SDs). The above data revealed excellent learning performance and paved the way for the disease classification validation stage.

3.4. The SVM Disease Classification Validation. Tables 3–5 present the various outcomes of the validation stages.

Table 3 presents the summary of groups' means (±SD) of the individual SVM disease classification outcome (probability estimation (%)).

Nonetheless, the level of the probability estimates varied widely within each group, signifying clinical heterogeneity regarding disease severity. The inclusion of participants with

Table 4: Performance summary of the SVM classification model.

Group	TP	FN	FP	TN
CHF	23	0	1	60
COPD	24	1	0	59
Healthy	36	0	0	48

CHF: chronic heart failure; COPD: chronic obstructive pulmonary disease; Healthy: healthy normal participants; TP: true positive; FN: false negative; FP: false positive; TN: true negative.

Table 5: Performance quantification of the SVM disease identification model (%).

Group	Sn (%)	Sp (%)	Acc (%)	Pr (%)
CHF	100	98	99	96
COPD	96	100	99	100
Healthy	100	100	100	100
Mean	**99**	**99**	**99**	**99**

CHF: chronic heart failure; COPD: chronic obstructive pulmonary disease; Healthy: healthy normal participants; Sn: sensitivity; Sp: specificity; Acc: accuracy; Pr: precision.

varying disease severity and fitness levels (peak VO_2/kg) reinforces the utilization of the proposed SVM classification models for patients with a wide range of disease severity and fitness levels.

Table 4 presents the confusion matrix of the SVM disease identification model and creates the basis for quantifying the performance of the SVM disease classification (Table 5).

Table 5 demonstrates the performance quantification of the SVM disease identification model.

The SVM multilabel model's sensitivity, specificity, accuracy, and precision for classifying the three studied groups are very high (Table 5). The disease classification results show that the overall predictive power of the model ranged from 96% to 100%, indicating very high predictive power.

4. Discussion

The goal of the current study was to develop and validate a computer-aided algorithm for automatically assessing CPET test results, thereby classifying three distinct groups of patients, clinically diagnosed as having CHF, COPD, or being healthy, by using machine learning techniques (SVM).

In this study, we show that by uniquely converting CPET raw data of clinically/manually diagnosed CHF, COPD, and healthy patients (normalized % predicted values), and transmitting them through a machine learning process, we can discriminate between individuals suffering from CHF, COPD, or, are genuinely healthy, with very high accuracy. Therefore, the study's hypothesis was confirmed.

The proposed module combines two novel approaches for the interpretation process of CPET results; the first one was the use of supervised machine learning techniques (SVM), and the second one was the use of normalized percent of predicted normal (% predicted), rather than absolute

CPET values. By doing so, it is possible to apply the proposed interpretive model to individuals with heterogeneous clinical, anthropometric, and demographic characteristics.

As shown in Figure 2, in all but four CPET features (WR, VO_2/kg, HR, and VE), the individual data points of the corresponding variables widely overlap among the three study groups. It makes manual interpretation highly complex, confusing, and to a certain extent, subjective. We, therefore, sought to demonstrate that by using machine learning-based analysis of all CPET data, it would be possible to reliably distinguish between COPD, CHF, and healthy participants, irrespective of their comorbidities, disease severity, age, gender, and fitness level.

The results demonstrate that using SVM-based learning and prediction approaches revealed strong agreement with common clinical disease diagnosis, made by expert cardiologists and pulmonologists (sensitivity of 99%, specificity 99%, and overall precision of 99%) (see Table 5).

The successful use of this algorithm in combining pulmonary function test (PFT) and CPET features (attributes) is, to the best of our knowledge, the only reported effort to combine such input features (% of predicted normal) for computerized diagnostic purposes.

So far, only one study has attempted to validate some CPET interpretive strategies [10] systematically. In this study, a newly proposed manual interpretive strategy was compared with a more conventional alternative [6] for evaluating CPET results. Although the consistency of the proposed interpretation method was relatively high (82%), it suffers from the previously mentioned disadvantages of most manually performed CPET interpretation schemes [12]. Moreover, in Schmid et al.'s study [10], blood gas analyses were performed during CPET, which is rarely used during routine CPETs.

Furthermore, in the single published attempt to computerize CPET interpretation, Ross and Corry [9] used absolute rather than relative (% of predicted) CPET values. Using "crude" CPET values refutes the use of such an interpretation strategy in heterogeneous populations (i.e., gender, age, pathologies, and fitness level). Also, the above computer-aided interpretation algorithm was never validated.

As it has in many sciences and other complex endeavors, interpretation software will undoubtedly become helpful in facilitating medical diagnoses and implementing appropriate therapies. A recent attempt to employ the machine learning (ML) technique in identifying cause/s for the unexplained reduced exercise capacity in lung transplant recipients using CPET data, and some additional external attributes (primarily subjective) showed promising results [31].

The present endeavor represents a novel and substantial addition in medical interpretive software to assist inpatient care.

The use of machine learning technology combined with a relative (% of predicted) rather than absolute input features opens up promising prospects for additional efforts to develop computer-aided modules to classify other pathologies, causes, and severity of exercise intolerance.

4.1. Study Limitations. The main shortcoming of the current study is the inclusion of only three sample populations (COPD, CHF, and healthy). As noted, this was a proof-of-principle study, which will lead to broader applications of the SVM methods in future work.

Also, the accuracy and precision of using such analysis (SVM) will be limited by the quality of the CPET raw data. CPET data could be affected by device limitations (sensors' accuracy) and the quantification process. Quality problems in the CPET data could also arise from the dependence on technical limitations of the currently available devices, including the one used here.

4.2. Conclusions. In this research work, the SVM classification process was used to identify, based on CPET data, three distinct sample populations, CHF, COPD, and healthy. Comparisons of SVM prediction outcomes with the respective conventional clinical diagnoses were made based on classifying each study participants' performance accuracy. Our results demonstrate that the discriminative performance of the SVM model matched perfectly with the official conventional clinical diagnosis, with the latter involving various costly and time-consuming clinical and lab procedures. Using such computer-aided techniques will reduce complexity, increase objectivity, and economize on CPET interpretation in clinical settings.

To our knowledge, this is the first study demonstrating that an automated classification approach using SVM can be used successfully to detect common chronic diseases with a single, short, noninvasive, and relatively inexpensive laboratory test such as CPET.

It should be pointed out that the presented report is the first part (being proof-of-principle one) of a larger project aimed at using the SVM technique for classifying several additional clinical conditions as well as types and severity of exercise limitations.

Abbreviations

ACCP: American College of Clinical Pharmacy
ATS: American Thoracic Society
CHF: Chronic heart failure
COPD: Chronic obstructive pulmonary disease
CPET: Cardiopulmonary exercise testing
ECG: Electrocardiogram
SD: Standard deviation
ML: Machine learning
SVM: Support vector machine.

Authors' Contributions

Or I, Omri I, Mickey S, and HG conceived and designed research. Or I, Omri I, RR, and Michael S analyzed the data. Or I and Omri I wrote the manuscript. All authors read and approved the manuscript.

Supplementary Materials

Supplementary 1. s-Table 1: an example of measured normal peak HR and VE and their respective normal ranges, and the resulting limits of their % predicted values for a 62-year-old male COPD patient and a 62-year-old healthy male.

Supplementary 2. s-Table 2. Comparison between nonnormalized and normalized CPET attributes (% predicted) as features for the multilabel SVM interpretive model design.

Supplementary 3. s-Table 3. Comparisons of CPET results (actual and % of predicted) among the three studied groups—the learning stage.

Supplementary 4. s-Table 4. Comparisons of CPET results (actual and % of predicted) among the three studied groups—the validation stage.

References

[1] K. Albouaini, M. Egred, A. Alahmar, and D. J. Wright, "Cardiopulmonary exercise testing and its application," *Postgraduate Medical Journal*, vol. 83, no. 985, pp. 675–682, 2007.

[2] G. J. Balady, R. Arena, K. Sietsema et al., "Clinician's guide to cardiopulmonary exercise testing in adults: a scientific statement from the American Heart Association," *Circulation* vol. 122, no. 2, pp. 191–225, 2010.

[3] C. G. Irvin and D. A. Kaminsky, "Exercise for fun and profi joint statement on exercise by the American Thoracic Society and the American College of Chest Physicians," *Chest* vol. 125, no. 1, pp. 1–3, 2004.

[4] American Thoracic Society, "ATS/ACCP statement on cardiopulmonary exercise testing," *American Journal of Respiratory and Critical Care Medicine*, vol. 167, no. 2, pp. 211–277, 2003.

[5] Writing Committee, EACPR, M. Guazzi et al., "Clinical recommendations for cardiopulmonary exercise testing data assessment in specific patient populations," *European Heart Journal*, vol. 33, no. 23, pp. 2917–2927, 2012.

[6] K. Wasserman, J. E. Hansen, D. Y. Sue, W. W. Stringer, and B. J. Whipp, "Principles of exercise testing and interpretation: including pathophysiology and clinical applications," *Medicine and Science in Sports and Exercise*, vol. 37, no. 7, p. 1249, 2005.

[7] I. M. Weisman and R. J. Zeballos, "Clinical exercise testing," *Clinics in Chest Medicine*, vol. 22, no. 4, pp. 679–701, 2001.

[8] W. L. Eschenbacher and A. Mannina, "An algorithm for the interpretation of cardiopulmonary exercise tests," *Chest* vol. 97, no. 2, pp. 263–267, 1990.

[9] R. M. Ross and D. B. Corry, "Software for interpreting cardiopulmonary exercise tests," *BMC Pulmonary Medicine*, vol. 7, no. 1, p. 15, 2007.

[10] A. Schmid, D. Schilter, I. Fengels et al., "Design and validation of an interpretative strategy for cardiopulmonary exercise tests," *Respirology*, vol. 12, no. 6, pp. 916–923, 2007.

[11] M. Guazzi, R. Arena, M. Halle, M. F. Piepoli, J. Myers, and C. J. Lavie, "2016 focused update: clinical recommendations for cardiopulmonary exercise testing data assessment in specific patient populations," *European Heart Journal*, vol. 39, no. 14, pp. 1144–1161, 2018.

[12] M. Chacey, L. F. Goodman, J. A. Kynyk, C. Russell, U. Magalang, and M. J. Asif, "Analysis of interpretation practices of cardiopulmonary exercise tests: a quality initiative," *American Journal of Respiratory and Critical Care Medicine*, vol. 185, p. A5772, 2012.

[13] S. H. Yusuf, M. N. Ahmad, M. Ellis, H. Yousaf, T. E. Patrick, and K. A. Ammar, "Validation of a diagnostic algorithm for cardiopulmonary exercise testing: usefulness in clinical cardiology," *Journal of the American College of Cardiology*, vol. 63, no. 12, p. A1640, 2014.

[14] R. C. Deo, "Machine learning in medicine," *Circulation*, vol. 132, no. 20, pp. 1920–1930, 2015.

[15] A. L. Beam and I. S. Kohane, "Big data and machine learning in health care," *Journal of the American Medical Association*, vol. 319, no. 13, pp. 1317-1318, 2018.

[16] T. Srivastava, B. T. Darras, J. S. Wu, and S. B. Rutkove, "Machine learning algorithms to classify spinal muscular atrophy subtypes," *Neurology*, vol. 79, no. 4, pp. 358–364, 2012.

[17] V. N. Vapnik, "An overview of statistical learning theory," *IEEE Transactions on Neural Networks*, vol. 10, no. 5, pp. 988–999, 1999.

[18] W. Yu, T. Liu, R. Valdez, M. Gwinn, and M. J. Khoury, "Application of support vector machine modeling for prediction of common diseases: the case of diabetes and pre-diabetes," *BMC Medical Informatics and Decision Making*, vol. 10, no. 1, p. 16, 2010.

[19] I. Guyon and A. Elisseeff, "An introduction to variable and feature selection," *Journal of Machine Learning Research*, pp. 1157–1182, 2003.

[20] V. N. Vapnik, *The Nature of Statistical Learning Theory*, Springer-Verlag, New York, NY, 1995.

[21] M. R. Miller, R. Crapo, J. Hankinson et al., "General considerations for lung function testing," *The European Respiratory Journal*, vol. 26, no. 1, pp. 153–161, 2005.

[22] C. W. Yancy, M. Jessup, B. Bozkurt et al., "ACCF/AHA guideline for the management of heart failure: a report of the American College of Cardiology Foundation/American Heart Association task force on practice guidelines," *Journal of the American College of Cardiology*, vol. 62, no. 16, pp. 147–239, 2013.

[23] E. V. Brusasco, R. Crapo, G. Viegi et al., *Series "ATS/ERS task force: standardization of lung function testing"*, 2005.

[24] O. Inbar, A. Oren, M. Scheinowitz, A. Rotstein, R. Dlin, and R. Casaburi, "Normal cardiopulmonary responses during incremental exercise in 20- to 70-yr-old men," *Medicine and Science in Sports and Exercise*, vol. 26, no. 5, pp. 538–546, 1994.

[25] C.-W. Hsu, C.-C. Chang, and C.-J. Lin, "ACM transactions on intelligent systems and technology," *IEEE Transactions on Neural Networks and Learning Systems*, pp. 1396–1400, 2003.

[26] M. Awad, L. Khan, F. Bastani, and I. L. Yen, "An effective support vector machines (SVMs) performance using hierarchical clustering," in *16th IEEE International Conference on Tools with Artificial Intelligence*, pp. 663–667, Boca Raton, FL, USA, 2004.

[27] B. E. Boser, I. M. Guyon, and V. N. Vapnik, "A training algorithm for optimal margin classifiers," in *Proceedings of the 5th Annual ACM Workshop on Computational Learning Theory*, pp. 144–152, 1992.

[28] C. C. Chang and C. J. Lin, "LIBSVM: a library for support vector machines," *ACM Transactions on Intelligent Systems and Technology (ACM TIST)*, vol. 2, no. 3, p. 27, 2011.

[29] R. E. Fan, K. W. Chang, C. J. Hsieh, X. R. Wang, and C. J. Lin, "LIBLINEAR: a library for large linear classification," *Journal of Machine Learning Research*, vol. 9, pp. 1871–1874, 2008.

[30] J. Platt, "Probabilistic outputs for support vector machines and comparisons to regularized likelihood methods," *Advances in Large Margin Classifiers*, vol. 10, no. 3, pp. 61–74, 1999.

[31] F. Braccioni, D. Bottigliengo, A. Ermolao et al., "Dyspnea, effort and muscle pain during exercise in lung transplant recipients: an analysis of their association with cardiopulmonary function parameters using machine learning," *Respiratory Research*, vol. 21, no. 1, pp. 267–278, 2020.

17

Establishment of Reference Norms for Lung Function Parameters of Healthy Sri Lankan Tamils

Mathanki Sooriyakanthan [1] Savithri Wimalasekera,[2] and Sivapalan Kanagasabai[1]

[1]*Department of Physiology, Faculty of Medicine, University of Jaffna, Jaffna, Sri Lanka*
[2]*Department Physiology, Faculty of Medical Sciences, University of Sri Jayewardenepura, Nugegoda, Sri Lanka*

Correspondence should be addressed to Mathanki Sooriyakanthan; mathu1481@yahoo.com

Academic Editor: Kazuyoshi Kuwano

Spirometry and Peak Expiratory Flow Rate (PEFR) are important measurements in diagnosing and monitoring of COPD and asthma. Ethnic specific reference equations are necessary in interpretation of these parameters. However, equations for Sri Lankan Tamil adults are not available. This study aims to establish reference equations for lung function parameters of Sri Lankan Tamils. A descriptive cross sectional study was carried out in all 5 districts of Northern Sri Lanka. Participants were selected by cluster sampling. Base line data were obtained by a questionnaire. Height, sitting height, weight, arm span, mid arm circumference, and chest expansion were measured. Respiratory functions were assessed by a calibrated spirometer (Cosmed Micro Quark, Italy) and Wright compatible peak expiratory flow meter. Means, and standard deviations for Vital Capacity (VC), Forced Vital Capacity (FVC), Forced Expiratory Volume in the first second (FEV_1), FEV_1%, Peak Expiratory Flow Rate (PEFR) and for other forced expiratory parameters of 775 males and 687 females were determined. Lung function parameters have significant ($p < 0.05$) positive correlations with most of the anthropometric measures. Age had a significant ($p < 0.05$) negative correlation with lung function parameters in adults >20 years and positive correlation ($p < 0.05$) in 14–20 years group. Step wise multiple regression analysis was used to determine the prediction equations. Also equations based on age, height and age, arm span were derived. Age, height based equations were retested in the same population. Predicted values by the developed equations had better agreement than that of GLI 2012 equations. This can be useful in assessing the respiratory function in Sri Lankan Tamil population as there are no already existing equations.

1. Introduction

Prevalence of preventable chronic respiratory diseases is increasing worldwide and affects the quality of life of affected individuals [1]. Early diagnosis is important to reduce mortality due to respiratory diseases. Spirometry is the gold standard for diagnosing COPD [2]. Spirometry and Peak Expiratory Flow Rate (PEFR) are important measurements in diagnosing asthma [3].

In Sri Lanka, spirometry was not used very much in clinical practice due to inconvenience of using the manual spirometers. The introduction of flow and volume sensing turbine flow meters which are portable and generate computerized data sheets immediately upon measurements greatly facilitate the use of modern spirometers as a useful assessment tool in primary and secondary respiratory care. Ethnic specific reference equations are necessary in interpreting lung function parameters (LFP) as ethnic variations have been reported by previous studies [4–7]. Considering the Sri Lankans studies, reference norms are available for Sinhalese ethnic group [7], for children aged 8–16 years [8] and for Sri Lankan Tamil young adults aged 20–28 years [9]. Using these equations in interpretations is also not appropriate as study in Sinhalese ethnic group was done nearly two decades before with outdated spirometers. Other equations do not cover a wide age range of representative samples. Hence, Sri Lankan equations are not incorporated into modern pulmonary function machines and at present, in Sri Lanka, South Indian values are compared to find the predicted percentage of these parameters in computerized lung function reports. Global Lung Initiative (GLI) produced spirometric prediction equations that can be used in all ages globally. Data from South Asians are scarce in GLI data source [10]. Equations derived for South East Asians over predict the values for Sri Lankans children [11]. Hence, establishment of reference norms with new turbine spirometers and validating the spirometry in Sri Lanka is essential. Therefore, this study is undertaken with the aim of establishing reference norms for LFP of Sri Lankan Tamils. As Northern Province has the highest percentage of Sri Lankan Tamils than other provinces in Sri Lanka, this study was carried out in Northern Province.

2. Materials and Methods

A population based descriptive cross sectional study was carried out among Sri Lankan Tamils above age 13 years in Northern Sri Lanka. Ethical clearance for the study was obtained from Ethical review committee, Faculty of Medical Sciences, University of Sri Jayewardenepura, Sri Lanka. Cluster sampling method was applied to Grama Niladhari (GN) divisions: the smallest administrative division, in all 5 districts. Number of clusters in each district was determined according to the population proportion in those districts. Altogether 24 clusters were selected; and the number of clusters in each district was according to the population proportion in those districts. Calculated sample size was 1344 byusing the formula for population mean: $n = Z^2\gamma^2/d^2$. It was decided to have participants in each age from 14–20 years as this is growing period. Thereafter, participants were grouped into age groups of half decades (21–25, 26–30, 31–35, 36–40, 41–45, 46–50, 51–55, 56–60, >60) to have participants in each group. About 50–65 participants were recruited from each cluster.

Total population in the district was divided by number of clusters to be included in that district, to find the sampling interval. The first GN division in the district was selected randomly. Number of population in the consequent GN divisions was added until sampling interval is achieved to find the next cluster. The same procedure was followed to find the required number of clusters in each district.

Officers working in the GN divisions were contacted and explained about this study. They were requested to inform the target population about this study and to invite them to a common place in their GN division in a particular day. The officers were requested to invite nonsmoking healthy participants to minimize the failures at the screening on the study day as the research team has to travel up to 250 kms to reach the study centre in out stations. Arrangements were done to have about 30 participants in a day. Study was done for 2-3 days in a cluster until the required number is achieved.

If the participantshad their both parents and grandparents of both maternal and paternal sides as Sri Lankan Tamil, they were recruited. Once the participants attend the study centre, they were explained about the study by principal investigator. If they consented, they were given an interviewer administered questionnaire to decide on inclusion or exclusion. A physical examination was done by a pre intern medical officer of the same sex. According to the outcome of questionnaire and physical examination, participants with diagnosed cardio pulmonary diseases, symptoms suggestive of respiratory disorders, smokers, alcoholics, pregnant women, those who had thoraco abdominal surgery, physical deformities and occupation related to high exposure of dust were excluded. Informed written consent was obtained from the participants. To include children below 18 years old, written consent was obtained from one of the parents/or guardians and assent was obtained from the child.

Height, weight, sitting height (SH), chest expansion (CE), and mid arm circumference (MAC) were measured as per the standard guidelines [12]. The procedure done by Mohanty et al. [13] in 2001 was followed in measuring arm span (AS). PEFR was measured with mini Wright compatible asma Plan peak flow meter which has a range of 50–800 L/min with an accuracy of 10%. PEFR and spirometric measurements were done as per ATS criteria [14]. Cosmed micro quark (Italy) electronic spirometer was used. Turbine flow meter was calibrated daily with 3 L syringe. Temperature and humidity of the environment was entered to change the volumes in BTPS. The participant was sitting erect with nose clip, with both feet on the floor, and facing away from the monitor while doing the spirometry. They were explained the procedure clearly with demonstrations. When they made errors in each attempt it was corrected by giving instructions and demonstration to correct the error. All anthropometric and lung function measurements were carried out at the same occasion in a participant. The test was done before lunch and atleast after 30 minutes of resting at the study site.

Data was analyzed in SPSS. Student's t-test was used to compare the significance of difference between means. Pearson's correlation coefficient (r) was used to get the relationship of each lung function parameter to anthropometric measurements. Step wise multiple regression analysis was done to find out the statistically significant independent variables and to devise the regression equations for lung function parameters.

To validate the equations, another 70 (38 males, 32 females) participants aged >20 years from the same population were recruited and spirometric measurements were carried out. The procedures and equipments used were same. VC, FVC and FEV_1 of the new population were predicted by using the equations based on height and age. Also, the values were predicted as per the South East Asian reference values of GLI 2012. Correlation analysis was done to find the Pearson correlation between measured and predicted values. Bland Altman analysis was done to determine the limits of agreement between measured and predicted values.

3. Results

Out of 2088 participants attended for the study, 1711 of them were enrolled as nonsmoking healthy Sri Lankan Tamils. After screening, 28 of the participants withdrew from the study on their own due to difficulty in doing the spirometry. Among the participants, 221 of participants (94 males, 127 females) were excluded from the analysis due to poor spirometry reports after 8 attempts. Exclusion of spirometry reports were mainly due to poor efforts in performing forced expiratory manuevere, leak at the beginning of forced expiration, blowing errors, sudden or early termination during forced expiration and nonrepeatable attempts. Finally data of 775 males and 687 females were included in the analysis.

TABLE 1: Mean ± SD of anthropometric characters of males and females in each age group.

Age group (*n*)	Height (cm)	Weight (kg)	SH (cm)	AS (cm)
		Males		
14 (77)	157.7 ± 7.0	43.8 ± 9.6	74.9 ± 4.1	163.0 ± 8.8
15 (53)	166.3 ± 7.3	54.6 ± 12.7	79.2 ± 4.2	174.1 ± 9.0
16 (68)	168.4 ± 7.2	54.1 ± 11.8	80.4 ± 3.8	176.5 ± 8.9
17 (56)	169.2 ± 6.6	53.6 ± 7.2	81.5 ± 3.4	177.0 ± 8.0
18 (57)	169.3 ± 6.7	58.0 ± 11.2	81.5 ± 4.6	177.5 ± 8.7
19 (47)	170.5 ± 7.7	63.8 ± 16.1	83.4 ± 3.5	179.5 ± 9.5
20 (48)	169.7 ± 7.4	60.6 ± 12.1	81.9 ± 4.3	179.1 ± 8.3
21–25 (38)	169.4 ± 6.9	62.7 ± 12.8	82.4 ± 3.2	178.2 ± 8.5
26–30 (37)	170.5 ± 7.4	72.8 ± 11.0	82.6 ± 3.4	179.5 ± 9.1
31–35 (49)	169.7 ± 5.3	72.8 ± 11.1	82.4 ± 3.2	177.8 ± 8.4
36–40 (56)	168.0 ± 7.0	74.1 ± 12.1	82.4 ± 3.2	177.8 ± 8.4
41–45 (48)	168.1 ± 6.1	74.1 ± 9.7	82.4 ± 3.0	177.3 ± 8.3
46–50 (45)	166.6 ± 8.3	72.8 ± 14.1	81.2 ± 3.9	174.2 ± 8.5
51–55 (42)	167.4 ± 6.2	69.8 ± 9.2	80.8 ± 3.6	178.4 ± 8.4
56–60 (33)	166.6 ± 7.2	71.4 ± 13.3	80.6 ± 3.7	177.5 ± 9.6
>60 (21)	164.4 ± 6.5	65.7 ± 9.8	79.4 ± 3.0	176.6 ± 8.3
		Females		
14 (45)	156.5 ± 4.4	45.9 ± 8.2	75.4 ± 2.3	161.1 ± 6.5
15 (49)	157.6 ± 6.1	48.0 ± 6.6	75.8 ± 3.4	162.6 ± 7.0
16 (44)	157.9 ± 6.7	47.3 ± 9.6	76.2 ± 3.6	162.5 ± 7.2
17 (49)	156.4 ± 5.6	48.4 ± 7.1	75.6 ± 2.5	161.0 ± 5.3
18 (46)	157.1 ± 5.7	49.9 ± 7.1	76.1 ± 2.6	162.4 ± 5.8
19 (49)	156.2 ± 5.5	53.0 ± 9.8	76.1 ± 2.5	162.9 ± 7.0
20 (55)	158.9 ± 6.2	55.5 ± 13.4	77.4 ± 3.9	164.5 ± 7.8
21–25 (43)	157.9 ± 6.4	53.8 ± 13.3	77.2 ± 3.5	162.7 ± 8.1
26–30 (52)	158.0 ± 5.8	58.9 ± 12.2	77.0 ± 2.8	164.2 ± 8.6
31–35 (49)	154.5 ± 5.1	60.0 ± 10.5	75.7 ± 2.4	161.8 ± 6.5
36–40 (49)	156.0 ± 6.4	64.4 ± 12.0	76.0 ± 3.0	163.2 ± 7.0
41–45 (40)	156.4 ± 6.8	63.4 ± 13.8	75.7 ± 3.1	164.1 ± 8.0
46–50 (40)	155.2 ± 6.2	65.5 ± 14.1	75.2 ± 2.9	163.4 ± 7.2
51–55 (37)	155.0 ± 5.9	66.2 ± 9.8	75.1 ± 2.3	161.6 ± 7.6
56–60 (20)	154.9 ± 5.2	64.8 ± 14.5	74.5 ± 2.5	162.9 ± 5.2
>60 (20)	152.4 ± 6.0	57.9 ± 8.5	72.9 ± 2.2	159.1 ± 4.5

SH-sitting height, AS-arm span.

The age ranges of participants were 14–85 years in males and 14–76 years in females. The height and weight ranges were 136.2–186.5 cm, 28.4–126.8 kg in males and 138.0–181.0 cm, 31.6–111.6 kg in females respectively. Table 1 summarizes the mean, SD of height, weight, SH and AS of males and females of each group.

In males, all mentioned parameters increased from 14 to 19 years of age, but remarkable higher rate ($p \le 0.001$) of increase was noticed between 14 and 15 years. Thereafter, changes are not significant but with age slow reduction occurs. After 20 years of age, weight increased up to 41–45 years age group and then followed by gradual reduction. SH and AS did not change significantly ($p \le 0.05$) from one age group to the next. In females, changes in these parameters are not significant.

As shown in Table 2, in males, Vital Capacity (VC) increased from 14 to 19 years of age with a significant increase of 580 ml ($p \le 0.001$), 300 ml ($p \le 0.01$) from 14 to 15 years and 15 to 16 years respectively. Then it decreased by 260 ml ($p \le 0.05$) from 19 to 20 years. It was followed by nonsignificant increase of about 70 ml in 21–25 years of age. Thereafter as the age increases VC reduced gradually. The mean Forced Vital Capacity (FVC) of 2.68 L in 14 years of age increased with age and reached 4.1 L in 19 years of age. The increases from 14 to 15 years ($p \le 0.001$), 15 to 16 years ($p \le 0.05$), 18 to 19 years ($p \le 0.05$) were significant. After 19 years of age, FVC decreased slowly with age. Changes in Forced Expiratory Volume in the first second (FEV_1) were same as that of FVC. Slight increases and reductions occurred in an irregular pattern in FEV_1% with age. Force expiratory Flow Rate at 25–75% (FEF_{25-75}) generally increases from 14 to 20 years. After 20 years of age, FEF_{25-75} reduces with age. Mid expiratory flow rates at 75%, 50%, 25% (MEF_{75}, MEF_{50}, MEF_{25} and PEFR) increased initially and peak values were observed at 20 years. These parameters in females are summarized in Table 3.

Unlike males, the changes in VC and FVC, FEV_1, $FEF_{25-75}$of females from 14 to 20 years were very minimal but the maximum mean values were observed in 20 years of age. Then it decreased slowly with age. Slight changes in FEV_1% were noticed between consequence age groups. Irregular increases and reductions were observed in MEF_{75}, MEF_{50} and $MEF_{25}$and after 41–45 years these values continuously reduced. PEFR did not show much difference from one age group to the next.

Correlation coefficient of lung function parameters with anthropometric measurements are summarized in Tables 4 and 5.

In 14–20 years population, VC, FVC and FEV_1 showed statistically significant ($p \le 0.05$) positive correlations with all anthropometric characters except SHHR in females. The highest correlation was observed with height and it is nearly strong positive (0.747) with FVC of males. Correlations with SH and AS are moderately positive ($p \le 0.001$). In >20 years adults also VC and FVC showed higher correlation (moderately positive) with height, SH and arm span of males. While lung volumes correlate better with height, flow rates like FEF_{25-75}, MEF_{75}, MEF_{50}, MEF_{25} and PEFR have the highest correlation with SH of 14–20 year group. In contrast to that, in >20 years of age group, flow rates correlate better with height. From 14 to 20 years, age correlated positively with lung parameters. But this was significant ($p \le 0.05$) only in males. After 20 years, age correlated negatively ($p \le 0.05$) with all parameters; but the correlations were moderate with FVC and FEV_1 while other correlations were mild. Although these observations were noticed in both sexes, correlation co-efficient were higher in males than in females and also in 14 to 20 year population compared to >20 years population.

Regression equations derived by step wise regression analysis for VC, FVC, and FEV_1 with highest R^2 values (0.517–0.683 in males and 0.379–0.503 in females) consisted of anthropometric characters such as age, height, weight, SH, BMI, CE, SHHR, AS and MAC in different combinations. As all these parameters are not measured routinely in clinical practice, and

TABLE 2: Mean ± SD of lung function parameters of males in each age group.

Age group	VC (L)	FVC (L)	FEV_1 (L)	FEV_1%	FEF $_{25-75}$ (L/S)	MEF_{75} (L/S)	MEF_{50} (L/S)	MEF_{25} (L/S)	PEFR (L/min)
14	2.61 ± 0.51	2.68 ± 0.53	2.35 ± 0.46	88.56 ± 4.15	2.85 ± 0.59	4.79 ± 0.98	3.26 ± 0.69	1.52 ± 0.36	327.01 ± 62.15
15	3.17 ± 0.57	3.28 ± 0.59	2.92 ± 0.5	87.78 ± 4.19	3.35 ± 0.91	5.85 ± 1.22	3.80 ± 1.05	1.83 ± 0.63	377.5 ± 68.63
16	3.48 ± 0.62	3.60 ± 0.6	3.18 ± 0.51	88.97 ± 5.76	3.85 ± 0.94	6.49 ± 1.25	4.26 ± 1.07	2.13 ± 0.68	419.56 ± 62.13
17	3.59 ± 0.49	3.72 ± 0.50	3.29 ± 0.41	88.77 ± 5.56	4.00 ± 0.84	6.77 ± 1.32	4.58 ± 0.96	2.13 ± 0.5	429.64 ± 64.69
18	3.64 ± 0.52	3.80 ± 0.56	3.23 ± 0.48	86.17 ± 6.17	3.69 ± 0.86	6.54 ± 1.56	4.23 ± 1.03	1.92 ± 0.49	445.6 ± 65.57
19	3.91 ± 0.66	4.10 ± 0.65	3.54 ± 0.54	87.17 ± 5.2	4.02 ± 0.85	6.84 ± 1.23	4.59 ± 1.05	2.16 ± 0.54	454.26 ± 65.89
20	3.65 ± 0.52	3.86 ± 0.58	3.45 ± 0.52	89.47 ± 5.20	4.27 ± 0.97	7.40 ± 1.29	4.82 ± 1.07	2.34 ± 0.67	469.58 ± 60.24
21–25	3.72 ± 0.58	3.88 ± 0.55	3.30 ± 0.48	85.03 ± 5.6	3.57 ± 0.89	6.57 ± 1.45	4.09 ± 1.08	1.83 ± 0.48	446.84 ± 73.92
26–30	3.69 ± 0.51	3.82 ± 0.49	3.26 ± 0.40	85.20 ± 4.07	3.61 ± 0.70	7.14 ± 1.41	4.24 ± 0.88	1.71 ± 0.37	480.81 ± 76.03
31–35	3.57 ± 0.55	3.70 ± 0.56	3.15 ± 0.48	85.09 ± 4.36	3.59 ± 0.88	7.18 ± 1.48	4.26 ± 1.14	1.66 ± 0.42	476.33 ± 60.19
36–40	3.43 ± 0.53	3.5 ± 0.54	3.02 ± 0.44	86.354 ± 4.48	3.66 ± 0.81	7.16 ± 1.47	4.39 ± 1.07	1.67 ± 0.38	467.1 ± 66.0
41–45	3.47 ± 0.55	3.54 ± 0.55	2.99 ± 0.43	84.56 ± 5.26	3.47 ± 0.94	7.09 ± 1.58	4.15 ± 1.12	1.58 ± 0.50	481.04 ± 67.32
46–50	3.19 ± 0.52	3.24 ± 0.52	2.75 ± 0.46	84.8 ± 4.59	3.2 ± 0.83	6.39 ± 1.39	3.90 ± 1.05	1.46 ± 0.42	449.33 ± 79.44
51–55	3.11 ± 0.59	3.17 ± 0.58	2.67 ± 0.50	84.22 ± 5.29	3.05 ± 0.86	6.32 ± 1.64	3.68 ± 1.23	1.38 ± 0.44	448.57 ± 78.44
56–60	3.05 ± 0.69	3.08 ± 0.68	2.56 ± 0.57	83.46 ± 5.76	2.86 ± 0.99	5.96 ± 1.76	3.52 ± 1.23	1.29 ± 0.47	438.18 ± 106.69
>60	2.62 ± 0.71	2.63 ± 0.73	2.15 ± 0.56	82.65 ± 5.95	2.30 ± 0.72	5.07 ± 1.42	2.91 ± 0.90	0.99 ± 0.38	367.14 ± 75.10

TABLE 3: Mean ± SD of lung function parameters of females in each age group.

Age group	VC (L)	FVC (L)	FEV_1 (L)	FEV_1%	FEF_{25-75} (L/S)	MEF_{75} (L/S)	MEF_{50} (L/S)	MEF_{25} (L/S)	PEFR (L/min)
14	2.54 ± 0.37	2.66 ± 0.31	2.39 ± 0.28	90.00 ± 4.22	3.00 ± 0.62	4.90 ± 0.74	3.47 ± 0.68	1.73 ± 0.51	310.67 ± 37.38
15	2.53 ± 0.40	2.63 ± 0.43	2.40 ± 0.35	91.60 ± 4.77	3.16 ± 0.63	4.94 ± 0.86	3.55 ± 0.74	1.80 ± 0.43	316.33 ± 46.66
16	2.49 ± 0.38	2.59 ± 0.43	2.38 ± 0.40	91.87 ± 4.29	3.17 ± 0.67	4.98 ± 0.75	3.57 ± 0.71	1.82 ± 0.51	311.14 ± 41.27
17	2.56 ± 0.30	2.65 ± 0.31	2.42 ± 0.30	91.35 ± 5.31	3.19 ± 0.75	5.09 ± 1.06	3.59 ± 0.79	1.83 ± 0.53	316.33 ± 47.06
18	2.67 ± 0.48	2.75 ± 0.50	2.48 ± 0.44	90.43 ± 5.64	3.22 ± 0.77	5.18 ± 1.04	3.57 ± 0.93	1.78 ± 0.54	331.3 ± 62.7
19	2.54 ± 0.31	2.67 ± 0.33	2.42 ± 0.32	90.8 ± 4.29	3.16 ± 0.79	5.11 ± 1.10	3.60 ± 0.89	1.74 ± 0.57	309.59 ± 42.47
20	2.67 ± 0.49	2.82 ± 0.49	2.54 ± 0.41	90.19 ± 5.36	3.23 ± 0.71	5.16 ± 1.21	3.65 ± 0.80	1.82 ± 0.49	324.91 ± 58.01
21–25	2.52 ± 0.52	2.69 ± 0.52	2.43 ± 0.41	90.65 ± 4.42	3.19 ± 0.68	5.32 ± 0.92	3.61 ± 0.75	1.83 ± 0.68	333.72 ± 42.09
26–30	2.45 ± 0.42	2.58 ± 0.41	2.25 ± 0.34	87.94 ± 4.83	2.74 ± 0.66	4.83 ± 1.05	3.20 ± 0.83	1.39 ± 0.36	322.69 ± 50.41
31–35	2.48 ± 0.37	2.60 ± 0.36	2.27 ± 0.29	87.33 ± 3.95	2.74 ± 0.51	5.10 ± 0.90	3.22 ± 0.65	1.34 ± 0.30	334.08 ± 53.26
36–40	2.39 ± 0.40	2.46 ± 0.40	2.13 ± 0.35	86.89 ± 4.92	2.63 ± 0.65	4.83 ± 1.04	3.13 ± 0.81	1.30 ± 0.38	317.76 ± 44.21
41–45	2.38 ± 0.30	2.45 ± 0.34	2.15 ± 0.30	87.66 ± 4.59	2.78 ± 0.63	5.31 ± 1.11	3.34 ± 0.78	1.36 ± 0.48	332.25 ± 55.35
46–50	2.18 ± 0.45	2.23 ± 0.45	1.93 ± 0.35	86.92 ± 4.20	2.42 ± 0.62	4.83 ± 1.37	2.95 ± 0.88	1.11 ± 0.26	311.75 ± 53.44
51–55	2.06 ± 0.43	2.13 ± 0.43	1.86 ± 0.36	87.54 ± 3.94	2.44 ± 0.67	4.50 ± 1.03	2.96 ± 0.77	1.14 ± 0.39	298.38 ± 51.93
56–60	1.87 ± 0.42	1.95 ± 0.45	1.69 ± 0.39	86.6 ± 3.79	2.13 ± 0.66	4.31 ± 1.31	2.65 ± 0.86	1.97 ± 0.30	272.5 ± 28.26
>60	1.70 ± 0.32	1.77 ± 0.33	1.51 ± 0.27	85.39 ± 5.09	1.93 ± 0.57	3.71 ± 0.92	2.39 ± 0.70	0.90 ± 0.30	263.00 ± 42.43

Global Lung Initiative equations [10] are also based on age and height, equations were derived based on these parameters (Table 6). R^2 values of both equations did not show much difference (0.034–0.064) except in females of 14 to 20 years (about 0.1 difference).

Mean, SD of the measured and predicted lung values of retesting population are summarized in Table 8.

Pearson correlations between measured and predicted values are shown in Table 9. Bland Altman analysis revealed 95% Confidence Interval (CI) for the differences between measured and predicted values of VC, FVC, and FEV_1 (Table 10).

The limits of agreement for differences between measured and predicted values were smaller with the present equations than the GLI equations except FVC in males. Predicted FVC and FEV_1 using present equations had higher correlations with measured values than the predicted values of GLI equations in both males and females. This shows that the new equation developed by this study has better agreement between measured and predicted values.

4. Discussion

Marked changes in lung function parameters of males from 14 to 15 years is associated with changes in anthropometric characters between these age groups. But the changes were minimal in females. This agrees with the findings of Neve et al. that the lung development in males occurred until

TABLE 4: Correlation co-efficient between lung function parameters & anthropometric characters in 14–20 years.

	Age	Height (cm)	Weight (kg)	BMI (kg/m^2)	SH (cm)	AS (cm)	MAC (cm)	SHHR	CE (cm)
				Females					
VC	0.107*	0.529*	0.408*	0.223*	0.525*	0.521*	0.284*	0.054	0.153*
FVC	0.130*	0.558*	0.437*	0.240*	0.546*	0.553*	0.312*	0.046	0.153*
FEV_1	0.114*	0.549*	0.393*	0.197*	0.539*	0.526*	0.278*	0.048	0.157*
FEV_1%	−0.048	−0.057	−0.161*	−0.147*	−0.053	−0.110*	−0.126*	0.000	0.009
FEF_{25-75}	0.074	0.241*	0.178*	0.094	0.240*	0.224*	0.144*	0.027	0.077
MEF_{75}	0.095	0.222*	0.245*	0.170*	0.236*	0.246*	0.240*	0.046	0.109*
MEF_{50}	0.058	0.229*	0.232*	0.157*	0.253*	0.223*	0.202*	0.060	0.090
MEF_{25}	0.014	0.206*	0.033	−0.045	0.181*	0.152*	−0.003	−0.011	0.050
PEFR	0.072	0.305*	0.282*	0.174*	0.311*	0.307*	0.239*	0.043	0.143*
				Males					
VC	0.527*	0.725*	0.632*	0.426*	0.694*	0.708*	0.549*	0.142*	0.109*
FVC	0.564*	0.747*	0.635*	0.420*	0.710*	0.728*	0.544*	0.138*	0.104*
FEV_1	0.560*	0.692*	0.573*	0.369*	0.689*	0.675*	0.487*	0.180*	0.096
FEV_1%	−0.029	−0.143*	−0.251*	−0.236*	−0.107*	−0.159*	−0.227*	0.018	−0.052
FEF_{25-75}	0.425*	0.439*	0.302*	0.163*	0.456*	0.430*	0.256*	0.141*	0.047
MEF_{75}	0.511*	0.510*	0.414*	0.267*	0.534*	0.502*	0.389*	0.171*	0.050
MEF_{50}	0.423*	0.414*	0.303*	0.178*	0.431*	0.410*	0.270*	0.135*	0.042
MEF_{25}	0.355*	0.383*	0.206*	0.071	0.395*	0.361*	0.156*	0.117*	0.020
PEFR	0.570*	0.575*	0.465*	0.299*	0.609*	0.565*	0.454*	0.203*	0.025

*$p \le 0.05$, SH-sitting height, AS-arm span, MAC-mid arm circumference, SHHR-sitting height to height ratio, CE-chest expansion.

TABLE 5: Correlation co-efficient between lung function parameters & anthropometric characters in >20 years.

	Age	Height (cm)	Weight (kg)	BMI (kg/m^2)	SH (cm)	AS (cm)	MAC (cm)	SHHR	CE (cm)
				Males					
VC	−0.464*	0.582*	0.254*	−0.032	0.548*	0.536*	0.109*	−0.014	0.240*
FVC	−0.513*	0.572*	0.235*	−0.048	0.545*	0.516*	0.107*	−0.005	0.213*
FEV_1	−0.551*	0.541*	0.247*	0.014	0.501*	0.475*	0.136*	0.025	0.197*
FEV_1%	−0.140*	−0.101	0.061	0.137*	−0.117*	−0.133*	0.111*	−0.026	−0.037
FEF_{25-75}	−0.367*	0.273*	0.136*	0.227*	0.236*	0.216*	0.199*	−0.035	0.093
MEF_{75}	−0.292*	0.329*	0.288*	0.154*	0.306*	0.292*	0.235*	−0.013	0.117*
MEF_{50}	−0.282*	0.234*	0.232*	0.145*	0.200*	0.184*	0.196*	−0.033	0.085
MEF_{25}	−0.437*	0.265*	0.167*	0.054	0.234*	0.207*	0.137*	−0.023	0.112*
PEFR	−0.241*	0.407*	0.379*	0.217*	0.412*	0.393*	0.290*	0.036	0.191*
				Females					
VC	−0.470*	0.504*	0.135*	−0.066	0.443*	0.476*	−0.049	−0.073	0.226*
FVC	−0.523*	0.498*	0.095	−0.106*	0.445*	0.467*	−0.081	−0.064	0.218*
FEV_1	−0.581*	0.476*	0.084	−0.107*	0.442*	0.430*	−0.091	−0.034	0.226*
FEV_1%	−0.223*	−0.198	−0.048	0.016	−0.008	−0.130*	−0.045	0.114*	0.026
FEF_{25-75}	−0.420*	0.258*	0.119*	0.016	0.249*	0.219*	0.005	−0.013	0.150*
MEF_{75}	−0.290*	0.302*	0.194*	0.079*	0.296*	0.285*	0.062	−0.004	0.077
MEF_{50}	−0.328*	0.256*	0.189*	0.093*	0.243*	0.228*	0.085	−0.018	0.107*
MEF_{25}	−0.469*	0.197*	−0.021	−0.108*	0.218*	0.112*	−0.106*	0.024	0.207*
PEFR	−0.344*	0.329*	0.255*	0.140*	0.360*	0.304*	0.162*	0.042	0.050

*$p \le 0.05$, SH-sitting height, AS-arm span, MAC-mid arm circumference, SHHR-sitting height to height ratio, CE-chest expansion.

TABLE 6: Reference equations lung function parameters based on age & height.

Parameter	Males			Females		
	Equation	SEE	Adj. R^2	Equation	SEE	Adj. R^2
		14–20 years				
VC (L)	0.051H + 0.091age − 6.565	0.451	0.579	0.036H − 3.153	0.340	0.277
FVC (L)	0.054H + 0.108age − 7.363	0.448	0.126	0.039H + 0.021age − 3.864	0.342	0.317
FEV_1 (L)	0.041H + 0.1age − 5.486	0.417	0.559	0.034H − 2.964	0.304	0.299
PEFR (L/min)	3.847H + 15.76age − 493.558	59.007	0.455	2.577H − 87.954	49.33	0.090
		>20 years				
VC (L)	0.046H − 0.018age − 3.677	0.469	0.453	0.033H − 0.015age − 2.234	0.365	0.396
FVC (L)	0.046H − 0.022age − 3.311	0.469	0.481	0.033H − 0.018age − 1.985	0.364	0.436
FEV_1 (L)	0.036H − 0.021age − 2.192	0.398	0.485	0.026H − 0.018age − 1.186	0.306	0.469
PEFR (L/min)	4.28H − 1.023age − 220.293	71.489	0.185	2.34H − 1.252age + 1.128	47.32	0.186

*H-height in cm. As height can not be measured accurately in people who have spinal disorders, another set of equations based on arm span and age also were derived (Table 7).

TABLE 7: Reference equations for lung function parameters based on age & arm span.

Parameter	Males			Females		
	Equation	SEE	Adj. R^2	Equation	SEE	Adj. R^2
		<20 years				
VC (L)	0.040AS + 0.091age − 5.105	0.463	0.554	0.031AS + 0.009age − 2.545	0.341	0.269
FVC (L)	0.042AS + 0.109age − 5.719	0.465	0.599	0.033AS + 0.013age − 2.971	0.345	0.305
FEV_1 (L)	0.032AS + 0.101age − 4.260	0.427	0.536	0.028AS + 0.01age − 2.266	0.309	0.275
PEFR (L/min)	3.009AS + 15.84 age − 379.033	59.68	442	2.199AS + 0.888age − 55.094	46.83	0.090
		>20 years				
VC (L)	0.036AS − 0.022age − 2.16	0.468	0.456	0.028AS − 0.017age − 1.632	0.361	0.412
FVC (L)	0.035AS − 0.025age − 2.971	0.470	0.479	0.028AS − 0.019age − 1.421	0.358	0.453
FEV_1 (L)	0.027AS − 0.023age − 0.943	0.400	0.481	0.022AS − 0.019age − 0.738	0.301	0.483
PEFR (L/min)	3.393AS − 1.327age − 90.520	71.22	0.191	1.991AS − 1.381age + 47.031	47.18	0.191

*AS-arm span (cm).

TABLE 8: Mean (SD) of measured and predicted values of males and females.

	Males (n = 38)			Females (n = 32)		
	FVC (L)	FEV_1 (L)	VC (L)	FVC (L)	FEV_1 (L)	VC (L)
Measured values	3.05 ± 0.52	2.52 ± 0.53	2.97 ± 0.48	2.31 ± 0.5	2.02 ± 0.46	2.21 ± 0.43
Predicted values (present equations)	3.3 ± 0.50	2.10 ± 0.48		2.28 ± 0.34	1.99 ± 0.32	2.16 ± 0.43
Predicted values (GLI 2012)	2.92 ± 0.52	2.4 ± 0.53		2.62 ± 0.32	2.22 ± 0.33	

TABLE 9: Correlation co-efficient between measured and predicted values.

	Males (n = 38)			Females (n = 32)		
	VC (L)	FVC (L)	FEV_1 (L)	VC (L)	FVC (L)	FEV_1 (L)
Present equation	0.690*	0.750*	0.705*	0.656*	0.723*	0.752*
GLI 2012		0.728*	0.685*		0.637*	0.747*

$p < 0.05$.

the end of puberty while lung development in females completed at menarche [15]. As females attend puberty earlier than males and this study population did not have participants <14 years, the changes were not observable. This is also in consistent with Uduphille [7] who pointed out that males achieving pulmonary maturity 5 years later than females.

Correlations of lung function parameters with anthropometric characters and the highest correlations with height were in agreements with other findings [16, 17].

Comparison of lung function parameters with other ethnic groups adjusted for age and height are shown in Table 11.

Comparison of lung function parameters with other ethnic groups shows a wide range of variation between different ethnic groups. The above studies were done in healthy population as per standard guidelines. Different types of instruments used would have slightly contributed to the variations. Although smoking males were included in the Pakistani study and South Indian study, lung volumes were higher than the present values. South Indian study did not include older adults >40 years

Table 10: 95% CI (range) for the differences between measured and predicted values.

	Males (n = 38)			Females (n = 32)		
	FVC (L)	FEV_1 (L)	VC (L)	FVC (L)	FEV_1 (L)	VC (L)
Present equation	−0.973 to 0.678 (1.651)	−0.189 to 1.131 (1.32)	−0.855 to 0.680 (1.535)	−0.647 to 0.708 (1.355)	−0.576 to 0.644 (1.22)	−0.599 to 0.689 (1.288)
GLI 2012	−0.636 to 0.899 (1.535)	−0.716 to 0.966 (1.682)		−1.0681 to 0.445 (1.5131)	−0.808 to 0.419 (1.227)	

Table 11: Comparison of lung function parameters of adults of different ethnic group.

Ethnicity	Males (predicted for 45 years, 170 cm height)					Females (predicted for 45 years age, 160 cm height)				
	VC	FVC	FEV_1	FEV_1%	PEFR	VC	FVC	FEV_1	FEV_1%	PEFR
Present study	3.33	3.52	2.98		461.27	2.37	2.48	2.16		319.18
Sinhalese [7]		3.5	2.85		571.44		2.27	2.03		400.74
Calcutta [18, 19]	3.70	3.73	2.99	78.77	527.51	2.23	2.30	1.89	75.25	399.40
South Indians [20]		3.68	3.03	77.88			2.71	2.26	79.29	
North Indians [21]			3.05				3.34	2.49	77.38	
Pakistanian [22]		3.80	2.86				2.72	1.98		
Malaysian [23]		3.22	2.88				2.35	2.08		
Chinese [6]		3.95	3.22				2.86	2.35		
Brazilian [24]		4.02	3.35	82.13	478.51		3.03	2.54	84.16	359.80
Jordanian [25]		4.78	3.92				3.49	2.8		
Canadian [26]		4.63	3.67	79.25			3.42	2.76	80.29	
GLI 2012 [10]		3.98	2.57	74.00			2.32	1.92	74.00	

of age. This may partly contribute to the higher lung volumes of the population.

Caucasians had wider chest circumference than other ethnic groups and longer chests than that of Chinese and Indians [27]. This could be the reason for higher lung volume amongst Caucasians. Sri Lankans are smaller in size than Caucasians which explain a smaller lung and therefore lower lung volumes.

Genetic, nutritional, environmental and socio economical factors and physical activity play role in development and growth of lung. Variation in these factors among the above ethnic groups could explain the differences in lung volumes.

Males in the present study have closer lung volumes to Sri Lankan Sinhalese whereas females have little higher VC and FEV_1 than that of Sinhalese. PEFR is higher in Sinhalese population than Sri Lankan Tamils. Sri Lankan Tamils and Sinhalese had almost similar mitochondrial genetic pattern [28]. Sri Lankans have mainly rice based diet. Altitude does no play a role in Sri Lanka. This explains the closer lung volumes in males of both populations. The study in Sinhalese was done using a bellow type spirometer whereas in the present study flow volume sensing turbine flow meter was used. Sample selection was convenient sampling in Sinhalese study and it was done in 1995. In addition to these factors, environmental changes in 2 decades may also have contributed to the small differences observed in females.

Multi ethnic reference equations of GLI 2012 [10], for South East Asians did not accurately predict the lung function parameters of Sri Lankan Tamils. Lack of data from South Asians for GLI equations [10] may explain these differences.

5. Conclusions

In conclusion, need for the ethnic specific equations for lung function parameters are reinforced and equations for Sri Lankan Tamil population were formed by this study. The study was done by including samples from all over the Northern Sri Lanka and equations derived were retested. Although retesting was done in a small sample it showed better agreement than GLI 2012 equations. Hence, new equations will useful in assessing the respiratory function in Sri Lankan Tamil population. It is anticipated that these study results will provide the data for GLI equations too.

Acknowledgments

The authors acknowledge technical support from Mr. S.B. Rameshkumar.

References

[1] J. Bousquet, N. G. Khaltaev, A. A. Cruz, and World Health Organization, *Global Surveillance, Prevention and Control of Chronic Respiratory Diseases: A Comprehensive Approach*, World Health Organization, Geneva, 2007, https://www.who.int/gard/publications/en/

[2] GOLD, "Global strategy for the diagnosis, management and prevention of COPD, global initiative for chronic obstructive lung disease," 2018, https://goldcopd.org/gold-2017-global-strategy-diagnosis-management-prevention-copd.

[3] National Institute for Health Care Excellence, "Asthma: daiagnosis, monitoring and chronic asthma management," *NICE Guide Line*, 2017, https://www.nice.org.uk/guidance/ng80.

[4] A. Bandyopadhyay, "Pulmonary function studies in young healthy Malaysians of Kelantan Malaysia," *Indian Journal of Medical Research*, vol. 134, no. 5, pp. 653–657, 2011.

[5] M. T. Knudsen, O. Morkve, S. Mfinanga, and J. A. Hardie, "Predictive equations for spirometric reference values in a healthy adult suburban population in Tanzania," *Tanzania Journal of Health Research*, vol. 13, no. 3, pp. 1–10, 2011.

[6] M. S. Ip, F. W. Ko, A. C. Lau et al., "Updated spirometric reference values for adult chinese in Hong Kong and implications on clinical utilization," *Chest*, vol. 129, no. 2, pp. 384–392, 2006.

[7] M. Udupihille, "Spirometric and flow standards for healthy adults nonsmoking Sri Lankans belonging to Sinhalese ethnic group," *Annals of Human Biology*, vol. 22, pp. 321–336, 1995.

[8] L. Guwani and B. D. W. Jayamanne, "Prediction of spirometry parameters using chest circumference in Sri Lankan boys aged 8–16 years," *Journal of Health and Science*, vol. 2, pp. 273–278, 2017.

[9] M. Balasubramaniam, K. Sivapalan, and R. Thuvarathipan, "Lung function parameters of healthy Sri Lankan tamil young adults," *Ceylon Medical Journal*, vol. 59, no. 2, pp. 49–53, 2014.

[10] P. H. Quanjer, S. Stanojevic, T. J. Cole et al., "Multi-ethnic reference values for spirometry for the 3–95 year age range: the global lung function 2012 equations," *European Respiratory Journal*, vol. 40, no. 6, pp. 1324–1343, 2012.

[11] G. Liyanage, B. D. W. Jayamanne, and M. Aaqiff, "Comparison of different spirometry reference equations in predicting lung function in Sri Lankan school children," *Annals of Medicine Health Sciences Research*, vol. 7, pp. 383–387, 2017.

[12] National Health and Nutrition Examination Survey (NHANES), *Anthropometry Procedures Manual*, 2009.

[13] S. P. Mohanty, S. S. Babu, and N. S. Nair, "The use of arm span as a predictor of height: a study of South Indian women," *Journal of Orthopaedic Surgery*, vol. 9, no. 1, pp. 19–23, 2001.

[14] M. R. Miller, J. Hankinson, V. Brusasco et al., "Standardisation of spirometry, series "ATS/ERS task.force: standardisation of lung function testing"," *European Respiratory Journal*, vol. 26, pp. 319–338, 2005.

[15] V. Neve, F. Girard, A. Flahault, and M. Boule, "Lung and thorax development during adolescence: relationship with pubertal status," *European Respiratory Journal*, vol. 20, no. 5, pp. 1292–1298, 2002.

[16] J. Kivastik and P. H. Kingisepp, "Lung function in Estonian children: effect of sitting height," *Clinical Physiology*, vol. 15, no. 3, pp. 287–296, 1995.

[17] C. O. Nku, E. J. Peters, A. I. Eshiet, S. A. Bisong, and E. E. Osim, "Prediction formulae for function parameters in females of South Eastern Nigeria," *Nigerian Journal of Physiological Sciences*, vol. 21, pp. 43–47, 2006.

[18] S. Chatterjee and D. Saha, "Pulmonary function studies in healthy nonsmoking women of Calcutta," *Annals of Human Biology*, vol. 20, no. 1, pp. 31–38, 1993.

[19] S. Chatterjee, D. Saha, and B. P. Chatterjee, "Pulmonary function studies in healthy nonsmoking men of Calcutta," *Annals of Human Biology*, vol. 15, no. 5, pp. 365–374, 1998.

[20] V. K. Vijayan, K. V. Kuppurao, P. Venkatesan, K. Sankaran, and R. Prabhakar, "Pulmonary function in healthy young adult Indians in Madras," *Thorax*, vol. 45, no. 8, pp. 611–615, 1990.

[21] S. K. Chhabra, R. Kumar, U. Gupta, M. Rahman, and D. J. Dash, "Prediction equations for spirometry in adults from Northern India," *Indian Journal of Chest Disease Allied Sciences*, vol. 56, pp. 221–229, 2014.

[22] E. David, R. Williams, D. Miller, and W. F. Taylor, "Pulmonary function studies in healthy Pakistani adults," *Thorax*, vol. 33, no. 2, pp. 243–249, 1978.

[23] J. Gnanou, B. Caszo, W. H. W. Mohamad, H. Nawawi, K. Yusoff, and T. Ismail, "Prediction equations for lung function in healthy, life time never-smoking Malaysian population," *The Southeast Asian Journal of Tropical Medicine and Public Health*, vol. 42, pp. 965–976, 2011.

[24] N. A. Sliman, B. M. Dajani, and H. M. Dajani, "Ventilatory function test values of healthy adult Jordanians," *Thorax*, vol. 36, no. 7, pp. 546–549, 1981.

[25] R. Rufino, C. H. Costa, A. J. Lopes et al., "Spirometry reference values in the Brazilian population," *Brazilian Journal of Medical and Biological Research*, vol. 50, no. 3, p. e5700, 2017.

[26] W. C. Tan, J. Bourbeau, P. Hernandez et al., " Canadian prediction equations of spirometric lung function for Caucasian adults 20 to 90 years of age: results from the Canadian Obstructive Lung Disease (COLD) study and the Lung Health Canadian Environment (LHCE) study," *Canadian Respiratory Journal*, vol. 18, no. 6, pp. 321–326, 2011.

[27] P. M. Donnelly, T. S. Yang, J. K. Peal, and A. J. Wool Cock, "What factors explain racial differences in lung volumes?" *European Respiratory Journal*, vol. 4, pp. 829–838, 1991.

[28] L. Ranaweera, S. Kaesutthi, A. W. Tun, H. Boonyarit, S. Poolsuwan, and P. Lertrit, "Mitochondrial DNA history of Sri Lankan ethnic people: their relations within island and with the Indian subcontinental populations," *Journal of Human Genetics*, vol. 59, no. 1, pp. 28–36, 2014.

iNOS Inhibition Reduces Lung Mechanical Alterations and Remodeling Induced by Particulate Matter in Mice

Carla Máximo Prado[1] **Renato Fraga Righetti**[2,3]
Fernanda Degobbi Tenorio Quirino dos Santos Lopes[2] **Edna Aparecida Leick**[2]
Fernanda Magalhães Arantes-Costa[2] **Francine Maria de Almeida,**[2]
Paulo Hilário Nascimento Saldiva,[2] **Thais Mauad,**[2]
Iolanda de Fátima Lopes Calvo Tibério[2] **and Mílton de Arruda Martins**[2]

[1]*Department of Bioscience, Federal University of Sao Paulo, Santos, Rua Silva Jardim 136, 11015-020 Santos, SP, Brazil*
[2]*Faculdade de Medicina FMUSP, Universidade de São Paulo, Av. Dr. Arnaldo 455, Sala 1210, 01246-903 São Paulo, SP, Brazil*
[3]*Hospital Sírio-Libanês, Rua Adma Jafet 115, 01308-060 São Paulo, SP, Brazil*

Correspondence should be addressed to Carla Máximo Prado; cmaximoprado@gmail.com

Academic Editor: Kazuyoshi Kuwano

Background. The epidemiologic association between pulmonary exposure to ambient particulate matter (PM) and acute lung damage is well known. However, the mechanism involved in the effects of repeated exposures of PM in the lung injury is poorly documented. This study tested the hypotheses that chronic nasal instillation of residual oil fly ash (ROFA) induced not only distal lung and airway inflammation but also remodeling. In addition, we evaluated the effects of inducible nitric oxide inhibition in these responses. For this purpose, airway and lung parenchyma were evaluated by quantitative analysis of collagen and elastic fibers, immunohistochemistry for macrophages, neutrophils, inducible nitric oxide synthase (iNOS), neuronal nitric oxide synthase (nNOS), and alveolar septa 8-iso prostaglandin F2α (8-iso-PGF-2α) detection. Anesthetized *in vivo* (airway resistance, elastance, H, G, and Raw) respiratory mechanics were also analyzed. C57BL6 mice received daily 60ul of ROFA (intranasal) for five (ROFA-5d) or fifteen days (ROFA-15d). Controls have received saline (SAL). Part of the animals has received 1400W (SAL+1400W and ROFA-15d+1400W), an iNOS inhibitor, for four days before the end of the protocol. A marked neutrophil and macrophage infiltration and an increase in the iNOS, nNOS, and 8-iso-PGF2 α expression was observed in peribronchiolar and alveolar wall both in ROFA-5d and in ROFA-15d groups. There was an increment of the collagen and elastic fibers in alveolar and airway walls in ROFA-15d group. The iNOS inhibition reduced all alterations induced by ROFA, except for the 8-iso-PGF2 α expression. In conclusion, repeated particulate matter exposures induce extracellular matrix remodeling of airway and alveolar walls, which could contribute to the pulmonary mechanical changes observed. The mechanism involved is, at least, dependent on the inducible nitric oxide activation.

1. Background

In the last few years, special attention has been devoted to the associations between levels of ambient particulate matter (PM) and health effects [1]. It is known that people that live in high polluted places may develop exacerbations of respiratory diseases [2]. However, less is known about the pathophysiology of chronic effects of high PM exposures, although such exposures are also associated with respiratory hospitalizations, including increases in cardiopulmonary mortality and in the rates of lung cancer and in respiratory exacerbations [3, 4].

Significant risks for the development of chronic bronchitis and obstructive airways disease were associated with increased exposure to ambient PM<10 and PM<2.5 μm in diameters (PM10 and PM2.5, respectively) [5]. In addition, Liu et al. [6] demonstrated that PM2.5 exposure decreased small airway function in asthmatic children and inhaled corticosteroid reverted this response improving lung function.

Accordingly, several animal models that mimic susceptible segments of the population are currently being used to elucidate physiological mechanisms [7]. Experimental studies have shown effects of PM exposure to lung function [8, 9]; however, most of them focused in acute effects of PM in the lung. In addition, scarce studies evaluated the effects of air pollution on lung remodeling [10, 11]. Although the extensive studies have evaluated effects of air pollution in health, the mechanisms involved in the lung injury induced by particulate matter were poorly investigated.

Most of the effects of air pollution, including particulate matter exposures, were related to oxidative stress activation [12, 13]. It is also known that a lot inflammatory cascade and modulators released in the inflammatory process are responsible for connective tissue and functional lung alterations observed in an experimental model of chronic lung inflammation and patients with asthma [14–17]. Moreover, is important to note that efficacy of current pharmacological treatments, including inhaled glucocorticoids and cysteinyl leukotriene type 1 receptor antagonists, is partial effective in patients with asthma [18].

Nitric oxide (NO) was associated with a modulation of many physiological effects. NO can be derived either from neuronal nitric oxide synthase (nNOS) and endothelial nitric oxide synthase (eNOS), or from other NO-adduct molecules (nitrosothiols) and it is associated with the airway and vascular tone control. On the other hand, NO derived from inducible nitric oxide synthase (iNOS) seems to be mainly involved in a modulation of immune system [19].

During inflammation, iNOS expression has been described in several types of cells, such as macrophages, neutrophils, and eosinophils, as well as in airway epithelial cells [20, 21]. NO derived from iNOS contributes to airway and distal lung parenchyma response, inflammatory process and extracellular matrix remodeling [22, 23]. Some evidence suggest that nitric oxide can control airway remodeling by interaction with some proteases and antiproteases, such as MMP (metalloproteinase)-12, MMP-9, or growth factors such as TGF (transforming growth factor)-β [24, 25], mediators strongly involved in lung remodeling.

Our hypothesis is that repeated PM could induce structural pulmonary changes related to inflammatory response, extracellular matrix remodeling, and oxidative stress activation. In addition, we considered that these alterations are modulated by iNOS activation. Also considering the health effects of air pollution above described, the clinical relevance of this study is related to the possibility that nitric oxide derived from iNOS is involved on lung injury associated with chronic particulate matter exposures since it may represent an important mechanism.

Therefore, our study aims in evaluate the effects of repeated nasal instillations of low dose of residual oil fly ash (ROFA), a concentrate of air pollution resulting from the burning of oil, on pulmonary mechanics and lung inflammation and remodeling. In order to investigate the effects of iNOS activation, we evaluated the effects of the treatment with a highly selective inhibitor of iNOS activity, 1400W, in pulmonary alterations induced by repeated ROFA instillations.

2. Methods

All mice received humane care in compliance with the "Guide for Care and Use of Laboratory Animals" (NIH publication 85-23, revised 1985). Animals were housed (12-h light/dark cycle) in plastic cages and received food and water *ad libitum*). All protocols performed in this study were approved by the institutional review board of University of São Paulo (São Paulo, Brazil).

2.1. Particulate Material (PM). Residual oil fly ash (ROFA) was collected from a solid waste incinerator, which is powered by combustible oil, from University Hospital from School of Medicine of University of São Paulo. Characterization of ROFA particles used in this investigation was previously performed [10, 26] by neutron activation to determine the elemental composition, as well as by gas chromatography and high performance liquid chromatography for organics. It was previously determined and detailed described in previous studies [10, 26]. Presence of toxic elements, such as As, Co, Li, and Zn, and several polycyclic aromatic hydrocarbons (PAHs) such as naphthalene, acenaphthylene, fluorene, acenaphthene, anthracene, fluoranthene, pyrene, B[a]anthracene, B[k]fluoranthene, B[a]pyrene, DB[ah]anthracene, B[ghi]perylene, and ind[123cd] were detected and previously detailed [10, 26]. The ROFA used is homogenous in relation to the particles diameter, since more than 80% of the material has particles less than 2.5 μm of diameter [26].

2.2. ROFA Instillation. All animals have received 10uL of ROFA solution (concentration of 6mg/mL) daily during the day 1 to 15th by intranasal instillations (Final dose of 60ug/animal/daily) [10]. This dose mimics a mice exposed to 24 hs in a high pollution day of a city as São Paulo, Brazil. Control animals received the same volume of saline intranasal. We did only the control group with 15 days of saline since we have unpublished data showing that five or fifteen instillation of saline did not affect lung inflammation.

2.3. 1400W Treatment. To investigate the effects of iNOS inhibition in lung inflammation induced by ROFA instillations, animals were treated for four days with 1400W i.p., in a dose of 2mg/Kg/daily, as previously described [25]. This approach was chosen based in previous studies that have shown that this dose is effective and selective for iNOS and did not cause toxic effects [25, 27]. Control animals were treated with saline solution.

2.4. Experimental Design. To investigate the time effects of air pollution in lung, mice received either

(a) intranasal ROFA daily for five days (ROFA-5, n=8);

(b) intranasal ROFA daily for fifteen days (ROFA-15, n=8);

(c) intranasal saline for fifteen days (SAL, n=8);

(d) intranasal ROFA daily for fifteen days and 1400W treatment (ROFA-15+1400W, n=8); or

(e) intranasal saline for fifteen days and 1400W treatment (SAL+1400W, n=8).

2.5. Pulmonary Mechanics Evaluation. Twenty-four hours after the last instillation, the animals were anesthetized with thiopental sodium (80 $mg.kg^{-1}$, i.p.), tracheostomized, and connected to a ventilator to small animals (FlexiVent, SCIREQ, Montreal, Canada). Animals were ventilated at 100 breaths/min with a tidal volume of 20 $mL.kg^{-1}$. This high value of tidal volume is to avoid inefficient ventilation due to an increase in the anatomic death space induced by the inhalation apparatus attached to the ventilator. A dose response curve was performed using 6.125; 12.5; 25; and 50 mg/mL of methacholine inhalation. Methacholine was inhaled for 1 minute and the data was collected 30 sec after the end of inhalation. There was an interval of 3 minutes between the administrations of each dose. The impedance of respiratory system (Zrs) was calculated for each animal and the perturbation volume of 16 sec was used. The same perturbation volume was used after each inhalation. Mechanical ventilation was stopped only to the perturbation application. The cylinder position (Vcyl) and the internal pressure of the cylinder (P cyl) were registered during the 16 sec of perturbation. We used a perturbation of 16 sec, composed by assertions of solenoids with frequencies between 0.25 and 19.625 Hz, avoiding the harmonic distortion [23]. To avoid the lost related to gases, some corrections were performed. Vcyl was correct to obtain a volume that really arrives in the animals (V) and P cyl was correct to the values of Pao, open airways pressure. By the derivation in the time of V, we get the flow (V'). To analyze the impedance, we used the model of constant phase: where the Raw is the airway resistance, Iaw is the inertance, G characterized the energy dissipated to the lung tissue, H characterized the energy accumulated in the lung tissue, and f is the frequency. Results were expressed as percentage of maximal increase (%) after methacholine challenge [23].

2.6. Lung Histology. At the end of pulmonary mechanics, the anterior chest wall was opened, animals were exsanguinated via the abdominal aorta and lungs were removed *en bloc*. The lungs were fixed in 10% formaldehyde for 24h in a constant pressure of 20 cmH2O. Sections representing peripheral areas of the lung were cut and processed for paraffin embedding. Five micron sections were stained with Sirius Red collagen and Weigert's technique for elastic fibers quantifications. To analyze collagen and elastic fibers content in airways and lung parenchyma, we measured the total area of airway wall or lung parenchyma tissue, and the collagen or elastic fibers (μm^2) area in a nine-ten airways or lung parenchyma fields, at a magnification of x10 for airways and x40 for lung parenchyma, in an image analysis system (Image ProPlus 4.6v). Collagen or elastic content (%) in peribronchiolar and alveolar wall was expressed as a relation between the area of collagen or elastic fibers in a specific frame and the total area of the frame [17].

Immunohistochemistry was performed with the following antibodies: Anti-Macrophage-2 (Clone M3/M38, Cedarlane Lab, Burlington, Canada), anti-Neutrophils (MCA771G, Abd Serotec, Oxford, UK), anti-nNOS (nNOS/NOS type I-N31020; BD Transduction Laboratories, San Diego, CA), anti-iNOS (IgG2a–iNOS/NOS type 2–N32020; BD Transduction Laboratories, San Diego, CA) anti-actin (nNOS/NOS type I-N31020; BD Transduction Laboratories, San Diego, CA), anti-8-iso-PGF2α (Oxford Biomedical Research, Oxford, UK), goat polyclonal anti-mouse MMP12 (1:200, Santa Cruz Biotechnology, USA), and rabbit polyclonal anti-transforming growth factor-β1 (TGF-β1) IgG (1:1200, Santa Cruz Biotechnology, USA). Secondary antibodies anti-goat, rat, or rabbit antibodies (Vectastain Abc Kit, Vector Laboratories, USA) were used in accordance with the manufacturer's instructions. Sections were counterstained with hematoxylin.

With a 50-line and 100-point grid connected to the ocular of the microscope, peribronchiolar and alveolar wall density of macrophages, neutrophils, iNOS, and nNOS, TGF-β and MMP-12 positive cells were assessed using a point counting technique [28]. Counting was performed in 5 airways (peribronchiolar area) and in 10 parenchyma fields (area of alveolar septa) in each animal at x1,000 magnification by a blinded investigator. The results were expressed as cell/$10^4$$um^2$. The 8-iso-PGF2$\alpha$ area was evaluated by image analysis as described above for collagen and elastic fibers. The 8-iso-PGF2α-positive area was expressed as a percentage of the total area in both peribronchiolar and alveolar wall [28].

2.7. Statistical Analysis. Statistical analysis was performed using SigmaStat software (SPSS Inc, Chicago, IL). Data were analyzed with One-way Analysis of Variance (ANOVA) followed by the *Holm-Sidak* method for multiple comparisons and data are presented as mean ± SE. To evaluate the effects of iNOS inhibition in ROFA-induced lung alterations, we used Two-way Analysis of Variance, considering one factor the ROFA and the other the 1400W treatment. $P<0.05$ values were considered significant.

3. Results

3.1. ROFA Increased the Lung Mechanics Alterations. We noted an increase in the maximal percentage of increase of Rrs and Ers as well as in Gtis and Htis in both ROFA-5 and ROFA-15 compared to saline ($P<0.05$) as shown in Table 1. There were no significant differences between ROFA-5 and ROFA-15 in all the mechanical parameters.

3.2. ROFA Increased Lung Inflammation. ROFA instillations (ROFA-5 and ROFA-15) induced an increase in the number of neutrophils in both peribronchiolar and alveolar wall compared to saline ($P<0.05$) (Table 2). The number of macrophages was increased only in ROFA-15 in both bronchiolar and alveolar wall compared to saline ($P<0.05$).

3.3. ROFA Increased Oxidative Stress. ROFA instillations (ROFA-5 and ROFA-15) increased the number of iNOS and nNOS-positive cells and the expression of fractional area of 8-iso-PGF2α in both peribronchiolar and alveolar wall compared to saline ($P<0.05$). The expression of 8-iso-PGF2α was increased in ROFA-15 group only at airway level (Table 3). Although the iNOS and nNOS-positive cells in airways were

TABLE 1: *ROFA instillation-induced lung mechanics alterations*: after both five (ROFA-5d) and fifteen instillations (ROFA-15d), mice presented an increase in the percentage of respiratory system resistance (%Rrs) and elastance (%Ers) as well as in lung tissue impedance (%Htis) and lung tissue resistance (%Gtis) compared to control that received only saline. ∗p<0.05 compared to saline (SAL group).

GROUPS	%Rrs	%Ers	%Gtis	%Htis
SALINE	67.05±16.99	39.70±10.51	40.36±6.65	33.23±7.47
ROFA-5d	213.58±29.06∗	149.62±42.57∗	124.93±20.72∗	74.72±10.26∗
ROFA-15d	214.18±31.97∗	175.95±59.21∗	106.56±42.25∗	104.99±12.56∗

TABLE 2: *ROFA-induced lung inflammation*: after both five (ROFA-5d) and fifteen instillations (ROFA-15d), mice presented an increase in the number of neutrophils and inflammatory cells that express nNOS and iNOS around airways and in distal lung parenchyma. The macrophages were significantly increased only in ROFA-15d groups compared to saline. ∗P<0.05 compared to saline.

	Airway		Distal lung parenchyma	
	Macrophage	Neutrophils	Macrophage	Neutrophils
SAL	3.9±0.5	3.2±1.1	7.8±0.98	9.4±1.5
ROFA-5d	10.7±6.5	8.3±1.4∗	8.3±1.4	18.9±1.8∗
ROFA-15d	9.0±1.0∗	8.3±1.9∗	14.16±1.71∗	22.3±1.9∗

TABLE 3: *ROFA-induced oxidative stress*: after both five (ROFA-5d) and fifteen instillations (ROFA-15d), mice presented an increase in the number of neutrophils and inflammatory cells that express nNOS and iNOS around airways and in distal lung parenchyma. The macrophages were significantly increased only in ROFA-15d groups compared to saline. ∗P<0.05 compared to saline; #P<0.05 compared to ROFA-5d.

	Airway			Distal lung parenchyma		
	iNOS	nNOS	8-iso-PGF2α	iNOS	nNOS	8-iso-PGF2α
SAL	3.3±0.6	3.13±1.20	10.42±0.98	9.30±1.70	10.80±3.20	8.71±1.36
ROFA-5d	44.5±5.0∗	20.01±3.65∗	8.73±1.51	33.0±7.4∗	33,40±5.50∗	13.53±0.87∗
ROFA-15d	27.82±3.14∗,#	10.83±1.9∗#	20.30±1.51∗	32.43±5.04∗	32.40±5.00∗	15.39±1.05∗

increased in ROFA-15 compared to saline group, these values were lower than those obtained in ROFA-5 group (P<0.05). There were no differences in nNOS, iNOS-positive cells and 8-iso-PGF2α in alveolar wall between ROFA 5 and ROFA-15 groups.

3.4. ROFA Increased Extracellular Matrix Remodeling. Collagen and elastic fibers were increased only in ROFA-15 compared to saline in peribronchiolar and alveolar wall compartments (P<0.001). We also analyzed the number of metalloproteinase 12 (MMP-12) and TGFβ-positive cells in the lung. There was an increase in TGFβ-positive cells in both peribronchiolar and alveolar wall in ROFA-5 group and ROFA-15 group compared to saline group (P<0.001). There was a decrease in the expression of TGF-β in peribronchiolar wall in ROFA-15d group compared to ROFA-5d group. Considering MMP-12-positive cells, the expression of MMP-12 was higher in AW only in ROFA-15 and in DLP in both ROFA-5 group and ROFA-15 group compared to saline (P<0.001) (Table 4).

3.5. Effects of 1400W in the Lung Mechanics Alterations Induced by Fifteen Instillations of ROFA. The 1400W treatment in animals that received ROFA instillations for 15 days reduced the maximal percentage of increase of Rrs and Ers compared to those received the vehicle (ROFA-15-W compared to ROFA-15d, P<0.05), as shown in Figure 1. There were no significantly effects of 1400W treatment in ROFA-induced an increase in Gtis [ROFA-W: 115.77± 32.22] and Htis [ROFA-W: 77.43± 20.88] values compared to those animals that received ROFA and vehicle (ROFA-15, values of ROFA-15 were shown in Table 1).

3.6. Effects of 1400W in the Lung Inflammation Induced by Fifteen Instillations of ROFA. The iNOS inhibition in ROFA-instilled animals (ROFA-15-W) reduced the number of neutrophils and macrophages in both peribronchiolar and alveolar wall compared with those animals that received vehicle (P<0.05) (Figure 2).

3.7. Effects of 1400W in the Oxidative Stress Induced by Fifteen Instillations of ROFA. We observed that in ROFA-15-W there was a decrease in the number of iNOS-positive cells in peribronchiolar and alveolar wall compared to ROFA-15 (P<0.05). As expected, the iNOS inhibition did not affect the nNOS-positive cells in animals that received ROFA-1400W compared to those that received vehicle (Figures 2(a) and 2(b)). The iNOS inhibition reduced the 8-iso-PGF2α content in ROFA-15 animals only in airways (P<0.05) (Figure 3).

3.8. Effects of 1400W in the Extracellular Matrix Remodeling by Fifteen Instillations of ROFA. Considering pulmonary remodeling (Figure 4), iNOS inhibition reduced both collagen and elastic content in airways and in lung distal parenchyma comparing to those animals that received vehicle (P<0.05). The iNOS inhibition reduced the TGF-β (Figure 5) and MMP-12 (Figure 6) positive cells only in peribronchiolar area, not affecting the alveolar wall positive cells (P<0.05).

TABLE 4: *ROFA-induced extracellular matrix remodeling*: after both five (ROFA-5d) and fifteen instillations (ROFA-15d), mice presented an increase in the number of neutrophils and inflammatory cells that express nNOS and iNOS around airways and in distal lung parenchyma. The macrophages were significantly increased only in ROFA-15d groups compared to saline. *P<0.05 compared to saline; **P<0.05 compared to ROFA-5d.

	Airway				Distal lung parenchyma			
	Collagen fibers	Elastic fibers	MMP-12	TGF-β	Collagen fibers	Elastic fibers	MMP-12	TGF-β
SAL	15.7±2.9	13.5±1.6	29.5±4.4	9.7±1.5	20.7±2.5	9.5±0.7	17.4±5.4	18.1±3.2
ROFA-5d	13.9±3.2	11.1±1.7	46.6±17.4*	34.6±3.7*	20.9±2.6	17.74±1.6	55.7±10.1*	46.3±4.5*,
ROFA-15d	26.7±1.9*, **	25.4±2.4*, **	79.5±5.3*	37.2±3.2*	37.2±3.2*, **	23.9±3.4*	36.7±4.4*	30.1±2.5*, **

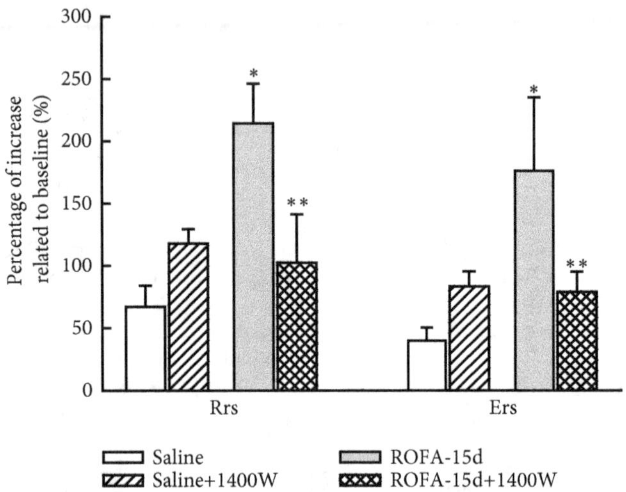

FIGURE 1: Lung mechanics. This figure represents the mean and SEM percentage of maximal increase of respiratory system resistance (Rrs) and elastance (Ers) relative to baseline. The animals that received fifteen instillations of ROFA presented higher values of both Rrs and Ers compared to control and 1400W treatment reduced this response. *p<0.05 compared with saline groups; **p<0.05 compared with animals that received ROFA and vehicle treatment.

3.9. Qualitative Analysis. Figure 7 shows representative photomicrographs of airway stained with immunohistochemistry to detect neutrophils, iNOS, isoprostane, and collagen fibers in all experimental groups. Peribronchiolar of ROFA-15 animals presented a prominent neutrophil infiltration including iNOS-positive cells and fractional area of the 8-iso-PGF2α and collagen fibers. Peribronchiolar sections from animals instilled with ROFA-15 and treated 1400W presented attenuation in neutrophil infiltration including iNOS-positive cells and fractional area of the 8-iso-PGF2α and collagen fibers (Scale bar = 30 μm).

4. Discussion

In this study we showed that repeated exposures to levels of PM induced significant changes on lung mechanics, lung inflammation, and extracellular matrix remodeling which occurred in both distal airways and lung parenchyma. The inflammatory response was characterized by macrophages and neutrophils and could be observed early after five instillations, while extracellular matrix remodeling associated with increase in MMP-12 and TGF-β expression occurred only after fifteen instillations. We also showed that repeated instillations of ROFA induced an increment in the number of nNOS and iNOS-positive inflammatory cells as well as in 8-iso-PGF2α expression around peribronchiolar and alveolar wall. This was a feasible and reproducible experimental model for studies of pathophysiological mechanisms involved in lung injury induced by air pollution. The effects of inhaled toxicants and allergen challenge on airway inflammation and oxidative stress has also been studied in well established in vitro experimental animal models [29, 30].

Several pathophysiological mechanisms may be involved in lung injury induced by air pollution [31, 32]. In order to investigate the hypothesis of NO involvement in the pathophysiology of lung inflammation induced by particulate matter, we evaluated the effects of specific iNOS inhibitor in this experimental model. We used 1400W, a highly selective and specific iNOS inhibitor, as previously shown in other experimental studies [25, 27, 33]. The effectiveness of this treatment was assessed by immunohistochemical detection of both nNOS and iNOS. We observed that 1400W treatment only reduced the number of iNOS-positive cells, not affecting the nNOS expression. The most important finding was related to the fact that NO, mainly originated from iNOS activation, was involved in the inflammatory and extracellular matrix remodeling, acting as proinflammatory modulator, since the treatment with 1400W, a high specific inhibitor, reduced the most of the features observed in this model. There were few studies evaluating experimental models of inflammation induced by repeated exposure to air pollution that had mapped the changes induced by chronic exposure of particulate matter not only in the lung parenchyma, but also in the airways [34]. Most of them have combined air pollution exposure to allergic inflammation or tobacco exposure.

It is well know that repeated exposures to irritants such as particulate matter, diesel, cigarette smoke results in bronchial epithelial damage, mucous hypersecretion, fibrosis and narrowing of the airways, destruction of parenchyma and vascular changes [35]. ROFA (residual oil fly ash) is a metal-rich particulate material, with little organic component derived from combustion processes at high temperatures [36]. Due to its high toxicity, it is used as a substitute for experimental environmental studies to assess the biological effects of particulate matter [37–39]. The element composition of ROFA used in the present study was previously characterized [26].

Repeated intranasal instillation of ROFA in mice induced an increased resistance and elastance of the respiratory

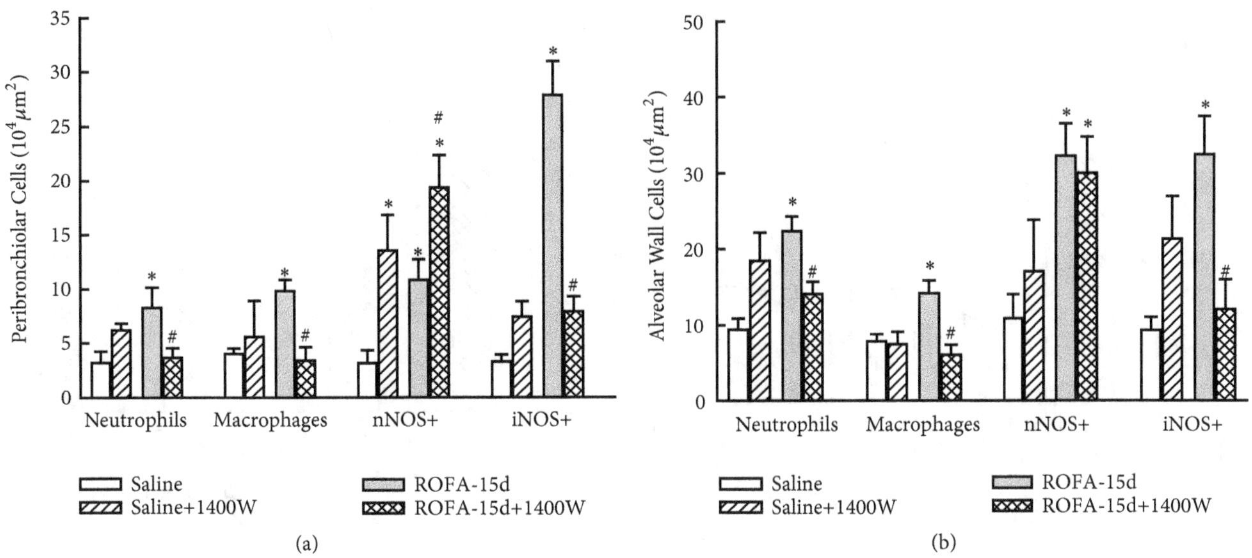

FIGURE 2: Lung inflammation and nitric oxide synthase expression. This figure represents the mean and SEM values of macrophages, neutrophils, nNOS, and iNOS-positive cells in peribronchiolar (a) and alveolar (b) wall. The animals that received fifteen instillations of ROFA presented higher values of all cells, and 1400W reduced inflammation and iNOS-positive cells, not interfering with nNOS expression. $*p<0.05$ compared with saline groups; $\#p<0.05$ compared with animals that received ROFA and vehicle treatment.

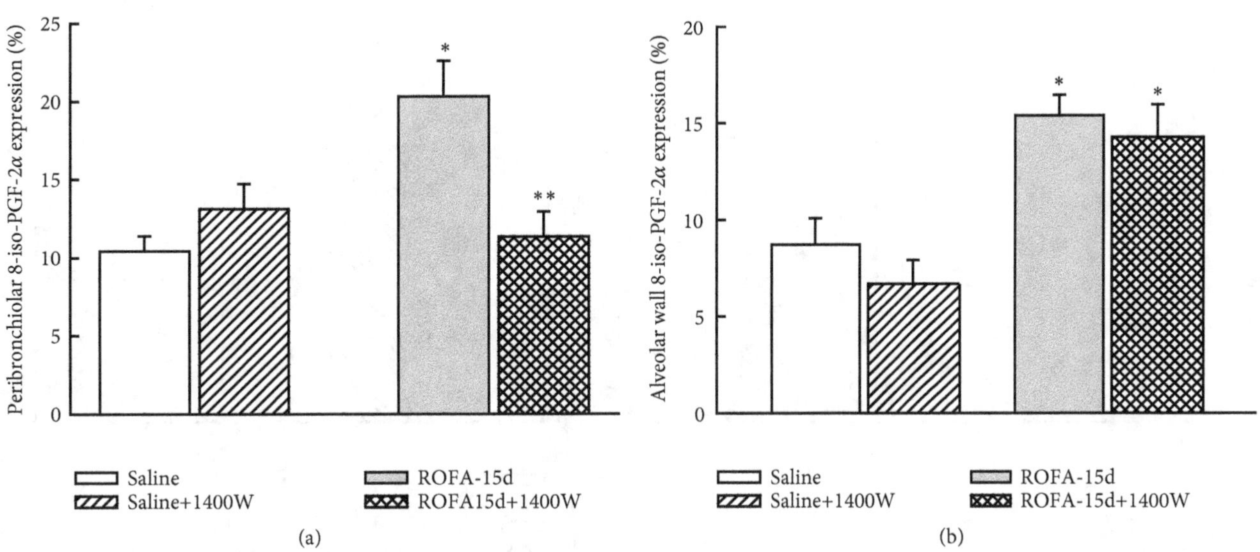

FIGURE 3: Oxidative stress: this figure represents the mean and SEM values of 8-iso-PGF-2a expression (%) in peribronchiolar and alveolar wall. The ROFA instillations increased the positive area and the iNOS inhibition reduced it only around bronchioles. $*p<0.05$ compared with saline groups; $**p<0.05$ compared with animals that received ROFA and vehicle treatment.

system as well as the strength and elasticity of lung tissue. Other authors had already demonstrated that ROFA exposures affected bronchial responsiveness. In this sense, Gavett et al. [40] demonstrated that single intratracheal instillation of ROFA in Balb/C altered the total resistance of the respiratory system in response to low doses of methacholine, and induced an accumulation of neutrophils in airways and alveolar walls. Arantes-Costa et al. [10] demonstrated that sensitized animals worsened mucus production when received ROFA after the sensitization period.

The alterations in lung function observed in animals that received ROFA may be secondary to pulmonary morphological alterations found. It is well known that airway extracellular matrix remodeling seen over the years may be associated with the irreversibility of pulmonary function, at least in asthmatic patients [41]. Thus, inflammation and extracellular matrix remodeling observed in ROFA-instilled group may, by itself, lead to increased responses of pulmonary mechanics. Inflammatory cell recruitment is associated with a release of several mediators/modulators, among them nitric oxide, which are also involved in the control of airway smooth muscle contractility and lung parenchyma mechanical responses [16, 25, 42].

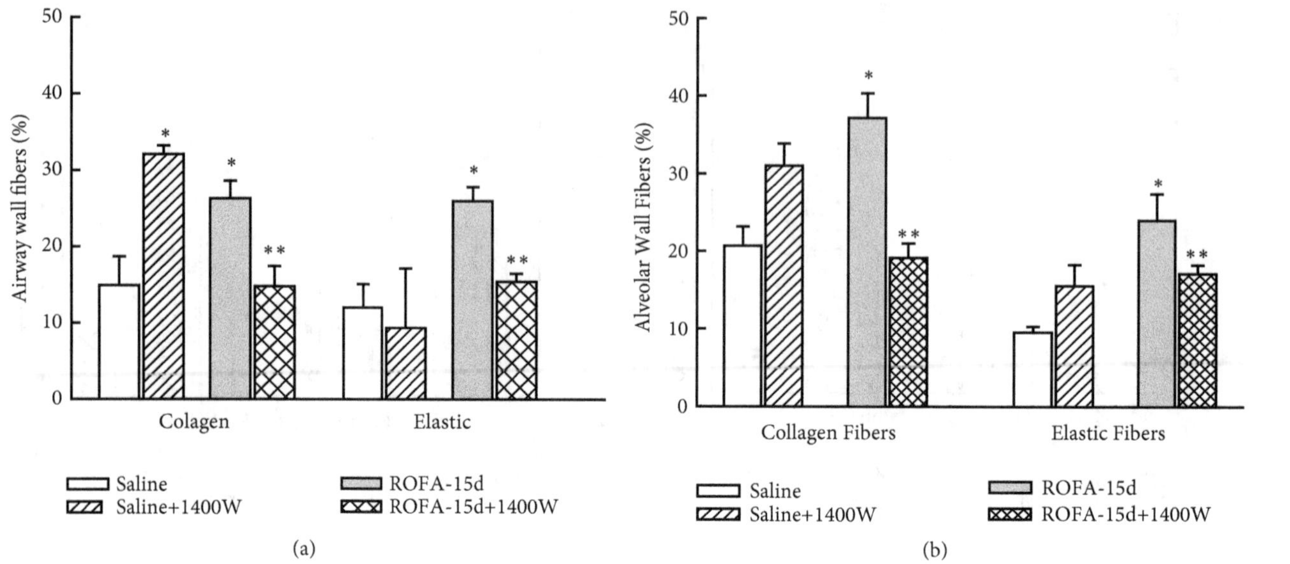

FIGURE 4: Lung remodeling: this figure represents the mean and SEM values of both collagen and elastic fibers content around airways (a) and in alveolar wall (b). The ROFA instillations increased the airway and parenchyma extracellular matrix fibers deposition compared to control, and the iNOS inhibition reduced these responses. $*p<0.05$ compared with saline groups; $**p<0.05$ compared with animals that received ROFA and vehicle treatment.

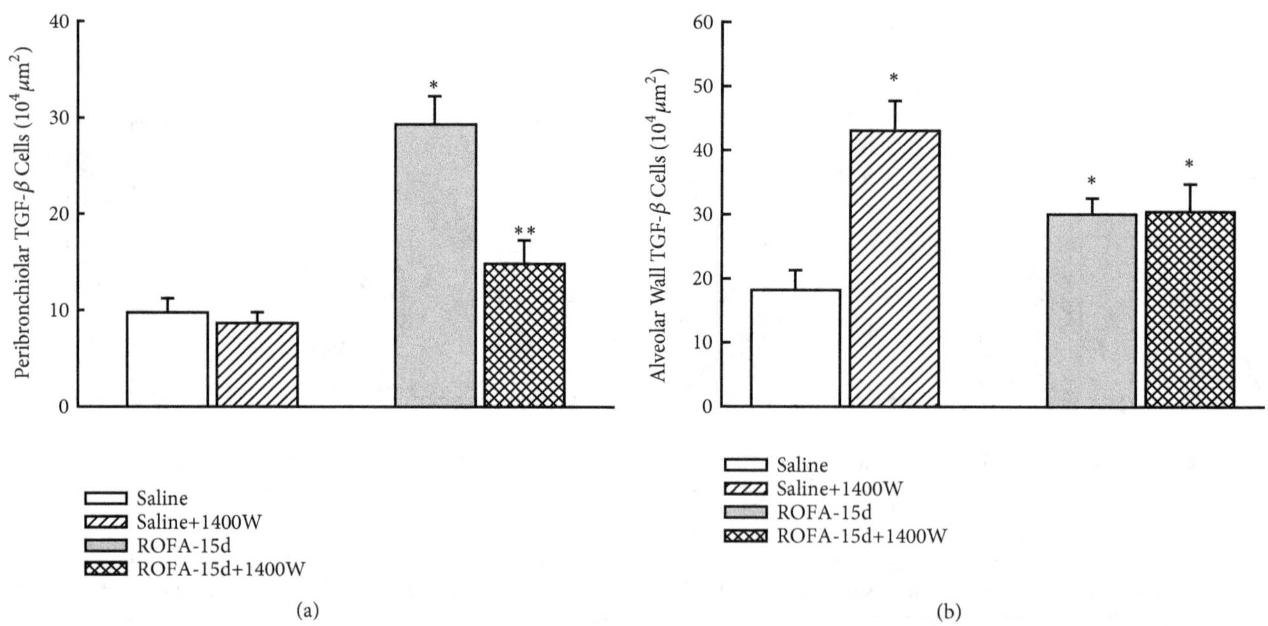

FIGURE 5: TGF-β expression: this figure represents the mean and SEM values of TGF-β expression in both peribronchiolar (a) and alveolar (b) wall. The ROFA instillations increased the number of TGF-β-positive cells in both airways and alveolar wall and iNOS inhibition reduced this response only in airways. $*p<0.05$ compared with saline groups; $**p<0.05$ compared with animals that received ROFA and vehicle treatment.

In addition, an increased 8-iso-PGF-2α in peribronchiolar and alveolar wall could be associated with the responsiveness observed. 8-iso-PGF2α concentrations were measurable in exhaled breath condensate (EBC) (Montuschi et al., 2010), a noninvasive technique for sampling airway secretions, and it has been found elevated in patients with COPD compared with healthy ex-smokers [43]. Although previous studies have evaluated the effects of PGE2, which was more potent as a constrictor than PGF2α, the latter isoprostane is considered the predominant form generated during free radical attack of cell membranes [44]. Jourdan et al. [45] showed that L-NAME treatment greatly inhibits 8-iso-PGF2α and also that pulmonary artery smooth muscle can release this isoprostane. This class of substances induces contractions of the smooth muscle of airways and vessels operating in the Rho tyrosinase and Rho-kinase, leading to increased activity of phosphorylated myosin [16, 22, 46]. Shiraki et al. [47] showed studying tracheal smooth muscle

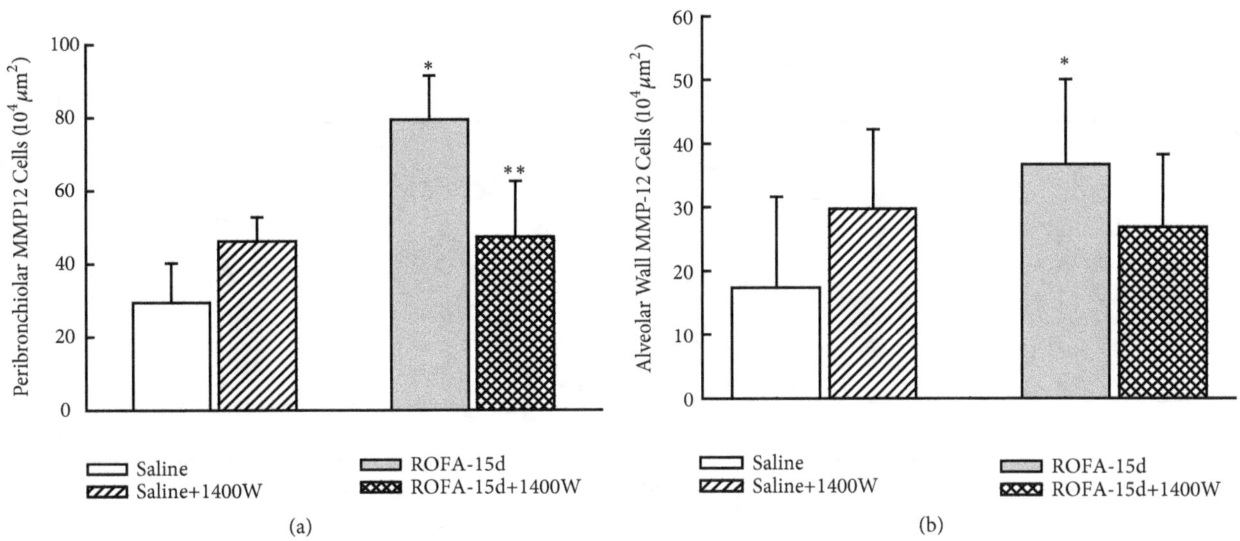

FIGURE 6: Metalloproteinase 12 expression. This figure represents the mean and SEM values of MMP-12 expression in both peribronchiolar (a) and alveolar (b) wall. The ROFA instillations increased the number of MMP-12-positive cells and iNOS inhibition significantly reduced this response only in airways. $*p<0.05$ compared with saline groups; $**p<0.05$ compared with animals that received ROFA and vehicle treatment.

contraction that 8-isoPGF2α increased the isometric tension and they concluded that 8-isoPGF2α causes airway smooth muscle contraction. However, few studies have evaluated the specific effects of 8-isoPGF2α in smooth muscle contraction. Our group also have demonstrated that the inhibition of 8-isoPGF2α by different agents reduced the airway hyperresponsiveness [48–50].

Furthermore, collagen and elastic fibers remodeling in the airways and distal lung parenchyma occurred only in ROFA-15 day group. Alterations in the elastic fibers content are known to occur in the pathophysiology of lung disease such as asthma and COPD, a major shortfall of elastic fibers followed by loss of elasticity and elastic recoil occurs in a second stage regeneration of these fibers, making them thicker. It would be expected that an increase in neutrophilic recruitment may reduce the elastic fiber content. However, corroborating our results, other authors have found an increase in elastic fibers [42, 49], probably because of the turnover processes of elastic fibers that involves the function of smooth muscle promoting elastin formation and the elastolytic effects of inflammation, particularly related to neutrophils, which was prominent in both peribronchiolar and alveolar wall in the present study.

In an attempt to understand some of the mechanisms involved in these responses, we evaluated the 8-iso-PGF-2α expression in the lung, a marker of oxidative stress pathway activation. The formation of peroxynitrite leads to lipid peroxidation and generation of isoprostanes such as 8-iso-PGF2 α, which is one of the predominant forms generated during the attack of free radicals in the cell membrane [50]. After both 5 and 15 days of ROFA exposures there was an increase in the oxidative stress pathway activation in the lung and an increase in the number of nNOS and iNOS-positive inflammatory cells in peribronchiolar and alveolar wall. As NO has a short half-life, the reactive oxygen (ROS) and reactive nitrogen species (RNS) can act as NO carriers, culminating with oxidative stress activation.

In addition, it is well known that NO modulates bronchial smooth muscle contractility and also lung parenchyma. In this regard, 1400W treated animals had a significant reduction in the resistance and elastance of the respiratory system compared to vehicle treated groups, suggesting an effect of this inhibitor attenuating the response of lung mechanics induced by ROFA in proximal and distal airways. However, there were no differences in Htis and Gtis, which reflects more lung distal parenchyma response.

Donors of nitric oxide (nitrovasodilator) are relaxing the smooth muscles, including airway smooth muscle [51, 52]. The effects of NO as a bronchodilator is well recognized, however various studies emphasized that the effects of NO on bronchodilation depends on the enzyme type that is producing NO. When NO was produced by iNOS in high quantities, it could induce bronchoconstriction [24]. Besides the direct effects of NO in smooth muscle is important to note that the control of inflammation and remodeling by the treatment of iNOS inhibition can also contribute to the improvement of lung function.

We found that iNOS inhibition reduced the infiltration of neutrophils and macrophages and deposition of collagen and elastic fibers. This effect was similar in airways and lung parenchyma. Some mechanisms may explain how nitric oxide acts on inflammatory cells. High levels of NO act as effectors molecule of the immune system and can inhibit DNA synthesis by inactivation of ribonucleic reductase and by direct deamination of DNA [24]. The activation of apoptosis can be induced by nitric oxide since it can influence DNA fragmentation and prolong cell survival [53]. However, Chung et al. [54] suggest that NO may have effects, both apoptotic and antiapoptotic, and that these responses depend on nitric oxide levels and also the producing cell.

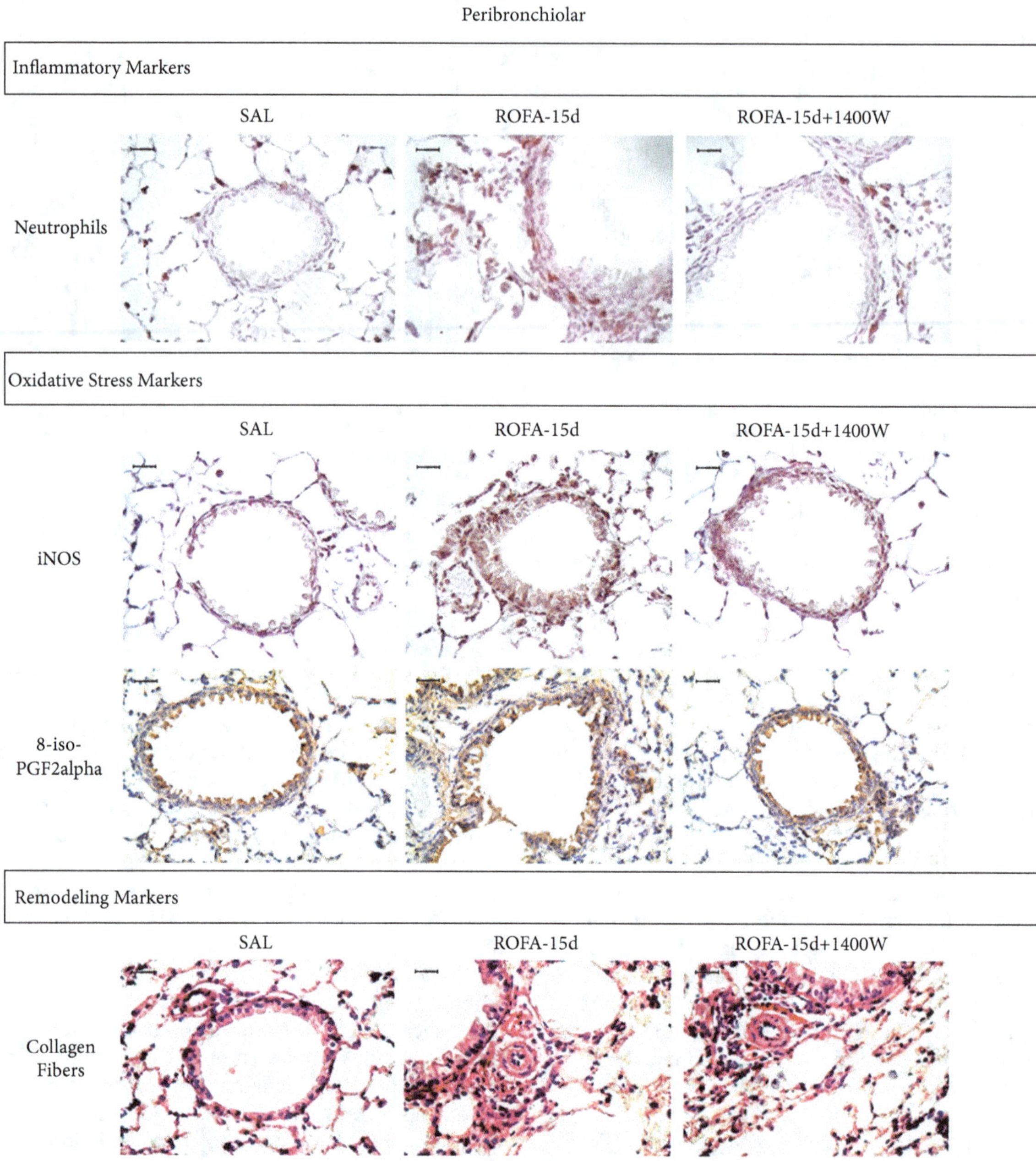

FIGURE 7: Representative photomicrographs of airway stained with immunohistochemistry to detect neutrophils, iNOS, isoprostane, and collagen fibers in all experimental groups.

Corroborating the present findings, we recently showed that iNOS inhibitor attenuates lung vascular remodeling in an asthma model [24]. Some evidence tried to explain how NO affect the collagen deposition. Horstman et al. [55] suggested that nitric oxide may attenuate vascular remodeling secondary to hypoxia in rats. Aristoteles et al. [25] studied a model of chronic allergic inflammation and demonstrated that nitric oxide inhibition derived from the inducible isoform modulates the extracellular matrix remodeling.

Other possible explanations are the role of nitric oxide in the modulation of metalloproteinases synthesis and activation as well as in their inhibitors [56]. Metalloproteinases are families of enzymes that are involved in the degradation of collagen and other extracellular matrix proteins [16].

We evaluated the MMP-12 since this metalloproteinase is able to degrade extracellular matrix components and is involved in lung tissue remodeling observed in inflammatory pulmonary diseases such as chronic obstructive pulmonary diseases (COPD). We observed that the number of MMP-12-positive cells was increased in both peribronchiolar and alveolar wall after fifteen ROFA instillations. Corroborating the idea that nitric oxide influences metalloproteinases, we observed that 1400W treatment reduced the number of MMP-12 positive cells only around peribronchiolar area, suggesting that iNOS is involved in MMP-12 upregulation induced by particulate matter, and it could be one of the mechanisms in which iNOS acts in lung remodeling. These results are in accordance with previous studies [17, 27, 57].

Another important mechanism involved in lung remodeling is the profibrotic cytokine TGF- β. It is produced by a number of cells, including macrophages, epithelial cells, and fibroblasts and is involved in most of the cellular biological processes of airway remodeling [58]. In the present study, we observed that both five and fifteen instillations of ROFA induce an increase in both peribronchiolar and alveolar wall TGF- β.-positive cells. The iNOS inhibition reduced this response only in peribronchiolar cells, not affecting alveolar wall.

1400W treatment reduces the 8-iso-PGF-2α only around airways, suggesting that oxidative stress is one important mechanism involved in air pollution-induced lung alterations, as extensively discussed in the literature [59–61]. Other studies of our group have shown this same effect of iNOS inhibition in oxidative stress using an animal model of chronic allergic lung inflammation [62, 63].

The major limitation of the present study was related to the fact that ROFA is a tool to study the effects of particulate matter in lung and may be not representative of particulate matter present in air pollution. However, its exact composition is known and makes the experiments reproducible which is important to elucidate mechanisms involved. The clinical relevance is related to two important views: First, we developed an experimental model to study air pollution with repeated instillations that can be used to investigate physiopathological mechanisms. Second, we clearly showed that iNOS is involved in lung inflammation induced by particulate matter. Further studies involved other mechanics such as the role of oxidative stress, IL-17 and cholinergic anti-inflammatory system, as recent studies suggested [64].

Collectively, ROFA instillation induced lung mechanics, inflammatory, and extracellular matrix remodeling alterations in lungs of C57BL mice. These changes are associated with an increased in the oxidative stress pathway, metalloproteinase, and TGF-β activation. NO, derived mainly from iNOS, is involved in proinflammatory and profibrotic alterations induced by particulate matter.

Acknowledgments

This study was supported by Fundação de Amparo à Pesquisa do Estado de São Paulo (FAPESP), Conselho Nacional de Desenvolvimento Científico and Tecnológico (CNPq), and HC-FMUSP, Brazil.

References

[1] K. Adams, D. S. Greenbaum, R. Shaikh, A. M. van Erp, and A. G. Russell, "Particulate matter components, sources, and health: Systematic approaches to testing effects," *Journal of the Air & Waste Management Association*, vol. 65, no. 5, pp. 544–558, 2015.

[2] M. Lippmann, K. Ito, A. Nádas, and R. T. Burnett, "Association of particulate matter components with daily mortality and morbidity in urban populations," *Research Reports Health Effects Institute*, vol. 95, pp. 5–72, 2000.

[3] A. Valavanidis, K. Fiotakis, and T. Vlachogianni, "Airborne particulate matter and human health: toxicological assessment and importance of size and composition of particles for oxidative damage and carcinogenic mechanisms," *Journal of Environmental Science and Health, Part C: Environmental Carcinogenesis and Ecotoxicology Reviews*, vol. 26, no. 4, pp. 339–362, 2008.

[4] A. Gawda, G. Majka, B. Nowak, and J. Marcinkiewicz, "Air pollution, oxidative stress, and exacerbation of autoimmune diseases," *Central European Journal of Immunology*, vol. 42, no. 3, pp. 305–312, 2017.

[5] S. Ling and S. F. van Eeden, "Particulate matter air pollution exposure: role in the development and exacerbation of chronic obstructive pulmonary disease," *International Journal of Chronic Obstructive Pulmonary Disease*, vol. 4, pp. 233–243, 2009.

[6] L. Liu, R. Poon, L. Chen et al., "Acute effects of air pollution on pulmonary function, airway inflammation, and oxidative stress in asthmatic children," *Environmental Health Perspectives*, vol. 117, no. 4, pp. 668–674, 2009.

[7] X. Lu, H. Fu, F. Han et al., "Lipoxin A4 regulates PM2.5-induced severe allergic asthma in mice via the Th1/Th2 balance of group 2 innate lymphoid cells," *Journal of Thoracic Disease*, vol. 10, no. 3, pp. 1449–1459, 2018.

[8] X. Zhang, W. Zhong, Q. Meng et al., "Ambient PM2.5 exposure exacerbates severity of allergic asthma in previously sensitized mice," *Journal of Asthma*, vol. 52, no. 8, pp. 785–794, 2015.

[9] H. Liu, X. Fan, N. Wang, Y. Zhang, and J. Yu, "Exacerbating effects of PM2.5 in OVA-sensitized and challenged mice and the expression of TRPA1 and TRPV1 proteins in lungs," *Journal of Asthma & Allergy Educators*, vol. 54, no. 8, pp. 807–817, 2017.

[10] F. M. Arantes-Costa, F. D. T. Q. S. Lopes, A. C. Toledo et al., "Effects of residual oil fly ash (ROFA) in mice with chronic allergic pulmonary inflammation," *Toxicologic Pathology*, vol. 36, no. 5, pp. 680–686, 2008.

[11] X. Xu, H. Wang, S. Liu et al., "TP53-dependent autophagy links the ATR-CHEK1 axis activation to proinflammatory VEGFA production in human bronchial epithelial cells exposed to fine particulate matter (PM2.5)," *Autophagy*, vol. 12, no. 10, pp. 1832–1848, 2016.

[12] P. Montuschi, J. A. Nightingale, S. A. Kharitonov, and P. J. Barnes, "Ozone-induced increase in exhaled 8-isoprostane in healthy subjects is resistant to inhaled budesonide," *Free Radical Biology & Medicine*, vol. 33, no. 10, pp. 1403–1408, 2002.

[13] G. D. Thurston, H. Kipen, I. Annesi-Maesano et al., "A joint ERS/ATS policy statement: what constitutes an adverse health effect of air pollution? an analytical framework," *European Respiratory Journal*, vol. 49, no. 1, Article ID 1600419, 2017.

[14] P. Montuschi, "Leukotrienes, antileukotrienes and asthma," *Mini-Reviews in Medicinal Chemistry*, vol. 8, no. 7, pp. 647–656, 2008.

[15] M. L. Manni, J. B. Trudeau, E. V. Scheller et al., "The complex relationship between inflammation and lung function in severe asthma," *Mucosal Immunology*, vol. 7, no. 5, pp. 1186–1198, 2014.

[16] R. F. Righetti, P. A. da Silva Pigati, and S. S. Possa, "Effects of Rho-kinase inhibition in lung tissue with chronic inflammation," *Respiratory Physiology & Neurobiology*, vol. 192, pp. 134–146, 2014.

[17] L. Camargo, R. F. Righetti, L. R. Aristóteles et al., "Effects of anti-IL-17 on inflammation, remodeling, and oxidative stress in an experimental model of asthma exacerbated by LPS," *Frontiers in Immunology*, vol. 8, article 1835, 2018.

[18] P. Montuschi and P. J. Barnes, "New perspectives in pharmacological treatment of mild persistent asthma," *Drug Discovery Therapy*, vol. 16, no. 23-24, pp. 1084–1091, 2011.

[19] U. Förstermann and W. C. Sessa, "Nitric oxide synthases: regulation and function," *European Heart Journal*, vol. 33, no. 7, pp. 829–837, 2012.

[20] S. S. Possa, E. A. Leick, C. M. Prado, M. A. Martins, and I. F. L. C. Tibério, "Eosinophilic inflammation in allergic asthma," *Frontiers in Pharmacology*, vol. 4, article 46, 2013.

[21] G. G. King, A. James, L. Harkness, and P. A. B. Wark, "Pathophysiology of severe asthma: We've only just started," *Respirology*, vol. 23, no. 3, pp. 262–271, 2018.

[22] P. A. Pigati, R. F. Righetti, S. S. Possa et al., "Y-27632 is associated with corticosteroid-potentiated control of pulmonary remodeling and inflammation in guinea pigs with chronic allergic inflammation," *BMC Pulmonary Medicine*, vol. 15, article 85, 2015.

[23] O. A. Theodoro-Junior, R. Fraga Righetti, R. Almeida-Reis et al., "A plant proteinase inhibitor from enterolobium contortisiliquum attenuates pulmonary mechanics, inflammation and remodeling induced by elastase in mice," *International Journal of Molecular Sciences*, vol. 18, no. 2, article 403, 2017.

[24] C. M. Prado, M. A. Martins, and I. F. Tibério, "Nitric oxide in asthma physiopathology," *ISRN Allergy*, vol. 2011, Article ID 832560, 2011.

[25] L. R. Aristoteles, R. F. Righetti, N. M. Pinheiro et al., "Modulation of the oscillatory mechanics of lung tissue and the oxidative stress response induced by arginase inhibition in a chronic allergic inflammation model," *BMC Pulmonary Medicine*, vol. 13, no. 1, article 52, 2013.

[26] R. Carvalho-Oliveira, M. Saiki, R. C. Pires-Neto, G. Lorenzi-Filho, M. MacChione, and P. H. N. Saldiva, "Anti-oxidants reduce the acute adverse effects of residual oil fly ash on the frog palate mucociliary epithelium," *Environmental Research*, vol. 98, no. 3, pp. 349–354, 2005.

[27] C. M. Prado, E. A. Leick-Maldonado, L. Yano et al., "Effects of nitric oxide synthases in chronic allergic airway inflammation and remodeling," *American Journal of Respiratory Cell and Molecular Biology*, vol. 35, no. 4, pp. 457–465, 2006.

[28] M. I. Bittencourt-Mernak, N. M. Pinheiro, F. P. R. Santana et al., "Prophylactic and therapeutic treatment with the flavonone sakuranetin ameliorates LPS-induced acute lung injury," *American Journal of Physiology-Lung Cellular and Molecular Physiology*, vol. 312, no. 2, pp. L217–L230, 2017.

[29] G. Ciabattoni, P. Montuschi, D. Curró, and P. Preziosi, "In vitro testing for lung toxicity," *Toxicology in Vitro*, vol. 7, no. 5, pp. 581–585, 1993.

[30] G. Ciabattoni, P. Montuschi, D. Currò, G. Togna, and P. Preziosi, "Effects of vasoactive intestinal polypeptide on antigen-induced bronchoconstriction and thromboxane release in guinea-pig lung," *British Journal of Pharmacology*, vol. 109, no. 1, pp. 243–250, 1993.

[31] P. Montuschi, P. Del Cecato, and G. Ciabattoni, "In vitro testing for lung toxicity: A method for distinguishing between immune- and non-immune-mediated reactions to xenobiotics," *Environmental Toxicology and Pharmacology*, vol. 2, no. 2-3, pp. 201–205, 1996.

[32] S. Esposito, R. Tenconi, M. Lelii et al., "Possible molecular mechanisms linking air pollution and asthma in children," *BMC Pulmonary Medicine*, vol. 14, no. 1, article 31, 2014.

[33] M.-Y. Lee, K.-H. Sun, C.-P. Chiang et al., "Nitric oxide suppresses LPS-induced inflammation in a mouse asthma model by attenuating the interaction of IKK and Hsp90," *Experimental Biology and Medicine*, vol. 240, no. 4, pp. 498–507, 2015.

[34] M. S. Happo, R. O. Salonen, A. I. Hlinen et al., "Inflammation and tissue damage in mouse lung by single and repeated dosing of urban air coarse and fine particles collected from six European cities," *Inhalation Toxicology*, vol. 22, no. 5, pp. 402–416, 2010.

[35] F. Xu, M. Luo, L. He et al., "Necroptosis contributes to urban particulate matter-induced airway epithelial injury," *Cellular Physiology and Biochemistry*, vol. 46, no. 2, pp. 699–712, 2018.

[36] A. J. Ghio, H. B. Suliman, J. D. Carter, A. M. Abushamaa, and R. J. Folz, "Overexpression of extracellular superoxide dismutase decreases lung injury after exposure to oil fly ash," *American Journal of Physiology-Lung Cellular and Molecular Physiology*, vol. 283, no. 1, pp. L211–L218, 2002.

[37] G. M. Carvalho, L. K. Nagato, S. d. Fagundes et al., "Time course of pulmonary burden in mice exposed to residual oil fly ash," *Frontiers in Physiology*, vol. 5, article 366, 2014.

[38] F. Gao, A. Barchowsky, A. A. Nemec, and J. P. Fabisiak, "Microbial stimulation by Mycoplasma fermentans synergistically amplifies IL-6 release by human lung fibroblasts in response to residual oil fly ash (ROFA) and nickel," *Toxicological Sciences*, vol. 81, no. 2, pp. 467–479, 2004.

[39] T. Marchini, D. Wolf, N. A. Michel et al., "Acute exposure to air pollution particulate matter aggravates experimental myocardial infarction in mice by potentiating cytokine secretion from lung macrophages," *Basic Research in Cardiology*, vol. 111, no. 44, 2016.

[40] S. H. Gavett, S. L. Madison, M. A. Stevens, and D. L. Costa, "Residual oil fly ash amplifies allergic cytokines, airway responsiveness, and inflammation in mice," *American Journal of Respiratory and Critical Care Medicine*, vol. 160, no. 6, pp. 1897–1904, 1999.

[41] H. Fehrenbach, C. Wagner, and M. Wegmann, "Airway remodeling in asthma: what really matters," *Cell and Tissue Research*, vol. 367, no. 3, pp. 551–569, 2017.

[42] C. P. P. Sakoda, A. C. de Toledo, A. Perini et al., "Sakuranetin reverses vascular peribronchial and lung parenchyma remodeling in a murine model of chronic allergic pulmonary inflammation," *Acta Histochemica*, vol. 118, no. 6, pp. 615–624, 2016.

[43] G. Santini, N. Mores, R. Shohreh et al., "Exhaled and non-exhaled non-invasive markers for assessment of respiratory inflammation in patients with stable COPD and healthy smokers," *Journal of Breath Research*, vol. 10, no. 1, article 017102, 2016.

[44] P. Montuschi, P. J. Barnes, and G. Ciabattoni, "Measurement of 8-isoprostane in exhaled breath condensate," *Methods in Molecular Biology*, vol. 594, pp. 73–84, 2010.

[45] K. B. Jourdan, J. A. Mitchell, and T. W. Evans, "Release of isoprostanes by human pulmonary artery in organ culture: A cyclo-oxygenase and nitric oxide dependent pathway," *Biochemical and Biophysical Research Communications*, vol. 233, no. 3, pp. 668–672, 1997.

[46] S. S. Possa, H. T. Charafeddine, R. F. Righetti et al., "Rho-kinase inhibition attenuates airway responsiveness, inflammation, matrix remodeling, and oxidative stress activation induced by chronic inflammation," *American Journal of Physiology-Lung Cellular and Molecular Physiology*, vol. 303, no. 11, pp. L939–L952, 2012.

[47] A. Shiraki, H. Kume, T. Oguma et al., "Role of Ca2+ mobilization and Ca2+ sensitization in 8-iso-PGF2α-induced contraction in airway smooth muscle," *Clinical & Experimental Allergy*, vol. 39, no. 2, pp. 236–245, 2009.

[48] T. M. Dos Santos, R. F. Righetti, L. d. Camargo et al., "Effect of Anti-IL17 antibody treatment alone and in combination with rho-kinase inhibitor in a murine model of asthma," *Frontiers in Physiology*, vol. 9, article 1183, 2018.

[49] A. C. Toledo, C. P. P. Sakoda, A. Perini et al., "Flavonone treatment reverses airway inflammation and remodelling in an asthma murine model," *British Journal of Pharmacology*, vol. 168, no. 7, pp. 1736–1749, 2013.

[50] T. J. van 't Erve, F. B. Lih, M. B. Kadiiska, L. J. Deterding, T. E. Eling, and R. P. Mason, "Reinterpreting the best biomarker of oxidative stress: The 8-iso-PGF2α / PGF2α ratio distinguishes chemical from enzymatic lipid peroxidation," *Free Radical Biology & Medicine*, vol. 83, pp. 245–251, 2015.

[51] J. F. Perez-Zoghbi, Y. Bai, and M. J. Sanderson, "Nitric oxide induces airway smooth muscle cell relaxation by decreasing the frequency of agonist-induced Ca2+ oscillations," *The Journal of General Physiology*, vol. 135, no. 3, pp. 247–259, 2010.

[52] B. S. Steinhorn, J. Loscalzo, and T. Michel, "Nitroglycerin and nitric oxide—a rondo of themes in cardiovascular therapeutics," *The New England Journal of Medicine*, vol. 373, no. 3, pp. 277–280, 2015.

[53] F. L. M. Ricciardolo, P. J. Sterk, B. Gaston, and G. Folkerts, "Nitric oxide in health and disease of the respiratory system," *Physiological Reviews*, vol. 84, no. 3, pp. 731–765, 2004.

[54] H. T. Chung, H. O. Pae, B. M. Choi, T. R. Billiar, and Y. M. Kim, "Nitric oxide a bioregulator of apoptosis," *Biochemical and Biophysical Research Communications*, vol. 282, no. 5, 2001.

[55] D. J. Horstman, L. G. Fischer, P. C. Kouretas, R. L. Hannan, and G. F. Rich, "Role of nitric oxide in heparin-induced attenuation of hypoxic pulmonary vascular remodeling," *Journal of Applied Physiology*, vol. 92, no. 5, pp. 2012–2018, 2002.

[56] T. Ichikawa, H. Sugiura, A. Koarai et al., "TLR3 activation augments matrix metalloproteinase production through reactive nitrogen species generation in human lung fibroblasts," *The Journal of Immunology*, vol. 192, no. 11, pp. 4977–4988, 2014.

[57] B. T. Martins-Olivera, R. Almeida-Reis, O. A. Theodoro-Júnior et al., "The plant-derived *Bauhinia bauhinioides* kallikrein proteinase inhibitor (rBbKI) attenuates elastase-induced emphysema in mice," *Mediators of Inflammation*, vol. 2016, Article ID 5346574, 12 pages, 2016.

[58] R. Halwani, S. Al-Muhsen, H. Al-Jahdali, and Q. Hamid, "Role of transforming growth factor-β in airway remodeling in asthma," *American Journal of Respiratory Cell and Molecular Biology*, vol. 44, no. 2, pp. 127–133, 2011.

[59] L. J. Janssen, "Isoprostanes: an overview and putative roles in pulmonary pathophysiology," *American Journal of Physiology-Lung Cellular and Molecular Physiology*, vol. 280, no. 6, pp. L1067–L1082, 2001.

[60] P. Montuschi, D. Currò, E. Ragazzoni, P. Preziosi, and G. Ciabattoni, "Anaphylaxis increases 8-iso-prostaglandin F2α release from guinea-pig lung in vitro," *European Journal of Pharmacology*, vol. 365, no. 1, pp. 59–64, 1999.

[61] P. J. C. Biselli, F. D. T. Q. S. Lopes, H. T. Moriya et al., "Short-term exposure of mice to cigarette smoke and/or residual oil fly ash produces proximal airspace enlargements and airway epithelium remodeling," *Brazilian Journal of Medical and Biological Research*, vol. 44, no. 5, pp. 460–468, 2011.

[62] P. Angeli, C. M. Prado, D. G. Xisto et al., "Effects of chronic L-NAME treatment lung tissue responses induced by chronic pulmonary inflammation mechanics, eosinophilic and extracellular matrix," *American Journal of Physiology-Lung Cellular and Molecular Physiology*, vol. 294, no. 6, pp. L1197–L1205, 2008.

[63] C. M. Starling, C. M. Prado, E. A. Leick-Maldonado et al., "Inducible nitric oxide synthase inhibition attenuates lung tissue responsiveness and remodeling in a model of chronic pulmonary inflammation in guinea pigs," *Respiratory Physiology & Neurobiology*, vol. 165, no. 2-3, pp. 185–194, 2009.

[64] F. P. Santana, N. M. Pinheiro, M. I. Bittencourt-Mernak et al., "Vesicular acetylcholine transport deficiency potentiates some inflammatory responses induced by diesel exhaust particles," *Ecotoxicology and Environmental Safety*, 2019.

19

Pulmonary Vein Occlusion and Lung Infarction after Radiofrequency Ablation of Atrial Fibrillation

Julyan Al Fori,[1] **Maryam Al Belushi,**[1] **Mohammed Al Shuraiqi,**[1] **Ghalia Al Mohanny,**[2] **Rashid Al Umairi,**[3] **and Nasser Al Busaidi**[1]

[1]*Department of Chest Medicine, The Royal Hospital, Muscat, Oman*
[2]*Department of Cardiology, The Royal Hospital, Muscat, Oman*
[3]*Department of Radiology, The Royal Hospital, Muscat, Oman*

Correspondence should be addressed to Julyan Al Fori; dr.julyan@hotmail.com

Academic Editor: Akif Turna

Background. Pulmonary vein (PV) radiofrequency ablation (RFA) is an effective technique for a selected group of patients with atrial fibrillation (AF) refractory to antiarrhythmic drugs (Alfudhili et al., 2017). However, pulmonary vein occlusion is a potentially rare, sometimes severe, complication which may present clinically as nonspecific respiratory symptoms, signifying pulmonary vein stenosis, that are often underrecognized or misdiagnosed, leading to progression of the low-grade stenosis to complete occlusion if not treated with timely intervention (Alfudhili et al., 2017). *Case Presentation.* We report the first case of haemoptysis, three months postradiofrequency ablation (i.e., late complication) secondary to pulmonary vein occlusion that was diagnosed by computed tomography angiogram (CTA), which showed occlusion of 2 out of 4 native pulmonary veins. *Conclusion.* The cause of haemoptysis in this patient was pulmonary vein occlusion, secondary to radiofrequency ablation, as demonstrated in the CTA.

1. Case Report

A 33-year-old male presented with refractory AF, nine months postradiofrequency ablation. The patient developed symptomatic palpitations due to atrial fibrillation, and he was prescribed flecainide and bisoprolol. Despite the antiarrhythmic therapy, the patient continued to have significant symptomatic atrial fibrillation. Hence, the patient was taken for a second RFA.

The preablation echocardiogram demonstrated normal ventricular function and pulmonary pressures. During the RFA procedure, the left atrium and all four PVs were individually isolated and mapped using the CARTO-3 advanced 3D cardiac mapping system. It was noticed that the patient has left common pulmonary veins. Then, voltage mapping was done revealing a connection between the superior pulmonary veins and the anterior wall of the atrium. Antral ablation lesions were done, electrical isolation was created and performed with energy (35-40 watts) applied on both superior veins, and complete pulmonary vein isolation was achieved and verified by pacing attempts and verification of exit block in both veins. Remapping by the voltage map was done to assure complete isolation between the veins and the Lt.atrium, and it confirmed complete isolation.

Echocardiography done post procedure showed no pericardial effusion. After the curative ablation therapy, the patient was kept on aspirin and rivaroxaban to prevent AF recurrence as well as pulmonary venous and/or arterial thrombosis.

However, two months later, the patient presented to the emergency department with cough associated with haemoptysis and mild left-sided pleuritic chest pain. He underwent computed tomography pulmonary angiogram (CTPA), which showed multiple patches of consolidation as well as ground glass opacities in the left upper lobe and lingula with minimal left pleural effusion, as shown in Figures 1(a) and 1(b); differentials were either an infective process or lung

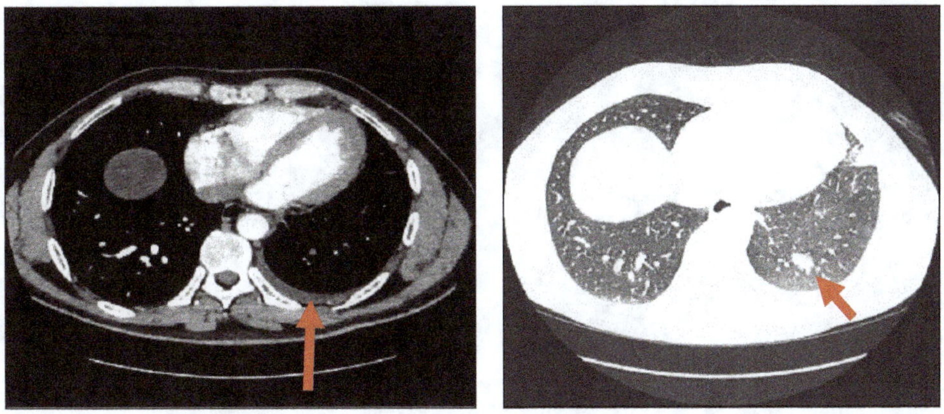

(a) (b)

FIGURE 1: Computed tomography: (a) left pleural effusion (arrow); (b) consolidation and GGO in LUL (arrow). GGO: ground glass opacity; LUL: left upper lobe.

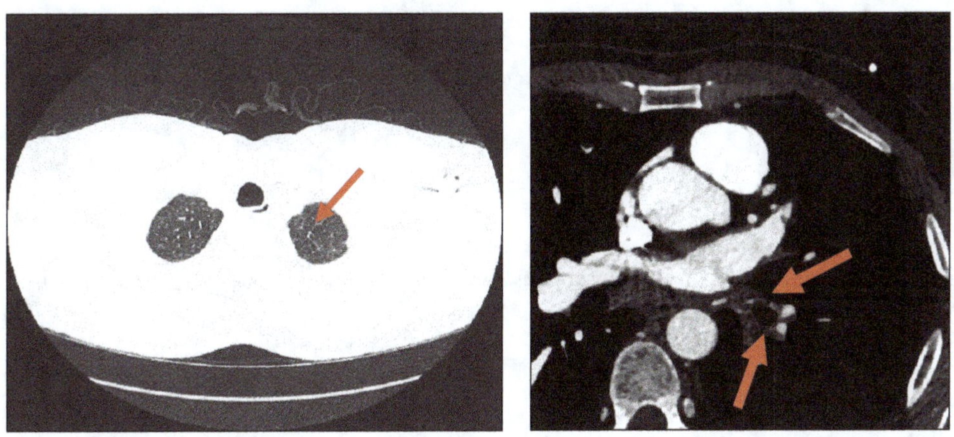

(a) (b)

FIGURE 2: CTPA: (a) unilateral pulmonary edema with interlobular septal thickening (arrow); (b) Lt.PVsO (arrow). CTPA: computed tomography pulmonary angiogram; Lt.PVsO: left pulmonary vein occlusion.

infarction. The patient was given broad spectrum antibiotics and referred to the pulmonology clinic for further investigation. Meanwhile, he was seen in cardiology OPD for follow-up, and he was advised to stop rivaroxaban as his CHA2DS2-VASc score was noted to be zero, in the setting of active haemoptysis. However, despite this, his haemoptysis persisted. Therefore, a contrast-enhanced CTPA was performed that showed features of unilateral left pulmonary venous congestion, and the left superior and inferior pulmonary veins were not visualized (as shown in Figures 2(a) and 2(b)), both signifying occlusion, most likely due to the prior ablation. In addition to that, he also underwent a coronary CTA which revealed that the right superior and inferior pulmonary veins are well-opacified with contrast; however, both left superior and inferior pulmonary veins are not visualized in the arterial phase (as shown in Figure 3). These findings of coronary CTA were consistent with the CTPA finding of left pulmonary vein occlusion. The patient also had a lung perfusion study, which showed absent perfusion in the left lung field in all perfusion views. In the ventilation images,

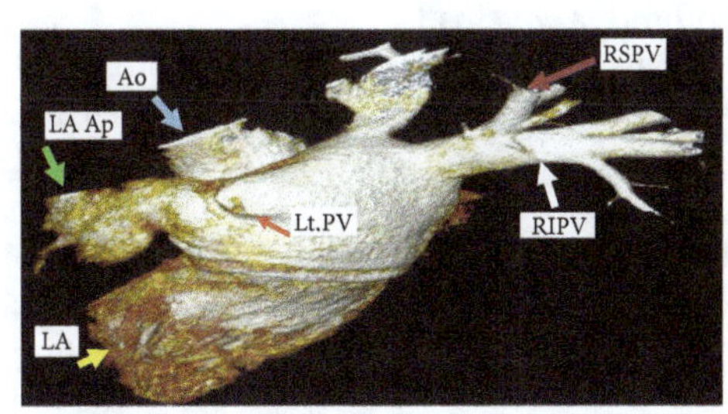

FIGURE 3: Three-dimensional cardiac CT reconstruction images: absent of left pulmonary veins following AF ablation (red arrow). CT: computed tomography; Ao: aorta (blue arrow); LA Ap: left atrial appendage (green arrow); LA: left atrium (yellow arrow); RSPV: right superior pulmonary vein (brown arrow); RIPV: right inferior pulmonary vein (white arrow); AF: atrial fibrillation.

there was adequate ventilation of the left lung, though it was lower compared to the right lung (as shown in Figure 4). A bronchoscopy was done as well and reported to be normal (no bleeding).

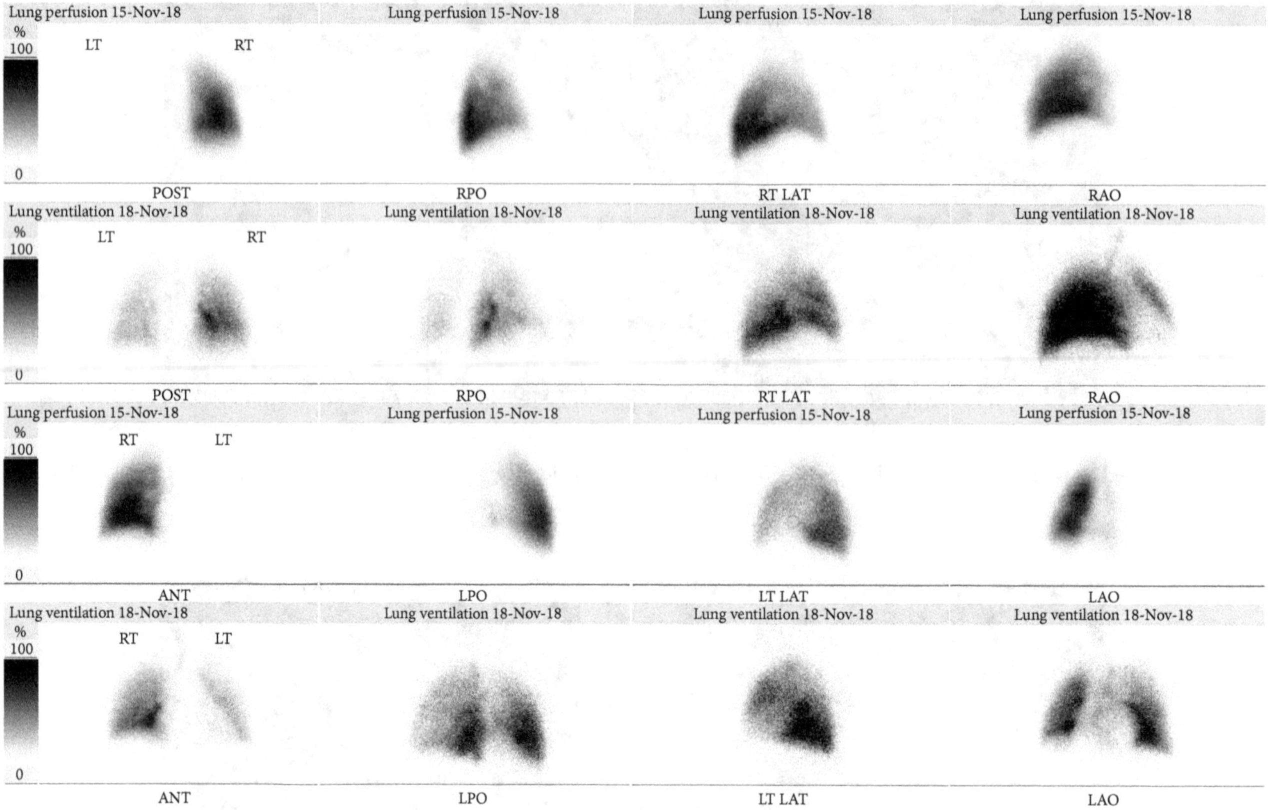

Figure 4: Absent perfusion in the left lung field in all perfusion views; in ventilation images, there is adequate ventilation of the left lung which is lower compared to the right lung.

2. Discussion

AF is one of the most common forms of cardiac arrhythmias and represents a major cause of stroke. The prevalence of AF increases with age; in people older than 65 years, it reaches up to 5%. Over 90% of ectopic beats that cause AF arise in the pulmonary veins and nearly 50% of them originate in left superior pulmonary veins [1].

Catheter-based radiofrequency ablation for AF is an effective treatment for patients with symptomatic AF refractory to therapy with antiarrhythmic drugs and has been increasingly performed worldwide [2]. The frequency of PV occlusion, a well-recognized complication following an AF ablation of pulmonary veins, has been declining due to the improvement of technique and operator experience [3]. Pulmonary vein occlusion is defined as more than 95% stenosis or complete loss of patency of a pulmonary vein as seen on chest CT [4]. The incidence rates vary from 1.3% to 15.6% in the reported articles, but the true incidence of PV occlusion following an AF radiofrequency ablation is still controversial [5]. The pathophysiology of progression of the injury in time was demonstrated in animal data showing intimal proliferation, collagen replacement of necrotic myocardium, endovascular contraction, and proliferation of the elastic lamina [6]. Both the arterial systems and pulmonary venous are well known to be interrelated. It has been shown that sudden occlusion of a pulmonary vein is soon followed by gradual decrease and then cessation of the arterial flow to the affected segment, and this is related to a decline in the arteriovenous gradient as well as compression by the developing tissue edema. Consequently, the involved alveoli are affected by the resulting ischemia and tissue edema, leading to atelectasis, infarction, or infection [7].

PV occlusion acquired after AF ablation varies in severity from asymptomatic to nonspecific symptoms, including persistent cough, haemoptysis, shortness of breath, and pleuritic chest pain [3]. Symptoms of PV occlusion depend on many factors, such as the number of veins involved, the time course of disease, and the severity of stenosis. Almost all patients with mild (<50%) or moderate PVS (50–70%) have no symptoms [1].

Chest X-ray finding can be nonspecific such as pulmonary and interstitial opacities and pleural effusion, so the final diagnosis is obtained with transoesophageal echocardiogram, magnetic resonance imaging, or CTPA after injection of intravenous contrast in the late phase to reduce flow artifacts [8].

PV occlusion can be treated acutely with balloon dilatation of the PV, although the long-term outcome is doubtful. Thus, treatment options are limited currently, and restenosis after PV intervention has been described and considered relatively frequent [9]. In the limited cases with irreversible occlusion with significant symptoms, dilation and stenting can be ineffective, and eventually, they require lung resection [10]. Hence, patients with PV occlusion need careful assessment and follow-up because of the risk of recurrence, which

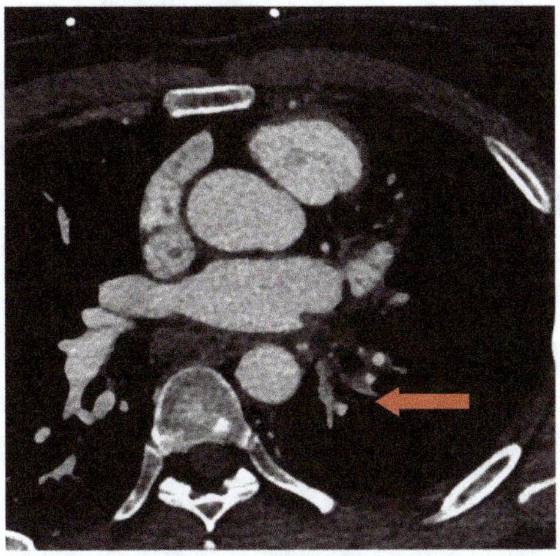

Figure 5: Left PV post balloon angioplasty (red arrow).

occurs in 50% of patients within 1 year [9]. Prevention of PV occlusion is mainly related to placing the ablation site from inside to outside the orifice of the PV and reducing the ablation temperature and energy applied [9]. This strategy helps to decrease the risk of PV occlusion to less than 1% [9].

Our patient was treated initially as pneumonia, based on his symptoms and imaging findings; however, he showed no improvement in the haemoptysis. He had CTPA which showed complete occlusion of the left superior and inferior pulmonary veins. Later, he underwent bronchoscopy which showed no active bleeding, and bronchial washing was negative for bacterial growth. Ventilation/perfusion scan showed no perfusion in whole left lung. Based on the diagnosis of left pulmonary vein occlusion in CTPA, the patient underwent balloon angioplasty of the same as shown in Figure 5; the procedure was complicated by arrhythmia and pericardial effusion which was drained successfully. Repeated ECHO showed normal ventricular function with no pericardial effusion.

References

[1] K. M. Alfudhili, H. H. Hassan, H. Abdullah, and M. Sherbiny, "Pulmonary vein occlusion and lung infarction complicating non-treated moderate single pulmonary vein stenosis after radiofrequency ablation of atrial fibrillation," *BJR|case reports*, vol. 3, no. 3, article 20160091, 2017.

[2] A. V. L. Sarabanda, L. C. Beck, L. G. G. Ferreira, W. L. Gali, F. Melo Netto, and G. U. Monte, "Treatment of pulmonary vein stenosis after percutaneous ablation of atrial fibrillation," *Arquivos Brasileiros de Cardiologia*, vol. 94, no. 1, pp. e7–e10, 2010.

[3] J. J. Lee, D. Weinberg, and R. Anand, "Asymptomatic pulmonary vein stenosis: hemodynamic adaptation and successful ablation," *Case Reports in Cardiology*, vol. 2016, 4 pages, 2016.

[4] N. A. Papakonstantinou, C. Zisis, C. Kouvidou, and G. Stratakos, "Lobectomy due to pulmonary vein occlusion after radiofrequency ablation for atrial fibrillation," *The Korean Journal of Thoracic and Cardiovascular Surgery*, vol. 51, no. 4, pp. 290–292, 2018.

[5] H.-W. Lu, P. Wei, S. Jiang et al., "Pulmonary vein stenosis complicating radiofrequency catheter ablation: five case reports and literature review," *Medicine*, vol. 94, no. 34, article e1346, 2015.

[6] D. Nehra, M. Liberman, P. A. Vagefi et al., "Complete pulmonary venous occlusion after radiofrequency ablation for atrial fibrillation," *The Annals of Thoracic Surgery*, vol. 87, no. 1, pp. 292–295, 2009.

[7] L. di Biase, T. S. Fahmy, O. M. Wazni et al., "Pulmonary vein total occlusion following catheter ablation for atrial fibrillation: clinical implications after long-term follow-up," *Journal of the American College of Cardiology*, vol. 48, no. 12, pp. 2493–2499, 2006.

[8] R. López-Reyes, A. García-Ortega, A. Torrents et al., "Pulmonary venous thrombosis secondary to radiofrequency ablation of the pulmonary veins," *Respiratory Medicine Case Reports*, vol. 23, pp. 46–48, 2018.

[9] S. Spadaro, S. Saturni, D. Cadorin et al., "An unusual case of acute respiratory failure in a patient with pulmonary veins stenosis late after catheter ablation of atrial fibrillation: a case report and the review of the literature," *BMC Pulmonary Medicine*, vol. 15, no. 1, 2015.

[10] C.-M. Lo, H.-I. Lu, Y.-Y. Chen, and J.-P. Chang, "Thoracoscopic lobectomy for pulmonary vein occlusion after radiofrequency catheter ablation of atrial fibrillation," *Journal of Cardiothoracic Surgery*, vol. 11, no. 1, 2016.

20

Lymphomatoid Granulomatosis in a Patient with Chronic Lymphocytic Leukemia and Rapidly Progressing Peribronchovascular Pulmonary Infiltrates

Shahab Rezvani,[1] Marie Tominna,[1] Sayf Al-Katib,[1] Marc D. Smith,[2] Craig Cousineau,[2] and Ayad Al-Katib[3]

[1]*Beaumont Health, Oakland University William Beaumont School of Medicine, Department of Diagnostic Radiology and Molecular Imaging, 3601 W 13 Mile Rd, Royal Oak, MI 48073, USA*
[2]*Beaumont Health, Oakland University William Beaumont School of Medicine, Department of Clinical Pathology, 3601 W 13 Mile Rd, Royal Oak, MI 48073, USA*
[3]*Wayne State University School of Medicine, Lymphoma Research Laboratory, 540 E Canfield Room No. 8829, Detroit, MI 48202, USA*

Correspondence should be addressed to Shahab Rezvani; shahab.rezvani@beaumont.edu

Academic Editor: Akif Turna

Lymphomatoid granulomatosis (LG) is an EBV-associated angiodestructive lymphoproliferative disease with multiorgan involvement that predominantly affects the lungs. We present a case of a 72-year-old man with a history of chronic lymphocytic leukemia who presented with upper respiratory symptoms and multiple erythematous skin papules. Chest CT showed ill-defined, irregular solid pulmonary nodules with peripheral ground-glass opacities in a peribronchovascular distribution. The differential for this pattern of lung disease is vast which includes but is not limited to infection, vasculitis, sarcoidosis, lymphoma, and Kaposi sarcoma. Subsequent PET/CT showed rapid progression of lung opacities and marked FDG uptake of pulmonary opacities and skin nodules, which raised the question of Richter syndrome. Wedge biopsy under video-assisted thoracoscopic surgery was performed. Pathology showed an extensive lymphoid infiltrate involving lymphatic and bronchovascular bundles and consisting of a mixture of large lymphocytes and inflammatory cells. Special stains showed that the large lymphocytes expressed B-cell markers and EBV virus. Overall, the findings were consistent with LG.

1. Case

A 72-year-old male with a long standing history of chronic lymphocytic leukemia (CLL) presented with upper respiratory symptoms including mild productive cough and dyspnea. An outpatient chest CT showed innumerable bilateral ill-defined solid pulmonary nodules in a peribronchovascular distribution, which were new from a prior scan 6 months earlier (Figure 1). Many of the lesions had a peripheral ground-glass halo. Nonenlarged mediastinal and bilateral axillary lymph nodes were suspected to be related to the patient's history of CLL. The pulmonary nodules were not a typical manifestation of CLL and other etiologies were considered such as atypical pulmonary infection, sarcoidosis, Kaposi sarcoma, and metastasis, even though patient had no other known malignancy. He was treated with antibiotics and steroids for his symptoms; however there was progressive clinical decline over several weeks and thus the patient was admitted for further work-up.

At the time of admission, vital signs showed exertional hypoxia, mild tachycardia in the low 100's, and a fever up to 102.4, which raised the concern for an infection and septic emboli. However, there were no significant pulmonary findings on exam. Skin examination revealed erythematous/purple skin papules on both lower extremities which broadened the differential to also include autoimmune and vascular etiologies.

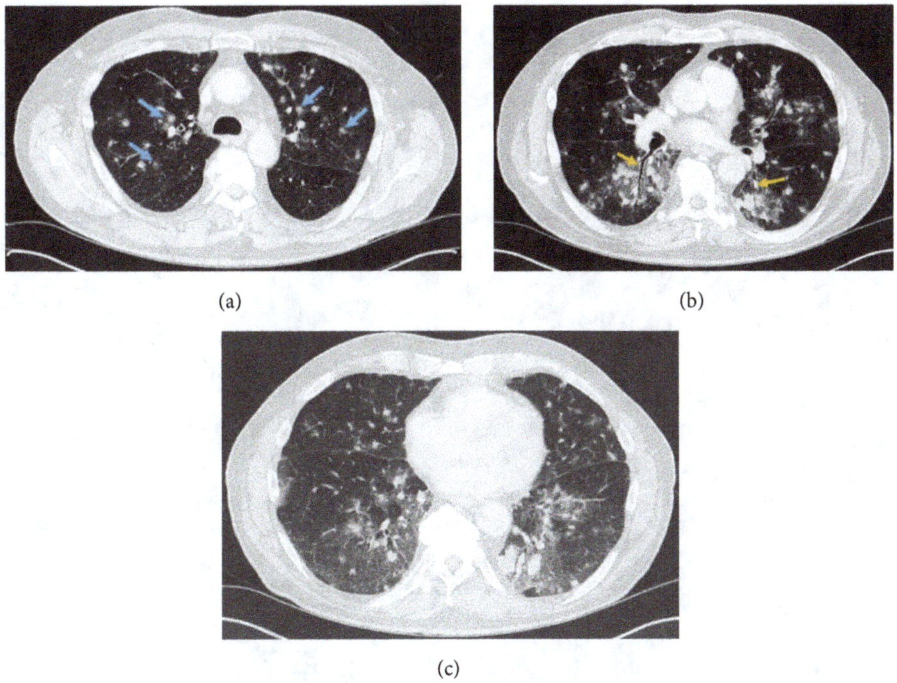

FIGURE 1: Axial lung window CT slices (a, b, c) at different levels demonstrate innumerable ill-defined solid nodules with peripheral ground-glass halos in a peribronchovascular distribution (blue arrows) and more prominent in the left lung. Air-bronchograms were seen (orange arrows).

Aside from normocytic anemia (Hb 11.6 mg/dL), initial laboratory evaluation with CBC and BMP showed no significant abnormalities. IgG levels were low. Blood and sputum cultures were negative. QuantiFERON was negative for tuberculosis. Serologies for aspergillus, blastomycosis, coccidioides, cryptococcus, histoplasma, HIV, and toxoplasma were negative. Bronchoalveolar lavage was negative for acid-fast bacilli, fungal organisms, and pneumocystis.

Immunologic evaluation was negative for ANCA, proteinase 3, and myeloperoxidase antibodies. This excluded granulomatosis with polyangiitis as a differential diagnosis. Bronchoalveolar lavage was negative for cytology.

Punch biopsy of one of the skin lesions demonstrated poorly circumscribed granulomas surrounding blood vessels and skin appendages, mild lymphocytic infiltration with no features to suggest cutaneous lymphoma, and no evidence of leukocytoclastic vasculitis. Stains for fungal and acid-fast bacilli were negative.

Left upper and lower lobe wedge biopsies of the nodules were taken through video-assisted thoracoscopic surgery (VATS) as the diagnosis was still unclear. The biopsies revealed EBV-positive DLBCL with features of LG grade 3 (Figure 2). The features that favor LG over DLBCL include a background that consisted predominantly of inflammatory cells with a minority of large B-cells and vascular invasion. In addition, lung involvement and EBV positivity are not exclusive to LG, but are almost always present in LG [1]. Flow cytometry did not detect the large B-cells which are sometimes too fragile to survive flow cytometric processing, but did detect rare, small monoclonal B-cells with a CLL/small lymphocytic lymphoma (SLL) phenotype. The flow cytometric findings are compatible with the morphology as no significant CLL/SLL population could be identified with CD5 and CD23 immunostaining (Figure 3). In this case, the source of rare CLL cells is likely peripheral blood, either physiologically through the inflammatory response or contamination during resection. Features of secondary organizing pneumonia were also present.

The patient underwent PET-CT 4 weeks following the initial chest CT (Figure 4). This showed significant progression and confluence of bilateral peribronchovascular lung opacities. The lung opacities had diffuse FDG uptake with a maximum SUV of 22.3. The PET/CT also demonstrated intense uptake in the cutaneous lesions of the lower extremities.

Bone marrow biopsy was consistent with hypercellular marrow with 20-30% marrow involvement by CLL/SLL cells. The patient was started on R-CHOP chemotherapy with Neupogen support. IVIG was also given for hypogammaglobulinemia.

2. Discussion

Lymphomatoid granulomatous (LG) is a rare EBV-associated B-cell lymphoproliferative disease with multiorgan involvement. It is most prevalent in men in the 4th through 6th decades [2]. The angiocentric and angiodestructive properties of lymphomatoid granulomatosis described by Liebow et al. are the hallmark of the disease [3]. LG can produce a spectrum of changes from inflammatory vasculitis

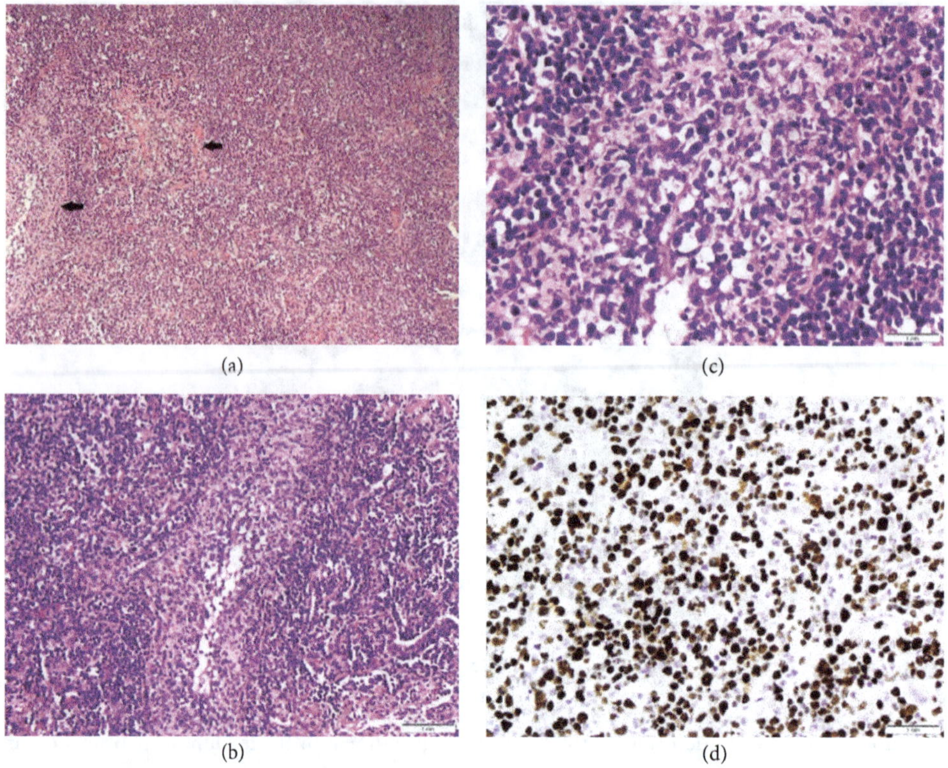

FIGURE 2: Low power section (a) from lung biopsy showing a diffuse neoplastic lymphoid cells (arrows) infiltrating the lymphatic and bronchovascular bundles. (H&E, 100x) Medium power view (b) showing neoplastic cells involving walls of pulmonary vessels. Small, reactive lymphocytes are seen in the background. (H&E, 200x) High power view (c) shows large, atypical B-cells with irregular nuclear membranes, open chromatin, and prominent nucleoli invading vessel walls (angioinvasion). (H&E, 500x) The neoplastic B-cells were positive for EBV (d).

to malignant lymphoma [4]. The diagnosis is made by a histologic triad of nodular polymorphic lymphoid infiltrates, angiitis, and granulomatosis [5]. The histologic grading scale ranges from 1-3 and is based on the degree of cytologic atypia and necrosis, and the number of EBV-positive cells correlates with the grade [2].

The lungs are affected in nearly all cases. Most patients will have symptoms of cough and dyspnea but can also have sputum production or hemoptysis. The predominant radiologic feature in LG is pulmonary nodules with irregular margins in a peribronchovascular distribution [6, 7]. The nodules may appear as diffuse infiltrates versus masses or areas of consolidation. Cavitation or necrosis can occur due to the angiodestructive properties [2]. A peripheral ground-glass halo and air-bronchograms have been reported with the pulmonary lesions, which were evident in our case. On PET-CT, the pulmonary lesions will be FDG-avid [8].

A pleural effusion may be present. Our case demonstrated nonenlarged mediastinal and axillary nodes, all of which were not FDG-avid and likely relate to underlying CLL. Lymph nodes, spleen, and bone marrow are not typically involved until later in the course of the disease, which differs from typical cases of lymphoma. Approximately 45% of individuals with LG have skin involvement such as patchy painful lesions or nodules that may ulcerate. CNS lesions are seen in 25-35% of cases and can present as a mass lesion or as various neurologic-type symptoms such as altered mental status or seizure [2]. Renal and liver involvement have been reported in autopsy cases although clinically significant disease is rare.

LG can be included in a long radiologic differential which often but not always includes pneumonia, malignant lymphoma, pseudolymphoma, lymphocytic interstitial pneumonia, metastasis, cryptogenic organizing pneumonia, granulomatosis with polyangiitis, and sarcoidosis. Wegener's granulomatosis is one of the mimickers of this diagnosis as it shares many features with LG including pulmonary nodules with cavitation or peripheral ground-glass halo, skin involvement, and renal involvement. The differential should also include other etiologies of cavitating lung nodules such as septic emboli. One may include sarcoidosis and Kaposi sarcoma in the differential given the peribronchovascular distribution of nodules.

Both CLL and LG are independently known to be associated with suppressed immunity, as evidenced in this case with hypogammaglobulinemia [9]. It is possible that the patient's history of CLL and immune suppression could be a risk factor for the development of LG.

CLL is known as an indolent type of lymphoma and should not demonstrate FDG activity. However, increased metabolic activity will occur in cases of Richter transformation, especially if the max SUV is greater than 5 [10]. The FDG negative mediastinal and axillary lymph nodes support the conclusion that the lymph nodes on CT are of CLL nature, as DLBCL of any subtype is FDG-avid.

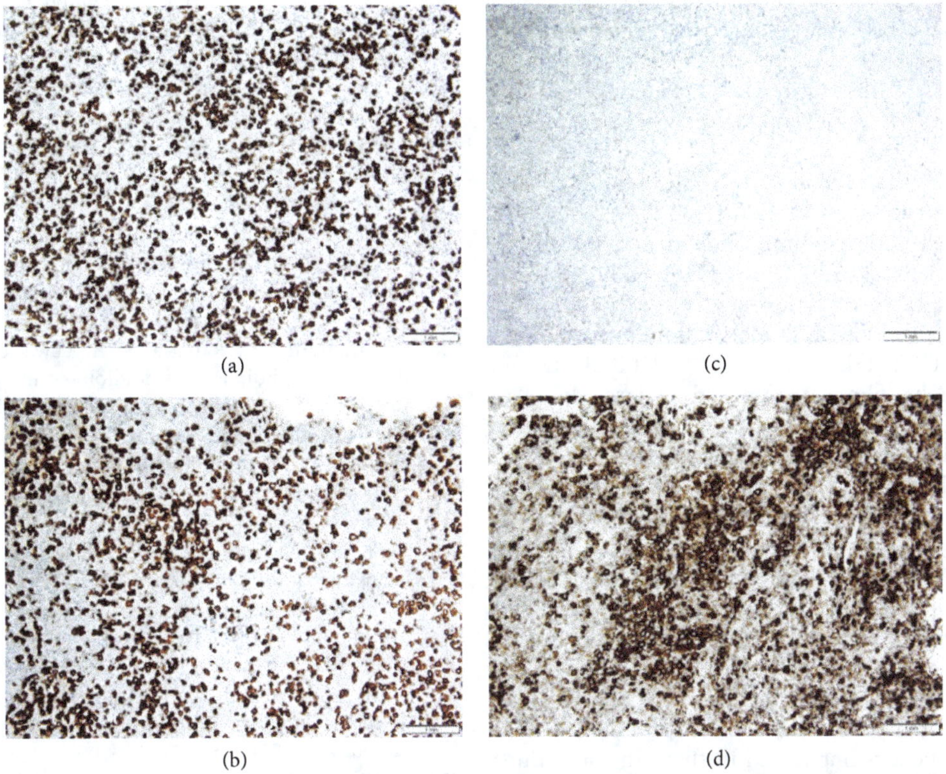

FIGURE 3: Immunostaining for CD3 (a) and CD5 (b) highlights background small, reactive T-cells. The large, atypical B-cells are negative. The large neoplastic B-cells are negative for CD5 and CD23 (c). CD20 is positive in large, atypical B-cells (d). The background small lymphocytes (reactive T-cells) are negative. The overall immunostaining pattern excludes both EBV+ CLL and EBV+ T-cell lymphoma as possible diagnoses.

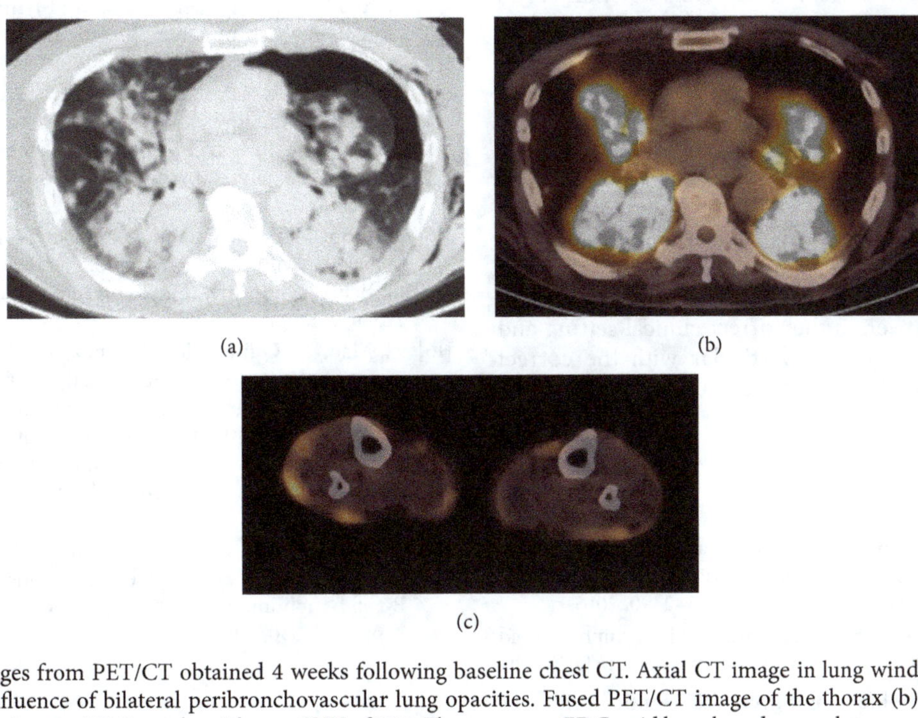

FIGURE 4: Axial images from PET/CT obtained 4 weeks following baseline chest CT. Axial CT image in lung windows (a) shows marked progression and confluence of bilateral peribronchovascular lung opacities. Fused PET/CT image of the thorax (b) shows the pulmonary abnormalities to have intense FDG uptake with max SUV of 22.3. There were no FDG-avid lymph nodes or splenomegaly. Left pneumothorax and subcutaneous emphysema were a result of the patient's recent VATS biopsy. Axial fused image of the lower extremities (c) shows FDG uptake within multiple subcutaneous nodules.

Lung nodules have a very low chance of being malignant if there is no uptake. There is a positive predictive value for malignancy of 90% if the SUV is above 2.5, and 80% if SUV is between 1.5 and 2.0 [11]. The highly FDG-avid lung lesions in our case with a max SUV of 22.3 support an aggressive tumor such as DLBCL.

Whether LG represents Richter syndrome or not is debatable. A minority of patients with CLL (2-10%) will develop a more aggressive second lymphoid malignancy, including prolymphocytic leukemia, DLBCL, and Hodgkin lymphoma [12–14]. Classically, Richter syndrome is associated with DLBCL, likely because DLBCL is most common histologic transformation of CLL [15]. But, similar to DLBCL, LG is a more aggressive lymphoma composed of large B-cells. The distinction between DLBCL and LG lies in the latter's characteristic localization (lung in>90%), histologic features (angiodestructive lesions in an inflammatory background), and EBV positivity [1]. DLBCL can also show any one of these features, but not as consistently as LG.

It is tempting to employ molecular studies to establish a clonal relationship between the LG and CLL in this case; however this has not been a requirement for the diagnosis of Richter syndrome. In fact, one study showed that 22% of patients with Richter syndrome had DLBCL and CLL components that were clonally unrelated [16].

Molecular risk factors implicated in the transformation of CLL to RS include germline genetic characteristics (BCL-2 GG genotype, CD38 GG genotype, and LRP4 TT genotype), biologic characteristics of CLL (unmutated IGHV, stereotyped B-cell receptors, telomere length less than 5000 base pairs, and the positive expression of CD38, CD49d and ZAP-70), somatic genetic events (CDKN2A deletion, TP53 disruption, C-myc activation, trisomy 12, Notch-1 mutation, and heterogenous genomic aberrations), disease stage, and possibly the type of CLL therapy. It is unclear if any of these risk factors played a role in this case [17].

Comparison of immunoglobulin gene rearrangements was not performed in this patient; however this would have no effect on diagnosis or treatment, as secondary aggressive lymphomas in these patients are typically treated like de novo malignancies.

The ability to diagnose LG strictly from radiologic findings is unlikely. However, in the correct clinical setting and in an EBV-positive patient in particular with the correct radiographic findings, it is a differential which should be considered.

References

[1] S. H. Swerdlow, E. Campo, S. A. Pileri et al., "The 2016 revision of the World Health Organization classification of lymphoid neoplasms," *Blood*, vol. 127, no. 20, pp. 2375–2390, 2016.

[2] R. Fernandez, E. Gonzalez, A. Fernandez et al., "Lymphomatoid Granulomatosis of Central Nervous System and Lung Driven by Epstein Barr Virus Proliferation: Successful Treatment with Rituximab," *Mediterranean Journal of Hematology and Infectious Diseases*, vol. 6, no. 1, Article ID e2014017, 2014.

[3] A. A. Liebow, C. R. B. Carrington, and P. J. Friedman, "Lymphomatoid granulomatosis," *Human Pathology*, vol. 3, no. 4, pp. 457–558, 1972.

[4] E. S. Jaffe and W. H. Wilson, "Lymphomatoid granulomatosis: Pathogenesis, pathology and clinical implications," *Cancer Surveys*, vol. 30, pp. 233–248, 1997.

[5] A. Ataya and E. Harman, *Rare and Interesting Cases in Pulmonary Medicine*, Academic Press, 2017.

[6] P. Hicken, J. C. Dobie, and E. Frew, "The radiology of lymphomatoid granulomatosis in the lung," *Clinical Radiology*, vol. 30, no. 6, pp. 661–664, 1979.

[7] J. S. Lee, R. Tuder, and D. A. Lynch, "Lymphomatoid granulomatosis: Radiologic features and pathologic correlations," *American Journal of Roentgenology*, vol. 175, no. 5, pp. 1335–1339, 2000.

[8] A. Sirajuddin, K. Raparia, V. A. Lewis et al., "Primary pulmonary lymphoid lesions: Radiologic and pathologic findings," *RadioGraphics*, vol. 36, no. 1, pp. 53–70, 2016.

[9] P. P. Sordillo, B. Epremian, B. Koziner, M. Lacher, and P. Lieberman, "Lymphomatoid granulomatosis. An analysis of clinical and immunologic characteristics," *Cancer*, vol. 49, no. 10, pp. 2070–2076, 1982.

[10] F. Shaikh, A. Janjua, F. Van Gestel, and A. Ahmad, "Richter Transformation of Chronic Lymphocytic Leukemia: A Review of Fluorodeoxyglucose Positron Emission Tomography–Computed Tomography and Molecular Diagnostics," *Cureus*, vol. 9, no. 1, Article ID e968, 2017.

[11] F. A. Mettler and M. J. Guiberteau, *Essentials of Nuclear Medicine Imaging*, Saunders/Elsevier, Philadelphia, Pa, USA, 5th edition, 2006.

[12] J. V. Melo, D. Catovsky, and D. A. G. Galton, "The relationship between chronic lymphocytic leukaemia and prolymphocytic leukaemia: II. patterns of evolution of 'prolymphocytoid' transformation," *British Journal of Haematology*, vol. 64, no. 1, pp. 77–86, 1986.

[13] K. Maddocks-Christianson, S. L. Slager, C. S. Zent et al., "Risk factors for development of a second lymphoid malignancy in patients with chronic lymphocytic leukaemia," *British Journal of Haematology*, vol. 139, no. 3, pp. 398–404, 2007.

[14] M. Solh, K. R. Rai, B. L. Peterson et al., "The impact of initial fludarabine therapy on transformation to Richter syndrome or prolymphocytic leukemia in patients with chronic lymphocytic leukemia: Analysis of an intergroup trial (CALGB 9011)," *Leukemia & Lymphoma*, vol. 54, no. 2, pp. 252–254, 2013.

[15] G. Fabbri, H. Khiabanian, A. B. Holmes et al., "Genetic lesions associated with chronic lymphocytic leukemia transformation to Richter syndrome," *The Journal of Experimental Medicine*, vol. 210, no. 11, pp. 2273–2288, 2013.

[16] Z. Mao, L. Quintanilla-Martinez, M. Raffeld et al., "IgVH mutational status and clonality analysis of Richter's transformation: Diffuse large B-cell lymphoma and hodgkin lymphoma in association with B-cell chronic lymphocytic leukemia (B-CLL) represent 2 different pathways of disease evolution," *The American Journal of Surgical Pathology*, vol. 31, no. 10, pp. 1605–1614, 2007.

[17] B. Timár, Z. Fülöp, B. Csernus et al., "Relationship between the mutational status of VH genes and pathogenesis of diffuse large B-cell lymphoma in Richter's syndrome," *Leukemia*, vol. 18, no. 2, pp. 326–330, 2004.

21

ECG Abnormalities in Patients with Acute Exacerbation of Bronchiectasis and Factors Associated with High Probability of Abnormality

Fatima Alhamed Alduihi

Department of Internal Medicine, Aleppo University, Aleppo, Syria

Correspondence should be addressed to Fatima Alhamed Alduihi; dr.duihi88@hotmail.com

Academic Editor: Yongchun Shen

Background. Bronchiectasis is an important reason for morbidity and mortality according to the last records that referred to high incidence rate of disease. Cardiovascular problems are common in pulmonary diseases, in general, and it can symptom by ECG abnormalities. The objective of this study was to define the most ECG abnormalities in patients with acute exacerbation of bronchiectasis and to study the correlation between the cardiac disorder and the other risk factors of the exacerbation. *Materials and Methods.* A prospective single-center observational cohort study was done at Aleppo University Hospital for patients with AEB between October 2017 and September 2018. They were divided into 2 groups (normal ECG vs. abnormal). Patients with COPD, cystic fibrosis, new diagnosis of ischemic accident through the last 6 months of the study, and treatment with macrolides or fluoroquinolones through the last 3 months of the study were excluded. We study the percent of abnormalities through the AEB and the percentage of the most common abnormalities. *Results.* 67 patients were included in the study (44 males and 23 females) with a mean age of 52.85 ± 21.456. ECG abnormalities were recorded in 43 patients, and it was more common in men (67.44% of cases). Advanced age and survival state had a statistical significance ($p = 0.003$, 0.023), respectively, between the 2 groups. Right axis deviation (RAD) is the most common abnormality (23.3%) followed by sinus tachycardia (20.9%), and it is close to T-depression (18.6%). AF was the most common arrhythmia from all recorded arrhythmias (6.98% from all cases). Positive sputum cultures were recorded in 55.8%, and the most common isolated pathogen factor was *Pseudomonas aeruginosa.* Recurrent pneumonia was seen in 30.2% of all patients with abnormal ECG. We find a high prevalence of ECG abnormalities in patients with Oximetry (90-95%, 39.5%), and the opportunity for abnormalities is equal in the 2 age groups (45–59 and more than 75) that reflexed the possibility of cardiac disorders in any age in patients with AEB. *Conclusions.* ECG abnormalities are common in AEB, and it can happen in any age and any value of Oximetry. It needs more attention because of the prognosis of the cardiac morbidity.

1. Introduction

Bronchiectasis is one of the most important reasons for attending the respiratory clinics.

Recent recodes refer to higher rates of prevalence in patients from all ages, and there is a notable peak on young ages [1–4].

The heart is the organ close to the lungs from anatomic side, so it will be affected by lesions that affected the lungs like COPD and bronchiectasis. This study is aimed at evaluating the function of the heart through bronchiectasis by performing a simple procedure which is usually applied to all patients admitted to hospital (electrocardiography (ECG)).

2. Patients and Methods

2.1. Patient Population. A prospective retrospective observational one-center study was applied to patients who were admitted with the diagnosis of acute exacerbation of bronchiectasis (AEB) in the period between October 2017 and September 2018 in Aleppo University Hospital, Aleppo, Syria.

They were divided into 2 groups (normal ECG and abnormal). Patients with COPD, cystic fibrosis, long treatment or treatment through the last 3 months with macrolide or fluoroquinolones, previous diagnosis of arrhythmia, and new ischemic accident (brain or cardiac infarction) through the last 6 months were excluded.

2.2. Data Collection. We reviewed and followed the patients' profiles and collected the following variables: demographics, smoking history, diagnosis of COPD or CF by a physician, sputum (and/or) tracheal cultures on admission, oxygen saturation on admission, medications, and morbidity.

The study is approved by the local ethical committee, and every patient agreed to continue participation in our study. Each patient gave his or her written consent for the collection and use of their clinical data.

2.3. Statistical Analysis. Demographic characteristics and variables of interest were summarized by the state of ECG (normal ECG vs. abnormal ECG) using descriptive statistics: mean (SD) for continuous variables and frequency (proportion) for categorical variables.

To assess the association between demographic characteristics and risk, logistic regression was used, and the results are reported as an odds ratio, with a 95% confidence interval.

A p value of less than 0.05 was used to detect the statistical significance. χ^2 is used as a test for statistical significance. Analysis was performed using IBM SPSS statistical software, V24.

3. Abbreviations Used in the Manuscript

The following abbreviations are used: ECG (electrocardiography), COPD (chronic obstructive pulmonary disease), CF (cystic fibrosis), RAD (right axis deviation), LAD (left axis deviation), LVH (left ventricle hypertrophy), HTN (hypertension), MAT (multifocal atrial tachycardia), PVC (premature ventricular complex), AEB (acute exacerbation of bronchiectasis), RBBB (right bundle-branch block), LBBB (left bundle-branch block), AF (atrial fibrillation), and AAA (acute asthma attack).

4. Results

67 patients were included in the study (44 males and 23 females) with a mean age of 52.85 ± 21.456 years old.

ECG abnormalities were recorded in 43 patients (64.17% of patients), and they were more common in men (29, 67.44% of all 43 cases).

Abnormal ECGs were recorded in patients with advanced age more than in younger ages. In a previous ischemic accident, cerebral or cardiac disorder was recorded in 20 cases (29.85%); 17 of them recorded abnormal ECGs (39.5%). Six of them have ages less than 60 years and 14 have ages more than 60 years.

Mean Oximetry (oxygen saturation) was 87.81 ± 10.123%, and it had higher values in patients with normal ECG.

40 patients were smokers (59.7%): 12 of them have normal ECG (30% of all smokers), and 28 of them have abnormal ECG (70%).

13 patients died through one year of follow-up; only one of them has normal ECG, while 12 have abnormal ECG. The mean age of dead patients was 68.15 years: the oldest one was 99 years old, and the youngest was 15 years old.

Positive sputum cultures were recorded in 42 patients (62.68% of all cases); 24 of them (55.8%) had abnormal ECG, and 8 (33.33%) of them showed *Pseudomonas aeruginosa* in the result of culture, the most isolated pathogen from all the positive cultures.

Recurrent pneumonia was the most common trigger factor of exacerbation in 23 patients (34.32%). 30.2% of the patients with abnormal ECG had recurrent pneumonia.

Pleural effusions were seen only in patients with abnormal ECGs (4 patients) and also autoimmune diseases (5 cases, 4 abnormal, and 1 normal).

Bronchitis was investigated in 7 patients (10.44%); 5 of them had normal ECG, while 2 had abnormal ECG.

Increased dyspnea was a stable variant in 65 patients (97% of all patients in the study); it was seen in all patients with normal ECG and in 41 patients with abnormal ECG.

Demographic characteristics and both the likelihood ratio and p value were calculated and are summarized in Table 1.

Right axis deviation (RAD) was the most common abnormality in 23.3% of cases followed by sinus tachycardia (20.9%), and it is close to T-depression (18.6%).

Both the left axis deviation (LAD) and left ventricle hypertrophy (LVH) recorded the same percent (4.7%) which reflexes the morbidity of hypertension (HTN) in such patients.

Less frequent abnormality was recorded equally for multifocal atrial tachycardia (MAT) and premature ventricular complex (PVCs) (2% for every abnormality).

Figure 1 shows the most common ECG abnormalities in patients who were included in our study with their percent of each abnormality.

What was really abnormal was a high prevalence of ECG abnormalities which was recorded in patients with oxygen saturation (90-95%, 39.5%), and the opportunity for abnormalities is equal in the 2 age groups (45–59 and more than 75), which reflexed the possibility of cardiac disorders in any age and in any value of saturation in patients with acute exacerbation of bronchiectasis (AEB).

Mortality, confirmed previous ischemic accident, and age had a statistical significance ($p = 0.023$, 0.025, and 0.003), respectively.

Figure 2 shows the graphs of the most common abnormalities according to the age.

5. Studying the Risk Estimate

To assess the association between demographic characteristics and risk of developing abnormal ECG, logistic regression

Table 1: Demographic characteristics for the patients of the study.

	All (*N*: 67)	Normal ECG (*N*: 24)	Abnormal ECG (*N*: 43)	Likelihood ratio	*p* value
Gender					
Male	44 (65.67%)	15 (62.5%)	29 (67.44%)	0.166	0.79
Female	23 (34.33%)	9 (37.5%)	14 (32.65%)		
Smoking	40 (59.70%)	12 (50%)	28 (65.11%)	1.454	0.3
Mortality (1 year)	13 (19.69%)	1 (4.16%)	12 (27.90%)	6.698	0.023
Previous ischemic accident	20 (29.85%)	3 (12.5%)	17 (39.53%)	5.888	0.025
Increased dyspnea	65 (62.68%)	24 (100%)	41 (95.34%)	1.808	0.533
Age (years)	52.85 ± 21.456.	43.33 ± 20.599	59.3 ± 19.939	45.46	0.003
Positive cultures	42 (62.68%)	18 (75%)	24 (55.81%)	2.501	0.187
Oximetry (%)	87.81 ± 10.123	90.38 ± 7.347	86.09 ± 11.196	8.758	0.227
Trigger factors					
AAA	6 (8.95%)	2 (8.33%)	4 (9.30%)	15.656	0.113
Recurrent pneumonia	23 (34.32%)	10 (41.66%)	13 (30.23%)		
Pleural effusion	4 (5.97%)	0	4 (9.30%)		
Autoimmune	5 (7.46%)	1 (4.16%)	4 (9.30%)		
Abscess	2 (2.98%)	1 (4.16%)	1 (2.32%)		
Exposure	6 (8.95%)	4 (16.66%)	2 (4.65%)		
Bronchitis	7 (10.44%)	5 (20.83%)	2 (4.65%)		
Another	14 (20.89%)	3 (12.5%)	11 (25.58%)		

p value of less than 0.05 was used to detect the statistical significance, and χ^2 is used as a test for statistical significance.

was used, and the results were reported as an odds ratio, with a 95% confidence interval.

We divided patients according to age (less than 60 years and more than 60 to be more accurate regarding the age, and we did not find an important statistical significance). We also studied the oxygen saturation between 2 values (less than 92% and more than 92%).

The odds ratios for the variants are printed on Table 2.

6. Discussion

The study highlighted the fact of the correlation between bronchiectasis and ECG abnormalities, as they were found in most of the patients with a high rate of 64.17%.

Cardiac disorders are common in respiratory disease in general and especially in chronic lung diseases [5]. There were many records about the increased risk of cardiovascular diseases in patients with bronchiectasis [6, 7].

The cardiac comorbidity can be a result of the disease itself because of anatomical correlation between the lung and the heart (as in the pulmonary hypertension for example) or because of the treatment of pulmonary diseases that may affect the heart; macrolides are used widely in the treatment of community-acquired pneumonia and bronchiectasis especially in cases of long-term treatment [8–10]. The fluoroquinolone group, another drug group used widely in the treatment of bacterial exacerbations of obstructive diseases, can increase the risk of arrhythmias [11–13].

ECG is a simple procedure. It can direct the physician or clinician to misdiagnosed cardiac comorbidity in patients with bronchiectasis or any other obstructive lung disease and hypertension in patients with marks of LVH on the ECG for example.

Male gender is a risk factor for developing abnormal ECG compared with women; however, there is no important statistical significance ($p = 0.79$) that refers the incidence of abnormalities as close between patients [14, 15]. Abnormal ECGs were more recorded in smokers, accepted in many studies in this field that confirmed the correlation between abnormalities and smoking [16, 17]. Mortality was higher between patients with abnormal ECGs, whose ages were advanced compared with those of young patients. This result confirmed the fact of the poor prognosis of patients with cardiac comorbidity compared with those who do not have this problem, especially in advanced ages. Age itself can be a risk factor for mortality in patients with AEB [1, 18, 19]. The likelihood ratio recorded the highest rate for age in our study (45.46). It suggested age as a reason for abnormalities by itself. It added another risk and enhanced the morbidity of the disease. Both cardiac morbidity and advanced age enhanced together the risk of mortality in such group of patients [20–22].

Oximetry (oxygen saturation) had high values in patients with normal ECG compared with those with abnormal ones, accepted in Kellett et al. [23] and Katz et al. [24], that suggested abnormalities in ECG as a result of hypoxemia in bronchoscopy, and it was so close to Romero and Jané's study [25] that suggested hypoxia as a reason for abnormalities in ECG. In a review, there were many studies suggesting hypoxia as a reason for ECG abnormalities in patients with obstructive pulmonary diseases [26, 27].

Dyspnea was a constant symptom in all patients, and there is no statistical significance between the 2 groups of

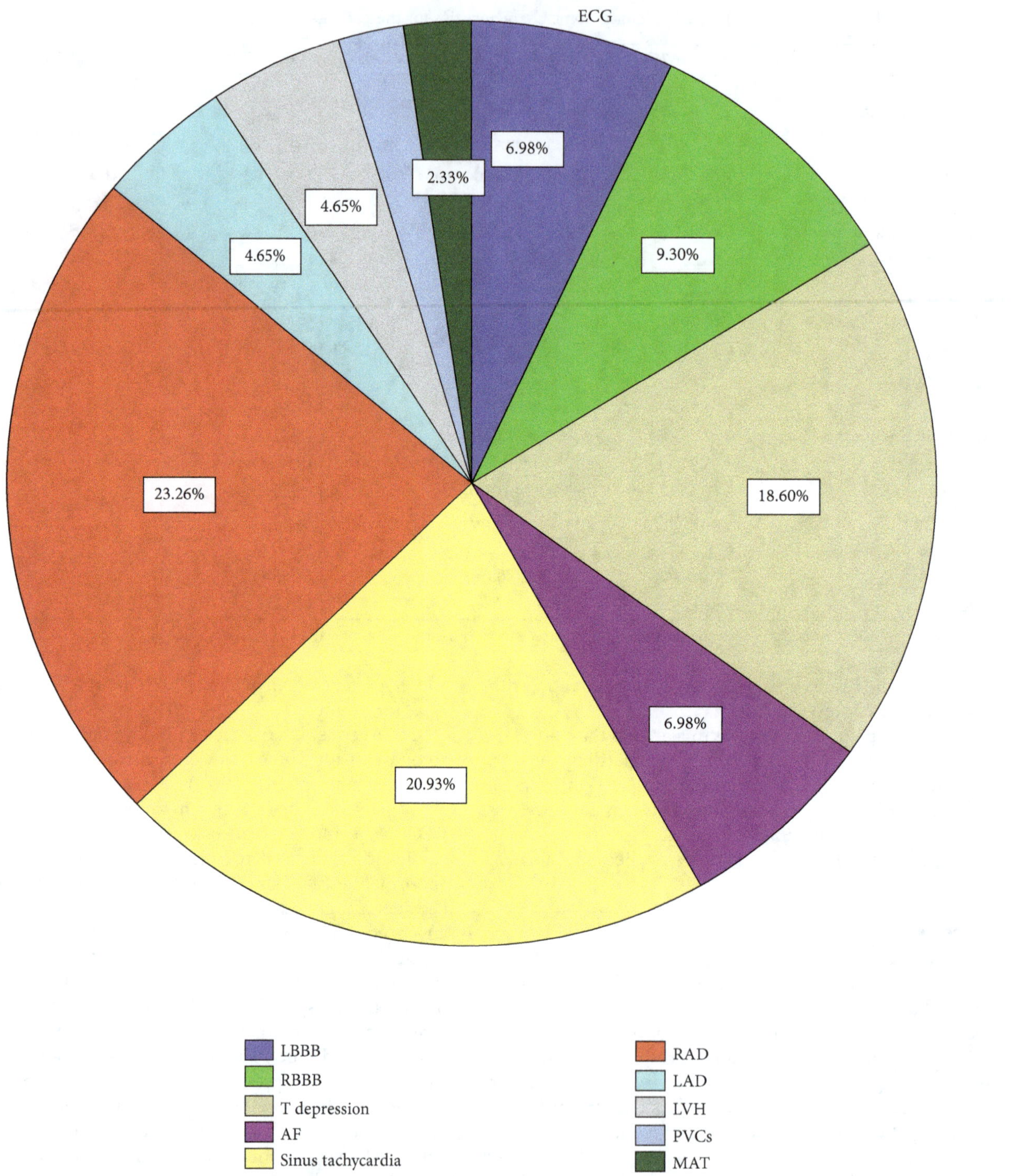

FIGURE 1: The most common ECG abnormalities in patients included in our study with their percent of each abnormality.

patients even though it had more risk to develop abnormalities on ECG (odds ratio, 1.585). Increased dyspnea had a likelihood of 1.808 for developing abnormal ECGs. Dyspnea can cause abnormalities in cases that lead to a metabolic acidosis [28]. Dyspnea induced by exercise in children and adolescents usually made a tachycardia, sinus, or ventricle [29, 30]. Our study showed that dyspnea was found in all patients with no differences between the 2 groups of study, normal and abnormal ECG. Nine patients with dyspnea had sinus tachycardia as the most common abnormality in the group of abnormal and also RAD.

Recurrent pneumonia triggers the exacerbation of bronchiectasis in 23 patients (34.32% of all cases, 30% of the abnormal ECG group), which confirms the etiology (postinfections) as a most common etiology in bronchiectasis [31].

Positive isolated cultures were more common in the group of abnormal ECGs, but there are no differences between the 2 groups. *Pseudomonas aeruginosa* was the most

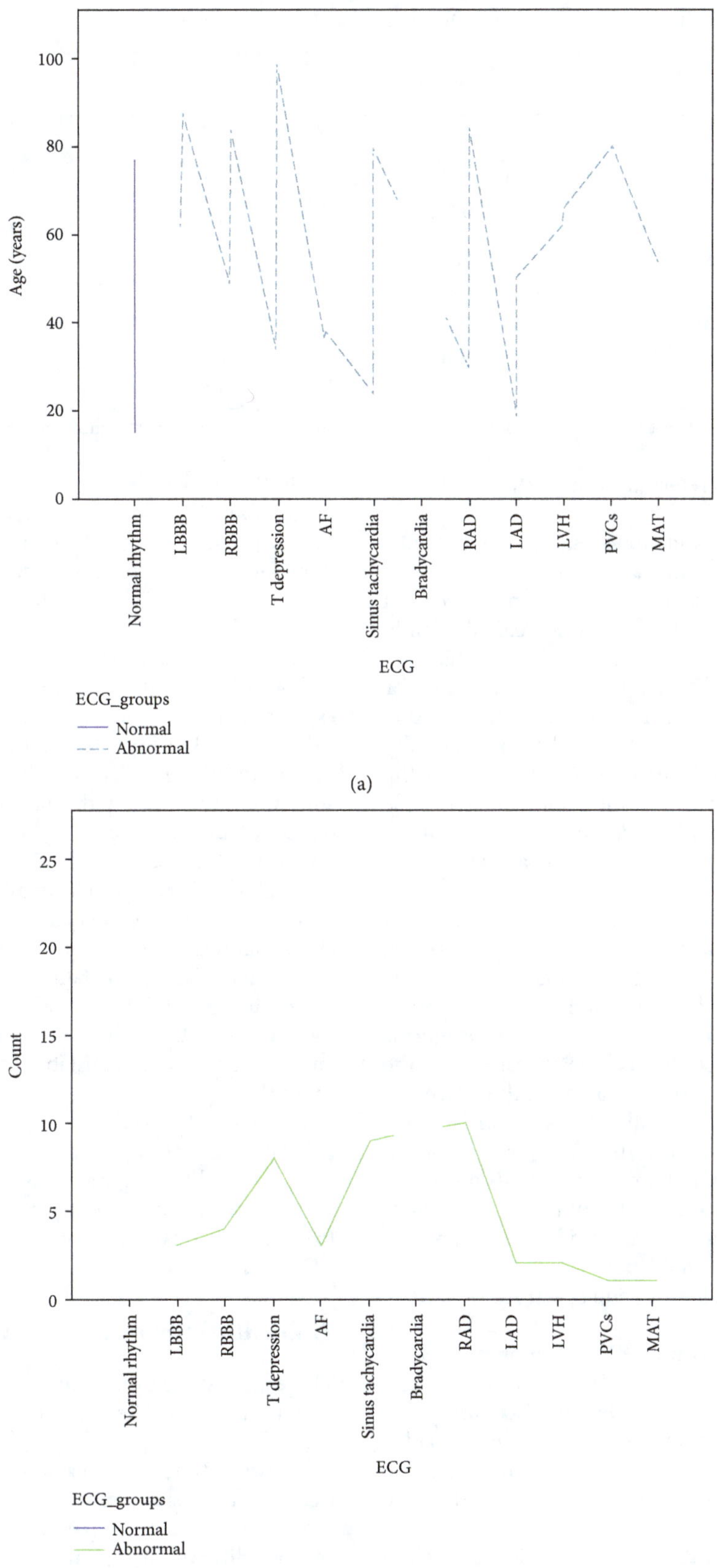

FIGURE 2: ECG records of the patients of study. (a) ECG changes according to the age. (b) ECG changes in all cases. MAT: multifocal atrial tachycardia; PVCs: premature ventricular contractions; LVH: left ventricle hypertrophy; LAD: left axis deviation; RAD: right axis deviation; AF: atrial fibrillation; RBBB: right bundle branch block; LBBB: left bundle branch block.

Table 2: Risk estimate in the study.

Variant	p value	Odd ratio	Confidence interval (95%) Low	Upper
Gender (man/women)	0.79	1.083	0.733	1.600
Smoking (smoking/nonsmoking)	0.3	1.260	0.850	1.868
Mortality (nonsurvivor/survivor)	0.023	1.329 0.149	1.084 0.021	1.630 1.097
Previous ischemic accident (yes/no)	0.025	1.564	1.133	2.159
Dyspnea (increased)	0.533	1.585	1.316	1.909
Age (less than 60/more than 60)	0.072	0.707	0.501	0.999
Oximetry (less than 92/more than 92)	0.109	1.422	0.900	2.247
Positive cultures (yes/no)	0.187	0.752	0.534	1.059

p value of less than 0.05 was used to detect the statistical significance, and χ^2 is used as a test for statistical significance.

common isolated pathogens referred by most studies all over the world [32–35].

RAD is the most common abnormality (10 patients, 23.3%); 9 of them 90% had dyspnea.

Right bundle-branch block (RBBB) had been recorded in 9.30% (4 patients). These abnormalities correlated mainly with disorders in the function of the right ventricle that carried a specific importance to have a right catheterization for pulmonary hypertension diagnosis after echocardiography was not enough in such patients [36, 37]. Another specialty of RAD is the correlation with the cases of PCD, as it is the most ECG abnormality in patients with Kartagener disease [38–40]. Three of the patients included in the study had the diagnosis of Kartagener disease, and some had a dextrocardia and RAD on ECG.

Sinus tachycardia was recorded in 9 cases (20.9%), all of them had dyspnea, and it was very close to T-depression (8, 18.6%) which reflexed the role of infectious state on the ECG, as tachycardia is a result of infection and high temperature [41]. It carries a bad predictor of poor prognosis especially in patients with severe asthma in cases that the exacerbation of asthma was a trigger factor of the exacerbation of bronchiectasis [42]. As asthma was recorded in 6 patients (8.95% of all cases in the study), it was important to suspect a severe infection and a poor prognosis outcomes in patients with sinus tachycardia as postinfection (recurrent pneumonia), and exacerbations of asthma had a high prevalence between the patients of the study.

T wave depression is a sign of wide spectrum of cardiac and noncardiac disease [43, 44]. It can be a sign of ischemic accident (ischemic heart disease [45], pulmonary edema [46], and heart failure in athletes [47]). T wave depression had its importance because of the underlying ischemic etiology, and in our study, 6 patients of the 8 patients had a previous ischemic accident. That really confirmed the comorbidity of ischemic accidents and patients with acute exacerbation of bronchiectasis.

Hypoxia is an important reason for inversion of T wave [48]. Patients with acute respiratory alkalosis present more danger than those with chronic because they are more likely to develop metabolic compensation [49], and as a final result, a case of uncompensated acidosis can cause inversion in T wave [50, 51].

Both the left bundle-branch block (LBBB) and atrial fibrillation (AF) have a 6.98 percentage for each one. LBBB was suspected to be a risk factor for cardiovascular morbidity in patients with chronic obstructive pulmonary diseases [52], so that will be a risk factor for cardiac disorders in patients with overlap syndrome (bronchiectasis-COPD).

Atrial fibrillation was the most common recorded arrhythmia in patients with chronic pulmonary diseases, especially those associated with pulmonary hypertension [53] and COPD [54]. It was one of the important findings of the study even with excluded patients with COPD; AF is still on the top of arrhythmias in patients with acute exacerbation of bronchiectasis. Other arrhythmias were less frequent like MAT and PVCs (2.3% for each one).

A study of arrhythmias in all the included patients shows that they were recorded in only 5 cases (11.62% from all abnormalities), so it was not common in our study compared with other ECG abnormalities.

Both the left axis deviation (LAD) and left ventricle hypertrophy (LVH) had a 4.65 percentage, which is correlated with an increased high risk of hypertension comorbidity in these patients [55].

As COPD correlated with a lot of cardiac disorders [56–58] and was suspected as a risk factor for cardiovascular comorbidity in patients with emphysema [59, 60] and at last was recorded to have a high rate of arrhythmias [61, 62], it was important to exclude the patients with COPD from the study.

7. Limitations of the Study

There are a small number of patients compared with international studies, as there is no registry for bronchiectasis in Syria.

It was difficult to exclude all patients with previous ischemic accidents because of the fact that there is a high prevalence in elderly patients and those who had much comorbidity in our region.

We did not assess the severity of AEB according to faced or BSI scores because not all patients accepted had lung function diseases, and we could not depend only to the previous records; the severity of disease was assessed by advanced lesions on HRCT.

8. Strong Points

This was the first study to suggest ECG abnormalities as a predictor of cardiovascular morbidity in patients with acute exacerbation of bronchiectasis. Patients of COPD were excluded to be more accurate and definite to bronchiectasis without overlap syndrome with COPD.

9. Conclusions

ECG abnormalities are common in patients with acute exacerbation of bronchiectasis. It can happen in any age and any value of oxygen saturation (Oximetry). Advanced age and survival state had a statistical significance ($p = 0.003$ and 0.023), respectively, between the 2 groups.

Male gender, smoking, and increasing dyspnea are factors with more likely opportunity for developing abnormalities on ECG.

References

[1] F. A. Alduihi and A. Khoury, "Factors affecting readmitted patients with acute exacerbation of bronchiectasis," *The Egyptian Journal of Internal Medicine*, vol. 31, no. 4, pp. 779–782, 2019.

[2] A. Khoury and F. A. Alduihi, "O'Donnell criteria as a sign of bad prognosis in hospitalized patients with bronchiectasis," *Journal of the Arab Board of Health Specializations*, vol. 3, 2019.

[3] M. Loeve, K. Gerbrands, W. C. Hop, M. Rosenfeld, I. C. Hartmann, and H. A. Tiddens, "Bronchiectasis and pulmonary exacerbations in children and young adults with cystic fibrosis," *Chest*, vol. 140, no. 1, pp. 178–185, 2011.

[4] S. Ginde and M. G. Earing, "When the heart is not to blame: managing lung disease in adult congenital heart disease," *Progress in cardiovascular diseases*, vol. 61, no. 3-4, pp. 314–319, 2018.

[5] C. Jenkins, "Cardiovascular comorbidity in chronic lung disease: gender differences," in *Cardiac Considerations in Chronic Lung Disease*, pp. 25–43, Springer International Publishing, 2020.

[6] A. D. Saleh, B. Kwok, J. S. Brown, and J. R. Hurst, "Correlates and assessment of excess cardiovascular risk in bronchiectasis," *European Respiratory Journal*, vol. 50, no. 5, p. 1701127, 2017.

[7] S. Chen, A. Qiu, Z. Tao, and H. Zhang, "Clinical impact of cardiovascular disease on patients with bronchiectasis," *BMC Pulmonary Medicine*, vol. 20, no. 1, 2020.

[8] J. D. Chalmers, W. Boersma, M. Lonergan et al., "Long-term macrolide antibiotics for the treatment of bronchiectasis in adults: an individual participant data meta-analysis," *The Lancet Respiratory Medicine*, vol. 7, no. 10, pp. 845–854, 2019.

[9] C. Kelly, D. J. Evans, J. D. Chalmers et al., "Macrolide antibiotics for non-cystic fibrosis bronchiectasis," *The Cochrane Database of Systematic Reviews*, vol. 10, 2016.

[10] D. Wang, W. Fu, and J. Dai, "Meta-analysis of macrolide maintenance therapy for prevention of disease exacerbations in patients with noncystic fibrosis bronchiectasis," *Medicine*, vol. 98, no. 17, 2019.

[11] X. Liu, J. Ma, L. Huang et al., "Fluoroquinolones increase the risk of serious arrhythmias: a systematic review and meta-analysis," *Medicine*, vol. 96, no. 44, 2017.

[12] L. A. Polgreen, B. N. Riedle, J. E. Cavanaugh et al., "Estimated cardiac risk associated with macrolides and fluoroquinolones decreases substantially when adjusting for patient characteristics and comorbidities," *Journal of the American Heart Association*, vol. 7, no. 9, 2018.

[13] F. Amati, M. Di Pasquale, M. I. Restrepo, J. Marin-Corral, S. Aliberti, and F. Blasi, "Cardiovascular side-effects of common antibiotics," in *Cardiovascular Complications of Respiratory Disorders (ERS Monograph)*, M. A. Martínez-García, J. L. Pépin, and M. Cazzola, Eds., pp. 264–278, European Respiratory Society, Sheffield, 2020.

[14] M. P. Czubryt, L. Espira, L. Lamoureux, and B. Abrenica, "The role of sex in cardiac function and disease," *Canadian journal of physiology and pharmacology*, vol. 84, no. 1, pp. 93–109, 2006.

[15] H. T. Shih, C. R. Webb, W. A. Conway, E. Peterson, B. Tilley, and S. Goldstein, "Frequency and significance of cardiac arrhythmias in chronic obstructive lung disease," *Chest*, vol. 94, no. 1, pp. 44–48, 1988.

[16] N. K. Sharma, K. K. Jaiswal, S. R. Meena et al., "ECG changes in young healthy smokers: a simple and cost-effective method to assess cardiovascular risk according to pack-years of smoking," *Journal of The Association of Physicians of India*, vol. 65, 2017.

[17] D. Domala Prasad, A. Berad, and T. V. Sagar, "Study of ECG changes in smokers compared to non smokers," *Scholars International Journal of Anatomy and Physiology*, vol. 2, no. 1, pp. 37–40, 2019.

[18] J. D. Finklea, G. Khan, S. Thomas, J. Song, D. Myers, and A. C. Arroliga, "Predictors of mortality in hospitalized patients with acute exacerbation of bronchiectasis," *Respiratory Medicine*, vol. 104, no. 6, pp. 816–821, 2010.

[19] F. A. Alduihi and A. Khoury, "Mario warning sign for mortality in acute exacerbation of bronchiectasis," *European respiratory and pulmonary diseases*, vol. 5, no. 1, pp. 20-21, 2019.

[20] M. J. McDonnell, S. Aliberti, P. C. Goeminne et al., "Comorbidities and the risk of mortality in patients with bronchiectasis: an international multicentre cohort study," *The lancet Respiratory medicine*, vol. 4, no. 12, pp. 969–979, 2016.

[21] W. J. Guan, Y. H. Gao, D. de la Rosa-Carrillo, and M. Á. Martínez-García, "Cardiovascular implications in bronchiectasis," *Cardiovascular Complications of Respiratory Diseases*, vol. 88, p. 96, 2020.

[22] V. Navaratnam, A. A. Root, I. Douglas, L. Smeeth, R. B. Hubbard, and J. K. Quint, "Cardiovascular outcomes after a respiratory tract infection among adults with non–cystic fibrosis bronchiectasis: a general population–based study," *Annals of the American Thoracic Society*, vol. 15, no. 3, pp. 315–321, 2018.

[23] J. Kellett, B. Deane, and M. Gleeson, "Derivation and validation of a score based on Hypotension, Oxygen saturation, low Temperature, ECG changes and Loss of independence (HOTEL) that predicts early mortality between 15 min and 24 h after admission to an acute medical unit," *Resuscitation*, vol. 78, no. 1, pp. 52–58, 2008.

[24] A. S. Katz, E. L. Michelson, J. Stawicki, and F. D. Holford, "Cardiac arrhythmias frequency during fiberoptic bronchoscopy and correlation with hypoxemia," *Archives of internal medicine*, vol. 141, no. 5, pp. 603–606, 1981.

[25] D. Romero and R. Jané, "Hypoxia-induced effects on ECG depolarization by time warping analysis during recurrent obstructive apnea," in *2020 42nd Annual International Conference of the IEEE Engineering in Medicine & Biology Society (EMBC)*, pp. 2626–2629, Montreal, QC, Canada, 2020.

[26] Gong H Jr, D. P. Tashkin, E. Y. Lee, and M. S. Simmons, "Hypoxia-altitude simulation test: evaluation of patients with chronic airway obstruction," *American Review of Respiratory Disease*, vol. 130, no. 6, pp. 980–986, 1984.

[27] K. G. Rosen and I. Kjellmer, "Changes in the fetal heart rate and ECG during hypoxia," *Acta Physiologica Scandinavica*, vol. 93, no. 1, pp. 59–66, 1975.

[28] A. S. Olson, A. Messersmith, and M. Robinson, "The patient with dyspnea," *Electrocardiogram in Clinical Medicine*, vol. 5, pp. 219–228, 2020.

[29] R. Bhatia, M. Abu-Hasan, and M. Weinberger, "Exercise-induced dyspnea in children and adolescents: differential diagnosis," *Pediatric annals*, vol. 48, no. 3, pp. e121–e127, 2019.

[30] B. Kessen and K. Williamson, "The ECG in clinical medicine," *Electrocardiogram in Clinical Medicine*, vol. 5, 2020.

[31] M. A. Martinez-García, C. Villa, Y. Dobarganes et al., "RIBRON: the Spanish online bronchiectasis registry. Characterization of the first 1912 patients," *Archivos de Bronconeumología (English Edition)*, vol. 57, no. 1, pp. 28–35, 2021.

[32] K. Dimakou, C. Triantafillidou, M. Toumbis, K. Tsikritsaki, K. Malagari, and P. Bakakos, "Non CF-bronchiectasis: aetiologic approach, clinical, radiological, microbiological and functional profile in 277 patients," *Respiratory Medicine*, vol. 116, pp. 1–7, 2016.

[33] R. Dhar, S. Singh, D. Talwar et al., "Bronchiectasis in India: results from the European multicentre bronchiectasis audit and research collaboration (EMBARC) and respiratory research network of India registry," *The Lancet Global Health*, vol. 7, no. 9, pp. e1269–e1279, 2019.

[34] S. K. Visser, P. T. Bye, G. J. Fox et al., "Australian adults with bronchiectasis: the first report from the Australian Bronchiectasis Registry," *Respiratory Medicine*, vol. 155, pp. 97–103, 2019.

[35] J. Rademacher, F. C. Ringshausen, H. Suhling et al., "Lung transplantation for non-cystic fibrosis bronchiectasis," *Respiratory Medicine*, vol. 115, pp. 60–65, 2016.

[36] G. Kovacs, A. Avian, V. Foris et al., "Use of ECG and other simple non-invasive tools to assess pulmonary hypertension," *PLoS One*, vol. 11, no. 12, article e0168706, 2016.

[37] S. Igata, N. Tahara, Y. Sugiyama et al., "Utility of the amplitude of RV1+ SV5/6 in assessment of pulmonary hypertension," *PLoS One*, vol. 13, no. 11, article e0206856, 2018.

[38] B. Ghewade, S. Cladius, S. Chaudhari, and A. Bhake, "A case of Kartagener syndrome with pulmonary hypertension," *Journal of Medical Cases*, vol. 7, no. 8, pp. 326–330, 2016.

[39] T. Martínez-Fernández, Y. Rivera-Sánchez, and P. Sharma, "Pulmonology," in *Pediatric Board Study Guide: A Last Minute Review*, pp. 691–730, Springer, 2020.

[40] V. Selvaraj, "Kartageners syndrome," *University Journal of Medicine and Medical Specialities*, vol. 2, 2017.

[41] S. A. Shabtaie, C. M. Witt, and S. J. Asirvatham, "Natural history and clinical outcomes of inappropriate sinus tachycardia," *Journal of cardiovascular electrophysiology*, vol. 31, no. 1, pp. 137–143, 2020.

[42] A. A. Mohammed and H. K. Salih, "A study of electrocardiographic changes in asthmatic patients attending Kirkuk General Hospital," *Journal of Kirkuk Medical College*, vol. 6, no. 1, p. 18, 2018.

[43] A. K. Bhoi, K. S. Sherpa, B. Khandelwal, and P. K. Mallick, "T wave analysis: potential marker of arrhythmia and ischemia detection-a review," in *Cognitive Informatics and Soft Computing: Proceeding of CISC 2017*, pp. 121–130, Springer, 2019.

[44] A. Cardona, K. M. Zareba, H. N. Nagaraja et al., "T-wave abnormality as electrocardiographic signature of myocardial edema in non-ST-elevation acute coronary syndromes," *Journal of the American Heart Association*, vol. 7, no. 3, 2018.

[45] D. J. Dzikowicz and M. G. Carey, "Cardiac cases. Myocardial ischemic induced non-sustained ventricular tachycardia in an older adult with pneumonia," *Medsurg Nursing*, vol. 29, 2020.

[46] T. M. Reed, "Immersion pulmonary edema in the setting of Takotsubo cardiomyopathy," *International Cardiovascular Forum Journal*, vol. 5, 2016.

[47] D. Akdis, C. Brunckhorst, F. Duru, Department of Cardiology, University Heart Center, Zurich, Switzerland, Center for Integrative Human Physiology, University of Zurich, Switzerland, and A. M. Saguner, "Arrhythmogenic cardiomyopathy: electrical and structural phenotypes," *Arrhythmia & electrophysiology review*, vol. 5, no. 2, pp. 90–101, 2016.

[48] D. A. Monteiro, E. W. Taylor, D. J. McKenzie, F. T. Rantin, and A. L. Kalinin, "Interactive effects of mercury exposure and hypoxia on ECG patterns in two neotropical freshwater fish species: matrinxã, *Brycon amazonicus* and traíra, *Hoplias malabaricus*," *Ecotoxicology*, vol. 29, no. 4, pp. 375–388, 2020.

[49] R. A. Johnson, "A quick reference on respiratory alkalosis," *Veterinary Clinics: Small Animal Practice*, vol. 47, no. 2, pp. 181–184, 2017.

[50] G. F. Glass, A. Sudhir, and A. A. Pandit, "The ECG and metabolic abnormalities," *Electrocardiogram in Clinical Medicine*, vol. 5, pp. 307–313, 2020.

[51] E. Barkoudah and C. L. Roy, "The many shades of dyspnea," *The American journal of medicine*, vol. 131, no. 1, pp. e5–e6, 2018.

[52] B. Lazović, N. Jovičić, V. Radlović et al., "Electrocardiographic predictors of five years mortality in chronic obstructive pulmonary disease patients," *Srpski arhiv za celokupno lekarstvo*, vol. 149, 2021.

[53] C. A. Vahdatpour, J. J. Luebbert, and H. I. Palevsky, "Atrial arrhythmias in chronic lung disease-associated pulmonary hypertension," *Pulmonary Circulation*, vol. 10, no. 1, p. 204589402091068, 2020.

[54] K. Milne and D. D. Sin, "Acute exacerbations of chronic lung disease: cardiac considerations," in *Cardiac Considerations in Chronic Lung Disease*, pp. 229–245, Springer International Publishing, 2020.

[55] X. Yu, Y. Xue, B. Bian et al., "NLR-A simple indicator of inflammation for the diagnosis of left ventricular hypertrophy in patients with hypertension," *International Heart Journal*, vol. 61, no. 2, pp. 373–379, 2020.

[56] P. Rogliani, B. L. Ritondo, R. Laitano, A. Chetta, and L. Calzetta, "Advances in understanding of mechanisms related to increased cardiovascular risk in COPD," *Expert Review of Respiratory Medicine*, vol. 15, no. 1, pp. 59–70, 2021.

[57] M. Shnoda, K. Gajjar, and V. Ivanova, "COPD and cardiovascular disease: a review of association, interrelationship, and basic principles for integrated management," *Critical Care Nursing Quarterly*, vol. 44, no. 1, pp. 91–102, 2021.

[58] D. A. McAllister, J. D. Maclay, N. L. Mills et al., "Diagnosis of myocardial infarction following hospitalisation for exacerbation of COPD," *European Respiratory Journal*, vol. 39, no. 5, pp. 1097–1103, 2012.

[59] H. Müllerova, A. Agusti, S. Erqou, and D. W. Mapel, "Cardiovascular comorbidity in COPD: systematic literature review," *Chest*, vol. 144, no. 4, pp. 1163–1178, 2013.

[60] K. Onishi, "Total management of chronic obstructive pulmonary disease (COPD) as an independent risk factor for cardiovascular disease," *Journal of Cardiology*, vol. 70, no. 2, pp. 128–134, 2017.

[61] T. Rusinowicz, T. M. Zielonka, and K. Zycinska, "Cardiac arrhythmias in patients with exacerbation of COPD," in *Clinical Management of Pulmonary Disorders and Diseases*, pp. 53–62, Springer, 2017.

[62] T. Konecny, J. Y. Park, K. R. Somers et al., "Relation of chronic obstructive pulmonary disease to atrial and ventricular arrhythmias," *The American journal of cardiology*, vol. 114, no. 2, pp. 272–277, 2014.

Interstitial Emphysema as a Rare Radiographic Presentation of Bronchial Dehiscence after Lung Transplant

Linda P. Vien,[1] Robert M. Marron,[2] Abbas Charlie,[3] Maruti Kumaran,[3] and James C. Brown[2]

[1]Department of Medicine, Temple University Hospital, 3401 North Broad Street, Philadelphia, PA 19140, USA
[2]Department of Thoracic Medicine and Surgery, Temple University Hospital, 3401 North Broad Street, Philadelphia, PA 19140, USA
[3]Department of Radiology, Temple University Hospital, 3401 North Broad Street, Philadelphia, PA 19140, USA

Correspondence should be addressed to Linda P. Vien; linda.vien@tuhs.temple.edu

Academic Editor: Inger F. Oey

Airway complications after lung transplantation are a major cause of morbidity and mortality. Bronchial dehiscence presents within a month of lung transplantation and is typically diagnosed radiographically as a sentinel gas pocket at the anastomotic site and confirmed with bronchoscopy. A 66-year-old man with idiopathic pulmonary fibrosis who underwent a right lung transplantation 4 weeks prior developed chest pain with palpable crepitus over his right chest wall. A chest X-ray revealed subcutaneous emphysema and a small right-sided pneumothorax. Computed tomography (CT) of the thorax without contrast revealed a gas pocket at the anastomotic site in the mediastinum as well as interstitial emphysema around the proximal bronchi of the right lung that had worsened when compared to CT from 11 days prior. A review of prior CT demonstrated interstitial emphysema without evidence of a sentinel gas pocket. These findings suggest that interstitial emphysema was the initial radiographic manifestation of the bronchial anastomotic site dehiscence. Interstitial emphysema is typically self-limiting, but severe cases can lead to major complications. Interstitial emphysema outside of the immediate postoperative period should be recognized as a possible early radiographic sign of bronchial dehiscence in lung transplant patients with vigilant monitoring of potential complications and strong consideration for early bronchoscopic investigation.

1. Introduction

Bronchial anastomotic site dehiscence typically occurs 2-4 weeks after lung transplantation and occurs in 1-10% of patients [1, 2]. It occurs as a result of bronchial ischemia and extreme mucosal necrosis due to disruption of native bronchial circulation and lack of systemic blood supply to the anastomotic region immediately after transplantation; reestablishment of bronchial artery circulation through collateral formation can take up to four weeks [3]. The most common radiographic finding is a sentinel gas pocket at the anastomotic site on computed tomography (CT) imaging [1, 4]. Indirect signs of bronchial anastomotic site dehiscence include a persistent pneumothorax and subcutaneous emphysema [1]. Risk factors for bronchial dehiscence include right lung anastomoses, primary graft dysfunction, microbiological contamination of the donor lung, high-dose perioperative steroids, telescoped anastomoses, inadequate organ preservation, prolonged organ ischemia times, discrepancy in size between donor and recipient bronchi, prolonged donor or recipient mechanical ventilation, and immunosuppression, most notably sirolimus [2, 3, 5, 6]. We report an atypical presentation of bronchial anastomotic site dehiscence in a recent lung transplant patient presenting with an initial radiographic finding of interstitial emphysema rather than a sentinel gas pocket.

2. Case Presentation

A 66-year-old male with chronic hypoxemic respiratory failure secondary to advanced interstitial pulmonary fibrosis, coronary artery disease, pulmonary hypertension, systemic lupus erythematosus, hypertension, and obesity presented for a single right lung transplantation which was performed with end-to-end anastomosis. His operation was uneventful with no significant major intraoperative complications or use of extracorporeal membrane oxygenation. He was extubated within 24 hours posttransplant after an airway and anastomosis inspection via flexible bronchoscopy was unremarkable. The patient was treated with antibiotics for methicillin-sensitive *Staphylococcus aureus* of the donor lung; other cultures were negative. The patient was to receive tacrolimus, mycophenolate, and prednisone for immunosuppression and nebulized amphotericin and intravenous valganciclovir for fungal and cytomegalovirus prophylaxis. No primary graft dysfunction was reported in the first 72 hours after surgery. CT without contrast was obtained on postoperative day 5 to evaluate a right lung basilar opacity, which showed extensive ground-glass opacities in the transplanted right lung, concerning reperfusion edema versus acute rejection. The patient was given diuretics, and glucocorticoid dosing was increased from prednisone 5 mg daily to methylprednisolone 40 mg intravenously twice a day. His postoperative course was further complicated by hypoxemia, for which a CT angiography was performed and showed a small distal pulmonary embolism in the right lower lobe, decreased ground-glass opacities in the right lung, and increased patchy basilar platelike peribronchial opacities for which rejection could not be ruled out. The patient received three days of pulse glucocorticoid dosing of methylprednisolone 250 mg IV daily, which was subsequently decreased. Persistent abnormalities on chest radiography and continued hypoxemia led to additional imaging. CT of the thorax on postoperative day 15 showed right allograft opacities, for which glucocorticoids were continued out of concern for rejection. Subsequent bronchoscopy on postoperative day 17 showed an abnormal area of eschar around the anastomotic site with a pale yellow-brown mucosa suggestive of ischemia. Cultures from the bronchoscopy were negative. A transbronchial biopsy of the right lower lobe was performed, and pathology showed organizing pneumonia without evidence of rejection. Donor-specific antibody serology did not suggest antibody-mediated rejection. Steroids were continued and tapered in an attempt to balance treating his organizing pneumonia while hoping to avoid the complications given the presence of anastomotic eschar on bronchoscopy.

On postoperative day 26, the patient developed chest pain. Vital signs were as follows: temperature was 36.9 degrees Celsius, blood pressure was 108/61 mmHg, heart rate was 67 beats per minute, respiratory rate was 20 breaths per minute, and oxygen saturation was 97% on 20 liters of high-flow nasal cannula with fraction of inspired oxygen of 60%. On physical exam, the patient had rhonchi at the right base and right-sided subcutaneous emphysema on the anterior chest with no respiratory distress or accessory muscle use. A portable anterior-posterior chest X-ray showed right-sided subcutaneous emphysema with a small right-sided pneumothorax (Figure 1). CT of the thorax showed a moderate-sized right pneumothorax with spontaneous decompression into the anterior chest wall with subcutaneous emphysema, a sentinel pocket of air adjacent to the anastomotic site, and interstitial emphysema around the right lower lobe proximal bronchus,

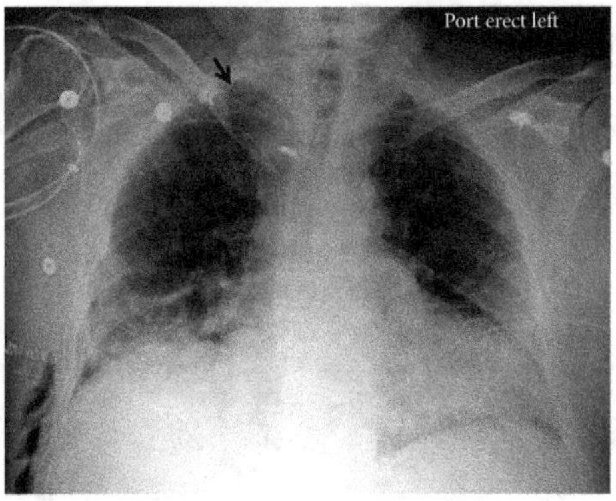

FIGURE 1: Chest X-ray showed right-sided subcutaneous emphysema (red caret) with a small right-sided pneumothorax (black arrow).

all of which were concerning bronchial dehiscence (Figure 2). The patient was transferred to the medical intensive care unit and was intubated for bronchoscopy for airway inspection. Bronchoscopy showed partial dehiscence of the right mainstem bronchus surgical anastomosis directly opposite to the right upper lobe orifice and distal to sutures with a surrounding stable hematoma and no bubbling apparent when flushed with saline (Figure 3). Retrospective evaluation of the prior CT thorax two weeks after transplantation showed air tracking along the bronchovascular bundle, suggestive of interstitial emphysema (Figure 4). Repeat bronchoscopy 32 days posttransplantation, seen in Figure 5, showed right mainstem bronchus surgical anastomotic dehiscence with the International Society for Heart and Lung Transplantation (ISHLT) grading as follows: ischemia and necrosis (extent I-a, location I-a), dehiscence (extent D-a, location D-c), stenosis (location S-a), and malacia (none). The right mainstem bronchus anastomotic dehiscence was managed conservatively with a reduction in glucocorticoid dosage, addition of prophylactic antibiotics, and serial bronchoscopy.

3. Discussion

Interstitial emphysema is defined as air dissecting into the interstitial space surrounding the bronchovascular bundles [7, 8]. This finding, typically seen in neonates with respiratory distress syndrome and positive pressure ventilation on mechanical ventilators, is rarely seen in adults [7, 8]. Interstitial emphysema is an atypical presentation of anastomotic site dehiscence after lung transplantation. Rare cases of interstitial emphysema have been reported after lung transplant [8, 9]. A retrospective study found that out of 17 patients with confirmed bronchial dehiscence after transplantation, there was one case of pulmonary interstitial emphysema in a patient with right bronchial dehiscence after undergoing bilateral lung transplantation [9].

Abnormal airway pressures can cause rupture of alveolar walls and subsequent transport of air from ruptured alveoli to the mediastinum via pulmonary vessels, leading to a pneumothorax and pneumomediastinum [10]. Physiologic and pathologic phenomena that are associated with interstitial emphysema are atelectasis, pneumonia, chest trauma,

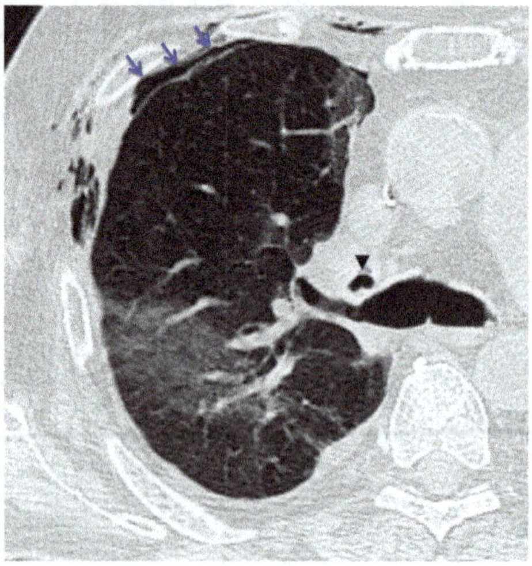

FIGURE 2: Axial chest CT showed a sentinel pocket of gas adjacent to the right bronchial anastomotic site (black caret); an anterior pneumothorax (blue arrows) is also seen.

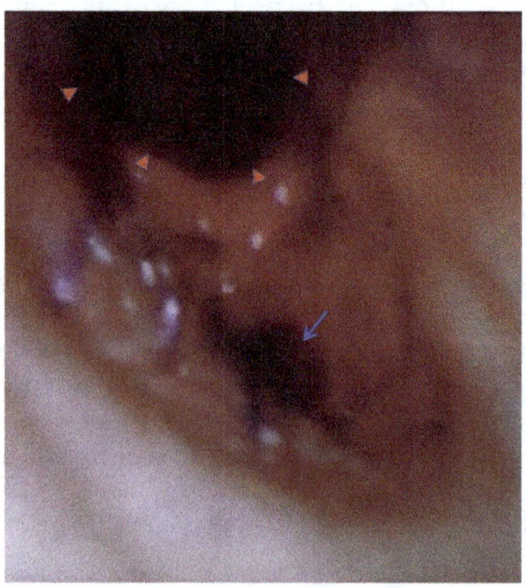

FIGURE 3: Bronchoscopy showed partial dehiscence of the right mainstem bronchus surgical anastomosis (blue arrow) directly opposite to the right upper lobe orifice (red carets) and distal to sutures.

bronchiolitis, asthma, and most commonly a need for mechanical ventilation. Interstitial emphysema has been reported in acute respiratory distress syndrome and positive pressure ventilation where peak airway pressures exceed 30-40-centimeter H_2O [11, 12]. Age also plays a factor. Neonates, particularly preterm babies, are at increased risk for interstitial emphysema due to reduced surfactant levels [12].

Mild interstitial emphysema is self-limiting. Severe interstitial emphysema can lead to complications including compression atelectasis, pneumomediastinum, pneumothorax, and hemodynamic effects from compression of the pulmonary vasculature [10, 12]. Management strategies include lateral decubitus positioning, inhaled helium or nitric oxide, mainstem bronchus intubation and occlusion for unilateral disease, high-frequency ventilation, extracorporeal membrane oxygenation, and lobectomy [12, 13].

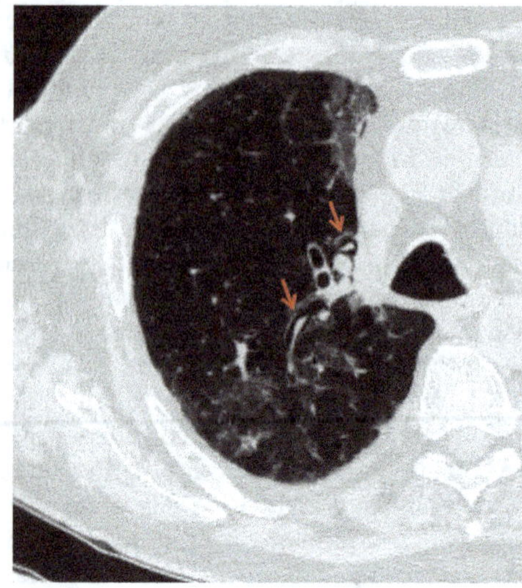

FIGURE 4: Initial axial chest CT two weeks prior shows interstitial emphysema along the bronchovascular bundle (red arrows).

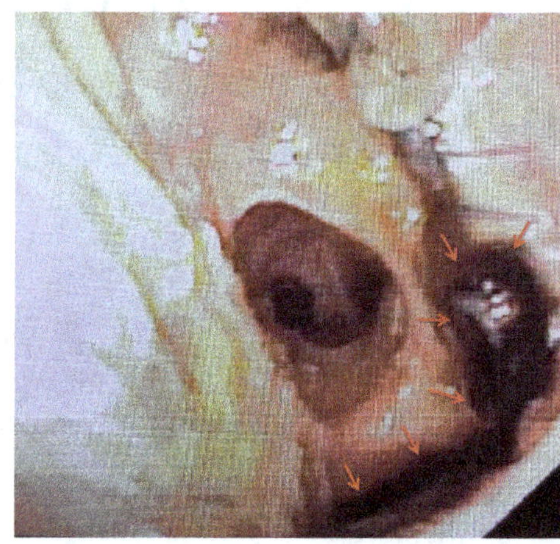

FIGURE 5: Repeat bronchoscopy 32 days posttransplantation showed right mainstem bronchial anastomotic site dehiscence (red arrows).

Interstitial emphysema on the CT thorax 11 days prior to the patient developing symptoms may have been evidence of an atypical radiographic presentation of bronchial anastomotic site dehiscence, which was later confirmed with the classic CT finding of a sentinel gas pocket. While interstitial emphysema can occur postoperatively and is self-limiting, persistent interstitial emphysema and subcutaneous emphysema warrant closer monitoring for possible bronchial anastomotic site dehiscence. Our patient had risk factors for bronchial anastomotic site dehiscence including right-sided anastomosis, microbial contamination of the donor lung, and high glucocorticoid dosing due to initial concerns for possible rejection.

Our patient received an end-to-end anastomosis. End-to-end anastomoses are associated with a lower risk of bronchial anastomotic complications as compared to telescoped anastomoses in patients who received single lung transplantation, with bronchial dehiscence seen in 25% of telescoped bronchial anastomoses compared to 2% of end-to-end bronchial anastomoses [14]. In a telescoped anastomosis, the donor bronchus is folded inwards into the recipient bronchus with sutures performed both anteriorly and posteriorly. Telescoped anastomoses also have an increased risk of stenosis due to a narrower airway and an increased risk of infection [15]. The end-to-end single running suture has also been associated with good results with airway healing [16]. Shorter length of the donor bronchus is preferred given risk of ischemia with excessive length [15]. Prolonged donor mechanical ventilation and donor-recipient bronchial size mismatch are also associated with airway complications.

Bronchial dehiscence should be suspected in patients with subcutaneous emphysema, worsening shortness of breath, pneumothorax, and infection within the first month of lung transplantation [3]. A chest X-ray and CT of the chest are initial noninvasive imaging modalities for diagnosis. Visualization with bronchoscopy confirms diagnosis. Routine management of dehiscence includes serial bronchoscopy for airway inspection, treatment of infections, reduction in glucocorticoid dosing to facilitate healing, and stent placement for extensive necrosis [2, 3]. Surgical repair is reserved for severe cases or complete dehiscence.

4. Conclusion

Recognition of interstitial emphysema outside of the immediate postoperative period on a chest X-ray and/or CT imaging as a sign of early bronchial dehiscence should prompt closer monitoring with serial exams, chest imaging, and bronchoscopy. Early diagnosis and treatment can prevent further complications.

Disclosure

This case was accepted as an abstract for presentation at the 2020 American Thoracic Society International Conference. This case was uploaded as a poster for a thematic poster session for the Virtual 2020 American Thoracic Society International Conference (https://cslide-us.ctimeetingtech.com/ats2020_eposter/attendee/eposter/poster/2131?s=a).

Authors' Contributions

LV and RM drafted the manuscript. RM and JB were involved in the patient's care. AC, MK, and LV prepared the images. All authors edited and approved the final manuscript.

Acknowledgments

Funding support for Open-Access was provided by the Micki Gitlin Lung Research Fund through the Department of Thoracic Medicine and Surgery at the Lewis Katz School of Medicine at Temple University.

References

[1] C. Habre, P. M. Soccal, F. Triponez et al., "Radiological findings of complications after lung transplantation," *Insights Imaging*, vol. 9, no. 5, pp. 709–719, 2018.

[2] M. M. Crespo, D. P. McCarthy, P. M. Hopkins et al., "ISHLT consensus statement on adult and pediatric airway complications after lung transplantation: definitions, grading system, and therapeutics," *The Journal of Heart and Lung Transplantation*, vol. 37, no. 5, pp. 548–563, 2018.

[3] A. K. Mahajan, E. Folch, S. J. Khandhar et al., "The diagnosis and management of airway complications following lung transplantation," *Chest*, vol. 152, no. 3, pp. 627–638, 2017.

[4] F. J. Schlueter, J. W. Semenkovich, H. S. Glazer, J. M. Arcidi Jr., E. P. Trulock, and G. A. Patterson, "Bronchial dehiscence after lung transplantation: correlation of CT findings with clinical outcome," *Radiology*, vol. 199, no. 3, pp. 849–854, 1996.

[5] J. Yserbyt, C. Dooms, R. Vos, L. J. Dupont, D. E. Van Raemdonck, and G. M. Verleden, "Anastomotic airway complications after lung transplantation: risk factors, treatment modalities and outcome-a single-centre experience," *European Journal of Cardio-Thoracic Surgery*, vol. 49, no. 1, pp. e1–e8, 2016.

[6] P. Moreno, A. Alvarez, F. J. Algar et al., "Incidence, management and clinical outcomes of patients with airway complications following lung transplantation," *European Journal of Cardio-Thoracic Surgery*, vol. 34, no. 6, pp. 1198–1205, 2008.

[7] D. M. Hansell, A. A. Bankier, H. MacMahon, T. C. McLoud, N. L. Muller, and J. Remy, "Fleischner society: glossary of terms for thoracic imaging," *Radiology*, vol. 246, no. 3, pp. 697–722, 2008.

[8] G. Rea, G. Scotto di Frega, and G. Fiorentino, "Pulmonary interstitial emphysema following spirometry in CPFE syndrome," *Archivos de bronconeumologia*, vol. 51, no. 11, pp. 602-603, 2015.

[9] J. W. Semenkovich, H. S. Glazer, D. C. Anderson, J. M. Arcidi Jr., J. D. Cooper, and G. A. Patterson, "Bronchial dehiscence in lung transplantation: CT evaluation," *Radiology*, vol. 194, no. 1, pp. 205–208, 1995.

[10] J. M. Unger, D. M. England, and G. A. Bogust, "Interstitial emphysema in adults: recognition and prognostic implications," *Journal of thoracic imaging*, vol. 4, no. 1, pp. 86–94, 1989.

[11] J. H. Woodring, "Pulmonary interstitial emphysema in the adult respiratory distress syndrome," *Critical care medicine*, vol. 13, no. 10, pp. 786–791, 1985.

[12] P. B. Sherren and T. Jovaisa, "Pulmonary interstitial emphysema presenting in a woman on the intensive care unit: case report and review of literature," *Journal of medical case reports*, vol. 5, p. 236, 2011.

[13] S. M. Barcia, J. Kukreja, and K. D. Jones, "Pulmonary interstitial emphysema in adults: a clinicopathologic study of 53 lung explants," *The American journal of surgical pathology*, vol. 38, no. 3, pp. 339–345, 2014.

[14] E. S. Garfein, M. E. Ginsberg, L. Gorenstein, C. C. McGregor, and L. L. Schulman, "Superiority of end-to-end versus telescoped bronchial anastomosis in single lung transplantation for pulmonary emphysema," *The Journal of Thoracic and Cardiovascular Surgery*, vol. 121, no. 1, pp. 149–154, 2001.

[15] L. Frye and M. Machuzak, "Airway complications after lung transplantation," *Clinics in Chest Medicine*, vol. 38, no. 4, pp. 693–706, 2017.

[16] C. Aigner, P. Jaksch, G. Seebacher et al., "Single running suture–the new standard technique for bronchial anastomoses in lung transplantation," *European Journal of Cardio-Thoracic Surgery*, vol. 23, no. 4, pp. 488–493, 2003.

23

Assessment of Bronchiectasis in HIV Patients among an Urban Population

Veena Dronamraju,[1] Navneet Singh,[1] Justin Poon,[1] Sachi Shah,[2] Joseph Gorga,[3] Hector Ojeda-Martinez,[4] and Samy McFarlane[1,5]

[1]*Department of Internal Medicine, SUNY Downstate Medical Center, USA*
[2]*Department of Infectious Disease, Montefiore Medical Center, USA*
[3]*Division of Pulmonary and Critical Care Medicine, New York Health and Hospitals Corporation, Kings County Hospital Center, USA*
[4]*Department of Infectious Disease, SUNY Downstate Medical Center, USA*
[5]*Department of Endocrinology, SUNY Downstate Medical Center, USA*

Correspondence should be addressed to Veena Dronamraju; vdronamraju@gmail.com

Academic Editor: Mortens Dahl

Bronchiectasis is characterized by permanent destruction of the airways that presents with productive cough, as well as bronchial wall thickening and luminal dilatation on computed tomographic (CT) scan of the chest; it is associated with high mortality. Accumulating data suggests higher rates of bronchiectasis among the HIV-positive population. This case series involves 14 patients with bronchiectasis and HIV followed at two major urban institutions from 1999 to 2018. Demographics, clinical presentation, microbiology, radiographic imaging, and outcomes were collected and compiled. Mean age was 42 years (range 12-77 years). 36% had a CD4 count greater than 500 cells/mm^3, 28% had a CD4 count between 200 and 500 cells/mm^3, and 36% had AIDS. 43% were treated for Pneumocystis jiroveci pneumonia (PJP) and 50% for Mycobacterium avium complex (MAC) infection. 21% had COPD, 7% had asthma, and 7% had a history of pulmonary aspergillosis. Two patients were followed up by pulmonary services after diagnosis of bronchiectasis on CT. The timeline of the follow-up in these cases was within months and after three years respectively. It is posited that the prevalence of bronchiectasis in HIV patients may be underestimated. Improving recognition and management of bronchiectasis could help diminish rehospitalization rates.

1. Introduction

Bronchiectasis is a permanent distortion of airways clinically characterized by productive cough and diagnosed with the presence of bronchial wall thickening and luminal dilatation on CT scan of the chest [1, 2]. There is a high prevalence of noncystic fibrosis bronchiectasis associated with underlying chronic lung diseases, rheumatoid arthritis, connective tissue disease, inflammatory bowel disease, and HIV [3]. The disease is difficult to recognize as its clinical features overlap with many other chronic lung diseases [4, 5]. Furthermore, even when the disease is properly identified, there is often inadequate treatment due the lack of understanding of the relationship between the underlying cause and bronchiectasis.

In the United States, there are currently no standardized treatment guidelines for the disease. British Thoracic Society guidelines recommend antibiotics for acute and maintenance therapy [6]. This approach to management presumes infectious origins of the disease, which may not be an accurate presumption. For instance, bronchiectasis in patients with HIV remains apparent despite availability of antiretroviral therapy and subsequent reduction of pulmonary infections.

Table 1: Patient characteristics and HIV/opportunistic infection history.

	Age	Gender	Congenital?	CD4	Viral load	Hx of PJP?	ARV	Prev tx of MAC?	Comorbidities
Pt 1	12	F	Yes	979	<50	No	TDF/FTC/ATV/r	No	None
Pt 2	17	F	Yes	4	68900	No	TDF/FTC/DRV/r	No	None
Pt 3	19	F	Yes	205	161	Yes	RAL/DRV/r	Yes	Esophageal/vaginal candidiasis, generalized seizures, anemia
Pt 4	22	F	No	6	40232	Yes	TDF/FTC/DTG	No	Squamous cell carcinoma in situ in skin, esophagitis, depression, oligomenorrhea, axillary abscess, seborrheic dermatitis, prurigo nodularis, postinflammatory hyperpigmentation
Pt 5	25	F	No	5	136	Yes	TDF/FTC/LPV/r	Yes	HIV-induced cardiomyopathy, CVA
Pt 6	35	F	No	715	5192	No	ETV/DRV/RAL	No	Asthma
Pt 7	41	F	No	2	1756	Yes	TDF/FTC/DRV/r	Yes	Aplastic anemia, recurrent HSV2 infections
Pt 8	48	M	No	797	29	No	TDF/FTC/RAL	Yes	CAD, BPH, pulmonary aspergillosis, metastatic rectal cancer
Pt 9	48	F	No	1	1942818	Yes	TDF/FTC/DTG	Yes	GERD, COPD, tobacco abuse, cocaine abuse, migraines, G6PD deficiency
Pt 10	54	F	No	319	N/A	No	ABC/EFV	No	Emphysema, HTN, marijuana use
Pt 11	55	F	No	333	40854	No	LPV/r/ATV	Yes	Stage IV metastatic cervical cancer s/p TAH (1999), recurrent UTI, HTN, hip replacement, osteoarthritis, CKD stage IV with nephrostomy tubes
Pt 12	62	F	No	211	<20	No	TDF/FTC/RPV	No	NHL (large B cell lymphoma s/p chemotherapy), hepatitis C, and substance abuse history on methadone, HTN
Pt 13	70	M	No	834	<48	No	ABC/AZT/LPV/r	Yes	COPD, DM
Pt 14	77	F	No	549	<20	Yes	AZT/3TC/DRV/r	No	HTN, HLD, CAD s/p PCI, left mastectomy (Ca buildup)

3TC: lamivudine; ABC: abacavir; AZT: zidovudine; FTC: emtricitabine; TDF: tenofovir; EFV: efavirenz; ETV: etravirine; RPV: rilpivirine; ATV: atazanavir; DRV: darunavir; LPV: lopinavir; r: ritonavir; RAL: raltegravir; DTG: dolutegravir.

To further understand the relationship between these two diseases, we present a case series of bronchiectasis in HIV-positive patients seen at two major urban institutions.

2. Subjects and Methods

A search of the electronic medical records at Kings County Hospital Center and SUNY Downstate Medical Center was completed looking for patients with both bronchiectasis and HIV infection identified by either ICD-9 (042 for HIV and 494.0 for bronchiectasis) or ICD-10 codes (B20 for HIV and J47 for bronchiectasis). Of approximately 3000 patients, 14 patients with both diagnoses were identified from 1999 to 2018. Demographics, clinical characteristics, diagnostic imaging, microbiology, and clinical course were obtained and are summarized in Tables 1 and 2.

2.1. Case Descriptions

2.1.1. Patient 1. A 12-year-old female with congenitally acquired HIV and a known history of bronchiectasis per patient survey presented with a productive cough that was treated with azithromycin. One year later, the patient reported purulent cough with rhinorrhea and nasal congestion. The patient had a repeat infection the next year, in which she had rhinorrhea and nasal congestion and completed a ten day course of amoxicillin. The patient moved to North Carolina later the same year and is presumed to be following there. Patient had no confirmatory CT scans obtained during her course.

2.1.2. Patient 2. A 17-year-old female with congenital AIDS arrived from Haiti with symptoms of productive blood-

Table 2: Distribution of bronchiectasis and microbiology data.

	Distribution of bronchiectasis	Sputum culture	PFT	Smoker?	Pack years
Pt 1	N/A	N/A	N/A	No	N/A
Pt 2	RML, lingula, B/L lower lobes	Candida albicans	N/A	No	N/A
Pt 3	RLL	Candida albicans	N/A	N/A	N/A
Pt 4	N/A	Normal throat flora	N/A	No	N/A
Pt 5	RU, RM, and B/L lower lobes	Normal throat flora	N/A	No	N/A
Pt 6	LLL, RLL, RUL, and RML, most severe in the RML	N/A	N/A	No	N/A
Pt 7	RML and inferior lingula	No growth	N/A	No	N/A
Pt 8	RUL, RML, RLL, LLL	Normal flora; Aspergillus (BAL)	Moderate obstructive	Yes	N/A
Pt 9	RU, RM, and B/L lower lobes	Candida	N/A	Yes	58
Pt 10	CT read does not specify distribution	N/A	N/A	Yes	15
Pt 11	RUL and LUL	Overgrown by non-AFB organisms	N/A	Yes	N/A
Pt 12	RUL and lingula	H. influenza, normal throat flora, overgrowth by non-AFB organisms	N/A	Yes	3
Pt 13	LUL, LLL	Morganella morganii, MRSA, strep viridans	Moderate obstructive	Yes	50
Pt 14	B/L lower lobe	N/A	N/A	No	N/A

streaked cough, rhinorrhea, and chest pains. The patient was hospitalized for pneumonia and was found to have evidence of bronchiectasis and air-filled bronchiectatic cysts in the left lower lobe on CT scan. Her previous history was significant for being hospitalized for six months because of a "lung problem" three years prior in Haiti. The patient presented to the chest clinic shortly after her initial hospitalization with another bout of dyspnea on exertion; she was started on albuterol treatments, which improved her symptoms. In the following year, the patient presented with cough productive of white sputum, fevers, and myalgias. She was subsequently admitted for a presumed exacerbation of bronchiectasis with PJP and viral syndrome on the differential. In the next two years, the patient was admitted several times for various infectious syndromes, including esophageal candidiasis, upper respiratory viral infection, pyelonephritis, and facial cellulitis.

2.1.3. Patient 3. A 19-year-old female with congenital AIDS was being followed in the pediatric immunology clinic for routine care. Over several years, she was treated for what was presumed to be recurrent bacterial sinusitis with symptoms of a dry cough and rhinorrhea with no fevers. She was prescribed several courses of amoxicillin/clavulanate. One year later, she was treated for oropharyngeal candidiasis several times and twice for esophageal candidiasis. During one of these admissions, she had a CT scan of the chest that demonstrated RLL bronchiectasis with scattered pneumatoceles. The next year, she was treated for otitis and then presumptively for PJP. The following year, she was admitted for anemia thought to be due to possible parvovirus in the background of a MAC infection. She was given IVIG and treated with anti-infectives for MAC. In subsequent years, she was treated two more times for presumed PJP (sputum negative) and MAC (sputum positive). This patient had several repeat chest CT scans over the course of her clinical picture which all remained stable.

2.1.4. Patient 4. A 22-year-old female with congenital AIDS who was intermittently compliant with ART) had a history of multiple hospital admissions for pneumonia, both community-acquired and PJP. Given the recurrence of infection, her primary care physician suspected bronchiectasis, but did not order chest imaging. One year later, the patient was seen in clinic for worsening cough and was treated with amoxicillin/clavulanate for bronchiectasis exacerbation. The patient had six admissions over the next year, one of which was for sepsis and the others for persistent cough in the absence of signs of pneumonia. She underwent multiple courses of antibiotic treatments over this time. This patient did not have diagnostic imaging to confirm her bronchiectasis during her course.

2.1.5. Patient 5. A 25-year-old female with congenital HIV who was noncompliant with ART and had a history of multiple admissions for severe pneumonia was admitted to the medical ICU for severe community-acquired pneumonia. Her hospital course was complicated with Haemophilus influenzae bacteremia and a pleural effusion. Her pleural fluid culture revealed MAC, and her symptoms improved with antibiotics. She was restarted on ART and PJP prophylaxis. During the admission, the patient had a CT scan that confirmed bronchiectasis in the right upper, right middle, and bilateral lower lobes. Sputum culture grew normal flora. The patient was discharged and remained noncompliant with HIV treatment. She did not follow up outpatient. The next year, she had three more admissions during which she received empiric treatment for both community-acquired pneumonia and PJP. The following year, the patient was admitted for severe pneumonia with confirmed PJP along with positive enterovirus and rhinovirus. The patient initially improved, however, she then developed a stroke that was thought to be secondary to disseminated MAC with HIV vasculitis on the differential. Her blood culture grew MAC, and she was treated accordingly. The patient's poor clinical condition persisted, and she decided to suspend treatment and transition to comfort care.

2.1.6. Patient 6. A 35-year-old female with history of congenital HIV and asthma was admitted to the hospital for persistent cough. The patient was diagnosed with likely bronchiectasis exacerbation with pneumonia on the differential. Her symptoms improved with a ten-day course of levofloxacin. Following this admission, the patient had a CT scan that showed bronchiectasis in the right upper, right middle, and bilateral lower lobes. The disease was most severe in the right middle lobe. The patient was never seen in the chest clinic. Of note, this patient had relatively well-controlled HIV, with no admissions related to PJP. She had multiple admissions for asthma in the past and once required intubation.

2.1.7. Patient 7. A 41-year-old female with AIDS who was noncompliant with ART and had a history for several admissions for recurrent pneumonias was admitted for presumed PJP. CT chest showed diffuse ground glass opacities, and bronchoalveolar lavage (BAL) was negative for PJP. The patient was still treated with prednisone and trimethoprim/-sulfamethoxazole for presumed PJP. Over the next year, the patient had three additional admissions for respiratory infections. During one of the admissions, the patient had an incidental finding of bulky adenopathy near the superior mesenteric artery. A biopsy of the node showed granulomatous lymphadenitis along with acid fast bacteria consistent with Mycobacterium species. The CT chest also demonstrated bronchiectasis of the right middle lobe and inferior lingula. The patient was discharged with treatment for tuberculous and MAC for one month. She was readmitted due to worsening of symptoms before completion of her treatment. The next year, the patient was admitted and treated for MAC bacteremia. Later that year, she was found to have worsening adenopathy throughout the body that was thought to be due to disseminated MAC. She was again admitted in 2016 for hypoxic respiratory failure with CT scan that showed worsening pleural effusion and tree-in-bud opacities. Broad spectrum antibiotics were initiated for septic shock, and the patient was transferred to the medical ICU where she expired.

2.1.8. Patient 8. A 48-year-old male with hypertension, COPD, and benign prostatic hyperplasia was admitted for weight loss with cough productive of yellow sputum for five weeks. He was diagnosed with pulmonary tuberculosis and HIV, and started on RIPE therapy. I patient clinically improved; however, he continued to have worsening radiographic consolidations that prompted concern for aspergillosis with resistant tuberculosis on the differential. The patient underwent bronchoscopy with bronchoalveolar lavage revealing Aspergillus species. His tuberculosis medications were discontinued, and the patient was started on Voriconazole to treat chronic necrotizing aspergillosis. The next year, the patient underwent right upper lobe wedge resection for persistent symptoms of pulmonary aspergilloma and proceeded to complete a seventeen-month course of Voriconazole. Two years later, the patient developed a chronic cough productive of clear sputum and was treated for an upper respiratory illness in the setting of a COPD exacerbation. An episode of hematuria brought the patient into the emergency department, where he was found to have new right lower lobe opacity caught on CT scan of the abdomen and pelvis. On further history, he was found to have severe cough with low-grade fevers. A CT chest showed interval progression of bronchiectasis and bronchial wall thickening in the right middle lobe and right lower lobe with mucus-filled airways as well as interval development of a peripheral airspace opacity. A repeat CT chest the next year showed widespread bronchiectasis with retained secretions. The patient was started on albuterol, and his symptoms improved. Almost two years later, the patient was diagnosed with poorly differentiated rectal adenocarcinoma and started on FOLFOX with palliative radiation. He was subsequently admitted for hypotension and expired.

2.1.9. Patient 9. A 48-year-old female with AIDS, a history of PJP complicated by pneumothorax, and a history of two admissions for community-acquired pneumonia who was admitted for one month of syncopal episodes. She was treated for MAC based on sputum and blood cultures. Two months later, the patient was admitted to the hospital for sepsis likely secondary to disseminated MAC with PJP on the differential. She was empirically treated for both MAC and PJP. CT scan of the chest was completed during this admission and showed bronchiectasis in right upper, right middle, and bilateral lower lobes. The patient had no further follow-up.

2.1.10. Patient 10. A 54-year-old female with HIV and previously documented bronchiectasis presented for fever, chill, and cough. The patient was admitted for community-acquired pneumonia. CT chest demonstrated that the patient had exacerbation of bronchiectasis with superimposed infection. She was discharged home with a seven-day course of levofloxacin.

2.1.11. Patient 11. A 55-year-old female with HIV and a remote history of tuberculosis was found to have metastatic cervical cancer to the pelvis, liver, and likely lung. Later that year, she was found to have reactivated tuberculosis with MAC on the differential. CT chest showed multiple cystic cavities, predominantly in the upper lobes, along with parenchymal scarring consistent with bronchiectasis. Despite optimal treatment with RIPE and clarithromycin, the patient had worsening hemoptysis secondary to disseminated intravascular coagulation and expired.

2.1.12. Patient 12. A 62-year-old female with history of large B cell lymphoma and HIV was admitted for pneumonia. The patient had a CT chest confirming bronchiectasis in the right upper lobe and lingula. Sputum culture grew Haemophilus influenzae. She clinically improved with antibiotics and was discharged. She subsequently had several admissions for community-acquired pneumonia and did not follow up outpatient.

2.1.13. Patient 13. A 70-year-old male with HIV, history of pulmonary tuberculosis and asthma/COPD presented to the emergency department with complaints of a productive cough and was treated for pharyngitis. Shortly after this episode, the patient was treated for an upper respiratory tract infection as an outpatient. Following a trip to the Dominican Republic, the patient began complaining of intermittent episodes of severe productive cough. Over the next few years, the patient had numerous hospitalizations for multiple recurrent upper respiratory tract infections, right hip cellulitis, and conjunctivitis. Five years after initial admission, the patient was recognized to have chronic bronchiectasis. CT chest showed an air-filled bronchiectatic cyst in the left lower lobe. He was started on azithromycin and advised to take it as needed during future episodes. Two years later, the patient was hospitalized twice, once for acute bronchitis for which he was treated with azithromycin and another time for hemoptysis. Three years after diagnosis of bronchiectasis, the patient was seen in the chest clinic for the first time.

2.1.14. Patient 14. A 77-year-old female with history of HIV was admitted for pneumonia. The patient was hypoxic and chest X-ray showed bilateral hazy opacities. CT scan of the chest showed bilateral mild bronchiectasis at the lung bases. During the admission, the patient had a repeat CT chest which showed radiographic signs suggestive of PJP. She received treatment for PJP empirically with trimethoprim/sulfamethoxazole and prednisone. The patient clinically improved.

3. Discussion

Bronchiectasis develops in the context of repeat occurrence of bronchial insult from infection or inflammation [1, 7]. The insult develops from pulmonic, oncologic, rheumatologic, infectious, or multifactorial disease [8–10]. Microbial toxins and increased inflammation compromise mucociliary clearance [9–12] causing patients to become susceptible to microbial colonization [2, 13]. This colonization then propagates further infection and inflammation, which creates a self-perpetuating cycle [14]. Bacterial colonization is therefore associated with increased airway damage and worsened severity of disease [2, 15, 16]. Most commonly, patients are colonized with Haemophilus influenzae and Pseudomonas aeruginosa [2, 13]. A Pseudomonas predominant lung microbiome has been associated with a worse clinical phenotype of bronchiectasis [16–18].

A minimal amount of research has been done in the field regarding bronchiectasis. A recent multisite study conducted under the Bronchiectasis Research Registry used a large sample size to characterize different aspects of the disease, identify prevalent medical comorbidities, and develop a microbiome of the lung in bronchiectasis [19]. Review of previous smaller-scale studies that focus on fewer aspects has shown differences in the microbiome of the lung based on age and gender [13].

Even less research has been done regarding the prevalence, etiology, and lung microbiome of patients with both bronchiectasis and HIV. One of the first descriptions of bronchiectasis in HIV patients was a case series published in 1992 [20], predating the availability of ART therapy. The exact etiology of bronchiectasis in HIV-positive patients remains unknown. It has been hypothesized that defective B lymphocyte and neutrophil function leads to decreased response to antigenic stimuli, which may predispose patients to increased lung infections that consequently act as a trigger for the above-mentioned cycle [21–23]. However, with the advent of newer antiretroviral therapy, there has been a decline in pulmonary infections due to an improved competency of the immune system.

HIV is now considered a chronic inflammatory disease that may have a different and even more direct role in the underlying pathogenesis of bronchiectasis [24]. A recent study on HIV-associated noninfectious lung disease suggests development of COPD in HIV patients due to a progressive loss of CD4 cells, which yields a persistent inflammatory state from CD8 T cell overexpression. It also suggests that HIV viral protein can exert direct effect on endothelial cells leading to pulmonary artery hypertension [25]. In this new age of understanding of the disease, there has been insufficient investigation regarding its association with bronchiectasis.

In our small sample, we noted that patients are routinely connected to the pulmonary service somewhat late in the course of their disease. Patients frequently did not receive adequate therapy and were often inappropriately treated for alternate and seemingly incorrect diagnoses.

As a result of these alternate diagnoses, patients routinely received broad-spectrum antimicrobial therapy that may have altered the respiratory flora. Instead of the typical organisms seen in patients with bronchiectasis such as Pseudomonas, nontuberculous mycobacterial and Aspergillus, we predominantly saw normal respiratory flora and colonizers, including Candida. Although our sputum samples were limited, there is research to suggest that the respiratory flora is altered in HIV-positive patients as compared to HIV-negative patients. The exact mechanism behind this finding is not understood [26].

Importantly, patients were uniformly not offered bronchodilator therapy for their bronchiectasis. They were diagnosed during an inpatient admission, and the results of their radiographic findings were not appropriately communicated to primary providers. As a result, referrals to the pulmonology clinic were rarely made. HIV-positive patients have been shown to have a higher independent risk of developing obstructive lung diseases [27], some of which may include bronchiectasis that is underrecognized. Referral to pulmonary subspecialists earlier in the clinical course may help to identify these patients sooner and provide them with more appropriate management.

The reason for lack of follow-through of care is hypothesized to be multifactorial. Beyond being high volume institutions with limited resources, both Kings County Hospital and Downstate Medical Center primarily serve the Central Brooklyn, East New York, and Flatbush populations; on average, these populations have lower education levels and higher poverty levels than those of New York City. Furthermore, there is a high percentage of uninsured patients [28]. All these factors contribute to limitations on health literacy, distrust of the system, and overall diminished access to care.

Another interesting observation to note in this study is that despite having access to almost 20 years of data from a very large cohort of HIV-positive patients, we were only able to identify these 14 patients with the concurrent diagnosis of bronchiectasis. While this may allude to a low prevalence of bronchiectasis in the HIV-positive population, given the underrecognition in our 14 patients, we instead posit that the prevalence of bronchiectasis in HIV patients may be grossly underestimated. This is understandable given its vague symptomatology that overlaps with other chronic pulmonary diseases. Unfortunately, many patients in our series were rehospitalized several times for vague respiratory symptoms that were thought to be due to an acute infectious process, but were more likely due to exacerbations of bronchiectasis. Improving recognition and management of bronchiectasis in our population could help diminish rehospitalization rates. It could also help to reduce the significant morbidity of repeated exposures to inappropriate therapy with antibiotics for presumed acute bacterial respiratory infections and instead allow focus on supportive therapy including bronchodilators and mucous clearance techniques. Better understanding the nature of bronchiectasis in the HIV-positive population can help to identify therapies better tailored to its more unique pathogenesis.

4. Conclusions

This case series highlights that bronchiectasis can carry a significant symptomatic burden in HIV-positive patients. With improvement in the life expectancy of HIV-positive patients, bronchiectasis will likely become a more important sequela of the disease that all primary providers and pulmonologists should be aware of and consider in their differential diagnosis for respiratory symptoms.

Disclosure

The data from this case series was previously presented at the SUNY Downstate Medical Center Annual Research Day on April 11, 2018.

References

[1] D. M. Hansell, "Bronchiectasis," *Radiologic Clinics of North America*, vol. 36, no. 1, pp. 107–128, 1998.

[2] J. Angrill, C. Agustí, and A. Torres, "Bronchiectasis," *Current Opinion in Infectious Diseases*, vol. 14, no. 2, pp. 193–197, 2001.

[3] J. K. Quint, E. R. C. Millett, M. Joshi et al., "Changes in the incidence, prevalence and mortality of bronchiectasis in the UK from 2004 to 2013: a population-based cohort study," *European Respiratory Journal*, vol. 47, no. 1, pp. 186–193, 2016.

[4] M. C. Pasteur, S. M. Helliwell, S. J. Houghton et al., "An investigation into causative factors in patients with bronchiectasis," *American Journal of Respiratory and Critical Care Medicine*, vol. 162, no. 4, pp. 1277–1284, 2000.

[5] J. R. Hurst, J. S. Elborn, A. de Soyza, and BRONCH-UK Consortium, "COPD–bronchiectasis overlap syndrome," *European Respiratory Journal*, vol. 45, no. 2, pp. 310–313, 2015.

[6] A. T. Hill, A. L. Sullivan, J. D. Chalmers et al., "British Thoracic Society guideline for bronchiectasis in adults," *BMJ Open Respiratory Research*, vol. 5, no. 1, article e000348, 2018.

[7] C. Olveira, A. Padilla, M. Á. Martínez-García et al., "Etiology of bronchiectasis in a cohort of 2047 patients. An analysis of the Spanish historical bronchiectasis registry," *Archivos de Bronconeumología (English Edition)*, vol. 53, no. 7, pp. 366–374, 2017.

[8] M. B. Nicotra, M. Rivera, A. M. Dale, R. Shepherd, and R. Carter, "Clinical, pathophysiologic, and microbiologic characterization of bronchiectasis in an aging cohort," *Chest*, vol. 108, no. 4, pp. 955–961, 1995.

[9] T. Isawa, T. Teshima, T. Hirano et al., "Mucociliary clearance and transport in bronchiectasis: global and regional assessment," *Journal of Nuclear Medicine*, vol. 31, no. 5, pp. 543–548, 1990.

[10] L. A. Smallman, S. L. Hill, and R. A. Stockley, "Reduction of ciliary beat frequency in vitro by sputum from patients with bronchiectasis: a serine proteinase effect," *Thorax*, vol. 39, no. 9, pp. 663–667, 1984.

[11] H. Tegner, K. Ohlsson, N. G. Toremalm, and C. von Mecklenburg, "Effect of human leukocyte enzymes on tracheal mucosa and its mucociliary activity," *Rhinology*, vol. 17, no. 3, pp. 199–206, 1979.

[12] R. Wilson, D. Roberts, and P. Cole, "Effect of bacterial products on human ciliary function in vitro," *Thorax*, vol. 40, no. 2, pp. 125–131, 1985.

[13] J. Angrill, C. Agustí, R. de Celis et al., "Bacterial colonisation in patients with bronchiectasis: microbiological pattern and risk factors," *Thorax*, vol. 57, no. 1, pp. 15–19, 2002.

[14] I. S. Patel, I. Vlahos, T. M. A. Wilkinson et al., "Bronchiectasis, exacerbation indices, and inflammation in chronic obstructive pulmonary disease," *American Journal of Respiratory and Critical Care Medicine*, vol. 170, no. 4, pp. 400–407, 2004.

[15] S. Fuschillo, A. De Felice, and G. Balzano, "Mucosal inflammation in idiopathic bronchiectasis: cellular and molecular mechanisms," *European Respiratory Journal*, vol. 31, no. 2, pp. 396–406, 2008.

[16] S. A. Evans, S. M. Turner, B. J. Bosch, C. C. Hardy, and M. A. Woodhead, "Lung function in bronchiectasis: the influence of *Pseudomonas aeruginosa*," *European Respiratory Journal*, vol. 9, no. 8, pp. 1601–1604, 1996.

[17] S. Aliberti, S. Lonni, S. Dore et al., "Clinical phenotypes in adult patients with bronchiectasis," *European Respiratory Journal*, vol. 47, no. 4, pp. 1113–1122, 2016.

[18] K. A. Miszkiel, A. U. Wells, M. B. Rubens, P. J. Cole, and D. M. Hansell, "Effects of airway infection by Pseudomonas aeruginosa: a computed tomographic study," *Thorax*, vol. 52, no. 3, pp. 260–264, 1997.

[19] T. R. Aksamit, A. E. O'Donnell, A. Barker et al., "Adult patients with bronchiectasis: a first look at the US Bronchiectasis Research Registry," *Chest*, vol. 151, no. 5, pp. 982–992, 2017.

[20] A. Holmes, B. Trotman-Dickenson, A. Edwards, T. Peto, and G. Luzzi, "Bronchiectasis in HIV disease," *QJM: An International Journal of Medicine*, vol. 85, no. 2-3, pp. 875–882, 1992.

[21] A. Verghese, M. Al-Samman, D. Nabhan, A. D. Naylor, and M. Rivera, "Bacterial bronchitis and bronchiectasis in human immunodeficiency virus infection," *Archives of Internal Medicine*, vol. 154, no. 18, pp. 2086–2091, 1994.

[22] E. C. Rosenow III, W. R. Wilson, and F. R. Cockerill III, "Pulmonary disease in the immunocompromised host (first of two parts)," *Mayo Clinic Proceedings*, vol. 60, no. 7, pp. 473–487, 1985.

[23] J. Beck and J. Shellito, "Effects of human immunodeficiency virus on pulmonary host defenses," *Seminars in Respiratory Infections*, vol. 4, no. 2, pp. 75–84, 1989.

[24] S. G. Deeks, S. R. Lewin, and D. V. Havlir, "The end of AIDS: HIV infection as a chronic disease," *The Lancet*, vol. 382, no. 9903, pp. 1525–1533, 2013.

[25] R. M. Presti, S. C. Flores, B. E. Palmer et al., "Mechanisms underlying HIV-associated noninfectious lung disease," *Chest*, vol. 152, no. 5, pp. 1053–1060, 2017.

[26] L. Cui, L. Lucht, L. Tipton et al., "Topographic diversity of the respiratory tract mycobiome and alteration in HIV and lung disease," *American Journal of Respiratory and Critical Care Medicine*, vol. 191, no. 8, pp. 932–942, 2015.

[27] M. B. Drummond and G. D. Kirk, "HIV-associated obstructive lung diseases: insights and implications for the clinician," *The Lancet Respiratory Medicine*, vol. 2, no. 7, pp. 583–592, 2014.

[28] Kings County Hospital Center, *2013 Community Health Needs and Assessment Implementation Strategy*, New York City Health and Hospitals Corporation, New York, NY, USA, 2013.

24

A Case Series of Vaping-Induced Lung Injury in a Community Hospital Setting

Mohammed Ali,[1] Kashmala Khan,[2] Mihir Buch,[1] Manuel Ramos- Ramirez,[1] Munish Sharma,[1] Seema Patel,[2] Saiara Choudhury,[2] Humayun Anjum,[1] Alamgir Khan,[1] and Salim Surani[1,3]

[1]*Department of Pulmonary Medicine, Corpus Christi Medical Center, Texas, USA*
[2]*Department of Internal Medicine, Corpus Christi Medical Center, Texas, USA*
[3]*Department of Pulmonary, Critical Care & Sleep Medicine, Texas A&M University, Health Science Center, Texas, USA*

Correspondence should be addressed to Salim Surani; srsurani@hotmail.com

Academic Editor: Mortens Dahl

Acute and subacute injury to the lung parenchyma can be caused by multiple products. Over the past few years, vaping (also known as E-cigarettes) has become a popular trend and has been considered "safer" alternative to smoking cigarettes, especially among young adults. The use of E-cigarettes has rapidly increased, and according to the most recent report by CDC released at the end of December 2019, 2,506 cases and more than 54 associated deaths due to vaping/E-cigarette-associated lung injury were reported. Though vitamin E acetate and tetrahydrocannabinol (THC) have been found in most of the bronchoalveolar lavage samples, there are still small numbers of cases that have not reported to using THC-containing compounds. Research looking into other possible constituents in E-cigarettes that can account for the etiology of disease and effects of vaping as it relates to pulmonary physiology still remains limited and uncertain. We hereby present a case series of 5 patients who were admitted primarily for respiratory symptoms of cough, dyspnea, and fevers and were diagnosed with vaping-induced pulmonary injury.

1. Introduction

"Vaping is safer than smoking traditional cigarettes," according to the literature that seems to be the rationale behind the steady rise in the use of E-cigarettes [1]. The average users are young adults who either use vaping or E-cigarettes as a bridge to quit smoking cigarettes, or they believe that they are making the healthier and smarter choice [2]. Vaping was introduced in the United States (US) market in 2007 [3]. It has gained popularity over the past few years, with celebrities and Instagram influencers endorsing its use and making it a preferred choice than regular cigarettes. E-cigarettes containing nicotine and other substances, for example marijuana, vaporizes or produces aerosols, which are then inhaled by the user. There are many flavors available in the vaping cartridges, which are particularly appealing to the younger users. Both traditional and E-cigarettes use nicotine, and some researchers have shown vaping to be just as addictive as smoking traditional cigarettes [4]. The extent of potential harmful effects of vaping is still not fully understood and is an area of much interest with public health researchers and physicians. We hereby present the 5 cases of vaping-induced lung injury, which we encountered during the very early phase of this disease process labeling.

2. Case 1

A 34-year-old male without any significant past medical history presented with the complaint of shortness of breath, fever, chills, and cough with mucoid sputum for a 6-day duration. He has initially been evaluated at an emergency department (ED) 2 days prior and was discharged home with the diagnosis of pneumonia on oral levofloxacin. His oxygen saturation on presentation to our ED was 84% on room air. He required 15 L/minute of oxygen via a nonbreather mask to maintain saturations over 90%. The initial arterial blood

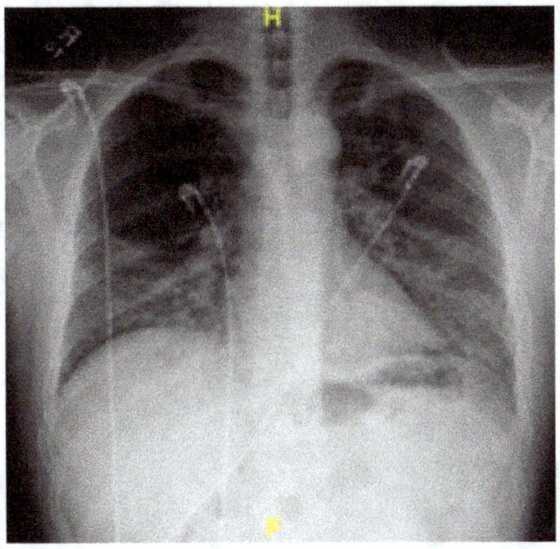

FIGURE 1: Initial chest X-ray showing bilateral patchy infiltrates with lower lobe predominance.

gas (ABG) revealed a pH of 7.47, PO_2 of 41 mmHg, and PCO_2 of 30.8 mmHg. His initial white cell count was 15.6×10^3 cells/μL (range: 4000-11000). Chest X-ray showed bilateral patchy infiltrates and consolidation with lower lobe predominance (Figure 1). Computed tomography (CT) with contrast of the chest was negative for pulmonary embolism but showed extensive bilateral airspace disease (Figure 2). Bronchoscopy revealed a moderate amount of thick mucoid secretions bilaterally with diffuse bronchial mucosal hyperemia.

Bronchoalveolar lavage (BAL) fluid analysis revealed increased WBC with lymphocytic predominance. Fluid culture did not grow any organisms, and cytology was negative for malignancy. Clinical improvement was seen after starting intravenous methylprednisolone 40 mg every 12 hours, ceftriaxone, and azithromycin. Antibiotics were discontinued once bronchoscopy cultures did not show any organisms. An echocardiogram showed a left ventricular ejection fraction of 55-60%. He was switched to oral prednisone 50 mg daily with significant improvement in his symptoms and oxygen requirements. He was subsequently discharged on a tapering dose of oral prednisone. On the fourth day after discharge, the patient presented to the ED once again with a complaint of sudden onset shortness of breath, right-sided chest pain, and cough productive of white sputum. Chest X-ray in the ED showed a right-sided tension pneumothorax along with bilateral parenchymal infiltrates (Figure 3). Emergent needle decompression was performed, and a small bore 12 French chest tube was inserted in the ED. The CT of the chest also revealed a right-sided pneumothorax, pneumomediastinum, right-sided subcutaneous emphysema, and parenchymal disease similar to previous imaging (Figure 4). The chest tube was removed on day 4. Repeat CT chest showed no pneumothorax, but a large bulla in the right lung adjacent to the major fissure with a few other bullae seen in the superior segment of the right lower lobe, pneumomediastinum, subcutaneous emphysema, and significant interstitial lung disease. The patient underwent blebectomy via video-assisted thoracic surgery. He did well and was discharged home and was doing well on room air on outpatient follow-up in one week.

3. Case 2

A 22-year-old male with a past medical history of substance abuse (marijuana vape pens daily), depression, and a history of suicidal ideation presented with a fever of 101°F and productive cough with white phlegm for 2 weeks. His symptoms were associated with nausea, vomiting, nonbloody diarrhea, night sweats, and headache. His blood pressure was 123/69 mmHg; heart rate 87 beats per minute; and oxygen saturation 93% on room air.

During the initial course in his hospitalization, he required 6 L of oxygen via a nasal cannula. His oxygen saturation began to decline, and he required 15 L of oxygen via an oxymask to maintain his oxygen saturation above 92%. Lung examination revealed wheezing bilaterally, while other systemic examinations remained unremarkable. He had white blood cell count of 14.31×10^3 cells/μL, with a neutrophil predominance of 94.3%, hemoglobin of 10 gm/dL, and platelet count of $487{,}000 \times 10^3/\mu$. ABG revealed pH 7.46, pCO_2 34.0 mmHg, pO_2 61.3 mmHg, and HCO_3 22.3. Chest X-ray showed bilateral airspace disease (Figure 5) and CT of the chest revealed scattered ground glass opacity in both lungs (Figure 6). We speculated the possibility of pneumonia versus pneumonitis caused by vaping. The patient was started on ceftriaxone, doxycycline, and oral prednisone at 60 mg daily. Bronchoscopy revealed inflammatory changes in bilateral upper lobes, more so on the right than the left. Bronchoalveolar lavage (BAL) sample analysis showed acute and chronic inflammatory cells with lymphocyte predominance and rare eosinophils. Cultures from BAL did not grow any organisms. Cytology did not reveal malignancy. His viral, fungal, and bacterial studies were negative. The patient improved and decided to leave against medical advice. However, upon reaching home, he had worsening dyspnea and subsequent syncopal episode prompting another visit to the ED. He was admitted once again and treated for both pneumonia and vaping-induced lung pneumonitis. He was restarted on prednisone 40 mg daily that was tapered over the next 2 weeks. The patient's symptoms completely resolved during follow-up in 2 weeks.

4. Case 3

A 42-year-old male with a past medical history of type 2 diabetes mellitus, hypertension, dyslipidemia, end-state renal disease on renal replacement therapy, and tobacco and marijuana use presented with an 8-day history of fever, cough productive of yellow sputum, myalgia, generalized weakness, multiple episodes of nausea, emesis, nonbloody diarrhea, and poor appetite. He was seen by his primary care physician two days prior to presentation in our ED and was prescribed levofloxacin. In the ED, the patient's white blood cell count was 13.0×10^3 cells/μL; chest X-ray showed diffuse bilateral infiltrates more pronounced on the right without pleural effusion (Figure 7). A CT chest without contrast was done which showed bilateral nonspecific ground glass opacity throughout the lungs without any pleural effusion or pneumothorax (Figure 8). Bronchoscopy showed mild clear secretions bilaterally. BAL washings had a hazy appearance with

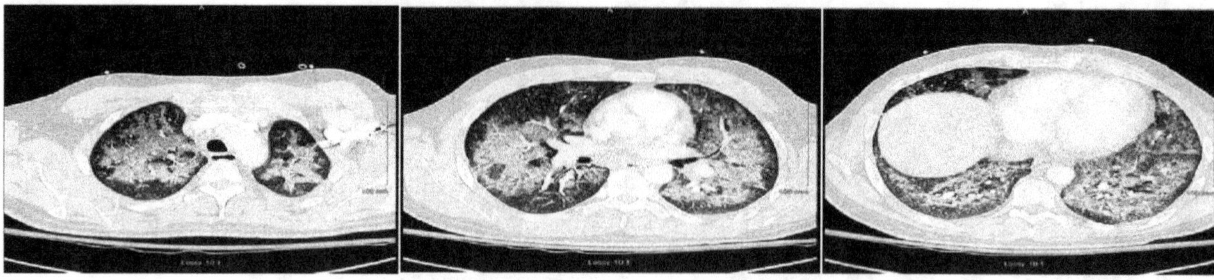

FIGURE 2: Chest CT showing bilateral airspace disease.

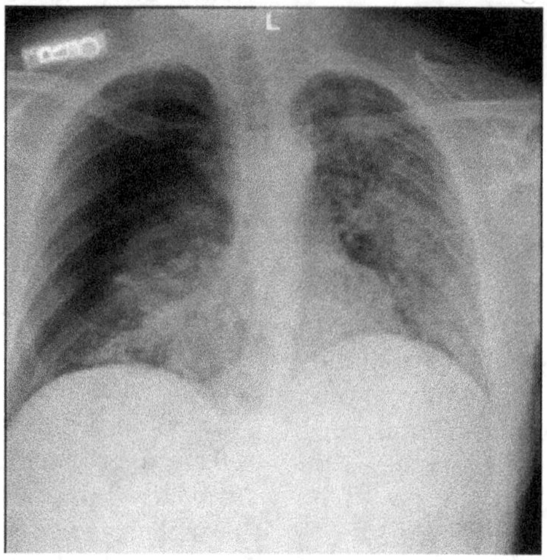

FIGURE 3: Chest X-ray showing bilateral parenchymal infiltrates and right-sided pneumothorax.

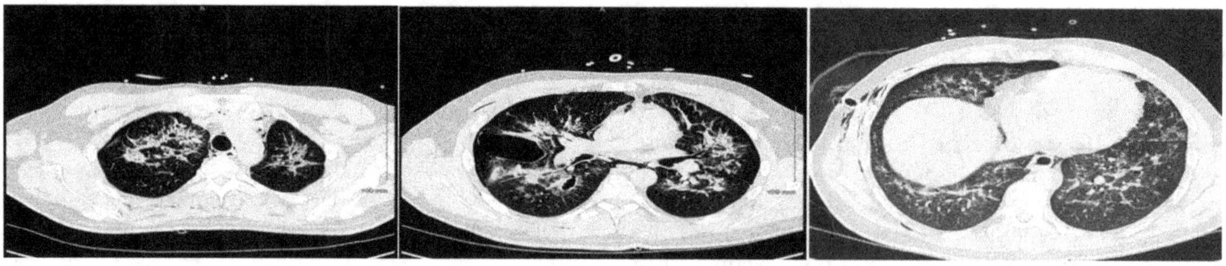

FIGURE 4: Chest CT showing a large bulla in the right lung adjacent to the major fissure with a few other bullae seen in the superior segment of the right lower lobe, pneumomediastinum, subcutaneous emphysema, and significant interstitial lung disease.

BAL fluid showing WBC 118, RBC of 3655, and 42 lymphocytes. Cultures and cytology were negative. Influenza A/B testing, human immunodeficiency virus (HIV) screen, fungal antibodies, autoimmune workup including antinuclear antibody, rheumatoid factor, anti-Ro antibody, anti-La antibody, c- ANCA, anti-Jo antibody, and anti-Smith antibody were all negative. He was started on IV methylprednisolone 40 mg every 12 hours for vaping-induced pneumonitis. The patient's symptoms significantly improved with the resolution of weakness, cough, nausea, and emesis. He was subsequently discharged on prednisone 40 mg daily tapered over 2 weeks and counseled heavily on discontinuing the use of E-cigarettes.

5. Case 4

A 27-year-old male with no significant past medical history who presented with the complaints of shortness of breath, nausea, vomiting, and night sweats for 5 days. He reported using an E-cigarette for 6 months. He was using products containing both nicotine and tetrahydrocannabinol (THC). He stated that he had started using a "black market" cartridge containing THC 2 days before symptom onset. His vital signs showed a temperature of 100°F, heart rate of 115 beats per minute, blood pressure of 137/81 mmHg, and oxygen saturation of 98% on room air. Laboratory workup was significant for a WBC of 18.28×10^3 cells/μL. Chest X-ray showed

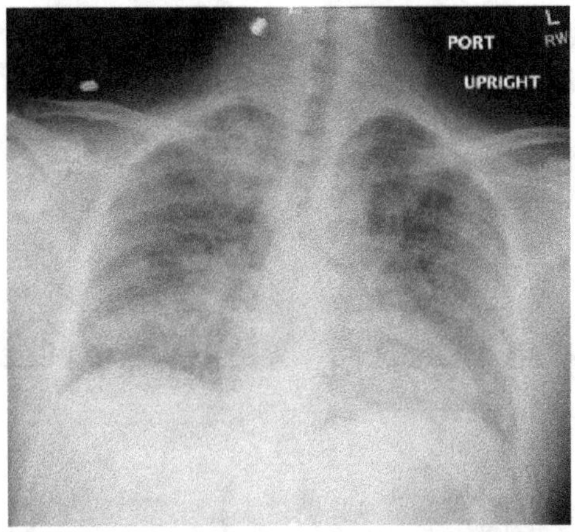

FIGURE 5: Chest X-ray showing bilateral infiltrates.

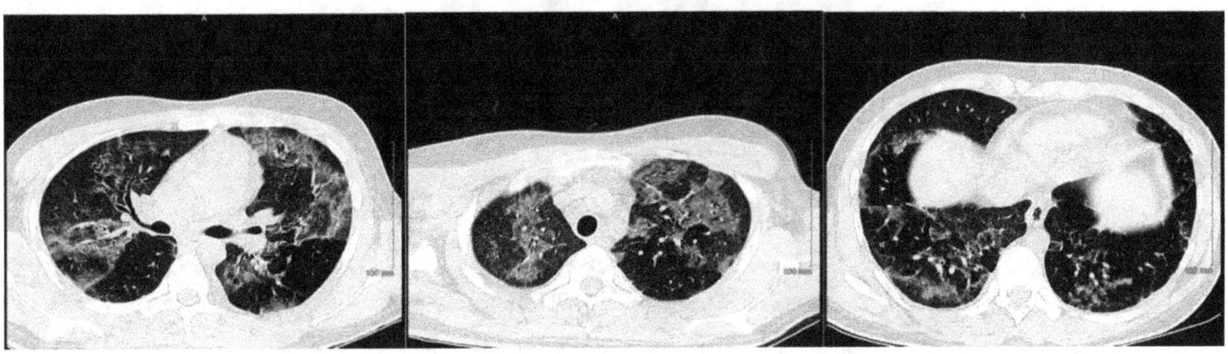

FIGURE 6: Chest CT showing bilateral scattered ground glass opacities.

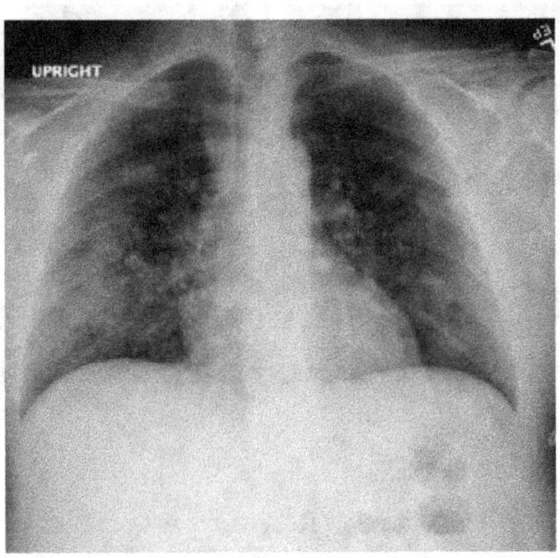

FIGURE 7: Chest X-ray showing diffuse bilateral infiltrates, more pronounced on the right side.

airspace opacities bilaterally (Figure 9). He was started on intravenous ceftriaxone and azithromycin and admitted to the hospital. He continued to have dyspnea; therefore, a CT chest without contrast was obtained which revealed diffuse infiltrates bilaterally (Figure 10). He was then initiated on IV methylprednisolone 40 mg every day. His symptoms continued to improve during the short hospital course, and after significant clinical improvement, he was discharged home on a prednisone 40 mg daily tapered over 2 weeks. He was counseled to avoid using E-cigarettes.

6. Case 5

A 21-year-old male with no past medical history presented with acute onset of left-sided chest pain. He stated he was at work and during his break was using an E-cigarette when he developed severe left-sided chest pain and shortness of breath. He reported using an E- cigarette for the past 3 years. He stated that he only used nicotine-containing cartridges and had never used any other cartridges containing THC. He went to an urgent care center where a chest X-ray was obtained which revealed a small left-sided pneumothorax. In the ED, a repeat chest X-ray was obtained which revealed a moderate sized pneumothorax (Figure 11). A left-sided chest tube was inserted. Laboratory workup was insignificant and did not reveal any abnormal findings. CT chest was obtained which revealed left-sided atelectasis (Figure 12). His pneumothorax resolved, and the chest tube was removed on hospital day 3 and he was discharged home with instructions to avoid vaping.

7. Discussion

The use of E-cigarettes or vaping has risen exponentially within the past few years. Although never officially approved by the FDA, there is a common misconception that their use is safe [5]. The majority of users are teens and young adults, which makes this latest phenomenon concerning. Popularity can be attributed to aggressive manufacturer campaigns

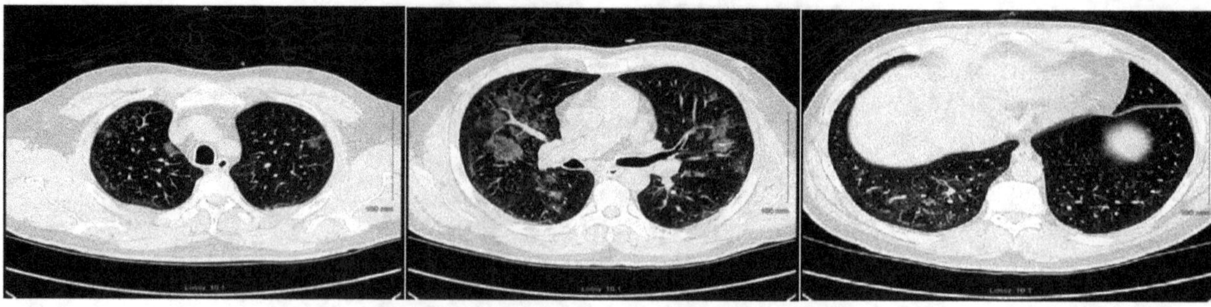

FIGURE 8: Chest CT showing nonspecific bilateral ground glass opacities.

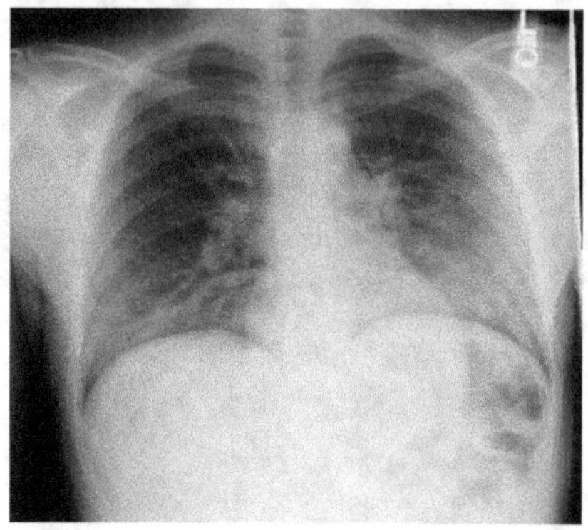

FIGURE 9: Chest X-ray showing bilateral airspace opacities.

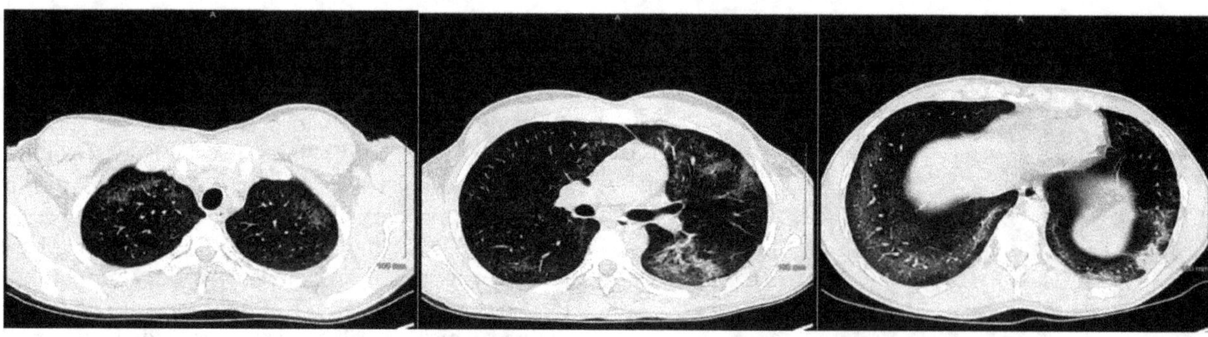

FIGURE 10: Chest CT showing bilateral diffuse infiltrates.

promoting these products and a sizable number of celebrities frequently seen using these products. Introduced to the US market in 2007, E-cigarettes visually mimic conventional cigarettes; however, they do not burn tobacco [3, 6]. Instead, they are battery-operated and vaporize an "E-liquid" at high temperatures producing aerosols. This liquid mixture contains nicotine and various compounds. The chemical composition of these liquids does vary, which includes, but not limited to, glycerin, propylene glycol, formaldehyde, acetaldehyde, acrolein, and various tobacco-specific nitrosamines. Propylene glycol and glycerin constitute about 66% and 24% of the liquid, respectively. One major factor at play is the numerous flavors that are available and readily added to the E-liquid.

They range from fruity flavors to unusual flavors like chocolate, coffee, etc. that are particularly appealing to the younger population [6, 7]. Recent reports of significant pulmonary illness from the use of vaping products have received significant attention. However, healthcare professionals remain at a disadvantage because there is a lack of complete understanding of how these products induce injury and cause significant symptoms.

According to the CDC, in 2015, among older E-cigarette users (aged 45 or older), 1.3% had never used traditional cigarettes. While in younger users (aged 18-24), 40% had never smoked traditional cigarettes. In 2018, more than 3.6 million US middle and high school students used E-cigarettes within the past 30 days [8]. In 2019, the CDC has reported 1299 cases, 70% of those were male, the median age was 24, and 80% of patients were under 35 years of age. On December 17, 2019, CDC published an updated document stating that

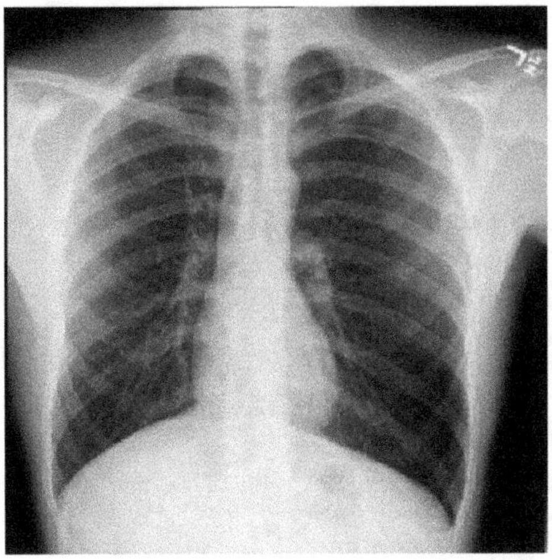

FIGURE 11: Chest X-ray showing moderate sized left-sided pneumothorax.

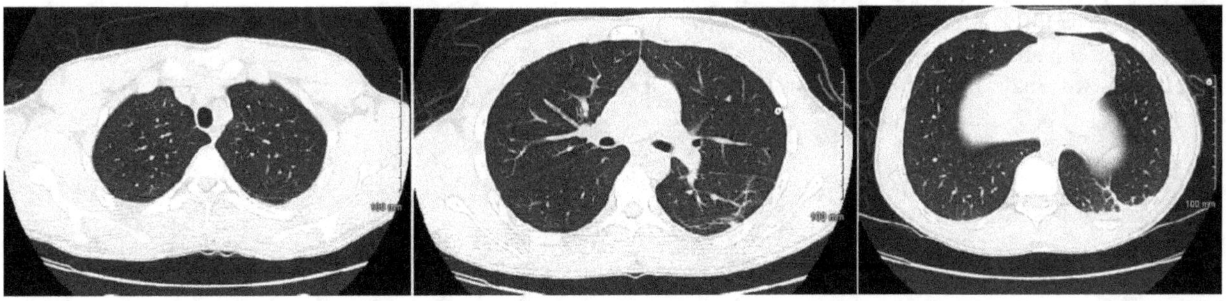

FIGURE 12: Chest CT showing left-sided atelectasis.

2,506 cases and more than 54 associated deaths due to vaping/E-cigarette-associated lung injury were reported [9]. We expect this data to change with the rising incidence of this disease. Initial data shows that most patients use E-cigarettes containing THC; some use nicotine while others used a combination of both nicotine and THC. Vitamin E acetate and THC were implicated as the most likely causative agents in the report released by CDC in December of 2019. Vitamin E acetate was detected in BAL samples of 48 of 51 samples collected by CDC. In this context, it is sensible to recommend avoidance of THC-containing vapes that are most likely laced with vitamin E acetate. But there are still a persistent small number of cases that have not reported the use of THC-containing compounds [9]. The FDA is analyzing samples collected from patients across the country that have suffered from this illness and is testing a variety of chemicals including but not limited to THC and nicotine. Interestingly, though vitamin E acetate and THC have been found to be the most likely culprit, no single chemical has been solely linked to these reports. We think that there might be more compounds playing the causative role that are yet to be unearthed. There is also scarcity of a definite clinical practice guideline in terms of the evaluation and management of the vaping-induced lung injury [10].

These case series of 5 patients that we presented were recently hospitalized with similar symptomology. These patients presented to the hospital between July and September of 2019, which encompass the early phase of this epidemic. They had symptoms of dyspnea, nausea, and vomiting as the most common presenting symptoms. Imaging showed diffuse bilateral ground glass opacities except in case 5, which predominantly showed pneumothorax only. Further understanding of the pathophysiology of vaping-induced lung injury is needed. To date, no absolute histopathologic findings have been linked to the use of E-cigarettes. In addition, BAL findings were nonspecific. With vaping being introduced almost a decade ago, the question that naturally arises is what changed? There is no conclusive evidence as to why so many people have suffered over the past few months. Studies need to be conducted to better understand the root cause of this challenge. Per our assessment, there must have been either an environmental change, change in the E-cigarette, or its components to have caused this serious epidemic. Another factors to take into consideration are genetic factors or common phenotype among the affected individuals. There are some limitations, which were noted in this case series. Not all patients underwent bronchoscopy, and therefore, we do not have BAL results. Lung biopsies were not done because they were not warranted at the time as the patients began to improve clinically. The treatment was not standardized as this was an emerging condition and the data on treatment was nonexistent.

8. Conclusion

We have presented the case series of 5 patients who were seen in the earlier stage of this disease emergence. Since our submission and revision process, the number of patients with this condition has drastically increased and the pathophysiology seems to have become little more apparent. We, as authors, still feel that there is much more to be learned in this condition, and we may not be surprised if pathophysiology and the inciting and exacerbating factors change over time as more patient data and information emerge. We feel that these early case reports will entice more vigilance among the readership to have an open mind as they come across the clinical vignette and urge them to be more proactive in reporting and studying this disease. It is prudent to continue reporting all the cases of vaping-induced lung injury and its subsequent complications in a relentless manner. Further data and evidence emanating from every possible stratum of the healthcare community will play a vital role in zeroing down on all the harmful compounds in the E-cigarettes. In the wake of recent data by CDC pertaining to vitamin E acetate and THC, we may be tempted to rest our case prematurely.

References

[1] K. Moore, H. Young II, and M. F. Ryan, "Bilateral pneumonia and pleural effusions subsequent to electronic cigarette use," *Open Journal of Emergency Medicine*, vol. 3, no. 3, pp. 18–22, 2015.

[2] P. Caponnetto, D. Campagna, F. Cibella et al., "Correction: Efficiency and safety of an electronic cigarette (ECLAT) as tobacco cigarettes substitute: a prospective 12-Month randomized control design study," *PLoS One*, vol. 9, no. 1, 2014.

[3] J. E. Layden, I. Ghinai, I. Pray et al., "Pulmonary illness related to E-cigarette use in Illinois and Wisconsin — preliminary report," *The New England Journal of Medicine*, 2019.

[4] C. K. Yamin, A. Bitton, and D. W. Bates, "E-cigarettes: a rapidly growing internet phenomenon," *Annals of Internal Medicine*, vol. 153, no. 9, pp. 607–609, 2010.

[5] J. F. Etter, C. Bullen, A. D. Flouris, M. Laugesen, and T. Eissenberg, "Electronic nicotine delivery systems: a research agenda," *Tobacco Control*, vol. 20, no. 3, pp. 243–248, 2011.

[6] R. Grana, N. Benowitz, and S. A. Glantz, "E-Cigarettes," *Circulation*, vol. 129, no. 19, pp. 1972–1986, 2014.

[7] R. M. Pellegrino, B. Tinghino, G. Mangiaracina et al., "Electronic cigarettes: an evaluation of exposure to chemicals and fine particulate matter (PM)," *Annali di Igiene*, vol. 24, no. 4, pp. 279–288, 2012.

[8] "Electronic cigarettes fact sheet," 2019, http://www.CDC.gov/.

[9] https://www.cdc.gov/media/releases/2019/t1220_telebriefing_update_lung_injury.html.

[10] A. Kalininskiy, C. T. Bach, N. E. Nacca et al., "E-cigarette, or vaping, product use associated lung injury (EVALI): case series and diagnostic approach," *The Lancet Respiratory Medicine*, vol. 7, no. 12, pp. 1017–1026, 2019.

25

Vaping and Commitment Flu-B Infection is a Deadly Combination for Spontaneous Pneumomediastinum

Md Didar Ul Alam,[1,2] **Khandakar Hussain**,[1,2] **Samsone Garedew**,[2] **and Muhammad imtiaz**[1]

[1]*Department of Internal Medicine, Conemaugh Medical Memorial Center, Johnstown, PA, USA*
[2]*Department of Hospital Medicine, Conemaugh Medical Memorial Center, Johnstown, PA, USA*

Correspondence should be addressed to Md Didar Ul Alam; didar.134@gmail.com

Academic Editor: Tun-Chieh Chen

Vaping or E-cigarettes were created to deliver nicotine-containing aerosol to users with a flavoring agent without agents such as tars, oxidant gases, and carbon monoxide smoke found in traditional tobacco cigarettes. The use of E-cigarettes is steadily increasing in the United States, especially among the young population. Electronic cigarettes seem capable of causing various injury patterns in the lungs, collectively called E-cigarettes or vaping-associated lung injury (EVALI). Spontaneous pneumomediastinum (SPM) is a rare finding in EVALI. Here, we report a case of spontaneous pneumomediastinum secondary to vaping in a young man with no past medical history except for daily vaping and a recent untreated influenza infection.

1. Introduction

Pneumomediastinum is defined as the presence of air or other gas in the mediastinum also known as mediastinal emphysema [1]. Pneumomediastinum can be categorized as spontaneous pneumomediastinum (SPM) and secondary pneumomediastinum. Secondary pneumomediastinum is caused by blunt or penetrating chest wall trauma, barotrauma from mechanical ventilation, underlying airway diseases, endobronchial, and esophageal perforation. Vaping or E-cigarettes gained popularity over the last few years. E-cigarettes containing nicotine and other substances vaporize or produce aerosols, which the users then inhale. Predisposing conditions or triggers are identified in some cases of pneumomediastinum in children. A respiratory illness that led to pneumomediastinum, especially during acute exaggeration with excessive coughing, i.e., in asthma and respiratory infections, is identified in children and adolescents [2–5]. The unique aspect was that the development of SPM was triggered by excessive coughing from untreated influenza infection in an otherwise healthy young man with concomitant lung injury from daily vaping.

2. Case Presentation

A 22-year-old male was brought to the emergency department (ED) for cough and progressive shortness of breath for the last six days. His past medical history is unremarkable except for daily vaping. A week ago he also tested positive for influenza B when he had chills, fatigue, and sore throat. He did not take oseltamivir due to a late prescription from his primary care physician. He had low-grade fever with nausea and vomiting with fierce cough four days before presentation to ED. He also felt crepitus in the neck. He did not have any prior chest surgical history or any history of illicit drug abuse. In the ED, his temperature was 99.1 degrees Fahrenheit, blood pressure of 150/95 mmHg, heart rate of 136 beats/min, and a saturation of 91% on 3 L nasal cannula (NC) oxygen. On physical examination, subcutaneous emphysema was noted in the anterior cervical region. Blood work showed leukocytosis of 18,000/mL and a procalcitonin level of 0.21 ng/mL. Chest X-ray (CXR) showed pneumomediastinum with subcutaneous emphysema extending into the cervical region with bilateral pneumonia (Figure 1).

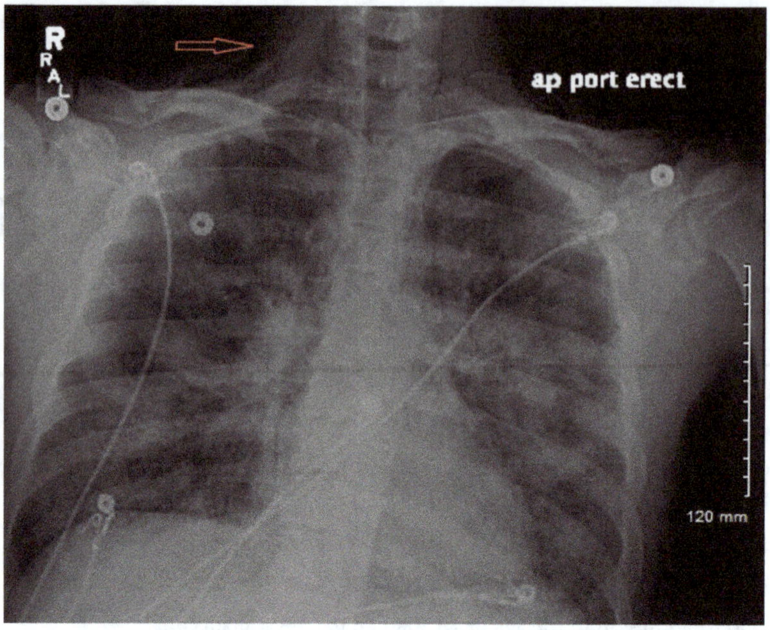

FIGURE 1: X-ray showing pneumomediastinum with subcutaneous emphysema (red arrow) extending to the cervical region with bilateral pneumonia.

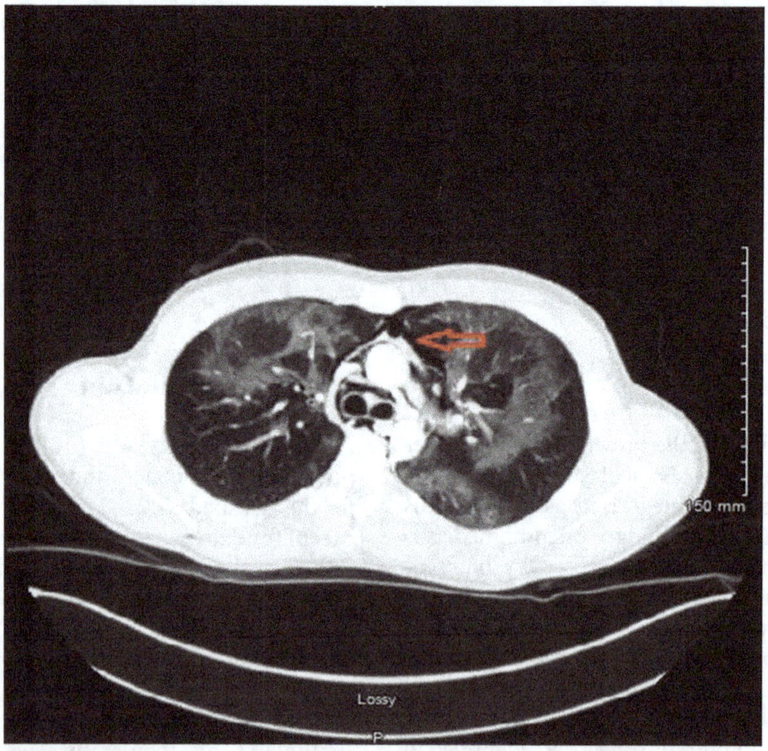

FIGURE 2: Computed tomography (CT) chest showing severe pneumomediastinum (red arrow) with diffuse pneumonitis.

Chest computed tomography (CT) showed severe pneumomediastinum with subcutaneous emphysema and diffuse pneumonitis (Figure 2).

The patient was admitted to the medical floor. He was treated with supplemental 3 L NC supplemental oxygen, and oseltamivir and antibiotics were discontinued. A gastrografin esophagogram was done, and esophageal rupture was ruled out. Repeat CXR two days later showed improvement of pneumomediastinum and subcutaneous emphysema (Figure 3). He was counseled extensively against vaping and was discharged home on room air.

3. Discussion

SPM occurs due to air leaks through small alveolar ruptures to the surrounding bronchovascular sheath.

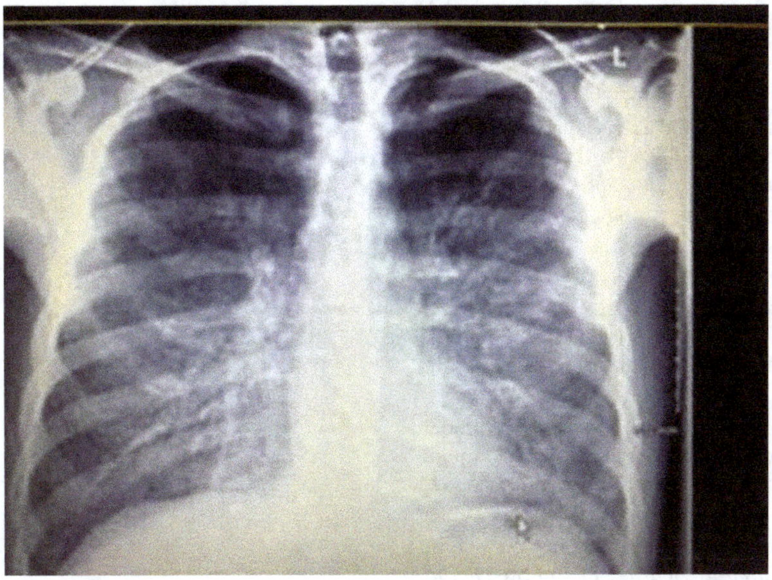

FIGURE 3: Improvement of pneumomediastinum and subcutaneous emphysema.

Pneumomediastinum also could result from air leaks from the gastrointestinal tract (esophageal rupture) and respiratory tract [1, 6]. The proposed mechanism occurs due to differential pressure gradient that develops between the alveoli and lung interstitium. This pressure gradient can occur either by increasing the alveolar pressure (Valsalva maneuver) or by decreasing the interstitial pressure (increased work of breathing). This leads to alveolar rupture and release of air into a mediastinal space with lower pressure (Macklin effect) [7]. As the mean pressure in the mediastinum is always negative than the pressure in the pulmonary parenchyma, the free air tends to move centripetally along the vascular sheaths, facilitated by the pumping action of breathing. The air spreads to the hilum and into the mediastinum or through the loose mediastinal fascia to the subcutaneous tissues of the thorax, upper limbs, and neck. Recently, postulated mechanisms by which vaping can lead to acute lung injury include airway remodeling, macrophage activation, and direct injury of airway epithelium [8].

In most cases, the movement of air into the subcutaneous tissues prevents the buildup of pressure in the mediastinum. Occasionally, air leaks into the pericardial space, causing pneumopericardium [9, 10]. In extremely rare cases, pressure accumulates in the mediastinal cavity, causing pneumothorax or compression of adjacent intrathoracic structure leading to tension pneumomediastinum or tension pneumopericardium [11–14].

The classic triad of pneumomediastinum is retrosternal pleuritic pain (with exacerbation during deep inspiration), subcutaneous emphysema, and dyspnea. Chest radiography including the cervical region should be the standard initial diagnostic procedure and shows lucent streaks or bubbles of gas that outline mediastinal structures [11]. Other radiologic evidence of SPM includes thoracic and cervical subcutaneous emphysema (which is most apparent on lateral neck radiographs). The diagnosis should be confirmed with a chest computed tomography scan. Gastrografin esophagogram and bronchoscopy should be performed if there is suspicion of esophageal and tracheobronchial tree rupture.

Uncomplicated SPM is managed conservatively with analgesia, rest, and avoidance of maneuvers that increase pulmonary pressure (Valsalva or forced expiration) [7, 15]. The complications of SPM include pneumothorax with pneumomediastinum (requires chest tube), esophageal perforation with secondary pneumomediastinum (requires intensive medical and surgical management), tension pneumomediastinum (requires limited mediastinotomy), and pneumopericardium (requires surveillance for pericardial tamponade) [9, 10, 12].

4. Conclusion

SPM is a rare presentation of EVALI. To our knowledge, this is the first reported case of spontaneous pneumothorax in a healthy young man with daily vaping with concomitant influenza infection. Treatment of uncomplicated SPM is supportive consists of analgesia, oxygen therapy, rest, and avoidance of maneuvers that increase pulmonary pressure. Most patients recover without sequelae within a few days, and recurrence is rare.

Acknowledgments

This case was presented in chest virtual meeting 2020. doi:10.1371/journal.pmed1000097

References

[1] R. Mason, "Pneumomediastinum and mediastinitis. In: Murray and Nadel's," in *Textbook of Respiratory Medicine*, Elsevier Health Sciences, 4th edition, 2005, Chapter 72.

[2] J. B. Jougon, M. Ballester, F. Delcambre, T. Mac Bride, C. E. H. Dromer, and J. F. Velly, "Assessment of spontaneous pneumomediastinum: experience with 12 patients," *The Annals of Thoracic Surgery*, vol. 75, no. 6, pp. 1711–1714, 2003.

[3] K. S. Wong, H. M. Wu, S. H. Lai, and C. Y. Chiu, "Spontaneous pneumomediastinum: analysis of 87 pediatric patients," *Pediatric Emergency Care*, vol. 29, no. 9, pp. 988–991, 2013.

[4] C. Y. Lee, C. C. Wu, and C. Y. Lin, "Etiologies of spontaneous pneumomediastinum in children in middle Taiwan," *Pediatric Pulmonology*, vol. 45, no. 9, pp. 869–873, 2010.

[5] K. Yamada, H. Shinmoto, M. Hamamoto et al., "Pneumonia induced by swine-origin influenza A (H1N1) infection: chest computed tomography findings in children," *Japanese Journal of Radiology*, vol. 29, no. 10, pp. 712–717, 2011.

[6] C. C. Macklin, "Transport of air along sheaths of pulmonic blood vessels from alveoli to mediastinum: clinical implications," *Archives of Internal Medicine*, vol. 64, no. 5, p. 913, 1939.

[7] I. Macia, J. Moya, R. Ramos et al., "Spontaneous pneumomediastinum: 41 cases," *European Journal of Cardio-Thoracic Surgery*, vol. 31, no. 6, pp. 1110–1114, 2007.

[8] J. R. Balmes, "Vaping-induced acute lung injury: an epidemic that could have been prevented," *American Journal of Respiratory and Critical Care Medicine*, vol. 200, no. 11, pp. 1342–1344, 2019.

[9] V. Vanzo, S. Bugin, D. Snijders, L. Bottecchia, V. Storer, and A. Barbato, "Pneumomediastinum and pneumopericardium in an 11-year-old rugby player: a case report," *Journal of Athletic Training*, vol. 48, no. 2, pp. 277–281, 2013.

[10] C. J. Allen, L. F. Teisch, and K. D. Stahl, "Spontaneous pneumomediastinum, pneumopericardium and epidural pneumatosis: insights on clinical management," *Acute Card Care*, vol. 17, no. 1, pp. 20–23, 2015.

[11] M. Chalumeau, L. le Clainche, N. Sayeg et al., "Spontaneous pneumomediastinum in children," *Pediatric Emergency Care*, vol. 31, no. 1, pp. 67–75, 2001.

[12] D. B. Herlan, R. J. Landreneau, and P. F. Ferson, "Massive Spontaneous Subcutaneous Emphysema: Acute Management with Infraclavicular "Blow Holes"," *Chest*, vol. 102, no. 2, pp. 503–505, 1992.

[13] I. S. I. Mohamed, Y.-H. Lee, S. Z. Yamout, S. Fakir, and A. M. Reynolds, "Ultrasound guided percutaneous relief of tension pneumomediastinum in a 1-day-old newborn," *Archives of Disease in Childhood. Fetal and Neonatal Edition*, vol. 92, no. 6, p. F458, 2007.

[14] K. L. Rao, S. Imamuddin, and A. P. Kumar, "Isolated tension pneumopericardium in a case of acute lymphoblastic leukemia," *Indian Heart Journal*, vol. 65, no. 6, pp. 705-706, 2013.

[15] J. W. Fitzwater, N. N. Silva, C. G. Knight, L. Malvezzi, C. Ramos-Irizarry, and C. A. Burnweit, "Management of spontaneous pneumomediastinum in children," *Journal of Pediatric Surgery*, vol. 50, no. 6, pp. 983–986, 2015.

26

Vaping-Induced Lung Injury: A Case of Lipoid Pneumonia Associated with E-Cigarettes Containing Cannabis

Bryno Gay,[1] Zachary Field,[1] Sachin Patel,[2] Rodrigo Murillo Alvarez,[3] Wael Nasser,[2] Mario Madruga,[1] and S. J. Carlan[4]

[1]*Department of Medicine, Orlando Regional Healthcare, Orlando, Florida, USA*
[2]*Department of Pulmonary, Critical Care and Sleep Medicine, Orlando Regional Healthcare, Orlando, USA*
[3]*Department of Pathology, Orlando Regional Healthcare, Orlando, USA*
[4]*Division of Academic Affairs and Research, Orlando Regional Healthcare, Orlando, USA*

Correspondence should be addressed to S. J. Carlan; stevecarlan@gmail.com

Academic Editor: Kenneth M Nugent

Electronic cigarette, or vaping product use-associated lung injury (EVALI), is a group of lung disorders associated with vaping and e-cigarette products that has previously been categorized as a diagnosis of exclusion and best described as an exogenous lipoid pneumonia or chemical pneumonitis. Here, we describe the onset of an exogenous cause of lipoid pneumonia in an otherwise healthy patient using cannabis-containing electronic cigarettes. We explore similarities in the clinical case, define a common clinical presentation with progression of disease, characteristic radiographic findings along with pathological diagnosis and management.

1. Introduction

Electronic cigarettes were introduced into the United States market in 2007. Since then, both nicotine-containing electronic cigarettes and cannabis-containing electronic cigarettes have seen a rapid rise in popularity [1, 2]. Frequently marketed as a less harmful alternative to conventional smoking, many chronic tobacco and cannabis smokers as well as new users have contributed to the rise in demand. In this paper, we will use the term "vape pen" to mean an electronic cigarette containing cannabis and "e-cigarette" to mean an electronic cigarette containing nicotine. Vape pens operate in the same way as e-cigarettes. However, unlike its nicotine counterpart, tetrahydrocannabinol is not widely available as a purified chemical. Instead, vape pens contain extracts of cannabis plant material. Known variously as cannabis extract, cannabis concentrate, THC oil, hash oil, and butane-hash oil, these extracts are not diluted in propylene glycol or glycerol like nicotine due to their hydrophobic properties. Instead, various forms of oils including vegetable oils, terpenes, and tocopheryl acetate (vitamin E acetate) have been reported as diluents. In most reported cases of EVALI, additional flavoring additives are also added to products [3].

Although many of these diluent agents and flavorings have been "generally recognized as safe" for oral ingestion by the FDA, recent research shows that when heated to form an aerosol and inhaled, conditions including bronchitis, bronchiolitis, acute hypoxic respiratory distress, lipoid-associated pneumonia, and pneumonitis may result [1, 4, 5]. As a relatively new product, the safety profile and long-term effects of vape pens and e-cigarettes remain largely undefined.

The outbreak of severe and acute pulmonary disease associated with the use of cannabis extract-containing vape pens and nicotine e-cigarettes has grown to 2,711 reported cases according to the most up-to-date data retrieved from the Center for Disease Control and Prevention (CDC) website posted on January 20, 2020 [6]. In fact, all 50 states, the District of Columbia, and two U.S. territories (Puerto Rico and the U.S. Virgin Islands) have reported severe and acute pulmonary disease associated with e-cigarettes with 27 confirmed associated deaths [6].

Although a definitive cause is postulated to be a chemical exposure, more specifically from substances within the cannabis vape pens [5, 7], the acute incidence of pulmonary disease has brought national attention to this epidemic and warrants a continued investigation into these products, their contents, and medical management for EVALI, especially those purchased from informal sources (i.e., black market products) as reported in the case below.

1.1. Case Report. A 46-year-old male with no significant medical history presented with shortness of breath and flu-like symptoms including generalized weakness, fatigue, chills, diaphoresis, fever, and cough. The patient denied any recent sick contacts, travel history, history of shortness of breath, or history of lung disease. The patient reported only smoking conventional marijuana for 20 plus years, smoking 2 to 3 times per day, and had approximately a 4-6-month history of vape pen usage, with and without flavor additives. The cannabis vape pens were purchased in bulk from an informal source. The patient reported a less than 1-year history of conventional cigarette use and quit over 20 years ago. He denied the use of chewing tobacco, electronic cigarettes containing nicotine, or any other nicotine-containing products during this time.

On arrival, the patient was afebrile with a respiratory rate of 20 breaths per minute, oxygen saturation was 96% on ambient air, blood pressure was 126/82 mmHg, and heart rate was 96 beats per minute. Over the next 4 hours, the patient rapidly deteriorated into acute hypoxic respiratory failure with hypoxia down to 86% while on 2 liters nasal cannula. The patient was increased to 13 liters high-flow nasal cannula, started on empiric antibiotics, and intravenous methylprednisolone 125 mg which corrected the hypoxia with sustained oxygen saturation of 94%.

Physical exam was remarkable for diaphoresis, tachypnea, labored breathing with accessory muscle use, and diffuse inspiratory crackles. An arterial blood gas showed a pH of 7.51 [7.35-7.45], pCO2 38 [35-45 mmHg], pO2 84 [80-100 mmHg], and HCO_3 of 30.3 mmol/L [22-26 mmol/L]. Lab work showed a venous lactic acidosis at 2.3 mmol/L [0.9-1.7 mmol/L], white blood cell count of $14.8 \times 10^3/\mu l$ [$4.4 - 10.5 \times 10^3/\mu l$], and a normal sedimentation rate. Chest X-ray noted diffuse, bilateral pulmonary consolidation sparing the apices, and bases with bronchopulmonary cuffing (Figure 1). Computed tomography (CT) imaging showed extensive bilateral airspace disease with increased reticulation, traction bronchiectasis, and ground glass opacities but noted sparing of apical spaces bilaterally (Figure 2).

Further lab work including blood and sputum cultures, HIV, urine Histoplasma, Legionella, Pneumococcal antigens, and respiratory viral panel were all negative. Serologies—-coccidiomycosis, histoplasmosis, and pneumocystis—were also negative. Bronchoscopy with transbronchial biopsies were performed and a sample from the right lower lobe was significant for intra-alveolar inflammation including foamy macrophages and activated type II pneumocytes (Figure 3). These findings were consistent with organizing pneumonia. A histopathology examination on bronchoalveolar lavage (BAL) sample stained with Oil red O showed numerous

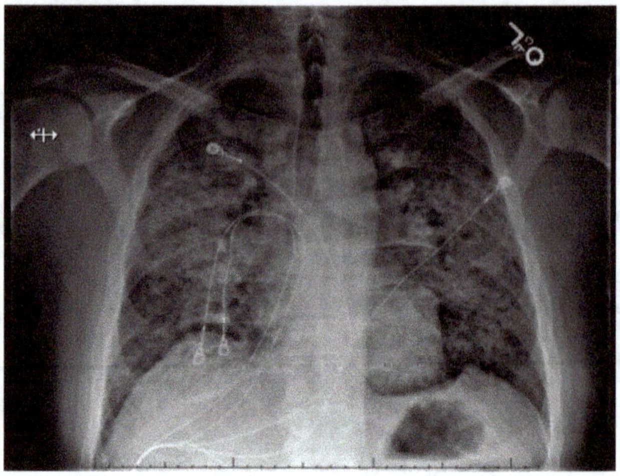

FIGURE 1: Chest X-ray showing extensive patchy bilateral consolidation.

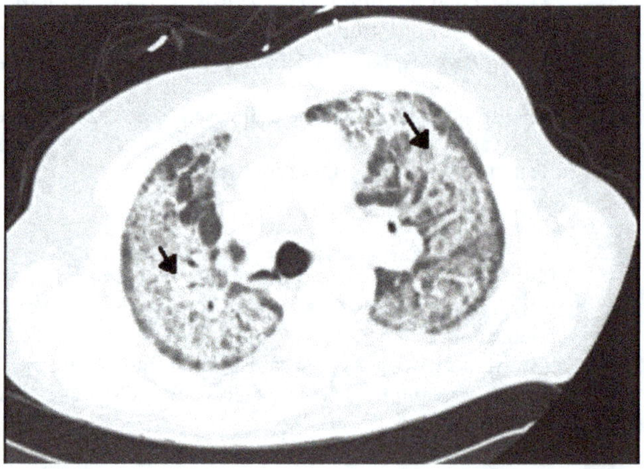

FIGURE 2: CT of the thorax showing extensive bilateral infiltrates and ground glass type densities (black arrow) sparing the periphery.

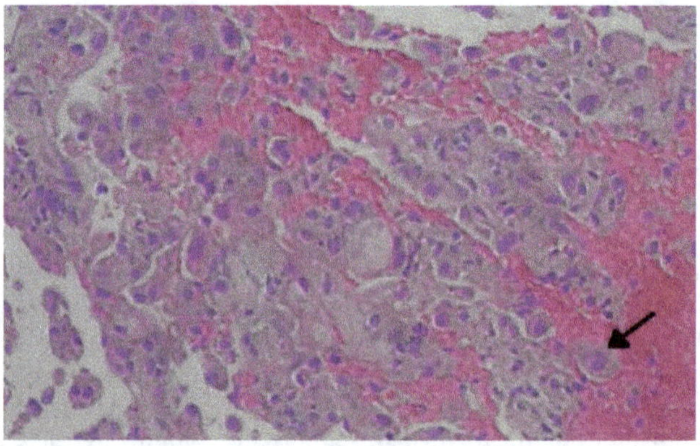

FIGURE 3: Lung biopsy showing organizing pneumonia and foamy macrophages (black arrow). (Hematoxylin-eosin, original magnification ×400).

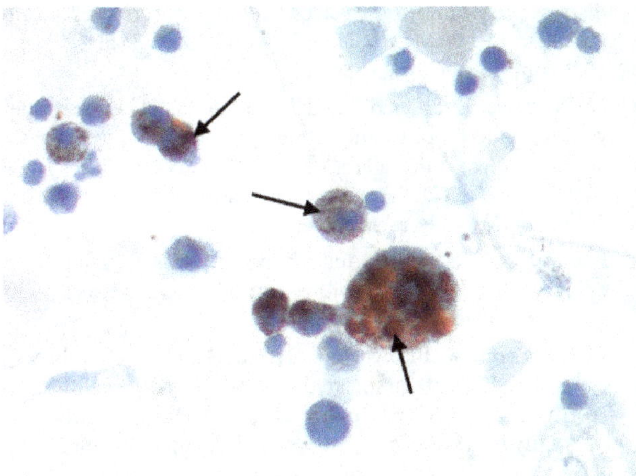

Figure 4: Bronchoalveolar lavage fluid stained with Oil red O highlights numerous macrophages containing lipid deposits, marked with black arrows (lipid-laden macrophages).

lipid-laden macrophages and intra-alveolar macrophages containing blackish-brown pigment (Figure 4). This was consistent with a diagnosis of lipoid pneumonia. Additional testing was negative for AFB stain, cytomegalovirus, herpes simplex antigen, and aspergillus antigen. During the hospital course, the patient improved over a six-day regimen of bronchodilators, steroids, and empiric antibiotics with supportive care of oxygen supplementation. He was discharged on the same regimen for 14 days with follow-up with pulmonology and repeat CT imaging in six weeks.

2. Discussion

Lipoid pneumonia is an unusual disease caused by the presence of lipids in the alveoli and is a chronic foreign body reaction to fat. It can be classified into two groups depending on an exogenous versus endogenous source of lipid or oil and host tissue reactions to the inhaled substances according to their chemical characteristics. The clinical presentation is unpredictable with progressive, subtle respiratory symptoms ranging from dyspnea and cough to severe life-threatening diseases [8–11].

Consequently, making a diagnosis of exogenous lipoid pneumonia requires a high degree of clinical suspicion. Radiographic findings consistent with EVALI include a crazy-paving pattern, interlobular septal thickening, diffuse infiltrates with a range of "ground glass" opacities, and nodular or "tree-in-bud" apical surfaces [12–14]. The presence of lipid-laden macrophages in the sputum or BAL specimen are also consistent with diagnosis of EVALI; however, high lipid-laden macrophages and high lipid-laden alveolar macrophage index (LLAMI) are nonspecific findings and can be found in various lung diseases [15]. Therefore, the addition of foamy macrophages, extracellular oily droplets, and macrophage with large cytoplasmic vacuoles contrasting to small vacuoles in the endogenous forms can guide a more specific diagnosis of exogenous lipoid pneumonia [16] which may also contain inflammatory cells similar to a foreign body reaction with a proliferative fibrosis and black pigmented dye in macrophages [17]. Lastly, vacuolated macrophages will stain orange with Sudan stain or red with Oil red O stain [15] as seen in BAL sample collected in this case (Figure 4).

THC-containing vape pens have become increasingly popular among adolescents. Current data from the Center of Disease Control (CDC) reports 27 deaths associated with EVALI. Interestingly, demographic data from a sample of 2,711 patients illustrated a majority of male patients (66%). Of the total reported cases 15% were below 18 years old, 37% were between 18 and 24 years old, 24% were between 25 and 34 years old, and 24% were 35 years old or older [6]. Approximately 82% reported using THC-containing products, 33% reported exclusive use of THC-containing products, 57% reported using nicotine-containing products, and 14% reported exclusive use of nicotine-containing products [6]. Of the EVALI patients who reported using THC-containing products, 78% reported acquiring products from informal sources while 69% of EVALI patients who reported using nicotine-containing products acquired theirs from an established business [6].

THC vape pens are a prefilled cartridge of cannabis extract, which may include diluents and flavorings, with a battery-operated heating system [7]. Although classified as "generally recognized as safe" by the Food and Drug Administration when ingested orally, these substances cause severe lung injury when heated to temperatures between 180 and 230°C and inhaled as an aerosol.

This disease outbreak is evolving rapidly. There appears to be some difference of opinion on whether e-cigarette, or vaping, product use-associated lung injury (EVALI) is best described as exogenous lipoid pneumonia or chemical pneumonitis [4]. However, the likely diagnostic path and treatment (trial and failure of albuterol and antibiotics, treatment with steroids, respiratory support and antibiotics to suppress secondary infections) remain the same. This case, with the positive oil red O staining for lipid vacuoles in macrophages, provides further evidence for the role of lipid. The patient described in this case disposed of his THC oil and vape pens after a diagnosis of EVALI was made; therefore, we were unable to collect samples for laboratory testing. Thus, this case does not inform the current debate over the role of tocopheryl acetate (vitamin E acetate) in the development of the disease.

3. Conclusion

The incidence of reported e-cigarette and vaping-induced lung injury has grown precipitously over the past year. Of the documented cases so far, the prevailing symptoms of THC-containing vape pens appears to be relatively consistent across many cases. While symptoms are nonspecific, including shortness of breath, asthenia, myalgias, fever, and cough, as clinicians, we must be vigilant to link this exposure and timing with lung diseases. Many patients are initially misdiagnosed and, therefore, continue using THC-containing vape pens. Our case demonstrates a common radiographic finding, diagnostic work-up, and histopathology to confirm our case for a vaping-induced lung disease, specifically exogenous lipoid pneumonia. While a definitive course of treatment remains undefined in these patients, treatment across many cases appears to show promise with conservative measures. Some patients recover with near baseline functioning in a week while others have taken months [7, 14].

The presumption that vaping is a completely safe alternative to conventional cigarette or marijuana smoking now appears to be challenged by the outbreak of EVALI. Because the patient disposed of his vape pens and cannabis extracts, we could not exclude the possibility that lung injury was caused by some contaminants. Other possible contributors to his severe adverse lung reaction include the methodology used to extract the cannabis, the heating temperature, and the diluents and flavorings. It is unclear whether or not our patient improved due to a cessation of the exposure or the medical therapy. Regardless, our patient survived with antibiotics, steroids, and supportive care. Further studies are needed to confirm our observation, to identify ingredients, and to better understand the pathophysiology of the disease.

References

[1] A. D. Osei, M. Mirbolouk, O. A. Orimoloye et al., "Association between e-cigarette use and cardiovascular disease among never and current combustible-cigarette smokers," *The American Journal of Medicine*, vol. 132, no. 8, pp. 949–954.e2, 2019, e2.

[2] T. Frohe, R. F. Leeman, J. Patock-Peckham, A. Ecker, S. Kraus, and D. W. Foster, "Correlates of cannabis vape-pen use and knowledge among U.S. college students," *Addictive Behaviors Reports*, vol. 7, pp. 32–39, 2018.

[3] Y. M. Butt, M. L. Smith, H. D. Tazelaar et al., "Pathology of vaping-associated lung injury," *The New England journal of medicine*, vol. 381, no. 18, pp. 1780-1781, 2019.

[4] MMWR Centers for Disease Control and Prevention, "Severe Pulmonary Disease Associated with Electronic-Cigarette–Product Use - Interim Guidance," September 2019, https://www.cdc.gov/mmwr/volumes/68/wr/mm6836e2.htm.

[5] L. F. Chun, F. Moazed, C. S. Calfee, M. A. Matthay, and J. E. Gotts, "Pulmonary toxicity of e-cigarettes," *American Journal of Physiology. Lung Cellular and Molecular Physiology*, vol. 313, no. 2, pp. L193–L206, 2017.

[6] Centers for Disease Control and Prevention, "Outbreak of Lung Injury Associated with E-Cigarette Use, or Vaping," January 2018, https://www.cdc.gov/tobacco/basic_information/e-cigarettes/severe-lung-disease.html.

[7] T. He, M. Oks, M. Esposito, H. Steinberg, and M. Makaryus, "Tree-in-Bloom: Severe Acute Lung Injury Induced by Vaping Cannabis Oil," *Annals of the American Thoracic Society*, vol. 14, no. 3, pp. 468–470, 2017.

[8] K. Moore, H. Young II, and M. F. Ryan, "Bilateral pneumonia and pleural effusions subsequent to electronic cigarette use," *Open Journal of Emergency Medicine*, vol. 3, no. 3, pp. 18–22, 2015.

[9] S. M. Frossard, P. M. Volansky, and A. S. Endara-Bravo, "A40 A HARD DAY'S NIGHT: DRUG INDUCED LUNG DISEASE: acute uvulitis secondary to electronic cigarette use," *American Journal of Respiratory and Critical Care Medicine*, vol. 191, p. 1, 2015.

[10] J. Kaslow, R. F. Brown, and M. Fazili, "Cookies and cream lung: hypersensitivity pneumonitis leading to acute respiratory distress syndrome after electronic cigarette use," in *C83. PEDIATRIC CLINICAL CHEST ROUNDS*, Dallas, Texas, 2019American Thoracic Society.

[11] N. Poponea, E. Shehada, and N. Freeman, "The dark side of vaping; acute dyspnea and granulomatous lung disease associated with electronic cigarettes," in *B51. CIGARETTES, E-CIGARETTES, AND HOOKAHS*, San Diego, CA, USA, 2018American Thoracic Society.

[12] J. Sturek and N. Malik, "Acute hypoxic respiratory failure with crazy paving associated with electronic cigarette use," *Chest*, vol. 152, no. 4, p. A746, 2017.

[13] K. Davidson, A. Brancato, P. Heetderks et al., "Outbreak of electronic-cigarette-associated acute lipoid pneumonia - North Carolina, July-August 2019," *MWR. Morbidity and Mortality Weekly Report*, vol. 68, no. 36, pp. 784–786, 2019.

[14] J. E. Layden, I. Ghinai, I. Pray et al., "Pulmonary illness related to e-cigarette use in Illinois and Wisconsin—Final report," *New England Journal of Medicine*, vol. 382, no. 10, pp. 903–916, 2020.

[15] S. Sung, H. D. Tazelaar, J. P. Crapanzano, A. Nassar, and A. Saqi, "Adult exogenous lipoid pneumonia: a rare and underrecognized entity in cytology—a case series," *Cytojournal*, vol. 15, no. 17, p. 17, 2018.

[16] G. Rossi, A. Cavazza, P. Spagnolo et al., "The role of macrophages in interstitial lung diseases," *European Respiratory Review*, vol. 26, no. 145, p. 170009, 2017.

[17] Z. Sheikh, P. J. Brooks, O. Barzilay, N. Fine, and M. Glogauer, "Macrophages, foreign body giant cells and their response to implantable biomaterials," *Materials*, vol. 8, no. 9, pp. 5671–5701, 2015.

27

E-Cigarette- and Vaping-Related Lung Injury (EVALI) at a Regional Hospital System in South Carolina

Daniel Temas and Armin Meyer

University of South Carolina School of Medicine-Greenville/Prisma Health-Upstate, 701 Grove Rd., Greenville, SC 29605, USA

Correspondence should be addressed to Daniel Temas; daniel.temas@prismahealth.org

Academic Editor: Shih-Yi Lee

We report on four cases of severe lung injury and respiratory failure attributed to E-cigarette use that presented between July and August, 2019. The patients described were relatively healthy without clinically significant history of lung disease. Each developed severe acute respiratory distress shortly following E-cigarette use. In each case, the patients initially presented with considerable hypoxia and infectious-appearing pattern with elevated inflammatory markers on laboratory values. Imaging studies demonstrated a consistent pattern of widespread bilateral interstitial infiltrates with a medial distribution. All but one of the cases involved the admitted use of THC oil in E-cigarettes. There was rapid progression of illness requiring increased supplemental oxygen and in two cases, requiring urgent intubation and mechanical ventilation. No infectious organism was isolated in any case, and patients improved rapidly with the initiation of steroids. These are among the first cases reported in South Carolina and are consistent with similar cases that have been reported around the country.

1. Introduction

E-cigarette use ("vaping") has exploded in popularity over the last 10 years. Now, approximately 2.8% of Americans are current E-cigarette users per CDC statistics [1]. Growth in use is particularly marked in youth demographics with 4.9% of middle school students and 20.8% of high school students reporting vaping within 30 days of the survey [1]. In spite of its rapid market growth, exploration of the short- and long-term health effects of E-cigarettes has been limited. However, initial data compiled by Klomparens et al. suggests an association between E-cigarette use and lung disease, as well as increased risk of cardiovascular disease [2]. Furthermore, due to the variations in manufacturing of these products and lack of regulatory oversight, there are wide variations in quality and composition of the products offered.

E-cigarettes are composed of a battery-powered heating element that heats a liquid substance ("e-juice") which generally contains propylene glycol, glycerine, flavoring, and nicotine in various concentrations, in addition to various other chemical components. This liquid is absorbed into a cotton wick. The cotton wick is then heated, and the absorbed liquids form an aerosol inhaled into the lungs.

In recent years, vaping of cannabis oil or other preparations of THC have increased in popularity as an alternative to traditional methods of consuming cannabis [3]. Many of these preparations are manufactured without uniform standards or quality control and sold illicitly or online from unverifiable sources. There has been at least one case report describing acute lung injury due to vaporized cannabis oil [4]. Several of the chemical components, including flavoring agents, have been identified as potentially toxic [5]. Vitamin E (alpha-tocopherol) acetate in particular has been implicated as a potential causative agent, based on BAL samples from affected patients [6].

This increase in the popularity of E-cigarette use has coincided with an increased number of reported cases of severe lung disease associated with or directly attributed to vaping. The first officially reported death attributed to E-cigarette use in America was reported in Illinois in August 2019 [7]. Subsequently, multiple additional cases of severe illness and mortality attributed to vaping have been reported around the country. This prompted the

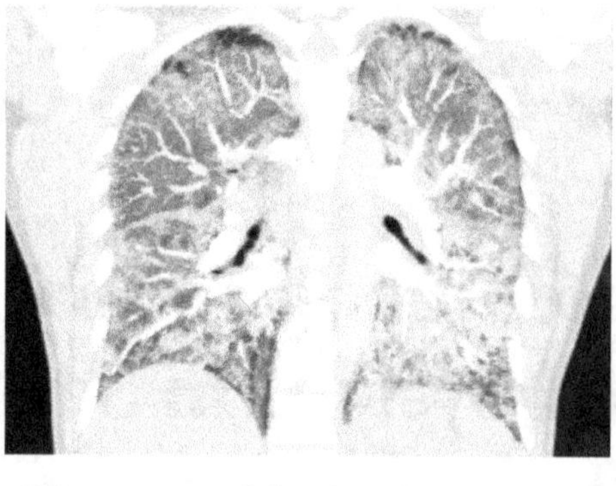

FIGURE 1: CT angiogram of the chest demonstrating widespread bilateral ground-glass opacities with some basilar and dependent predominance.

CDC to develop a case definition for E-cigarette-associated lung injury which includes the following criteria [8]:

(i) E-cigarette use within 90 days

(ii) With pulmonary infiltrates and ground-glass opacities on imaging

(iii) Negative respiratory viral panel and influenza screen and absence of any other identifiable disease-causing pathogen

Here, we present four cases of E-cigarette- and vaping-related lung injury (EVALI) in a regional health system in South Carolina treated between July and August 2019. Initial presentation, evaluation, and hospital treatment course are described.

2. Cases

2.1. Case 1. A 43-year-old female patient presented to the Emergency Department via EMS following 3-4 days of reported cough, confusion, and fever up to 38.9°C. Her prior medical history was significant for 1-pack-per-day cigarette smoking and polysubstance abuse. On EMS arrival, she was noted to have an O_2 saturation of 50% on room air. On physical exam at presentation, she was noted to have dry rales throughout bilateral lung fields. The patient was in possession of a vape pen, along with paraphernalia including a "Dank Vapes" THC oil cartridge labeled "92.33% THC." The patient denied any environmental exposures or significant sick contacts. She was emergently intubated in the Emergency Department due to hypoxia and altered mental status.

Initial lab studies were significant for white blood cell (WBC) of 11,100/mm^3 with 17% bands, lactate 5.35 mmol/L, C-reactive protein (CRP) 315.7 mg/L, and procalcitonin 5.14 ng/mL. Urine drug screen resulted positive for cannabinoids and benzodiazepines. B-natriuretic peptide (BNP) on admission was 326 pg/mL, which rose to 1195 pg/mL on the second day of hospitalization. Hemoglobin dropped from 11.4 g/dL to 8.4 g/dL on hospital day 3 without obvious evidence of bleeding. Arterial blood gas on 100% FiO_2 demonstrated pH 7.38, pCO_2 42 mmHg, and pO_2 65 mmHg. CT angiogram of the chest (Figure 1) demonstrated diffuse bilateral ground-glass opacities with some dependent and basilar predominance and no acute focal consolidation. Respiratory culture resulted with light growth yeast. Respiratory pathogen viral PCR (RPP) was negative for acute viral illness. Blood and urine cultures collected on admission were negative. HIV screen was nonreactive. Bronchoscopy demonstrated normal appearance of bilateral bronchioles to segmental levels with minimal secretions throughout. Bronchoalveolar lavage (BAL) cultures were negative. BAL cytology demonstrated WBC of 1195/mm^3 with neutrophilic predominance and 2900/mm^3 RBC. Pathology further noted presence of mixed leukocytes and alveolar macrophages.

The patient was initially treated empirically for sepsis with broad-spectrum antibiotics. She continued to require 100% FiO_2 on hospital day 2, and intravenous methylprednisolone 500 mg daily was initiated. Her respiratory status subsequently improved, and she was extubated on hospital day 3 to heated high-flow nasal cannula, initially at 60% FiO_2. Steroid treatment was transitioned to oral prednisone 60 mg twice daily. Oxygen requirement was progressively weaned to 6 L via nasal cannula over the subsequent 48 hours. Patient would ultimately leave against medical advice on hospital day 5 while still requiring 4-6 L supplemental oxygen.

2.2. Case 2. A 33-year-old male patient presented with a 2-day history of cough, shortness of breath, and fever. Medical history was significant for remote history of asthma as a child and hospitalization for uncomplicated community-acquired pneumonia 2 years prior to presentation. He was not taking any chronic medications. He reported smoking approximately 1 pack of cigarettes daily and regular e-cigarette use. He endorsed he had increased smoking due to stress over the preceding week and had vaped "all night" prior to presentation. He denied THC use.

Initial vital signs were significant for hypoxia, tachycardia, and temp of 38.0°C. There were decreased breath sounds bilaterally but no wheezes, rales, or rhonchi noted on physical exam. Patient was started on supplemental oxygen via nasal cannula at 4-5 L.

Initial labs were significant for WBC of 18,100/mm^3 and procalcitonin of 0.08 ng/mL. The patient's hemoglobin fell from 15.4 g/dL on initial labs to 12.1 on hospital day 3. Chest X-ray demonstrated bilateral infiltrates. CT angiogram of the chest demonstrated diffuse, multifocal bilateral ground-glass opacities with relative peripheral sparing. Reactive mediastinal/hilar lymphadenopathy along with bilateral pleural effusions was also noted (Figure 2). Urine toxicology screen was not performed. RPP was negative, as were blood and respiratory cultures. HIV screen was also negative. Bronchoscopy was not performed in this patient.

Patient was initially treated empirically with ceftriaxone and azithromycin. He became more dyspneic and hypoxic over the 24 hours following admission requiring increase in supplemental oxygen to high-flow nasal cannula at 8 L. On hospital day 3, he was started on methylprednisolone 125 mg IV daily. Clinical condition subsequently improved and supplemental O_2 requirement was weaned to room air on day of discharge (hospital day 6). He was discharged with

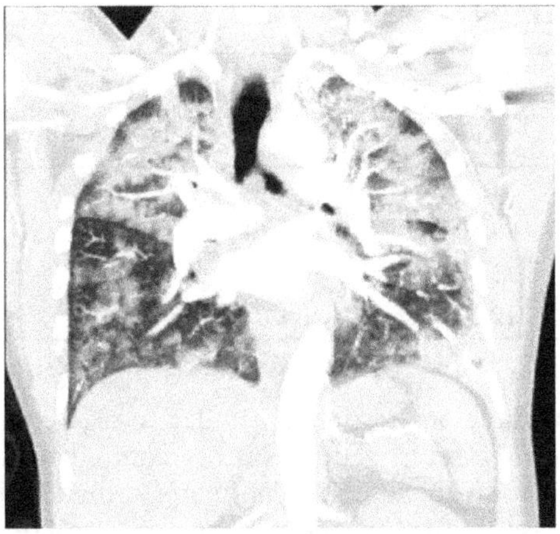

Figure 2: CT angiogram of the chest demonstrating diffuse multifocal ground-glass opacities with peripheral sparing and left pleural effusion.

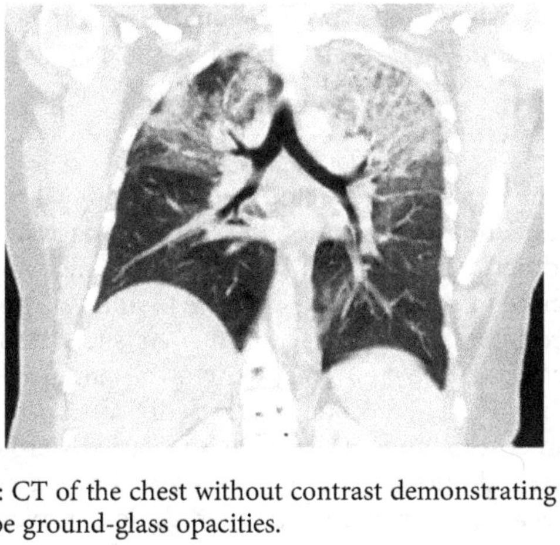

Figure 3: CT of the chest without contrast demonstrating bilateral upper lobe ground-glass opacities.

a 4-week prednisone taper, starting with 60 mg daily, and PRN albuterol inhaler.

2.3. Case 3. A 20-year-old male presented to the ED with epigastric pain and intractable nausea and vomiting. He also reported 3 days of nonproductive cough, shortness of breath, and fever for three days. There were no reported sick contacts or toxic exposures. Patient was a never-smoker and denied drug use but admitted to E-cigarette use.

On presentation, the patient was normotensive and tachycardic with a rate of 120 bpm, with O_2 saturation of 94% on room air. Physical exam was only remarkable for mild abdominal pain. Labs were significant for WBC of 15,800/mm^3, procalcitonin 0.86 ng/mL, and lactate 3.33 mmol/L. Hemoglobin dropped from 15.4 g/dL on presentation to 10.6 g/dL on hospital day 7 without evidence of frank bleeding. Urine drug screen was positive for cannabinoids. Blood cultures, respiratory cultures, and RPP were negative. HIV was also negative.

On hospital day 3, the patient became acutely febrile with temperature up to 39.1°C, tachycardic, short of breath, and hypoxic requiring up to 6 L O_2 via nasal cannula. CT of the chest (Figure 3) demonstrated bilateral upper lobe-predominant consolidations with overlying ground-glass opacities. Follow-up labs demonstrated an erythrocyte sedimentation rate (ESR) of 51 mm/hr and CRP > 320.0 mg/L. Arterial blood gas demonstrated pH 7.45, pCO_2 33 mmHg, and pO_2 52 mmHg. His supplemental O_2 was increased to heated high-flow nasal cannula at 70% FiO_2. He was subsequently started on steroid treatment with methylprednisolone 1000 mg IV daily.

Oxygen requirement was successfully weaned over the next several days. At time of discharge, the patient was maintaining adequate O_2 saturations on room air at rest but continued to require 2 L via nasal cannula with ambulation. Patient was discharged on hospital day 8 with a 6-week steroid taper, starting with Prednisone 60 mg PO daily.

On chart review follow-up, patient reported ongoing dyspnea on exertion and shortness of breath limiting daily activities 6 months following initial presentation and hospitalization. Further workup and testing are in the process at the time of this report.

2.4. Case 4. A 19-year-old male presented to the ED with 3 days of headache, malaise, abdominal pain, and nausea/-vomiting. He also reported shortness of breath and cough with occasional scant hemoptysis. He had no significant prior medical history and took no medications. He denied any significant sick contacts or exposures. Patient was reportedly a nonsmoker but admitted to vaping marijuana.

Vital signs are significant for tachycardia at a rate of 103 bpm and temp of 38.5°C. Oxygen saturation was 94% on 4-liter supplemental oxygen. Bibasilar rales were noted on auscultation. The initial labs were significant for WBC of 12,400/mm^3, procalcitonin 0.27 ng/mL, CRP > 320.0 mg/L, and ESR 100 mm/hr. Initial chest X-ray demonstrated bibasilar consolidations without definite focal infiltrate. Urine drug screen was positive for cannabinoids. Hemoglobin fell from 14.6 g/dL on the day prior to presentation to 11.0 g/dL on hospital day 3. Respiratory cultures and RPP were negative. Due to the severity of headache, a lumbar puncture was performed. Opening pressure within normal limits at 26 cm H_2O and spinal fluid analysis was unremarkable.

Patient was started on empiric antibiotics for suspected community-acquired pneumonia. He became progressively more hypoxemic over the next 4 days requiring escalation from 4 L O_2 via nasal cannula to high flow. He underwent bronchoscopy which demonstrated airways without noted structural abnormalities to segmental branches bilaterally and minimal secretions. BAL cytology demonstrated neutrophilic predominance. Pathology review noted acute inflammatory background with blood and numerous macrophages; occasional clusters of abnormal cells were also noted. Follow-up CT of the chest (Figure 4) demonstrated dense, patchy bilateral ground-glass opacities, bilateral lower lobe consolidations with air bronchograms, and small bilateral pleural effusions.

On hospital day 4, the patient became acutely hypoxic with increasing oxygen requirement. He was intubated for suspected Acute Respiratory Distress Syndrome (ARDS), requiring 100% FiO_2 to maintain adequate oxygen saturations.

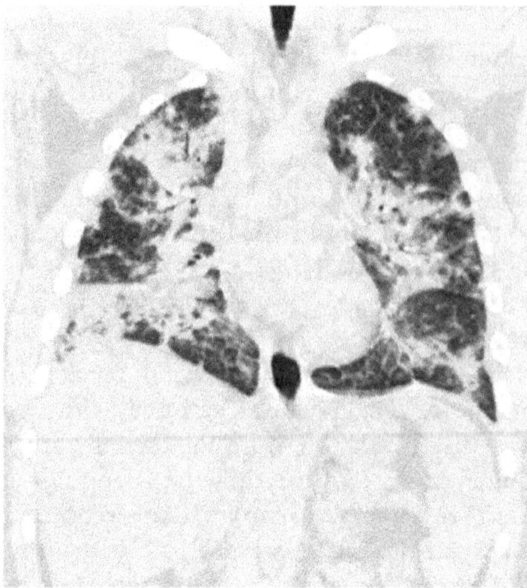

FIGURE 4: CT of the chest without contrast demonstrating patchy bilateral ground-glass opacities and small bilateral pleural effusions.

He was subsequently started on steroid therapy with methylprednisolone 250 mg IV twice daily. Respiratory status gradually improved on mechanical ventilation, and steroid dose was weaned to methylprednisolone 60 mg IV every 8 hours on day 3 of mechanical ventilation. The patient was extubated after a total of 4 days of mechanical ventilation. He was transitioned to prednisone 60 mg PO daily. Oxygen requirement and overall clinical status gradually improved over the next several days, and the patient was tolerating room air at time of discharge on hospital day 10. He was discharged on a prolonged steroid taper starting with prednisone 60 mg PO daily.

3. Discussion

In the cases described above, the patients presented with acute hypoxia, respiratory distress, and diffuse inflammatory pattern on imaging. Patient age ranged from 19 years old to 43 years old, three male and one female. All of the described patients admitted to E-cigarette use; all but one admitted to vaping THC. Initial presentation in all cases was concerning for infection with fever and leukocytosis, but in all cases, no organism was identified. The patients described were without significant prior pulmonary disease. In each case, the patients were found to have severe hypoxemia requiring significant supplemental oxygen to maintain adequate oxygenation. In two of the four cases, intubation and mechanical ventilation were required due to the severity of hypoxemia. All received steroids at varying doses with subsequent improvement in symptoms and hypoxia. Each of these cases fit the CDC case definition for EVALI [8] as described above.

Some other commonalities among these cases include modest elevation in WBC and significantly elevated CRP (Table 1). Procalcitonin was notably elevated in case 1 but the remaining cases had only modest elevations. Imaging studies in all cases demonstrated bilateral pulmonary opacities without focal consolidation. The elevated CRP and clinical response to steroids suggest a reactive inflammatory process. E-cigarette use has previously been described to cause inflammatory responses similar to cigarette smoking [2, 9]. Further investigation will be required to determine the correlation between inflammatory markers and E-cigarette use; however, measurement of C-reactive protein and other inflammatory markers may be warranted in suspected cases. Additionally, all patients experienced a significant drop in hemoglobin, averaging -3.675 g/dL drop in hemoglobin without evidence of bleeding. The significance of this is unclear; however, this could also be related to the acute inflammatory state suggested by the elevated CRP.

TABLE 1: Lab value similarities among observed cases.

Case	Leukocyte count (TH/mm^3)	Procalcitonin (ng/mL)	CRP (mg/L)	Change in hemoglobin (g/dL)
1	11,000	5.14	315.7	-3.0
2	18,100	0.08	~	-3.3
3	15,800	0.86	>320	-4.8
4	12,400	0.15	>320	-3.6

4. Limitations

There were several notable limitations to our evaluation. The evaluation and treatment of the patients described above occurred between July and August, 2019. This was early in the timeline of reported cases of EVALI and was not a commonly recognized clinical syndrome. As such, standards of care for evaluation and treatment of potential cases were not established. This accounts for lack of bronchoscopic evaluation in cases 2 and 3, as well as the varied steroid dosing regimens. Additionally, case 2 did not have a measured CRP level and, while there was a high clinical suspicion, there was no urine toxicology screen to confirm THC use. Furthermore, these cases were identified prior to the NEJM article published in December 2019 identifying vitamin E acetate as a potential causative agent [6]; as such, it was not measured on the BAL samples.

5. Conclusion

The cases described represent only a small sample of an alarming trend across the country. A growing number of cases are being described of severe and life-threatening pulmonary illness with E-cigarette use and more specifically THC-based products, as a potential culprit. This is further supported by the data surrounding the presence of vitamin E acetate in these products and its suspected role in contributing to EVALI [10]. Furthermore, of 2022 cases of EVALI identified by the CDC, 82% reported the use of THC-containing products [10].

With this growing incidence, appropriate and prompt identification of these cases and initiation of appropriate treatment will be essential to minimizing associated mortality. The infectious-appearing presentation and imaging findings as described above, along with the appropriate history, should raise clinical suspicion for this disease process. As we have reported, prompt initiation of high-dose corticosteroid treatment is associated with improvement in oxygenation and overall clinical condition.

While some initial strides have been made to identify the underlying etiology, further research will be essential to both identifying the agent (s) responsible for the lung injury and establishing standardized evaluation and treatment protocols. Furthermore, it remains to be seen what the long-term consequences of this clinical syndrome present for the affected patients. Outpatient follow-up and appropriate clinical monitoring with serologies, imaging, and pulmonary function testing would be warranted.

At the time of completion of this report, at least 10 additional cases of vaping-associated lung injury have been identified within the hospital system.

References

[1] Centers for Disease Control and Prevention, "About electronic cigarettes," https://www.cdc.gov/tobacco/basic_information/e-cigarettes/about-e-cigarettes.

[2] E. A. Klomparens and Y. Ding, "Potential health risks of long-term E-cigarette use," *Environmental Disease*, vol. 4, no. 1, pp. 1–5, 2019.

[3] K. F. Trivers, E. Phillips, A. S. Gentzke, M. A. Tynan, and L. J. Neff, "Prevalence of cannabis use in electronic cigarettes among US youth," *JAMA Pediatrics*, vol. 172, no. 11, pp. 1097–1099, 2018.

[4] T. He, M. Oks, M. Esposito, H. Steinberg, and M. Makaryus, "Tree-in-bloom: severe acute lung injury induced by vaping cannabis oil," *Annals of the American Thoracic Society*, vol. 14, no. 3, pp. 468–470, 2017.

[5] P. Clapp and I. Jaspers, "Electronic cigarettes: their constituents and potential links to asthma," *Current Allergy and Asthma Reports*, vol. 17, no. 11, p. 79, 2017.

[6] B. C. Blount, M. P. Karwowski, P. G. Shields et al., "Vitamin E acetate in bronchoalveolar-lavage fluid associated with EVALI," *The New England Journal of Medicine*, vol. 382, no. 8, pp. 697–705, 2020.

[7] R. Redfield, *CDC director's statement on the first death related to the outbreak of severe lung disease in people who use e-cigarette or "vaping" devices*, Centers for Disease Control and Prevention, 2019, https://www.cdc.gov/media/releases/2019/s0823-vaping-related-death.html.

[8] Centers for Disease Control and Prevention, *2019 lung injury surveillance primary case definition (CDC)*, Centers for Disease Control and Prevention, 2019, https://www.cdc.gov/tobacco/basic_information/e-cigarettes/severe-lung-disease/health-departments/index.

[9] G. Kaur, R. Pinkston, B. Mclemore, W. C. Dorsey, and S. Batra, "Immunological and toxicological risk assessment of E-cigarettes," *European Respiratory Review*, vol. 27, no. 147, article 170119, 2018.

[10] Centers for Disease Control and Prevention, *Outbreak of lung injury associated with E-cigarette use, or vaping*, Centers for Disease Control and Prevention, 2020, https://www.cdc.gov/tobacco/basic_information/e-cigarettes/severe-lung-disease.

28

Review of Cases of E-Cigarette or Vaping Product Use-Associated Lung Injury (EVALI) and Brief Review of the Literature

Amr Essa,[1] Jeffrey Macaraeg,[2] Nikhil Jagan,[2] Daniel Kwon,[3] Saboor Randhawa,[1] Matthew Kruse,[4] Stanley Thomas,[2] Manasa Velagapudi,[5] John Horne,[5] Shraddha Narechania,[2] Michael Kaster,[2] Carrie Valenta,[1] Venketraman Sahasranaman,[2] and Douglas Moore[2]

[1]*Creighton University School of Medicine, Department of Internal Medicine, Omaha, USA*
[2]*Creighton University School of Medicine, Department of Pulmonary, Critical Care, and Sleep Medicine, Omaha, USA*
[3]*Creighton University School of Medicine, Department of Pathology, Omaha, USA*
[4]*Creighton University School of Medicine, Department of Radiology, Omaha, USA*
[5]*Creighton University School of Medicine, Department of Infectious Diseases, Omaha, USA*

Correspondence should be addressed to Amr Essa; amressa@creighton.edu

Academic Editor: Takeshi Terashima

Since the appearance of the E-Cigarette in the early 2000s, its industry, popularity, and prevalence have risen dramatically. In the past, E-Cigarette use with the vaping of nicotine or cannabis products had been associated with a few reported cases of lung injury. However, in 2019, thousands of cases of E-Cigarette or vaping product use-associated lung injury (EVALI) were reported in the United States. Evidence linked this outbreak with vaping of tetrahydrocannabinol (THC). We report two confirmed cases of EVALI and their associated clinical, radiologic, and pathologic features. This report supports the growing body of information regarding EVALI. It also discusses various substances, particularly vitamin E acetate, which has been suggested as a causative agent.

1. Introduction

The E-Cigarette is a battery-operated device used to produce an aerosol that is inhaled into the lungs, the composition of which is determined by the content of the E-Liquid. It usually delivers nicotine; however, it can be used to deliver other substances such as tetrahydrocannabinol (THC), cannabidiol (CBD), and butane hash oils [1]. Since the introduction of E-Cigarette into the US market in 2007, there have been a few published and documented cases which describe lung disease in relation to vaping of nicotine or extracts of cannabis, with the earliest documented in 2012 [2–5]. The summer of 2019 witnessed an alarming upsurge in the number of vaping-induced lung injury cases. The increasing mortality and associated morbidity catapulted it to national attention and led to the coining of the term E-Cigarette or vaping product use-associated lung injury (EVALI) [6]. Despite the prevalence of vaping in the US and other developed countries, such as the United Kingdom, wherein 3.2 million people vape, an outbreak of this magnitude had never occurred previously [7]. Collaboration between the Centers for Disease Control and Prevention (CDC), state health departments, the medical communities, and the public is ongoing to further delineate the nature of this outbreak and the causative agents. An association between EVALI and non-nicotine-containing liquids has been suggested. Although it remains unclear which group of chemicals are involved, vitamin E acetate recently has been implicated. In this report, we highlight two cases of EVALI which were diagnosed and treated at our institution. We further discuss the clinical, radiologic, and pathologic features, with a brief review of the current body of published literature.

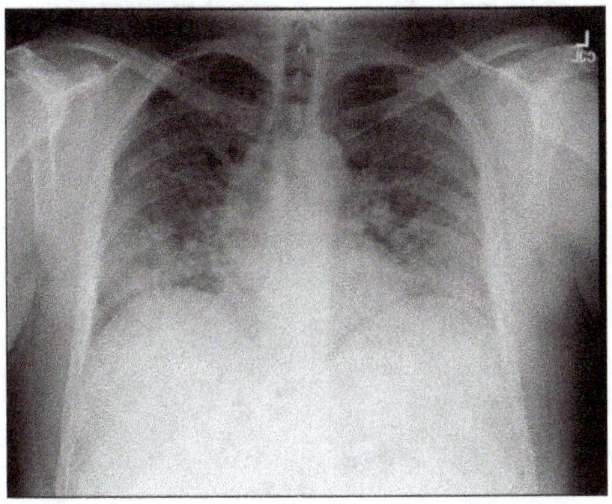

Figure 1: Case 1 CXR on presentation.

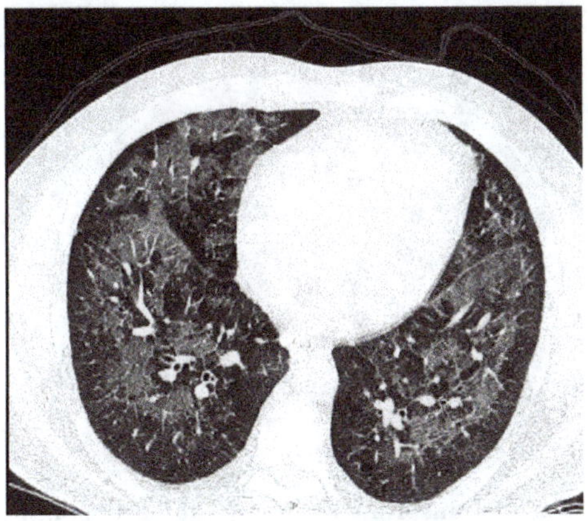

Figure 2: Case 1 chest CT scan on presentation (axial view).

2. Case Presentation

2.1. Case 1. A 42-year-old man with no underlying medical problems presented with a two-week history of worsening nonproductive cough, subjective fever, chills, and diaphoresis. The history was significant for vaping THC once or twice weekly for the last one year. He reported no use of tobacco, alcohol, or illicit drugs. He denied any recent travel, and he had a desk job with no reported occupational exposures. On presentation, he was hypoxic with an oxygen saturation of 85% on room air that improved with one liter of oxygen via nasal cannula. He was afebrile and hemodynamically stable. Physical exam was significant for diffuse bilateral rales. Chest radiograph (CXR) revealed diffuse interstitial prominence (Figure 1). A subsequent computed tomography (CT) scan of the chest revealed extensive symmetric ground-glass opacities in all lobes with interlobular septal thickening and subpleural sparing (Figures 2 and 3). He was started on broad-spectrum antimicrobial therapy with azithromycin, ceftriaxone, and levofloxacin to treat potentially bacterial pneumonia, all of which was discontinued after cultures were sterile (Table 1). Bronchoalveolar lavage (BAL) of the right middle lobe was performed. A transbronchial tissue biopsy of the left upper lobe (upper division and lingula) (Figures 4 and 5) revealed benign bronchial mucosa without significant pathologic abnormality. Since an infectious etiology was ruled out, he was discharged on prednisone 40 mg daily with tapering over four weeks. He reported improvement of symptoms within one week after discharge.

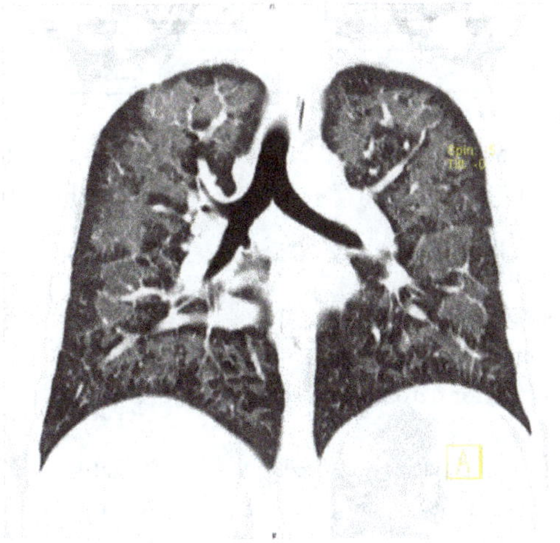

Figure 3: Case 1 chest CT scan on presentation (coronal view).

2.2. Case 2. A 21-year-old man with a history of exercise-induced asthma presented with a one-week history of worsening productive cough, dyspnea, nausea, vomiting, and malaise. He stated that he vaped THC once every hour while awake for the last three months and once daily for the previous year. He reported no use of tobacco products, alcohol, or other illicit drugs. He reported recent travel to the Southwestern United States and Minnesota the month prior to hospitalization. He denied any occupational exposure. On presentation, he was hypoxic with an oxygen saturation of 88%, which improved with two liters of oxygen via nasal cannula. He was afebrile and hemodynamically stable. Physical exam was significant for bibasilar crackles. CXR on admission showed patchy alveolar opacities in the mid and lower lungs bilaterally (Figure 6). CT chest demonstrated basal-predominant bilateral ground-glass opacities with subpleural sparing, in addition to pneumomediastinum and slightly prominent bilateral hilar lymph nodes (Figures 7 and 8). He was started on broad-spectrum antimicrobial therapy with vancomycin, piperacillin-tazobactam, azithromycin, and fluconazole with coverage to treat potential coccidioidomycosis and presumed bacterial pneumonia, all of which were discontinued after cultures were sterile (Table 1). BAL of the right lower lobe revealed macrophages with neutrophils and lymphocytes (Figure 9). A transbronchial tissue biopsy of the right lower lobe showed an acute fibrinous and organizing pneumonia pattern with no prominent eosinophils, granulomas, or malignancy (Figures 10–13). Six-minute walk before discharge was notable for oxygen desaturation with activity, and subsequently, he was discharged on one-liter oxygen via nasal cannula and prednisone 40 mg daily tapering over four weeks. He reported a resolution of his symptoms at the time of his clinic follow-up visit about six weeks following discharge. Repeat chest high-resolution CT (HRCT) at that time showed remarkable improvement in the aeration of his

Table 1: Lab work on admission.

	Case 1	Case 2
Infectious workup		
White cell count	11.3K/μl	14.3K/μl
Sedimentation rate (ESR)	80 mm/hr	91 mm/hr
Procalcitonin	0.21 ng/ml	0.40 ng/ml
Legionella urine antigen	Negative	Negative
Pneumococcal urine antigen	Negative	Negative
Histoplasma urine antigen	Negative	Negative
Blood culture for aerobic & anaerobic growth	Negative	Negative
Respiratory viral pathogen screen	Negative	Negative
Sputum culture	Negative	Negative
Sputum AFB smear	Negative	Negative
HIV AG/AB	Negative	Negative
ANCA	Negative	Negative
1,3-b-d-Glucan	Negative	Negative
BAL cell count and differentials	Normal	Normal
BAL total nucleated cells	440/μl	640/μl
BAL RBCs	<10.000/μl	<10.000/μl
BAL neutrophils	49%	39%
BAL lymphocytes	28%	5%
BAL monocytes	17%	8%
BAL phagocytes	6%	48%
BAL fungal culture with special	Negative	Negative
BAL vulture viral reflex	Negative	Negative
BAL bacterial culture	Negative	Negative
BAL Aspergillus antigen	Negative	Negative
Miscellaneous workup		
Lyme disease serology	Negative	
Rapid strep A	Negative	
West Nile antibodies	Negative	
Glomerular basement membrane (GBM) antibodies	Negative	
Mononucleosis screen	Negative	
Complement levels	Normal	
LDH level	Normal	
ProBNP	74 pg/ml	
CRP	>375 mg/l	
Coccidioides antibodies		Negative
Hypersensitivity pneumonitis panel		Negative
BAL AFP culture and smear	Negative	
BAL PCR for Legionella	Negative	

lungs and resolution of the bilateral ground-glass opacities (Figures 14 and 15).

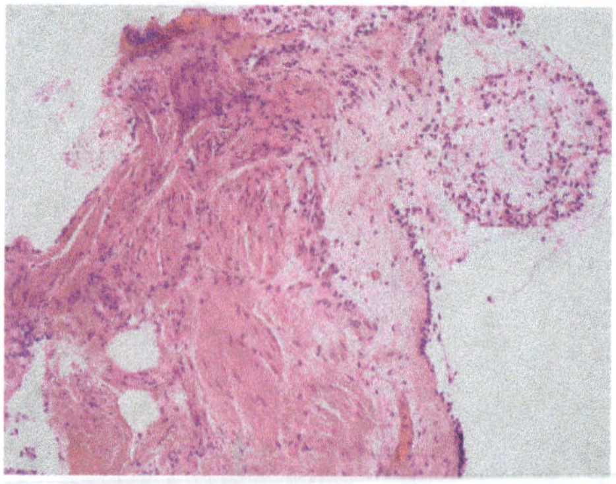

Figure 4: Case 1 transbronchial biopsy of upper division of left upper lobe with benign bronchial mucosa.

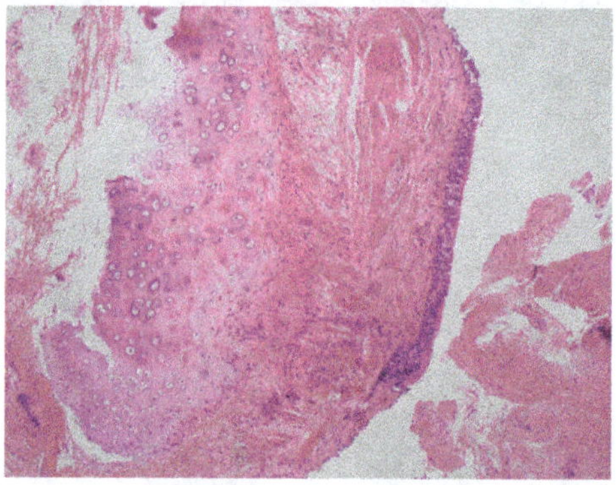

Figure 5: Case 1 transbronchial biopsy of left lingula with benign bronchial mucosa.

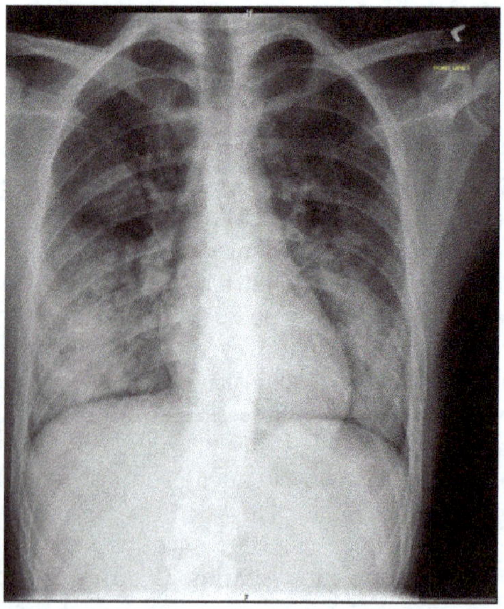

Figure 6: Case 2 CXR on presentation.

3. Discussion

Since the 2000s, when E-Cigarette made its initial appearance, the vaping industry has shown rapid emergence. Its popularity and prevalence have been driven by an apparent improved nicotine delivery system with attractive features for users and a wide variety of flavors. E-Cigarette marketing-related expenditure in the United States increased from \$3.6 million in 2010 to \$125 million in 2014 [7]. At the same time, the prevalence of vaping has been on the rise, with

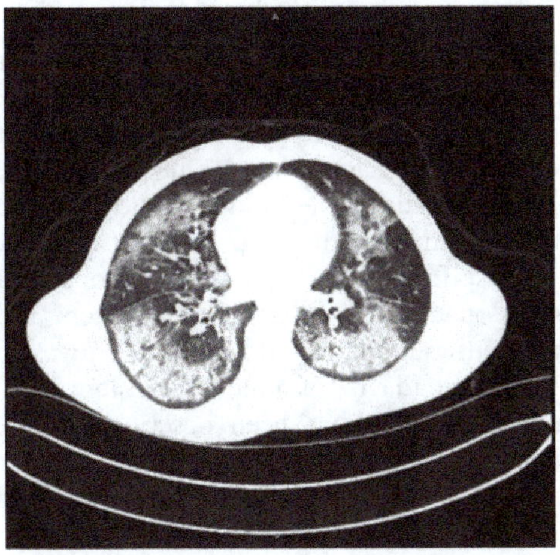

FIGURE 7: Case 2 chest CT scan on presentation (axial view).

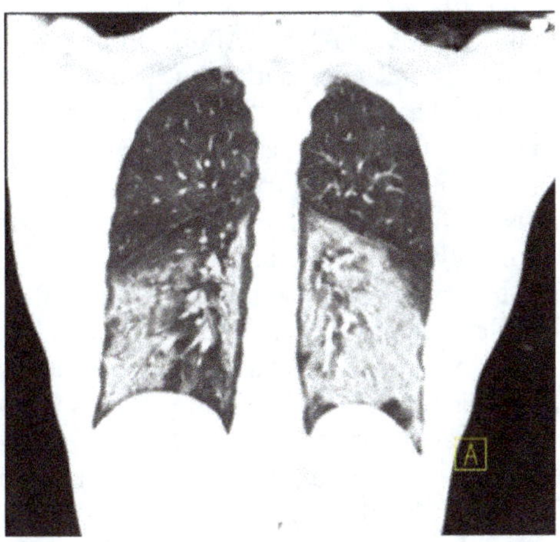

FIGURE 8: Case 2 chest CT scan on presentation (coronal view).

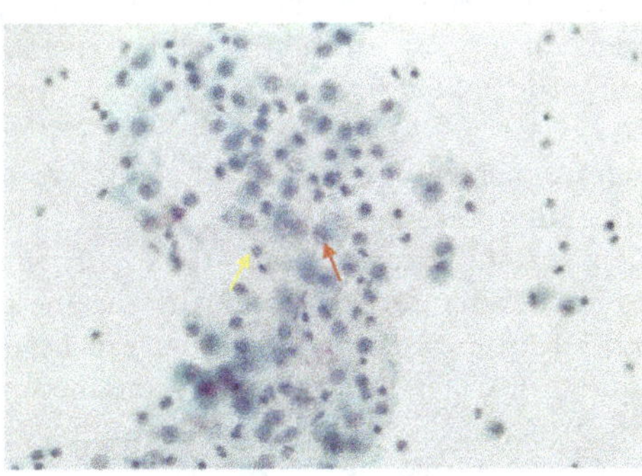

FIGURE 9: Case 2 bronchioalveolar lavage (BAL) of right lower lobe. Macrophages (red arrow) and neutrophils (yellow arrows).

more than a quarter (25.4%) of 12th-grade students in 2019 saying that they had vaped in the last 30 days, more than double the rate in 2017 [8]. A study developed to describe advertising claims made on branded E-Cigarette reported that it is marketed as a healthier and cheaper alternative to conventional smoking. And the appeal of the wide array of flavors, perception of modernity, enhanced social appearance and celebrity use, and avoidance of smoking policy were appealing to many [9].

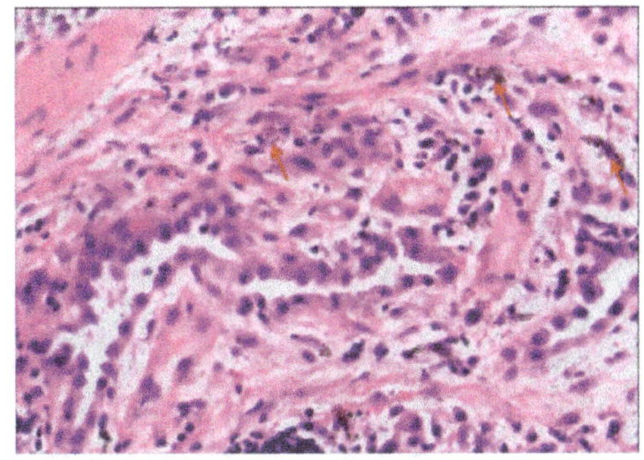

FIGURE 10: Case 2 transbronchial biopsy of right lower lobe. Macrophages containing blackish brown pigmented particles (red arrows).

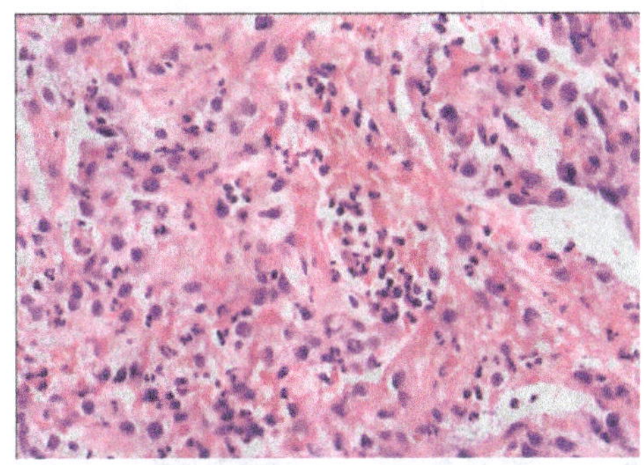

FIGURE 11: Case 2 transbronchial biopsy of right lower lobe with multiple neutrophils.

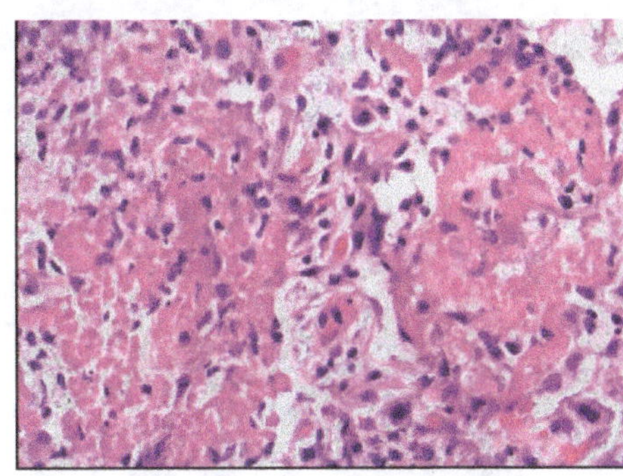

FIGURE 12: Case 2 transbronchial biopsy of right lower lobe. Eosinophilic fibrin exudate between cells, typical for pneumonia.

Based on largely observational data on the current outbreak, the majority of reported cases were young males [10–13]. The commonly reported clinical symptoms include fever, chills, and a headache. Respiratory symptoms include shortness of breath, cough, and chest pain. Gastrointestinal symptoms include nausea, vomiting, diarrhea, and abdominal pain [10–13]. Fever was present in 29%, tachycardia in 64%, and tachypnea in 43%, with oxygen saturation < 88% in 31% of the cases in one report [10]. There are no clear guidelines regarding the management of EVALI, although glucocorticoids and empiric systemic antimicrobial therapy have been prescribed in the majority of cases [10, 11, 13]. The improvement in respiratory symptoms has been attributed to glucocorticoids [10, 12].

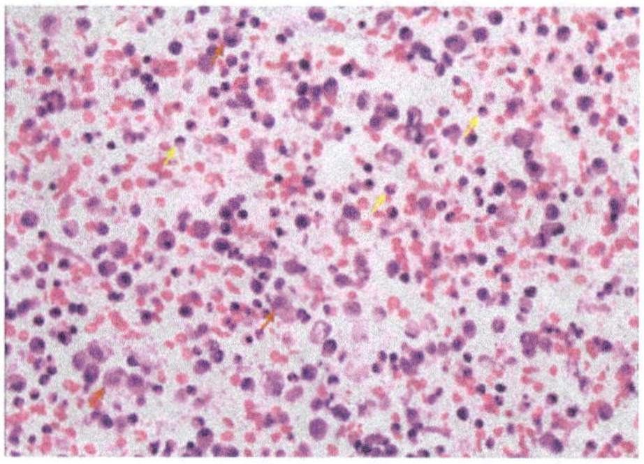

Figure 13: Case 2 transbronchial biopsy. Macrophages (red arrows) and neutrophils (yellow arrows) in a background of exudative material.

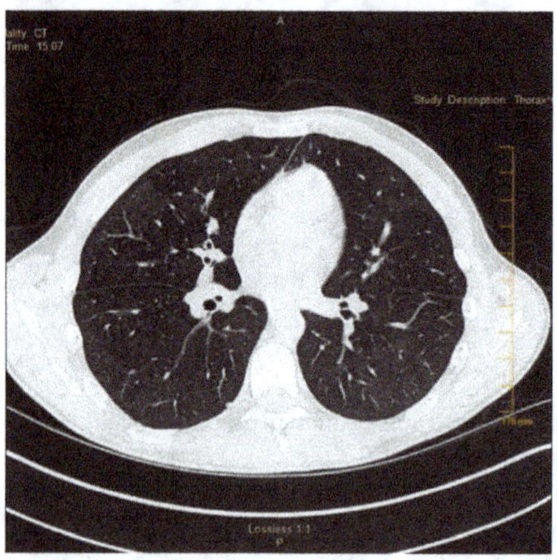

Figure 14: Case 2 chest CT scan 6 weeks post discharge (axial view).

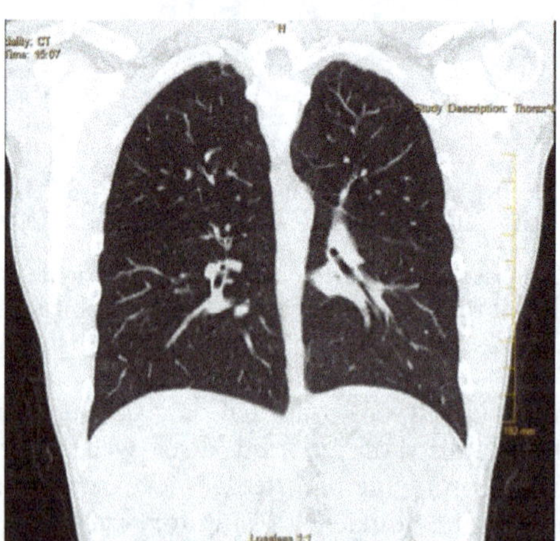

Figure 15: Case 2 chest CT scan 6 weeks post discharge (coronal view).

86% of the 867 EVALI patients report using THC-containing products in the three months preceding symptom onset with mild elevations in white cell count, sedimentation rate, and procalcitonin [14]. Both of our patients were young males who vaped THC and met a "confirmed" diagnosis of EVALI set by the CDC. The clinical characteristics and presentation were consistent with previously reported cases [15].

A wide range of imaging patterns has been described in EVALI [16, 17], including hypersensitivity pneumonitis, diffuse alveolar damage, acute lung injury, acute eosinophilic pneumonia, organizing pneumonia, lipoid pneumonia, and giant cell interstitial pneumonia. Imaging obtained during the acute phase for both our patients demonstrated diffuse ground-glass opacities slightly more prominent at the lower lung zones, with subpleural and peribronchovascular sparing. Our patients had a pattern most consistent with organizing pneumonia, which has been described in the EVALI literature. Peribronchovascular sparing, as was seen in our patients, is not a well-described feature that may represent clearing by the peribronchovascular lymphatics related to a subacute process with vaping. Of note, 100% of the cases in the report of 53 cases had bilateral infiltrates on chest radiograph or CT [10].

The pathology of EVALI continues to be poorly understood with no specific histopathological findings. A recent review described lung biopsies from 17 patients with either a "confirmed" or "probable" diagnosis of EVALI. All showed a pattern of acute lung injury, including acute fibrinous pneumonitis, diffuse alveolar damage, or organizing pneumonia. While other reports suggested an exogenous lipoid pneumonia-like process, the authors suggested that the patterns resemble a chemical pneumonitis [18]. Nevertheless, both findings do not provide clarity while making a histological diagnosis for EVALI. Our second patient showed similar histopathology, as described in the literature, with findings suggestive of acute pneumonia/inflammation with macrophages containing blackish brown pigmented material. Our first patient did not show any histological pattern of lung injury despite meeting a "confirmed" diagnosis of EVALI by the CDC [15]. However, the biopsy showed predominantly bronchial mucosa and not adequate alveolar tissues; thus, whether the patient had normal lung histopathology is inconclusive.

E-Cigarette aerosol contains different harmful substances, including carbonyls, volatile organic compounds, toluene, benzene, and heavy metals [19, 20]. Their constituents undergo thermal decomposition by the metallic coils, which then release new compounds that can be toxic [21]. In one study, E-Cigarette products contained microbial toxins, which included endotoxin concentrations above the limit of detection (LOD) in 17 of the 75 products tested and glucan concentrations greater than the LOD in 61 of 75 products tested [22]. Certain pesticides, such as chlorpyrifos ethyl and trifluralin, have been detected in high concentrations in some E-Liquid samples [23].

Triantafyllou et al. described several proposed mechanisms of EVALI, which include alteration in the expression of bronchial epithelial proteins, inducing airway remodeling, and macrophage activation [12]. Marijuana smoke inhalation has been associated with damage to the pulmonary epithelial barrier, and even the flavoring component has been linked to lung injury [23]. Compounds such as diacetyl, 2,3-pentanedione, and acetoin can impair ciliary function and have been evaluated and linked to bronchiolitis obliterans, the popular term being "popcorn lung," which causes severe respiratory diseases among workers inhaling these heated vapors [24–26].

Recently, samples of THC-containing products have been analyzed to identify the potential contributing substance resulting in harmful effects on the lung. Different substances were identified, which have included vitamin E acetate, medium-chain triglyceride oil (MCT oil), and other lipids [27] (Personal communication, D.T. Heitkemper, FDA Forensic Chemistry Center, November 2019). Vitamin E acetate, in particular, has been identified in the majority of the THC cartridge samples tested in various states and facilities [14, 28]. Vitamin E acetate is a compound that is used as an additive to E-Cigarette and as a thickening agent in THC products [29]. Vitamin E acetate was further implicated when a breakthrough report from CDC on November 8, 2019, showed that it was detected in 100% of the BAL samples of the 29 cases with EVALI that were sent to the CDC from 10 different states across the United States, while THC was identified in 82% and nicotine in 62% of the samples. Of note, no other suspected substances (plant oils, MCT oil, petroleum distillates, and diluent terpenes) were detected in those 29 BAL samples [30]. Inhaling vitamin E is not as benign as ingesting vitamin E, as it can impair lung function [31]. This provides strong evidence that vitamin E acetate might be a potential agent, though further studies are needed to validate this link.

4. Conclusion

EVALI can be devastating and even fatal, as was seen by the recent outbreak. Although various substances have been investigated, vitamin E acetate appears to be a risk factor. More data is needed to establish causality. With this report of two cases with radiologic and pathological findings, we hope to enrich the growing database and increase our knowledge of this disorder.

Abbreviations

EVALI: E-Cigarette or vaping product use-associated lung injury
THC: Tetrahydrocannabinol
CBD: Cannabidiol
CDC: Centers for Disease Control and Prevention
CXR: Chest X-ray
CT: Computed tomography
BAL: Bronchoalveolar lavage
HRCT: High-resolution computed tomography
ESR: Sedimentation rate
ANCA: Antineutrophil cytoplasmic antibody
AFB: Acid-fast bacillus
HIV: Human immunodeficiency virus
AG: Antigen
AB: Antibody
GBM: Glomerular basement membrane
LDH: Lactate dehydrogenase
BNP: B-Natriuretic peptide
PCR: Polymerase chain reaction
LOD: Limit of detection
MCT: Medium-chain triglyceride.

Acknowledgments

We thank Laurel Preheim, MD, for assistance with editing and formatting.

References

[1] A. K. Breitbarth, J. Morgan, and A. L. Jones, "E-cigarettes—an unintended illicit drug delivery system," *Drug and Alcohol Dependence*, vol. 192, pp. 98–111, 2018.

[2] L. McCauley, C. Markin, and D. Hosmer, "An unexpected consequence of electronic cigarette use," *Chest*, vol. 141, no. 4, pp. 1110–1113, 2012.

[3] C. R. Gilbert, M. Baram, and N. C. Cavarocchi, ""Smoking wet": respiratory failure related to smoking tainted marijuana cigarettes," *Texas Heart Institute Journal*, vol. 40, no. 1, pp. 64–67, 2013.

[4] H. R. T. Hashmi, R. Duncalf, and M. Khaja, "A case report of cannabis induced hemoptysis," *Medicine*, vol. 95, no. 13, p. e3232, 2016.

[5] M. Monfort, A. Larakeb, and F. Gouraud, "Hemoptysis in a young man smoking cannabis," *Archives de Pediatrie*, vol. 20, no. 6, pp. 637–639, 2013.

[6] US Centers for Disease Control and Prevention, *Investigation notice: outbreak of lung illness associated with using e-cigarette products*, 2019.

[7] S. A. Glantz and D. W. Bareham, "E-cigarettes: use, effects on smoking, risks, and policy implications," *Annual Review of Public Health*, vol. 39, pp. 215–235, 2018.

[8] G. Iacobucci, "Vaping among US teens has doubled since 2017," *BMJ*, vol. 366, article l5653, 2019.

[9] R. A. Grana and P. M. Ling, ""Smoking revolution": a content analysis of electronic cigarette retail websites," *American Journal of Preventive Medicine*, vol. 46, no. 4, pp. 395–403, 2014.

[10] J. E. Layden, I. Ghinai, I. Pray et al., "Pulmonary illness related to e-cigarette use in Illinois and Wisconsin — Final report," *New England Journal of Medicine*, vol. 382, no. 10, pp. 903–916, 2020.

[11] G. A. Triantafyllou, P. J. Tiberio, R. H. Zou et al., "Vaping-associated acute lung injury: a case series," *American Journal of Respiratory and Critical Care Medicine*, vol. 200, no. 11, pp. 1430-1431, 2019.

[12] S. D. Maddock, M. M. Cirulis, S. J. Callahan et al., "Pulmonary lipid-laden macrophages and vaping," *New England Journal of Medicine*, vol. 381, no. 15, pp. 1488-1489, 2019.

[13] N. Lewis, K. McCaffrey, K. Sage et al., "E-cigarette use, or vaping, practices and characteristics among persons with associated lung injury—Utah, April–October 2019," *Morbidity and Mortality Weekly Report*, vol. 68, no. 42, pp. 953–956, 2019.

[14] E. D. Moritz, L. B. Zapata, A. Lekiachvili et al., "Update: characteristics of patients in a national outbreak of e-cigarette, or vaping, product use–associated lung injuries—United States, October 2019," *Morbidity and Mortality Weekly Report*, vol. 68, no. 43, pp. 985–989, 2019.

[15] https://www.cdc.gov/tobacco/basic_information/e-cigarettes/assets/2019-Lung-Injury-Surveillance-Case-Definition-508.pdf.

[16] T. S. Henry, J. P. Kanne, and S. J. Kligerman, "Imaging of vaping-associated lung disease," *New England Journal of Medicine*, vol. 381, no. 15, pp. 1486-1487, 2019.

[17] T. S. Henry, S. J. Kligerman, C. A. Raptis, H. Mann, J. W. Sechrist, and J. P. Kanne, "Imaging findings of vaping-associated lung injury," *American Journal of Roentgenology*, vol. 214, no. 3, pp. 498–505, 2020.

[18] Y. M. Butt, M. L. Smith, H. D. Tazelaar et al., "Pathology of vaping-associated lung injury," *New England Journal of Medicine*, vol. 381, no. 18, pp. 1780-1781, 2019.

[19] R. Grana, N. Benowitz, and S. A. Glantz, "E-cigarettes: a scientific review," *Circulation*, vol. 129, no. 19, pp. 1972–1986, 2014.

[20] E. Kamilari, K. Farsalinos, K. Poulas, C. G. Kontoyannis, and M. G. Orkoula, "Detection and quantitative determination of heavy metals in electronic cigarette refill liquids using total reflection X-ray fluorescence spectrometry," *Food and Chemical Toxicology*, vol. 116, pp. 233–237, 2018.

[21] I. Burstyn, "Peering through the mist: systematic review of what the chemistry of contaminants in electronic cigarettes tells us about health risks," *BMC Public Health*, vol. 14, no. 1, p. 18, 2014.

[22] M.-S. Lee, J. G. Allen, and D. C. Christiani, "Endotoxin and (1→3)-β-D-glucan contamination in electronic cigarette products sold in the United States," *Environmental Health Perspectives*, vol. 127, no. 4, article 047008, 2019.

[23] N. Beauval, S. Antherieu, M. Soyez et al., "Chemical evaluation of electronic cigarettes: multicomponent analysis of liquid refills and their corresponding aerosols," *Journal of Analytical Toxicology*, vol. 41, no. 8, pp. 670–678, 2017.

[24] E. Gil, B. Chen, E. Kleerup, M. Webber, and D. P. Tashkin, "Acute and chronic effects of marijuana smoking on pulmonary alveolar permeability," *Life Sciences*, vol. 56, no. 23-24, pp. 2193–2199, 1995.

[25] J. G. Allen, S. S. Flanigan, M. LeBlanc et al., "Flavoring chemicals in e-cigarettes: diacetyl, 2, 3-pentanedione, and acetoin in a sample of 51 products, including fruit-, candy-, and cocktail-flavored e-cigarettes," *Environmental Health Perspectives*, vol. 124, no. 6, pp. 733–739, 2016.

[26] H.-R. Park, M. O'Sullivan, J. Vallarino et al., "Transcriptomic response of primary human airway epithelial cells to flavoring chemicals in electronic cigarettes," *Scientific Reports*, vol. 9, no. 1, pp. 1400–1411, 2019.

[27] https://fox17.com/news/nation-world/cdc-finds-vitamin-e-acetate-as-potential-cause-of-vaping-illnesses.

[28] L. Sun, *Vaping lung injuries top 1,000 cases as deaths rise to 18. The Washington Post*, 2019, https://www.washingtonpost.com/health/2019/10/03/vaping-lung-injuries-top-cases-deaths-rise.

[29] D. Downs, *Amid Vape Pen Lung Disease Deaths: What Exactly Is Vitamin E Oil?*, Seattle, WA, USA, Leafly, 2019.

[30] https://www.cdc.gov/mmwr/volumes/68/wr/mm6845e2.htm?s_cid=mm6845e2_w.

[31] J. B. Massey, H. S. She, and H. J. Pownall, "Interaction of vitamin E with saturated phospholipid bilayers," *Biochemical and Biophysical Research Communications*, vol. 106, no. 3, pp. 842–847, 1982.

Sequencing Alpha-1 MZ Individuals Shows Frequent Biallelic Mutations

Kimberly E. Foil,[1] **M. Gwen Blanton**,[1] **Chris Sanders**,[2] **Joannah Kim**,[2] **Haitham S. Al Ashry**,[1] **Suchit Kumbhare**,[1] **and Charlie Strange**[1]

[1]*Division of Pulmonary, Critical Care, Allergy and Sleep Medicine, Medical University of South Carolina, Charleston, SC, USA*
[2]*Biocerna LLC, Gaithersburg, MD, USA*

Correspondence should be addressed to Kimberly E. Foil; foilk@musc.edu

Academic Editor: Andrew Sandford

Rationale. Individuals with a single Z mutation in the *SERPINA1* gene that codes for alpha-1 antitrypsin (AAT) are at increased risk for COPD if they have ever-smoked. Whether additional variants alter the risk for COPD in this population remains unknown. *Objectives.* To determine whether additional *SERPINA1* variants impact COPD development in a previously identified MZ (carrier) cohort. *Methods.* Individuals with prior MZ results and AAT serum level <16uM were recruited from the Alpha-1 Coded Testing study and Alpha-1 Foundation Research Registry. Participants completed smoking history, demographics, and COPD Severity Score (Range 0-33) using REDCap data capture. At-home finger-stick tests were performed for next generation sequencing (NGS) at the Biocerna LLC laboratory. A genetic counselor reviewed records and interviewed participants with additional variants by NGS. A Wilcoxon Rank Sum test was used to assess correlation between variants and the COPD severity score. *Results.* A second *SERPINA1* variant of known or possible significance was identified in 6 (5.8%) participants. One each of ZZ, SZ, FZ, ZSmunich, ZM2obernburg, and Z/c.922G>T genotypes were identified. ZZ, SZ, and FZ are known pathogenic genotypes. Smunich is a likely pathogenic variant. M2obernburg and c.922G>T are variants of uncertain significance. The ZZ individual was on augmentation therapy when determined MZ by protease inhibitor (Pi) phenotyping; the others had limited targeted genotyping with MZ results. These six participants with biallelic variants had positive COPD severity scores >1. Presence of additional variants was not significantly associated with COPD symptoms in this small sample size. *Conclusions.* Some diagnosed MZ individuals instead have biallelic variants. Larger studies are needed to determine COPD-risk liability of variants. Accurate diagnosis impacts medical management and familial risk assessment. Pi phenotyping can be confounded by augmentation therapy and liver transplantation. Because a normal M allele may be reported in the absence of tested mutation(s) in AATD genotyping, clinicians should consider clinical circumstances and laboratory methods when selecting and interpreting AATD tests. Advanced testing, including NGS, may be beneficial for select individuals with prior MZ results. *Clinical Trial Registration.* This study was registered with clinicaltrials.gov (NCT NCT02810327).

1. Introduction

An increased risk for chronic obstructive pulmonary disease (COPD) exists for alpha-1 antitrypsin deficiency (AATD) MZ heterozygotes who have ever smoked [1]. Although excess risk is not established for MZ never-smokers, group mean lung function differences can hide the clinical observation that some MZ individuals present at a young age with panlobular emphysema similar to ZZ (classic, severe) AATD [2]. The genetic and/or environmental contributions to this advanced phenotype are incompletely understood.

Mechanisms to detect genetic signatures that predict clinical phenotypes would allow improved AATD diagnostics and therapeutics. Gene sequencing has not been routinely applied in AATD diagnostics. AATD testing methods commonly include one or more of AAT immunoassay (level), targeted genotyping, and proteinase inhibitor (Pi) phenotyping. The type of AAT testing should reflect the clinical circumstance (targeted detection versus screening) [3]. Conventionally, gene sequencing has been employed only when a rare or null allele is suspected after first tier tests [4].

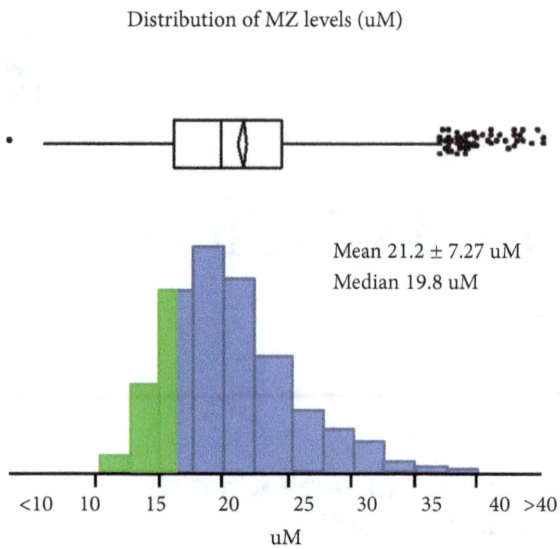

FIGURE 1: Distribution of AAT levels (uM) among MZ AATD individuals. Those in the lower quartile (less than or equal to 16uM) were included in this study.

Over 120 alleles of the AAT-encoding *SERPINA1* gene have been reported in the literature, and additional unpublished variants have been identified in proprietary laboratories [4, 5]. The Z mutation (c.1096G>A, p.Glu366Lys) is the most common clinically relevant allele, followed by the S mutation (c.863A>T, p.Glu288Val). Together, the S and Z alleles account for >95% of known cases of AATD. Most other alleles are rarely detected and their functional and clinical effects poorly understood. We were interested in using *SERPINA1* next generation sequencing (NGS) to assess whether additional sequence variants impact COPD presence and severity in a previously identified MZ cohort for AATD.

2. Methods

Inclusion criteria included age 18 and up and a prior MZ result for AATD with AAT level in the lower quartile for the MZ state (<16uM, 83mg/dL) because additional sequence variants may underlie these lower levels (Figure 1).

Three hundred and seventy eligible individuals from the Alpha-1 Coded Testing (ACT) study and the Alpha-1 Foundation Research Registry were invited to participate by phone and email. The Alpha-1 Coded Testing (ACT) Study is a research study that has tested over 20,000 individuals in the United States and Canada for AATD since 2001 to determine barriers to genetic testing. People with abnormal Alpha-1 genotypes are invited to join the Alpha-1 Foundation Research Registry. Participants in both programs have given permission for recontact for research purposes. This study was listed on clinicaltrials.gov (Registration number: NCT02810327). This research was approved by the Medical University of South Carolina (MUSC) Institutional Review Board.

All participants completed informed consent between June 2014 and June 2015. Following informed consent, participants completed survey questionnaires and reported demographic information, smoking history, and survey-based COPD severity score using a validated integrated measure of disease severity based on symptoms, treatments, and hospitalizations for COPD (range 0-33) [6]. A higher COPD severity score correlates with poorer FEV1 percentage predicted and health related quality of life. The surveys were constructed in REDCap allowing for web-based entry of data [7]. Participants were mailed a home testing kit to perform a finger-stick and submit blood spots for testing under a unique research code. Participants mailed their samples to the Biocerna LLC lab. NGS was performed blinded to the identity and symptomology of the participants with massively parallel high-throughput *SERPINA1* sequencing of coding and promoter regions by the Ion Torrent platform. These bioinformatics suites were used for sequencing and variant interpretation [8].

The genomic interpretations were matched to participant identity by researchers at MUSC and results were mailed to participants. A certified genetic counselor was available for questions. The genetic counselor contacted each participant who had additional findings by NGS. Clinical, laboratory, and patient-reported histories were reviewed to reconcile initial MZ designations with additional NGS findings for these participants.

The MUSC Bioinformatics Core used descriptive statistical analysis to perform means, standard deviations, medians, and percentages and analyzed group genomic data for variant association with COPD severity score using correlation analysis tools focused on keeping a false discovery rate <5%. These analyses included single variant associations and type of variant (e.g., promoter versus coding region) associations with symptoms. Variants found were correlated with symptoms in a Wilcoxon rank sum test using statistical package SAS 9.4 for Windows (SAS Institute Inc., Cary, NC, USA).

3. Results

One hundred and seventeen participants were consented (31.6%) and 103 (88.0%) completed the study. Fourteen (12.0%) consented participants did not return their study materials and were excluded from the analyses. Participants were 75.7% female, age range 18-73, and 39.8% ever-smokers. Participants had prior testing through the ACT study (57.3%) and other testing including clinical AATD testing by a clinician. Participant characteristics are shown in Table 1. Six participants (5.8%) had an additional *SERPINA1* sequence variant of known or possible significance. The remaining 94.2% had their MZ genotype confirmed by NGS. Frequency of additional variants did not vary by participant age, gender or smoking history. Each newly identified variant occurred in only one participant and no single variants correlated with COPD symptoms in this small sample size.

One each of ZZ, SZ, FZ, ZSmunich, ZM2obernburg, and Z/c.922G>T (p.Ala308Ser) genotypes were identified. ZZ, SZ, and FZ genotypes are of known clinical significance. Smunich is a likely pathogenic variant. M2obernburg and c.922G>T (p.Ala308Ser) are variants of uncertain significance (VUS) (Table 2).

TABLE 1: Participant characteristics, N= 103.

Gender	N (%)	Average Age (range)
Female	78 (75.7)	53.9 ± 12.2 (25-73)
Male	25 (24.3)	46.4 ± 15.9 (18-73)
Smoking History		
Ever-smoker	41 (39.8)	
Female	31	53 ± 12.0 (25-71)
Male	10	56 ± 10.7 (34-73)
Never-smoker	62 (60.2)	
Female	47	54 ± 12.1 (27-73)
Male	15	40 ± 14.9 (18-69)
Recruited From		
Alpha-1 Coded Testing Study	59 (57.3)	
Alpha-1 Foundation Research Registry or Clinicaltrials.gov	44 (42.7)	

TABLE 2

NGS *SERPINA1* Genotype	Variant Significance	Participant Age	Ever-Smoker	COPD Severity Score	AAT level (uM at enrollment)	RepeatAAT level (uM)
ZZ	Pathogenic	59	Yes	17	13.8*	31.1*
SZ	Pathogenic	18	No	2	12.3	9.3
FZ	Pathogenic	58	No	12	15	13
ZSmunich	Likely Pathogenic	67	Yes	4	13.6	11.3
ZM2Obernburg	Uncertain	34	Yes	3	15.5	14
Z/c.922G>T (p.Ala308Ser)	Uncertain	65	No	3	14.8	13

*On augmentation therapy at the time of testing.

All 6 participants with biallelic variants had positive COPD severity scores (>1). The distribution of COPD severity scores for all study participants is shown in Figure 2. The median COPD severity score was 3.0 for confirmed MZs (range = 0-24) in this sample and 3.5 for those with biallelic variants (range = 2-17). These were not statistically significant.

The initial mode of MZ assignment and relevance of new NGS findings are discussed by case below:

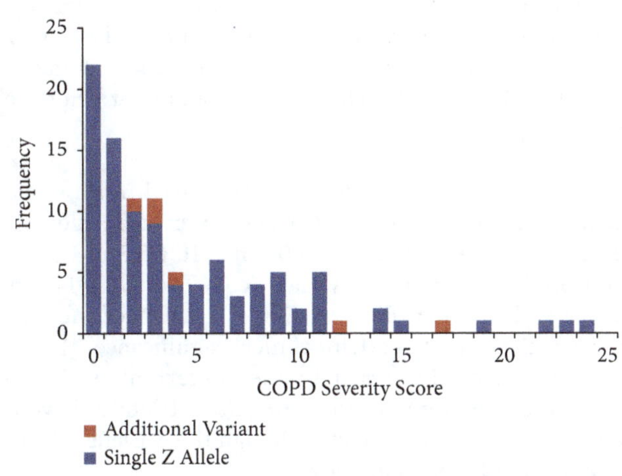

FIGURE 2: Biallelic variants all had COPD severity scores >1. The distribution of COPD severity scores for all study participants is shown.

3.1. Case 1, ZZ. A 59-year-old male was diagnosed with AATD in 1997 by AAT immunoassay (level) and began augmentation therapy in 2014. In 2015, Pi phenotyping yielded Pi MZ results and AAT level of 72mg/dL (13.8 uM). He was identified as a MZ heterozygote and informed his family members of MZ-associated familial risk. Two siblings had genotyping (MM, MZ) and two did not test. The participant received a double lung transplant during the study. The ZZ diagnosis explained his severe, progressive lung disease disproportionate to the MZ genotype. Augmentation therapy was appropriate for severely low pretreatment AAT level and clinical emphysema. The ZZ diagnosis is risk-raising for liver disease where evaluation and monitoring are recommended. The untested siblings have a risk for ZZ-AATD and should be tested.

3.2. Case 2, SZ. An 18-year-old male was referred to pulmonology with documented MZ status and AAT level of 64 mg/dL (12.3 uM). The participant's father died of ZZ-AATD disease. He had targeted familial genotyping, which identified a single Z allele as expected, and received consultation about MZ health and reproductive risks. The SZ result by NGS conferred higher health and reproductive risks that require follow-up. Should symptoms worsen in the future, augmentation therapy may be considered (whereas is not recommended for MZ heterozygotes). His results revealed that his mother carries an S allele, and the maternal half-siblings are at previously unknown increased risk.

3.3. Case 3, FZ. A 58-year-old female tested through the ACT study in 2014 due to pulmonary symptoms. Prior to 2015 the ACT study performed targeted genotyping for the S and Z mutations only and estimated AAT level. She received a MZ result with AAT level 78 mg/dL (15 uM). The F allele is a dysfunctional allele where the functional capacity to inhibit neutrophil elastase, rather than the quantity of AAT, is altered [9]. The FZ result by NGS diagnosed a rare form of AATD. In the presence of emphysema and fixed obstruction on spirometry, augmentation therapy may be indicated (whereas is not indicated for MZ heterozygotes with the same symptomology). Full siblings have a risk for FZ-AATD and should be tested. Familial testing should cover the F allele to ensure accurate results. Retesting may be recommended for relatives who tested before the F allele was commonly detected. Since 2015, the ACT study genotypes for the Z, S, F, and I mutations.

3.4. Case 4, ZSmunich. A 57-year-old male tested through the ACT study in 2016 after his brother was diagnosed with AATD-emphysema. He did not know his brother's genotype. ACT results reported the MZ genotype and level of 70.1 mg/dL (13.6 uM). NGS identified the Smunich variant (c.1061C>T, p.Ser330Phe) which was classified by Biocerna LLC as likely pathogenic [10, 11]. The ZSmunich genotype should be interpreted in the context of AAT level and clinical presentation. This result may alter surveillance and treatment for AATD disease. Genetic risks to relatives are altered by this result although the clinical implications are not well known.

3.5. Case 5, ZM2obernburg. A 34-year-old male tested through the ACT study in 2011 and received results with the MZ genotype and level of 80.6 mg/dL (15.5 uM). NGS identified the M2obernburg variant (c.710T>C, p.Gly148Trp) which was classified by Biocerna LLC as a variant of uncertain pathogenicity and uncertain clinical significance [11, 12]. Interpretation of this result in the context of AAT level and clinical symptoms is recommended. Relatives have an increased risk for this variant, although this variant's contribution to AATD risk is unknown.

3.6. Case 6, Z/c.922G>T (p.Ala308Ser). A 65-year-old female tested through the ACT study in 2013 and received results with the MZ genotype and level of 77.0 mg/dL (14.8 uM). NGS identified the c.922G>T (p.Ala308Ser) which was classified by Biocerna LLC as a variant of unknown clinical significance [11]. Interpretation of this result in the context of AAT level and clinical symptoms is recommended. Relatives have an increased risk for this variant, although this variant's contribution to AATD risk is unknown.

4. Discussion

Because AATD is a relatively rare condition in individuals who require testing because of COPD or liver disease, testing platforms have been constructed to be most cost effective. In this context, MZ AATD results did not reflect the true genotype in some individuals. Over 5% of previously assessed MZ individuals with AAT level in the lower quartile for the genotype had additional variants that were missed by previous testing. Accurate genotypic diagnosis guides AATD management and genetic risk assessment for family members. Testing limitations, clinical circumstances, and rare variants contribute to inaccurate MZ results. Advanced testing, including NGS, may be beneficial for select individuals with prior MZ results.

AATD testing algorithms and detection rates vary and best testing practice has changed with time [4]. Commercial and institutional labs employ a variety of algorithms, including one or more laboratory methodologies. Guidelines for the diagnosis of AATD (2016) recommend genotyping for at least the S and Z alleles for diagnostic testing of symptomatic individuals [3]. Advanced or confirmatory testing should include Pi-typing, AAT level testing, and/or expanded genotyping. AAT level alone should not be used for the primary diagnosis of AATD. The reasons that people undergo AATD testing are varied and include personal symptoms, family history and general screening. The most limited targeted genotyping detects only the most common clinically relevant Z mutation. Examples include select genetic carrier screens and targeted familial mutation testing. Expanded genotyping detects additional mutations, ranging from S and Z, to 4 or more alleles. The S, Z, F, and I alleles are thought to comprise >99% of AATD mutations, although the frequency and clinical relevance of many less common AATD alleles remains unknown.

AATD allele nomenclature was established based on electrophoretic migration of the alpha-1 proteinase inhibitor (AAT) before the encoding *SERPINA1* gene was identified. This lends to unconventional genomic nomenclature that persists due to wide use and acceptance in the literature. The genotypic designation "M" serves as an alias for the wild-type allele. AATD genotyping tests often report a normal M allele in the assessed genotype, even though genotyping detects specific mutations only and does not confirm a normal allele. One or more M alleles reported by genotyping (e.g., MZ, MM) should more precisely be interpreted as absence of mutation(s) tested. A small but real residual risk exists for patients who have fewer than two mutations identified by genotyping.

Pi phenotyping discriminates serum AAT variants by isoelectric focusing. A normal M protein (including subvariants of M1A, M1V, M2, and M3) and many abnormal AAT variants may be visualized. Pi-type and allelic genotype are the same in most cases and direct inferences can often be made between the two. However, Pi testing for patients on augmentation therapy results in detection of normal M-AAT in serum due to treatment, rather than biologic production.

Augmentation therapy is an FDA approved intravenous AAT replacement therapy indicated for select patients with

AATD-emphysema. Normal M-AAT pooled from healthy donor plasma is infused to raise serum AAT levels above the conventionally accepted protective threshold of 11uM. Augmentation slows progression of emphysema in patients with severe deficiency (<11uM) and FEV1 35-70% predicted [13] and has not been extensively studied in other serum level and lung function cohorts. Infused wild-type AAT does not impact DNA level testing for the patient (genotyping or sequencing) but has profound implications for interpretation of Pi phenotyping after therapy initiation, as the normal M-AAT will be detected after therapy as a direct result of the treatment. Serum AAT level will also be elevated as the therapeutic goal. AATD patients who have had a liver transplant have normal M-AAT and AAT level in serum, produced by the transplanted organ. Pi results for patients on augmentation therapy and postliver transplant do not determine the patient's germline genotype. Patient history may not be provided to a testing lab and not all clinicians are aware of these clinical interferences when interpreting results.

Although a majority of individuals with AATD will be ascertained by guideline-based testing, this study shows that some cases are missed. Improved diagnostics and interpretations could reduce error in MZ assignment and improve diagnostic yield. The utility of NGS in AATD diagnostics has not been studied in large series. NGS should be explored in other AATD cohorts and larger studies. NGS permits greater coverage of the *SERPINA1* gene for detection of both common and rare *SERPINA1* variants.

There are some limitations to this study. The individuals in this study were assessed MZ by mixed methodologies (genotyping and Pi-typing) at various points in the past. Therefore, the diagnostic error of any given test is not assessed by this study. Proper application and interpretation of current clinically available methods may reduce the error rate. This study enrolled only individuals with levels in the lower MZ quartile. The diagnostic error rates in MZ individuals with higher levels and individuals tested without a level may be different. The significance of individual variants was not determined by this study. Each additional variant in this study was found in only one participant. Identification of a VUS poses challenges to clinicians and patients/families alike. Variant interpretation is an evolving science. In some cases, laboratories do not agree on assignment of pathogenicity for a single variant (e.g., a VUS at one lab may be considered likely benign at another). Despite these limitations, recognition of sequence variants serves a step toward understanding their prevalence and effect on clinical risk through further research and data aggregation.

In this study NGS identified biallelic variants in over 5% of individuals previously assessed as MZ carriers. This impacts medical management and family risk assessment. These results remind clinicians to consider the clinical circumstances and laboratory methods when selecting and interpreting AATD tests and invite further evaluation of NGS in AATD diagnostics. Advanced or repeat testing, including NGS, may be beneficial for fully defining AATD in select cases.

Abbreviations

COPD:	Chronic obstructive pulmonary disease
AAT:	Alpha-1 antitrypsin
AATD:	Alpha-1 antitrypsin deficiency
ACT study:	Alpha-1 coded testing study
NGS:	Next generation sequencing.

Disclosure

The views expressed in this article do not communicate an official position of the Medical University of South Carolina, Biocerna LLC, or CSL Behring. Biocerna LLC receives funding from CSL Behring. A poster entitled *Sequencing Alpha-1 MZ Individuals Shows Frequent Biallelic Mutations* was presented at the 2017 American Thoracic Society International Conference; Washington DC, USA. Tatsiana Beiko, M.D., contributed to poster preparation and presentation.

Authors' Contributions

Charlie Strange and Chris Sanders made substantial contributions to conception and design. Charlie Strange, Chris Sanders, Kimberly E. Foil, M. Gwen Blanton, and Joannah Kim made substantial contributions to the acquisition of data. Charlie Strange, Kimberly E. Foil, M. Gwen Blanton, Joannah Kim, Suchit Kumbhare, and Haitham S. Al Ashry made substantial contributions to analysis and interpretation of data. Charlie Strange, Kimberly E. Foil, and M. Gwen Blanton made substantial contributions to the drafting of work and revising it critically for important intellectual content. Charlie Strange, Kimberly E. Foil, M. Gwen Blanton, Joannah Kim, Chris Sanders, Suchit Kumbhare, and Haitham S. Al Ashry are responsible for final approval of the version to be published. Charlie Strange, Kimberly E. Foil, M. Gwen Blanton, Joannah Kim, Chris Sanders, and Haitham S. Al Ashry contributed to agreement to be accountable for all aspects of the work in ensuring that questions related to the accuracy or integrity of any part of the work are appropriately investigated and resolved

Acknowledgments

This study was funded by CSL Behring with support to MUSC and Biocerna LLC. Data analysis was performed with the assistance of the MUSC Bioinformatics Core.

References

[1] K. Molloy, C. P. Hersh, V. B. Morris et al., "Clarification of the Risk of Chronic Obstructive Pulmonary Disease in α1-Antitrypsin Deficiency PiMZ Heterozygotes," *American Journal of Respiratory and Critical Care Medicine*, vol. 189, no. 4, pp. 419–427, 2014.

[2] D. L. Demeo, R. A. Sandhaus, A. F. Barker et al., "Determinants of airflow obstruction in severe alpha-1-antitrypsin deficiency," *Thorax*, vol. 62, no. 9, pp. 805–812, 2007.

[3] R. A. Sandhaus, G. Turino, M. L. Brantly et al., "The diagnosis and management of alpha-1 antitrypsin deficiency in the adult," *Chronic Obstructive Pulmonary Diseases: Journal of the COPD Foundation*, vol. 3, pp. 668–682, 2016.

[4] F. Kueppers and C. Sanders, "State-of-The-Art testing for alpha-1 antitrypsin deficiency," *Allergy and Asthma Proceedings*, vol. 38, no. 2, pp. 108–114, 2017.

[5] F. Rodriguez-Frias, M. Miravitlles, R. Vidal, S. Camos, and R. Jardi, "Rare alpha-1-antitrypsin variants: Are they really so rare?" *Therapeutic Advances in Respiratory Disease*, vol. 6, no. 2, pp. 79–85, 2012.

[6] M. D. Eisner, L. Trupin, P. P. Katz et al., "Development and validation of a survey-based COPD severity score," *CHEST*, vol. 127, no. 6, pp. 1890–1897, 2005.

[7] P. A. Harris, R. Taylor, R. Thielke, J. Payne, N. Gonzalez, and J. G. Conde, "Research electronic data capture (REDCap): a metadata-driven methodology and workflow process for providing translational research informatics support," *Journal of Biomedical Informatics*, vol. 42, no. 2, pp. 377–381, 2009.

[8] Ion Torrent Next-Generation Sequencing Technology, Available from: https://www.thermofisher.com/us/en/home/life-science/sequencing/next-generation-sequencing/ion-torrent-next-generation-sequencing-technology.html, 2018.

[9] N. J. Sinden, F. Koura, and R. A. Stockley, "The significance of the F variant of alpha-1-antitrypsin and unique case report of a PiFF homozygote," *BMC Pulmonary Medicine*, vol. 14, p. 132, 2014.

[10] D. N. Greene, M. Procter, P. Krautscheid, R. Mao, E. Lyon, and D. G. Grenache, "α_1-Antitrypsin deficiency in fraternal twins born with familial spontaneous pneumothorax," *CHEST*, vol. 141, pp. 239–241, 2012.

[11] D. W. Cox, G. D. Billingsley, and T. Mansfield, "DNA restriction-site polymorphisms associated with the alphal-antitrypsin gene," *American Journal of Human Genetics*, vol. 41, no. 5, pp. 891–906, 1987.

[12] J.-P. Faber, W. Poller, S. Weidinger et al., "Identification and DNA sequence analysis of 15 new alpha 1-antitrypsin variants, including two PI∗Q0 alleles and one deficient PI∗M allele," *American Journal of Human Genetics*, vol. 55, pp. 1113–1121, 1994.

[13] K. R. Chapman, J. G. W. Burdon, E. Piitulainen et al., "Intravenous augmentation treatment and lung density in severe $\alpha 1$ antitrypsin deficiency (RAPID): A randomised, double-blind, placebo-controlled trial," *The Lancet*, vol. 386, pp. 360–368, 2015.

30

Solid Indeterminate Nodules with a Radiological Stability Suggesting Benignity: A Texture Analysis of Computed Tomography Images Based on the Kurtosis and Skewness of the Nodule Volume Density Histogram

Bruno Max Borguezan,[1] Agnaldo José Lopes ,[1,2] Eduardo Haruo Saito ,[1,3] Claudio Higa,[3] Aristófanes Corrêa Silva ,[4] and Rodolfo Acatauassú Nunes [1,3,5]

[1]*Post-graduate Programme in Medical Sciences, School of Medical Sciences, State University of Rio de Janeiro, Rio de Janeiro, Brazil*
[2]*Rehabilitation Sciences Post-graduate Programme, Augusto Motta University Centre (UNISUAM), Rio de Janeiro, Brazil*
[3]*Division of Thoracic Surgery, Pedro Ernesto University Hospital, State University of Rio de Janeiro, Rio de Janeiro, Brazil*
[4]*Technology Centre, Federal University of Maranhão, São Luis, Brazil*
[5]*University Centre for Cancer Control, State University of Rio de Janeiro, Rio de Janeiro, RJ, Brazil*

Correspondence should be addressed to Agnaldo José Lopes; agnaldolopes.uerj@gmail.com

Academic Editor: Stefano Centanni

Background. The number of incidental findings of pulmonary nodules using imaging methods to diagnose other thoracic or extrathoracic conditions has increased, suggesting the need for in-depth radiological image analyses to identify nodule type and avoid unnecessary invasive procedures. *Objectives.* The present study evaluated solid indeterminate nodules with a radiological stability suggesting benignity (SINRSBs) through a texture analysis of computed tomography (CT) images. *Methods.* A total of 100 chest CT scans were evaluated, including 50 cases of SINRSBs and 50 cases of malignant nodules. SINRSB CT scans were performed using the same noncontrast enhanced CT protocol and equipment; the malignant nodule data were acquired from several databases. The kurtosis (KUR) and skewness (SKW) values of these tests were determined for the whole volume of each nodule, and the histograms were classified into two basic patterns: peaks or plateaus. *Results.* The mean (MEN) KUR values of the SINRSBs and malignant nodules were 3.37 ± 3.88 and 5.88 ± 5.11, respectively. The receiver operating characteristic (ROC) curve showed that the sensitivity and specificity for distinguishing SINRSBs from malignant nodules were 65% and 66% for KUR values >6, respectively, with an area under the curve (AUC) of 0.709 ($p < 0.0001$). The MEN SKW values of the SINRSBs and malignant nodules were 1.73 ± 0.94 and 2.07 ± 1.01, respectively. The ROC curve showed that the sensitivity and specificity for distinguishing malignant nodules from SINRSBs were 65% and 66% for SKW values >3.1, respectively, with an AUC of 0.709 ($p < 0.0001$). An analysis of the peak and plateau histograms revealed sensitivity, specificity, and accuracy values of 84%, 74%, and 79%, respectively. *Conclusions.* KUR, SKW, and histogram shape can help to noninvasively diagnose SINRSBs but should not be used alone or without considering clinical data.

1. Introduction

Smoking is the most preventable cause of death globally, followed by cancer and cardiovascular disease. Many case series have considered lung cancer as the leading cause of cancer mortality [1]. Fortunately, increased access to computed tomography (CT) and newly recommended low-dose CT screening has facilitated the detection of new cases and helped reduce mortality [2].

Solitary pulmonary nodules (SPNs) are masses ≤3 cm surrounded by normal tissue. SPNs are generally asymptomatic and an incidental finding on the imaging results of the chest or upper abdomen [3, 4]. In fact, dozens of diseases might present in the nodular form, including infections such as tuberculosis, benign masses (e.g., hamartomas), and malignancies (e.g., primary or metastatic lung cancer). Unfortunately, a significant proportion of these nodules are classified as indeterminate, with an intermediate density between fat and calcium [3, 5]. For this type of nodule, the clinical stability criteria and risk factors for cancer are particularly important for diagnosis and treatment. According to the recommendations of the Fleischner Society, at least 2 years of tomographic follow-up study are required without significant changes to classify the nodule as benign [3–5].

International guidelines suggest that the diagnostic investigation of peripheral pulmonary nodules can be performed with both invasive transthoracic biopsy techniques (e.g., CT-guided transthoracic needle aspiration) and bronchoscopic techniques [6, 7]. Endoscopic techniques are useful for diagnosing peripheral (also benign) lesions, particularly when guided by newer navigational methods such as endoscopic ultrasound radial probes, electromagnetic navigation bronchoscopy, and others as well as when specific predictors of success are present (e.g., CT bronchus sign) [8]. Unfortunately, fine-needle aspiration biopsies of suspected benign nodules are relatively low in sensitivity and specificity because this method often cannot reach an aetiological diagnosis of the benign process; furthermore, it generates technical difficulties and complications, especially with regard to smaller nodules located deep in the lung parenchyma [9]. Hence, the need exists to use three-dimensional imaging technology to establish new lung nodule evaluation methods for more in-depth analyses of the textural features of the nodule by analysing the histogram data obtained on CT imaging [10].

With the onset of CT, nodule growth is often visualised more accurately through its largest diameter. Although a nodule diameter measurement seems sufficient and is commonly used, it cannot determine the spatial growth of the nodule across its several axes, which can cause confusion with regard to a nodule that maintains its diameter in the X and Y axes but progresses in the Z axis perpendicular to the other axes [11]. Some studies have shown that thin CT sections (approximately 1 mm) in the region of interest (ROI) of the nodule can determine its growth through volumetry [12, 13]. However, volume is not the only parameter measured because the texture can be evaluated with or without the administration of contrast [14].

In clinical practice, the evaluation of densities is frequently and briefly performed by delimiting a generally circular or elliptical area within an image (i.e., the ROI). One of the most simplified forms of texture analysis is the use of first-order grey-level statistics, which by definition uses the volumetric version of the pixel (voxel), one at a time. The three-dimensional structure of the voxel that results from the incorporation of thickness into the pixel provides information about radiological density, enabling its study [15, 16]. A recent study analysed 60 CT sets and demonstrated the textural heterogeneity of SPN, concluding that this calculation is useful when differentiating malignant from benign nodules [17]. In addition to the mean (MEN), other statistics of texture corresponding to the first-order grey levels rarely used in clinical practice such as kurtosis (KUR) and skewness (SKW) can be studied throughout the volume of the pulmonary nodules [18, 19]. Thus, the present study evaluated solid indeterminate nodules with a radiological stability suggesting benignity (SINRSBs) through a texture analysis of CT images.

2. Materials and Methods

A total of 50 CT scans of SINRSBs and 50 CT scans of malignant nodules from two image databases were retrospectively analysed. The research ethics committee at our institution approved the protocol under the number CAAE-36881414.1.0000.5259, and our procedure complies with current national and international standards.

2.1. CT-Scan-Acquisition Protocol. CT scans were obtained at our institution (University Hospital Pedro Ernesto of the State University of Rio de Janeiro, Rio de Janeiro, Brazil) using a helical acquisition apparatus (HiSpeed LX; General Electric Medical Systems, Milwaukee, WI, USA). The acquisitions were performed along the axial plane with the patients in the dorsal decubitus position using the following parameters: 120 kV, 100–200 mA (which varied according to the biotype of the patient) with automatic exposure control, a slice thickness of 1 mm, and a pitch of 2 mm from the jugular notch to the xiphoid process at full inspiration. The gantry was inclined by 43 cm. No intravenous contrast enhanced was administered during any of the examinations. After the scan acquisition, the CT images were reconstructed using a standard soft tissue kernel. In addition, a high-resolution reconstruction with a matrix of 512 × 512 points was performed using a high-frequency algorithm, a window width of 1,500 HU, and a MEN centre level of −700 HU.

2.2. Database. The SINRSB image database consisted of CT scans from 50 patients treated at our institution who presented with solid SPNs that met the stability criteria (minimal volume variation and volume doubling time >2,000 days) after at least 3 years of observation. Scans with the following characteristics were excluded: nodules with findings suggestive of benignity (total, central, lamellar, or popcorn calcification) and those with characteristics suggestive of malignancy (spiculation, lobulation, or high irregularity); nodules with total or partial ground-glass opacity; scans with more than one nodule; and scans that did not include sections with a thickness between 0.90 and 1.25 mm for the ROI of that nodule.

The image database of malignant nodules consisted of 50 CT scans whose diagnoses were confirmed via invasive methods and histopathology. These images were acquired from two databases, including that of our institution and that of the projects of the development of nodule detection programmes stored by the Cancer Imaging Archive (https://www.cancerimagingarchive.net), which is a server maintained by Siemens Healthcare™ that includes data from unidentified patients. The Cancer Imaging Archive is a platform seeks to provide data for the research and development of image processing methods. CT scans are available in downloadable DICOM format, and the portal provides spreadsheets that contain various image-acquisition information. To maintain radiomics robustness, we selected CT scans with a configuration similar to that of our institution's database (including CT mode, no contrast enhancement, a section thickness between 0.9 and 1.25 mm, a matrix of 512 × 512 points, and a soft tissue reconstruction kernel).

2.3. Segmentation and Imaging Processing. The images were quantised in 12 bits (i.e., the equivalent of 12 grey levels) [15] and were later stored in DICOM format. The digital data were transferred to Bebúi software (Technological Centre, Federal University of Maranhão, São Luis, MA, Brazil) where the extraction of radiomic features based on the ROI was completed using in-house texture analysis algorithms. The images were evaluated using Bebúi software by fellowship-trained readers (B.M.B. and R.A.N. with 14 and 20 years of experience, respectively). An ROI was carefully drawn in the nodule avoiding contact with its edges using a semiautomated process. The software provides tools that digitally subtract vessels, bronchi, fibrosis scars, and other structures that do not belong to the nodule for all of the slices that correspond to its volume. The software also shows the region growing processing and segmentation algorithm installed through a "seed" to generate a database of that nodule with volume and histogram data. During this process, if motion, contrast streaking, or beam-hardening artefacts were noted on the image with maximal dimensions, then another "artefact-free" image demonstrating the lesion was chosen.

Using the software's dialog box, the interval was defined in Hounsfield units (HUs) between −450 and +1500. The seed voxel was placed within the nodule that analysed the neighbouring voxels using a 3D region growing algorithm [17] for inclusion based on the contrast intervals and number of slices determined in the dialog box. The location of the seed in the slice was automatically revealed based on the two-dimensional coordinates X and Y.

After SPN segmentation, the radiomics features were extracted for each nodule, including first-order statistics to assess the distribution of CT or voxel values. Using the CT scans, KUR and SKW were determined for the whole volume of each nodule. By definition, KUR is the property of a frequency distribution that characterises its flattening relative to the Gaussian curve (i.e., it determines the degree of flattening of a distribution curve) [18]. Thus, KUR measures the peakedness of the distribution of values and is considered as a marker of vascularity and tumour angiogenesis, which in turn are essential factors that determine tumour aggressiveness and overall survival [19]. High KUR is related to several outliers, whereas low KUR suggests a lack of outliers [18, 19]. A given curve is symmetrical when the distribution of values around the centre point is exact (i.e., the MEN, median, and mode coincide). The deviation from symmetry is measured as SKW, which indicates the asymmetry in the distribution of voxel intensities [18].

KUR is mathematically defined as the fourth moment of statistical distributions and, unlike the as the standard deviation, should not be considered as a measure of dispersion; rather, it is a distribution model. KUR is as a mass movement that does not affect the variance (VAR). Positive KUR is characterised as the presence of a peak with heavy tails, whereas negative KUR is characterised by lighter tails and a flatter peak than the normal distribution [20].

KUR and SKW were calculated using the following formulas:

$$\mathrm{KUR} = \frac{1}{\mathrm{VAR}^4} \sum_{i=0}^{G-1} (i - \mathrm{MEN})^4 \mathrm{HU} - 3, \tag{1}$$

$$\mathrm{SKW} = \frac{1}{\mathrm{VAR}^3} \left\{ \sum_{i=0}^{G-1} (i - \mathrm{MEN})^3 \mathrm{HU} \right\}^2, \tag{2}$$

where KUR = kurtosis, SKW = skewness, VAR = variance, MEN = mean, and HU = Hounsfield unit.

Additionally, CT scans were used to evaluate the histogram and obtaining data on the SPN texture patterns. Thus, Portable Network Graphics (PNG) files were generated using Python's Matplotlib tool (https://www.matplotlib.org).

Using Bebúi software, the inter-observer reliabilities of the images acquired were compared with 25 retrospectively segmented images for extraction of ROI-based morphological features by two independent readers (B.M.B. and R.A.N.) in a blinded form. These readers segmented the images and processed the histogram data for KUR and SKW without a front end. The semiautomatic calculation process minimized human intervention during the various histogram data processing events.

2.4. Statistical Analyses. Statistical analyses were performed using SPSS 16 (Chicago, IL, USA), which automatically generated the receiver operating characteristic (ROC) curve and calculated the best cut-off point by establishing test and state variables. The histograms were analysed and separated into two patterns: (1) the peak pattern (i.e., leptokurtic) in which the data are symmetrical or skewed but with a predominance of an increase in values; and (2) the plateau pattern (i.e., platykurtic) in which the MEN was distributed within regular intervals without a sudden increase of the data. Interclass correlation coefficients (ICCs) were employed to study the reliability of radiomic features, and an ICC was considered as acceptable if it was ≥0.85 [21]. Statistical significance was considered as $p < 0.05$.

3. Results

The interobserver reliabilities for KUR and SKW were high (ICCs of 0.87 ± 0.10 and 0.91 ± 0.12, respectively). Regarding the data extracted for analysis, however, we used the data agreed upon by both readers.

The MEN KUR of the 50 SINRSBs and malignant nodules were 3.37 ± 3.88 and 5.88 ± 5.11, respectively. The ROC curve was obtained, showing that when KUR >6, the sensitivity and specificity for distinguishing between malignant nodules and SINRSBs were 65% and 66%, respectively, with an area under the curve (AUC) of 0.709 and $p < 0.0001$ (Figure 1).

The MEN SKW of the 50 SINRSBs and malignant nodules were 1.73 ± 0.94 and 2.07 ± 1.01, respectively. The ROC curve enabled the establishment of a cut-off point that best fit the sensitivity and specificity values of the SKW, where 3.1 was the cut-off point for malignant nodules and SINRSBs. This value was associated with a sensitivity of 62.7%, a specificity of 69%, and an AUC of 0.705 ($p < 0.005$) to differentiate malignant nodules from SINRSBs (Figure 2).

Additionally, a histogram analysis was performed between the peak and plateau patterns. Typical aspects of SINRSBs and malignant nodules are shown in Figure 3. Among the 50

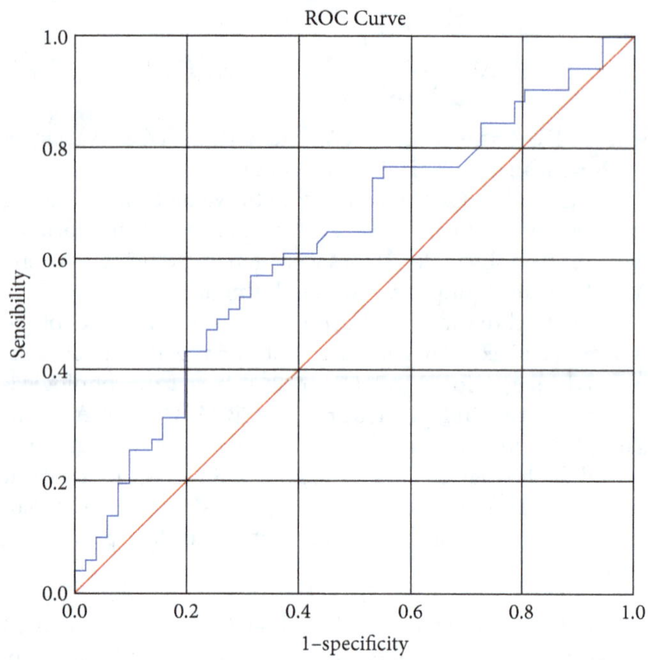

Figure 1: ROC curve for KUR, AUC=0.709 ($p < 0.0001$). The diagonal segments were produced by ties.

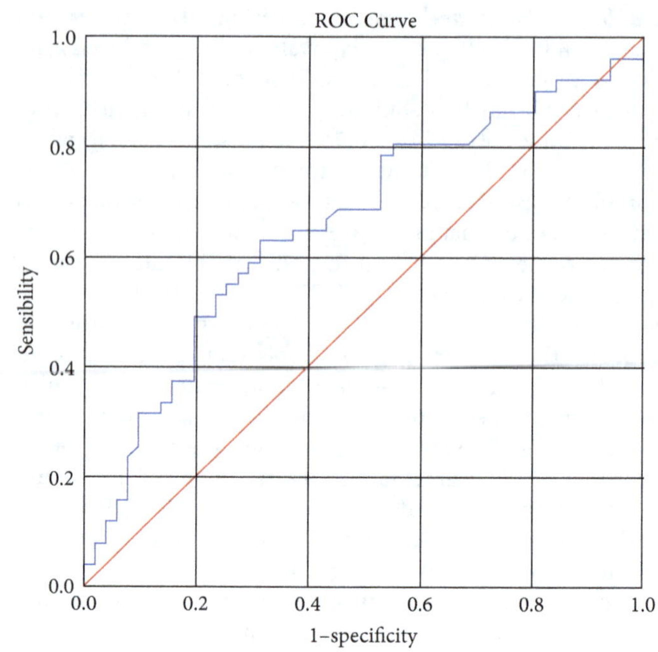

Figure 2: ROC curve for SKW, AUC=0.705 ($p < 0.0001$). The diagonal segments were produced by ties.

malignant nodules, 42 presented with the peak pattern, and only eight presented with the plateau pattern. Among the 50 SINRSBs, however, 37 presented with the plateau pattern, and only 13 showed the peak pattern. The histogram analysis between the peak and plateau patterns revealed a sensitivity of 84%, a specificity of 74%, and an accuracy of 79%.

4. Discussion

The present study revealed that a texture analysis of the CT images of patients with SINRSBs using easy-to-use software aids in the assessment the nature of the lesion. The KUR, SKW, and graphical analysis of histogram patterns might help differentiate SINRSBs from malignant nodules in these patients.

Radiomics (the study of extracting computerised, algorithm-based features to quantify the phenotypic characteristics of lesions using medical images) [22, 23] has been used to construct predictive models that relate image characteristics to tumour characteristics. Its four quantitative descriptive characteristics are morphological, statistical, regional, and model-based [23]. Several recent studies have used KUR and SKW as diagnostic indicators for various purposes, including to analyse liver fibrosis due to hepatitis C virus infection [24], central nervous system injuries with tumour differentiation [25], substantia nigra lesions due to carbon monoxide exposure [26], pancreatic tumour type differentiation [27, 28], and the association between metabolic patterns and several types of lesions in patients with cervical carcinoma [29]. Son et al. [30] collected tomographic measurements of lung tissue that included the KUR and SKW values associated with ground-glass nodules with or without solid components. These authors found that statistical analyses are a useful tool for differentiating invasive adenocarcinoma from pre-invasive and minimally invasive adenocarcinoma. More recently, Yagi et al. [31] performed a similar study that confirmed the potential of this method for differentiating minimally invasive adenocarcinoma from invasive adenocarcinoma [31].

Given the high morbidity and mortality associated with lung cancer, differentiating benign nodules from malignant nodules is crucial [22]. Alpert et al. [32] evaluated nodules with a lepidic pattern. In that study, 3D volumetry and first-order grey-level statistics obtained a sensitivity of 81% and a specificity of 76.7% when differentiating lepidic lesions from invasive lung adenocarcinoma. In another study, Kamiya et al. [33] examined the KUR and SKW of solid nodules to differentiate malignant from benign nodules. Similar to our results, those authors noted that KUR tends to be higher among malignant nodules than benign nodules. The AUC values of the ROC curve ranged from 0.71 to 0.83, and these results were similar to those of our study.

The CT pixels or voxels that comprise the image are the result of X-ray beam attenuation as it passes through a small portion of living tissue [2, 10]. The behaviours of the various attenuations are used to construct the histogram, and its study is only another step in the process of differentiating SINRSBs from malignant nodules, without ignoring the initial appearance (spicules, lobules, MEN diameter, and visceral pleural retraction) that, when combined with the radiologist's experience and the support of clinical data, contributes to the definition of probable malignancy. If doubt persists and the nodule is classified as indeterminate, then volumetric monitoring and the determination of the volume-doubling time are recommended [2–4]. In this context, the histogram that does not use a contrast can be useful, especially for patients who present with characteristics that prevent the administration of

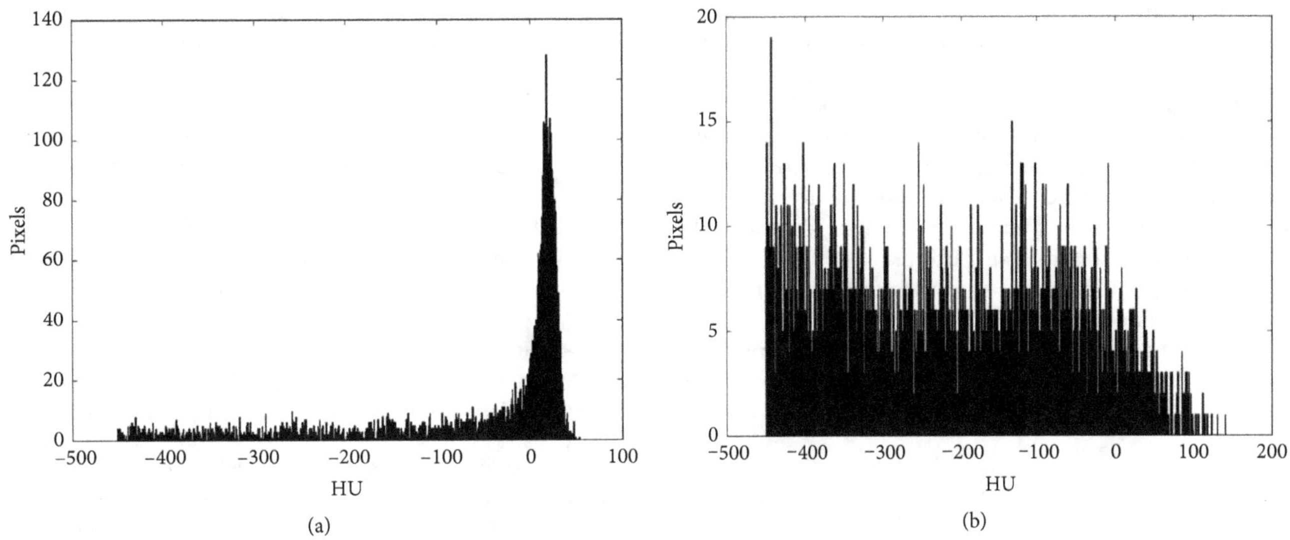

FIGURE 3: Histogram of a malignant nodule with a leptokurtic (i.e., resembling a peak) and negatively skewed distribution (a); histogram of a solid indeterminate nodule with a radiological stability suggesting benignity with a platykurtic distribution curve (i.e., resembling a plateau) and lower SKW (b).

radiological contrast and hinder follow-up assessment. Interestingly, the histogram plots presented in our study demonstrate that malignant nodules showed a spiculated pattern ranging from 0 to 100 HU, which corresponds to the range of predominant protein tissues such as soft tissue.

The present study found that KUR and SKW can be used to differentiate SINRSBs from malignant benign nodules. Because the sensitivity and specificity values were close to 65%, however, KUR and SKW should not be used alone; rather, they should be combined with other parameters. Therefore, volumetric assessment and volume doubling time remain key elements in the evaluation of indeterminate pulmonary nodules [34, 35]. More recently, Mao et al. [23] evaluated the usefulness of a radiomic predictive model developed from baseline low-dose CT screening. These authors observed that the sensitivity and specificity for predicting malignancy in SPNs were 81% and 92.2%, respectively. In that study, the benign nodules had greater SKW and less KUR compared with malignant nodules.

For efficient data processing, it was necessary to develop a specific tool that, in addition to aiding the calculation of KUR and SKW, generated PNG files using the Matplotlib tool for Python. Thus, it was possible to separate peak and plateau patterns. In addition to the calculating KUR and SKW, the graphical appearance of the histograms for these two patterns helped differentiate nodules into groups of SINRSBs and malignant nodules with an accuracy of 79%. The sensitivity and specificity values were encouraging in terms of the viable contribution of this method for identifying malignant lesions. However, it remains possible that the high protein level of the malignant nodules is related to increased protein synthesis by the cells (i.e., the small tissue portion that corresponds to a voxel in the image might also correspond to a group of cells with high protein synthesis). In this respect, positron emission tomography (PET) has demonstrated greater metabolic activity with protein synthesis in malignant lesions.

Obviously, benign nodules can exhibit high-density tissue masses (e.g., fat) and high-volume calcifications (e.g., hamartomas), thereby generating HU peaks. However, because the nodules in the present study were indeterminate and stable, their composition was likely more homogeneous and with less rich material in the cells. Naturally, this finding does not suggest that these nodules do not experience slower changes over longer periods [36]. Interestingly, recent studies have shown that tumour heterogeneity estimation using the distribution of pixel values with radiomic features can be used as a marker of tumour aggressiveness and treatment response in this patient population [37, 38]. In particular, KUR might be useful for predicting and assessing response to antiangiogenic treatment among patients with lung cancer [19]. More recently, Digumarthy et al. [19] demonstrated that a radiomics evaluation adds incremental value to one's clinical history and standard imaging features in predicting histology (i.e., distinguishing squamous and adenocarcinoma subtypes of nonsmall cell lung cancers) and epidermal growth factor receptor mutations.

One strength of our study is that we believe it is the first to show how histogram patterns differ between SINRSBs and malignant pulmonary nodules, likely contributing to the tomographic study of these lesions. As with any other study, however, ours also has limitations. First, the sample size was relatively small, although the size was justified by the strict imaging criteria used to exclude characteristically benign and malignant lesions to only evaluate indeterminate pulmonary nodules. Second, the benign nodules had no histological diagnoses, and these diagnoses were made only at the radiological level based on stability criteria; thus, we chose to call these cases "SINRSB". Third, the radiomics reproducibility likely depends on the amount of data and the consistency of the parameters used to produce the images; therefore, slight changes in the imaging dataset can greatly affect the robustness of the radiomic features [23, 39]. In our study, the SINRSB data comprised a single image database, whereas the malignant nodule dataset included several image databases obtained outside a follow-up setting. Although the chest CT protocol might affect the radiomics results, importantly, no recommendations exist for a standardised protocol to evaluate SPN radiomics, which limits our ability to compare studies and affects the generalisation of radiomic analysis [39]. Despite these limitations, we believe that our results justify additional research on the use of CT image texture analysis, especially with regard to peak and plateau patterns.

In conclusion, the present study shows that KUR, SKW, and the general appearance of the histogram contribute to the non-invasive diagnoses of SINRSBs and malignant nodules. However, these characteristics should not be used alone or without considering clinical data.

Abbreviations

AUC:	Area under the curve
ICC:	Interclass correlation coefficient
CT:	Computed tomography
DICOM:	Digital imaging communications in medicine
HU:	Hounsfield units
KUR:	Kurtosis
MEN:	Mean
PET:	Positron emission tomography
PNG:	Portable network graphics
ROC:	Receiver operating characteristic
ROI:	Region of interest
SINRSB:	Solid indeterminate nodules with a radiological stability suggesting benignity
SKW:	Skewness
SPN:	Solitary pulmonary nodule
VAR:	Variance.

Authors' Contributions

Bruno Max Borguezan, Agnaldo José Lopes, Eduardo Haruo Saito, Claudio Higa, Aristófanes Corrêa Silva, and Rodolfo Acatauassú Nunes contributed substantially to the study design, data analysis and interpretation, and the writing of the manuscript.

Acknowledgments

The Conselho Nacional de Desenvolvimento Científico e Tecnológico (CNPq, #304625/2016-7) and Fundação Carlos Chagas Filho de Amparo à Pesquisa do Estado do Rio de Janeiro (FAPERJ, #E-26/202.679/2018) partially funded this study.

References

[1] F. R. Hirsch, G. V. Scagliotti, J. L. Mulshine et al., "Lung cancer: current therapies and new targeted treatments," *The Lancet*, vol. 389, no. 10066, pp. 299–311, 2017.

[2] National Lung Screening Trial Research Team, D. R. Aberle, A. M. Adams et al., "Reduced lung-cancer mortality with low-dose computed tomographic screening," *The New England Journal of Medicine*, vol. 365, no. 5, pp. 395–409, 2011.

[3] C. J. Álvarez Martínez, G. Bastarrika Alemañ, C. Disdier Vicente et al., "Guideline on management of solitary pulmonary nodule," *Archivos de Bronconeumología*, vol. 50, no. 7, pp. 285–293, 2014.

[4] S. Quadrelli, G. Lyons, H. Colt, D. Chimondeguy, and A. Buero, "Clinical characteristics and prognosis of incidentally detected lung cancers," *International Journal of Surgical Oncology*, vol. 2015, Article ID 287604, 6 pages, 2015.

[5] S. Shinohara, T. Hanagiri, M. Takenaka et al., "Evaluation of undiagnosed solitary lung nodules according to the probability of malignancy in the American college of chest physicians (ACCP) evidence-based clinical practice guidelines," *Radiology and Oncology*, vol. 48, no. 1, pp. 50–55, 2014.

[6] M. P. Rivera, A. C. Mehta, and M. M. Wahidi, "Establishing the diagnosis of lung cancer: diagnosis and management of lung cancer, 3rd ed: American college of chest physicians evidence-based clinical practice guidelines," *Chest*, vol. 143, suppl. 5 pp. e142S–e165S, 2013.

[7] M. K. Gould, J. Donington, W. R. Lynch et al., "Evaluation of individuals with pulmonary nodules: when is it lung cancer? diagnosis and management of lung cancer, 3rd ed: American college of chest physicians evidence-based clinical practice guidelines," *Chest*, vol. 143, suppl. 5, pp. e93S–e120S, 2013.

[8] M. Mondoni, G. Sotgiu, M. Bonifazi et al., "Transbronchial needle aspiration in peripheral pulmonary lesions: a systematic review and meta-analysis," *The European Respiratory Journal*, vol. 48, no. 1, pp. 196–204, 2016.

[9] N. Tomiyama, Y. Yasuhara, Y. Nakajima et al., "CT-guided needle biopsy of lung lesions: a survey of severe complication based on 9783 biopsies in Japan," *European Journal of Radiology*, vol. 59, no. 1, pp. 60–64, 2006.

[10] J. J. Wang, H. F. Wu, T. Sun et al., "Prediction models for solitary pulmonary nodules based on curvelet textural features and clinical parameters," *Asian Pacific Journal of Cancer Prevention*, vol. 14, no. 10, pp. 6019–6023, 2013.

[11] Y. Wang, G. H. de Bock, R. J. van Klaveren et al., "Volumetric measurement of pulmonary nodules at low-dose chest CT: effect of reconstruction setting on measurement variability," *European Radiology*, vol. 20, no. 5, pp. 1180–1187, 2010.

[12] S. M. Barros Netto, A. Corrêa Silva, H. Lopes, A. Cardoso de Paiva, R. Acatauassú Nunes, and M. Gattass, "Statistical tools for the temporal analysis and classification of lung lesions," *Computer Methods and Programs in Biomedicine*, vol. 142, pp. 55–72, 2017.

[13] I. Petkovska, M. S. Brown, J. G. Goldin et al., "The effect of lung volume on nodule size on CT," *Academic Radiology*, vol. 14, no. 4, pp. 476–485, 2007.

[14] S. J. Swensen, R. W. Viggiano, D. E. Midthun et al., "Lung nodule enhancement at CT: multicenter study," *Radiology*, vol. 214, no. 1, pp. 73–80, 2000.

[15] R. Gonzalez and R. E. Woods, *Digital Image Processing*, Addison-Wesley, Reading, MA, USA, 3rd edition, 1992.

[16] J. R. Parker, *Algorithms for Image Processing and Computer Vision*, John Wiley & Sons, Hoboken, NJ, 2nd edition, 1997.

[17] M. Nishio and C. Nagashima, "Computer-aided diagnosis for lung cancer: usefulness of nodule heterogeneity," *Academic Radiology*, vol. 24, no. 3, pp. 328–336, 2017.

[18] G. Casella and R. Berger, *Statistical Inference*, Thomson Learning, Pacific Grove, CA, 2nd edition, 2010.

[19] S. R. Digumarthy, A. M. Padole, R. L. Gullo, L. V. Sequist, and M. K. Kalra, "Can CT radiomic analysis in NSCLC predict histology and EGFR mutation status?," *Medicine (Baltimore)*, vol. 98, no. 1, p. e13963, 2019.

[20] L. T. DeCarlo, "On the meaning and use of kurtosis," *Psychological Methods*, vol. 2, no. 3, pp. 292–307, 1997.

[21] L. I.-K. Lin, "A concordance correlation coefficient to evaluate reproducibility," *Biometrics*, vol. 45, no. 1, pp. 255–268, 1989.

[22] S. R. Digumarthy, A. M. Padole, S. Rastogi et al., "Predicting malignant potential of subsolid nodules: can radiomics preempt longitudinal follow up CT?," *Cancer Imaging*, vol. 19, no. 1, p. 36, 2019.

[23] L. Mao, H. Chen, M. Liang et al., "Quantitative radiomic model for predicting malignancy of small solid pulmonary nodules detected by low-dose CT screening," *Quantitative Imaging in Medicine and Surgery*, vol. 9, no. 2, pp. 263–272, 2019.

[24] M. G. Lubner, D. Jones, J. Kloke, A. Said, and P. J. Pickhardt, "CT texture analysis of the liver for assessing hepatic fibrosis in patients with hepatitis C virus," *The British Journal of Radiology*, vol. 2018, Article ID 20180153, 2018.

[25] W. Wang, J. Cheng, Y. Zhang, and C. Wang, "Use of apparent diffusion coefficient histogram in differentiating between medulloblastoma and pilocytic astrocytoma in children," *Medical Science Monitor*, vol. 24, pp. 6107–6112, 2018.

[26] M.-C. Chou, P.-H. Lai, and J.-Y. Li, "Early white matter injuries associated with dopamine transporter dysfunction in patients with acute CO intoxication: a diffusion kurtosis imaging and Tc-99m TRODAT-1 SPECT study," *European Radiology*, vol. 29, no. 3, pp. 1375–1383, 2019.

[27] J. Li, J. Lu, P. Liang et al., "Differentiation of atypical pancreatic neuroendocrine tumors from pancreatic ductal adenocarcinomas: using whole-tumor CT texture analysis as quantitative biomarkers," *Cancer Medicine*, vol. 7, no. 10, pp. 4924–4931, 2018.

[28] K. Sandrasegaran, Y. Lin, M. Asare-Sawiri, T. Taiyini, and M. Tann, "CT texture analysis of pancreatic cancer," *European Radiology*, vol. 29, no. 3, pp. 1067–1073, 2019.

[29] H. J. Meyer, S. Purz, O. Sabri, and A. Surov, "Cervical cancer: associations between metabolic parameters and whole lesion histogram analysis derived from simultaneous 18F-FDG-PET/MRI," *Contrast Media & Molecular Imaging*, vol. 2018, Article ID 5063285, 8 pages, 2018.

[30] J. Y. Son, H. Y. Lee, K. S. Lee et al., "Quantitative CT analysis of pulmonary ground-glass opacity nodules for the distinction of invasive adenocarcinoma from pre-invasive or minimally invasive adenocarcinoma," *PLoS One*, vol. 9, no. 8, Article ID e104066, 2014.

[31] T. Yagi, M. Yamazaki, R. Ohashi et al., "HRCT texture analysis for pure or part-solid ground-glass nodules: distinguishability of adenocarcinoma in situ or minimally invasive adenocarcinoma from invasive adenocarcinoma," *Japanese Journal of Radiology*, vol. 36, no. 2, pp. 113–121, 2018.

[32] J. B. Alpert, H. Rusinek, J. P. Ko et al., "Lepidic predominant pulmonary lesions (LPL): CT-based distinction from more invasive adenocarcinomas using 3D volumetric density and first-order CT texture analysis," *Academic Radiology*, vol. 24, no. 12, pp. 1604–1611, 2017.

[33] A. Kamiya, S. Murayama, H. Kamiya, T. Yamashiro, Y. Oshiro, and N. Tanaka, "Kurtosis and skewness assessments of solid lung nodule density histograms: differentiating malignant from benign nodules on CT," *Japanese Journal of Radiology*, vol. 32, no. 1, pp. 14–21, 2014.

[34] S. M. Barros Netto, A. C. Silva, R. A. Nunes, and M. Gattass, "Analysis of directional patterns of lung nodules in computerized tomography using getis statistics and their accumulated forms as malignancy and benignity indicators," *Pattern Recognition Letters*, vol. 33, no. 13, pp. 1734–1740, 2012.

[35] A. O. de Carvalho Filho, A. C. Silva, A. C. de Paiva, R. A. Nunes, and M. Gattass, "Computer-aided diagnosis system for lung nodules based on computed tomography using shape analysis, a genetic algorithm, and SVM," *Medical & Biological Engineering & Computing*, vol. 55, no. 8, pp. 1129–1146, 2017.

[36] S. M. Netto, A. C. Silva, R. A. Nunes, and M. Gattass, "Voxel-based comparative analysis of lung lesions in CT for therapeutic purposes," *Medical & Biological Engineering & Computing*, vol. 55, no. 2, pp. 295–314, 2017.

[37] L. Fan, M. Fang, Z. Li et al., "Radiomics signature: a biomarker for the preoperative discrimination of lung invasive adenocarcinoma manifesting as a ground-glass nodule," *European Radiology*, vol. 29, no. 2, pp. 889–897, 2019.

[38] Y. She, L. Zhang, H. Zhu et al., "The predictive value of CT-based radiomics in differentiating indolent from invasive lung adenocarcinoma in patients with pulmonary nodules," *European Radiology*, vol. 28, no. 12, pp. 5121–5128, 2018.

[39] J. Choe, S. M. Lee, K.-H. Do et al., "Deep learning-based image conversion of CT reconstruction kernels improves radiomics reproducibility for pulmonary nodules or masses," *Radiology*, vol. 292, no. 2, pp. 365–373, 2019.

Exercise Capacity in Unilateral Diaphragm Paralysis: The Effect of Obesity

Paul S. Richman[1] **Pomin Yeung,**[2] **Thomas V. Bilfinger,**[3]
Jie Yang[4] **and William W. Stringer**[5]

[1] *Pulmonary and Critical Care Division, Stony Brook University Health Sciences Center, Stony Brook, NY 11794-8172, USA*
[2] *Weill Cornell University Medical Center, 1300 York Ave, New York, NY 10065, USA*
[3] *Cardiothoracic Surgery Division, Stony Brook University Health Sciences Center, Stony Brook, NY 11794-8172, USA*
[4] *Department of Family, Population & Preventive Medicine, Stony Brook University Health Sciences Center, Stony Brook, NY 11794-8172, USA*
[5] *Los Angeles Biomedical Institute (LABIOMED) at Harbor-UCLA Medical Center, 1000 West Carson St, Torrance, CA 90509, USA*

Correspondence should be addressed to Paul S. Richman; paul.richman@stonybrookmedicine.edu

Academic Editor: Akio Niimi

Purpose. Healthy patients with unilateral diaphragm paralysis (UDP) are often asymptomatic; those with UDP and comorbidities that increase work of breathing are often dyspneic. We report the effect of obesity on exercise capacity in UDP patients. *Methods*. All obese and nonobese patients with UDP undergoing cardiopulmonary exercise testing (CPET) during a 32-month period in the exercise laboratory of an academic hospital were compared to a retrospectively identified cohort of obese and nonobese controls without UDP, matched for key features. CPET used a modified Bruce treadmill protocol with breath-to-breath expired gas analysis. O2 uptake, minute ventilation, exercise time, and work rate were recorded at peak exercise. Static pulmonary functions were measured. Kruskal-Wallis, Wilcoxon rank sum, and Fisher's exact tests were used to compare continuous and categorical variables, respectively. Stratified linear regression was used to quantify the effect of UDP and obesity on CPET variables. *Results*. Twenty-two UDP patients and 46 controls were studied. The BMI of obese and nonobese patients was 33.0±4.2 and 25.8±2.4 kg/m2, respectively. UDP subjects with obesity, compared to controls with neither condition, showed significantly reduced peak O2 uptake normalized to actual body weight (1.57±0.64 versus 2.01±0.88 L/min), shorter exercise time (5.7±2.0 versus 8.5±2.9 minutes), and lower peak ventilation. This was not observed in UDP alone or obesity alone. Peak work rate trended lower in the combined UDP-obesity group. *Conclusion*. Neither UDP nor obesity alone significantly reduced exercise capacity. Superimposed UDP and obesity interact to create a ventilatory limitation to exercise, with reduced peak-VO2, exercise time, and work rate.

1. Introduction

Patients with unilateral paralysis of the diaphragm (UDP) have near-normal static pulmonary function and are only mildly dyspneic during exercise, if there is no coexisting cardiopulmonary disease [1–3]. Cardiopulmonary exercise testing (CPET) in healthy subjects with UDP has shown mild or insignificant reduction in peak O2 uptake (VO2peak) and only mildly reduced total exercise time [2, 4], unlike those with bilateral diaphragm paralysis who have significant exercise limitation [2, 5]. However, many patients with UDP have comorbid disease of the heart or lungs; dyspnea on exertion has been commonly reported in such patients [1, 6, 7]. Thus, it seems likely that exercise limitation in UDP patients is magnified by any coexisting disorder that increases the work of breathing, such as chronic hyperinflation, V/Q mismatch, or poor compliance of the respiratory system.

Obesity is a common disorder that imposes a mechanical load during exercise, limiting the capacity to do external work. Prior studies have shown that peak work rate during cycle ergometry is reduced in healthy moderately obese subjects [8–12], despite generally normal values for peak VO2, O2 pulse, and anaerobic threshold (AT). This is referred to as mechanical inefficiency: O2 consumption is relatively

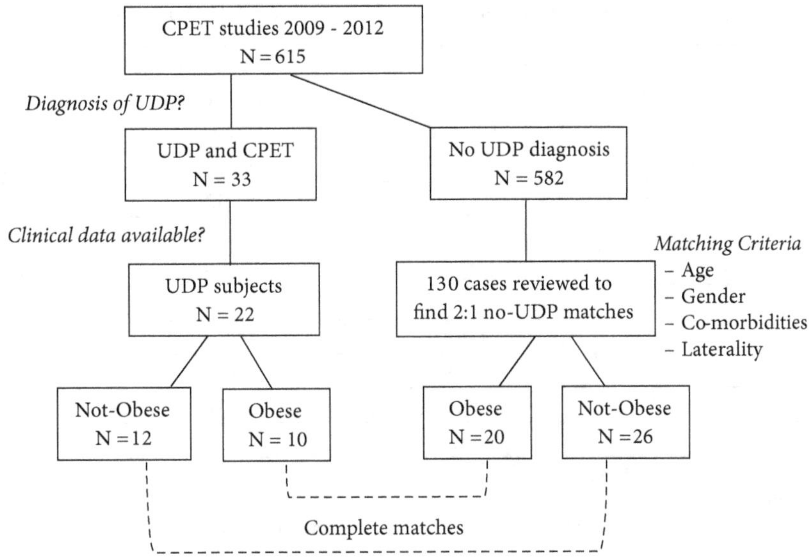

FIGURE 1: Flow diagram of the study.

high at any given level of external work, reflecting an excessive metabolic cost of moving heavy limbs [10, 12]. In addition, inertia and noncompliance of the obese chest wall may impose an intolerable load on the respiratory muscles causing dyspnea that limits exercise capacity [13].

We postulate that the generally mild exercise limitation among UDP patients is magnified by these mechanical loads due to obesity. No studies have specifically addressed this issue. The aim of this study was to determine the combined effects of obesity and UDP on exercise limitation in a cohort of patients undergoing CPET in our exercise laboratory.

2. Methods

2.1. Study Design. This was a matched-cohort study of patients with a confirmed diagnosis of UDP in the pulmonary practice of an academic medical center who performed CPET during a 32-month period from 2009 to 2013. Comorbidities were recorded from each subject's chart and placed in four disease categories: cardiovascular, pulmonary, neuromuscular, or joint/pain disorder. The definition of each type of comorbidity is detailed in the Supplementary Materials (available here). UDP subjects were categorized as obese (body mass index, BMI, ≥30) or nonobese (BMI<30). We matched each obese and nonobese UDP subject to 2 control subjects without UDP who underwent CPET in that timeframe. Controls were screened in batches of 10 until at least two matching controls were identified for every UDP patient. All screened controls were included; as a result, in two cases a UDP subject was matched to 3 controls. Eight matching criteria were utilized: age within 10 years, gender, presence of obesity, laterality of UDP, and presence of each of the above 4 comorbidities. This resulted in 4 distinct study subgroups: UDP/obese; UDP/nonobese; no-UDP/obese; no-UDP/nonobese (flow diagram, Figure 1).

2.2. Diagnosis of Unilateral Diaphragm Paralysis. UDP patients had all of the following: diminished unilateral breath sounds, PA and lateral upright chest X-ray demonstrating asymmetric elevation of one hemidiaphragm, and diaphragm fluoroscopy ("sniff testing") showing paradoxical upward motion of one hemidiaphragm [14]. We included only cases with paradoxical motion of a hemidiaphragm, not those with diminished or asynchronous descent of a hemidiaphragm, which may reflect only weakness or eventration. The sniff test was performed within 2 months prior to CPET. Duration of UDP at the time of CPET testing was estimated by the onset-time of symptoms, the date of the probable causative event (e.g., surgery) and prior X-rays.

2.3. Pulmonary Function (PFT) Tests. Subjects were tested in the sitting position (KoKo Px, NSpire Health, Longmont, CO, USA) with recording of maximal FEV1 and FVC during 3 forced expiratory maneuvers, following ATS/ERS guidelines [15]. The majority of patients had spirometry repeated while supine. NHANES-III reference equations [16] were used to calculate FVC as percent predicted (FVC %pred). Maximal inspiratory pressure (MIP) at RV and maximal expiratory pressure (MEP) at TLC were determined in the sitting position using a hand-held manometer (Instrumentation Industries Inc., Bethel Park, PA, USA).

2.4. Exercise Testing. Subjects performed symptom-limited exercise on an incremental treadmill protocol (modified Bruce protocol) with breath-to-breath analysis of minute ventilation (VE), O2 consumption, and CO2 excretion (Vmax Encore CPET System, Becton, Dickinson, USA). O2-hemoglobin % saturation by pulse oximetry and EKG tracings (CardioSoft, G.E. Healthcare, Chicago IL, USA) were measured continuously and recorded each minute. The duration of exercise and reason for stopping exercise were recorded. Predicted maximal O2 uptake was calculated by

TABLE 1: Demographic matching of UDP to non-UDP subjects.

	Obese		Non-Obese		
	UDP (n=10)	No-UDP (n=20)	UDP (n=12)	No-UDP (n=26)	P-value
Age, years (mean +/- SD)	59 +/- 11	60 +/- 6.4	64 +/- 9	61 +/- 11	P = 0.31
Male Gender, n (%)	6 (60)	12 (60)	11 (92)	22 (92)	P = 0.14
Right-Sided (proportion)	5/10	-	7/12	-	NS
Duration UDP (mean yrs)	2.8 +/- 1.6	-	2.2 +/- 1.3	-	NS
BMI (mean +/- SD)	34.2 +/- 6.3	33.0 +/- 2.7	26.9 +/- 1.5	25.4 +/- 2.6	<.0001*
Comorbidities, n (%)					
Cardiovascular	3 (30)	6 (30)	6 (50)	14 (54)	P = 0.41
Pulmonary	3 (30)	6 (30)	6 (50)	14 (54)	P = 0.41
Neuromuscular	0 (0)	0 (0)	0 (0)	0 (0)	-
Joint/Pain syndrome	1 (10)	2 (10)	1 (8)	2 (8)	P = 1.0

Numerical values are reported as mean +/- standard deviation.
UDP = unilateral diaphragm paralysis.
*For the difference between obese and nonobese groups, using Wilcoxon rank-sum test and Fisher's exact test as described in the Methods.

the equations: Women: VO_2 max/kg =42.83− (0.371 ∗ years). Men: VO_2 max/kg =50.02− (0.394 ∗ years) [11]. The equation of Jones [17] was used to estimate work rate during treadmill exercise: peak work rate (PWR, watts) = 9.81(m∗v∗i)/100, where m is mass (kg), v is velocity(m/sec), and i is %incline of the treadmill.

2.5. Statistical Analysis. The Kruskal-Wallis test was used to compare continuous clinical variables among the four groups. Wilcoxon rank sum test was used to compare the continuous demographic and clinical variables between obese DP and nonobese DP groups. Fisher's exact tests were used to compare categorical variables between obese DP and nonobese DP groups. To quantify the effect of obesity and UDP on exercise performance, a stratified linear regression was used to test the association of UDP, obesity, or their combination on six CPET variables: peak VO2 expressed as % predicted by actual and ideal body weight (VO2Max% ABW and VO2Max% IBW, respectively), Peak VE, breathing reserve, estimated PWR, and exercise time; the strength of the association is expressed by their estimated coefficients. Obesity (yes vs. no), UDP (yes vs. no), and their interaction were considered as explanatory variables. Statistical significance was set at 0.05. Analysis was done using SAS 9.3 (SAS Institute Inc., Cary, NC).

2.6. Human Subjects Protection. This study was conducted in accordance with the amended Declaration of Helsinki. The study was approved by Stony Brook University's Committee on Research Involving Human Subjects (CORIHS approval # 207533-1). It was exempted from the requirement of informed consent, because of its low-risk and deidentified data collection.

3. Results

3.1. Subject Characteristics. The study included 68 subjects in four groups as noted above. 22 subjects had UDP; 46 matched controls did not. By design of the matching process, there were no significant differences between UDP and control subjects with respect to demographic and clinical features (Table 1). The difference in BMI between obese and nonobese subjects was statistically significant and clinically meaningful: 33.3 +/- 4.2 kg/m2 versus 25.8 +/- 2.4 kg/m2 (mean +/- SD). Our obese subjects tended to be more female and have fewer cardiac and pulmonary comorbidities (nonsignificant differences).

3.2. PFTs and CPET Parameters (Table 2 and Figures 2(c) and 2(d)). Obesity alone was not associated with a restrictive PFT pattern (though FRC was reduced) and no decline in peak minute ventilation. The absolute value for peak O2 uptake and estimated peak work rate were observed to reach supranormal values in subjects with obesity alone. Conversely, UDP alone was associated with mild restriction, a trend to lower peak VE (coefficient estimate 16.9, p=0.06), absence of a breathing reserve, and slightly reduced absolute value for peak O2 uptake (p=.04). However, exercise capacity was not affected by UDP alone, as shown by preserved values for peak work rate and exercise time. The combination of obesity and UDP was associated with more pronounced restriction, a 29% reduction in peak minute ventilation, and a breathing reserve that was <12% of the predicted maximal VE, suggesting a respiratory limitation compared to non-UDP controls. With regard to exercise capacity, the regression model showed that UDP lowered exercise time significantly only for obese subjects, not for nonobese subjects. There was a similar trend for a combined effect of UDP and obesity on PWR, which did not reach statistical significance (p=0.13) (see Figures 2(c) and 2(d)).

3.3. Oxygen Uptake and Work Efficiency. Peak VO2 expressed as % predicted for *actual* body weight ($VO2_{Max}$% ABW) was significantly lower in the group with combined UDP and obesity compared to the other 3 groups (Figure 2(a), coefficient estimate: −28.2, p=.001). Peak VO2 expressed as % predicted for *ideal* body weight ($VO2_{Max}$% IBW) was higher in the group with obesity alone, compared to the other 3

Table 2: Effect of UDP, obesity, and their combination on static PFTs and exercise parameters.

	Not obese	Obese	UDP + Not obese	UDP + Obese	p-value*
Static PFT values					
FEV-1, absolute value Liters	2.57 +/- 0.93	2.74 +/- 0.65	1.96 +/- 0.80	1.91 +/- 0.58	p=.004
Forced vital capacity % predicted	91 +/- 17	99 +/- 12	67 +/- 17	62.9 +/- 13.5	p<.0001
Total lung capacity % predicted	97 +/- 18	94 +/- 15	74 +/- 14	66.1 +/- 14.0	p=.0002
Functional residual capacity % predicted	99 +/- 21	73 +/- 18	71 +/- 15	53.7 +/- 12.0	p<.0001
DLCO/Alveolar volume % predicted	84 +/- 26	98 +/- 16	103 +/- 14	111.7 +/- 20.3	p=.054
Exercise parameters					
O2 uptake, peak exercise ($VO2_{peak}$ L/min)	2.01 +/- 0.88	2.33 +/- 0.67	1.85 +/- 0.83	1.57 +/- 0.64	p=.04
Peak minute ventilation, VE (L/min)	76.4 +/- 35.3	78.4 +/- 21.0	66.2 +/- 24.0	54.4 +/- 23.2	p=.06
Breathing Reserve % of predicted VE (max)‡	16.1 +/- 22.0	15.4 +/- 18.4	-0.81 +/- 21.5	11.9 +/- 19.5	p=.16
Estimated peak work rate (PWR, watts)	132.4 +/- 76.6	149 +/- 74.7	130 +/- 75.8	93.9 +/- 66.2	p=.13
Total exercise time (minutes)	8.5 +/- 2.9	8.1 +/- 2.2	8.9 +/- 3.1	5.7 +/- 2.0	p=.008
Estimated work efficiency at peak exercise (watts/L/min)$	64.7 +/- 23.5	61.8 +/- 20.7	68.2 +/- 27.1	51.4 +/- 21.2	p=.23
Anaerobic Threshold† % of maximal predicted VO2	64 +/- 18	62 +/- 14	59 +/- 13	44 +/- 17	p=.03
SpO2, resting minus nadir (%)	3.0 +/- 3.6	2.0 +/- 1.9	4.3 +/- 3.3	2.9 +/- 3.8	p=.61

Numerical values are reported as mean +/- standard deviation.
UDP = unilateral diaphragm paralysis.
*P-values are based on the Kruskal-Wallis test.
$Estimated peak work efficiency is calculated as the ratio PWR/VO2peak.
‡Breathing reserve is expressed as the percent reduction in peak VE below the predicted maximal VE.
†No clear anaerobic threshold could be identified in 8 of the 46 subjects.

groups (Figure 2(b), coefficient estimate: 31.7, p<.001). The regression model showed that $VO2_{Max}$% IBW was reduced by UDP only in obese subjects, not in normal-weight subjects.

We estimated work efficiency at peak exercise, defined as peak work rate/peak-VO2. This variable was not affected by either UDP or obesity alone. However, subjects with combined obesity and UDP showed a trend toward lower exercise efficiency (p=0.12).

3.4. Oxygenation. All groups showed a small average decline in SpO2 at peak exercise, although <90% in only 7 subjects. Eight subjects experienced a >5% drop in SpO2. These subjects, compared to others, had a higher prevalence of concomitant cardiovascular disease (88% vs. 38%) and lower O2 pulse at peak exercise (10.9 vs. 16.0 ml/beat), though prevalence of concomitant respiratory disease and spirometric values were similar. DLCO was not substantially different between the groups (Table 2).

3.5. Other Findings. Thirty-eight of the 46 subjects achieved an anaerobic threshold (Table 2). The anaerobic threshold was normal (mean value >55% of predicted VO2-max) in all groups except the combined UDP- Obese group, which was mildly reduced at 44%. A subset of 12 UDP subjects performed both sitting and supine spirometry; the mean decline in FVC (sitting to supine) was 26%. Their mean maximal inspiratory and expiratory pressures (MIP and MEP) were -55 and +84 cmH2O, respectively. There was no between-group difference in FEV-1/FVC ratio.

4. Discussion

The main findings of our study are that obese subjects with UDP have markedly reduced peak O2 uptake when normalized to actual body weight, a lower peak minute ventilation, and exercise for a shorter time on an incremental treadmill protocol. Subjects with obesity alone or UDP alone did not show this reduction in peak VO2. The interactive effect of UDP and obesity on peak O2 uptake was evident whether VO2 is expressed in relation to the patient's actual or ideal body weight. Consistent with these findings, we also found a trend for a lower estimated peak work rate in the group with combined UDP and obesity. This would appear to support the idea that a subtle exercise limitation in UDP is magnified by both the excessive metabolic cost of moving heavy limbs and the inertia and noncompliance of the obese

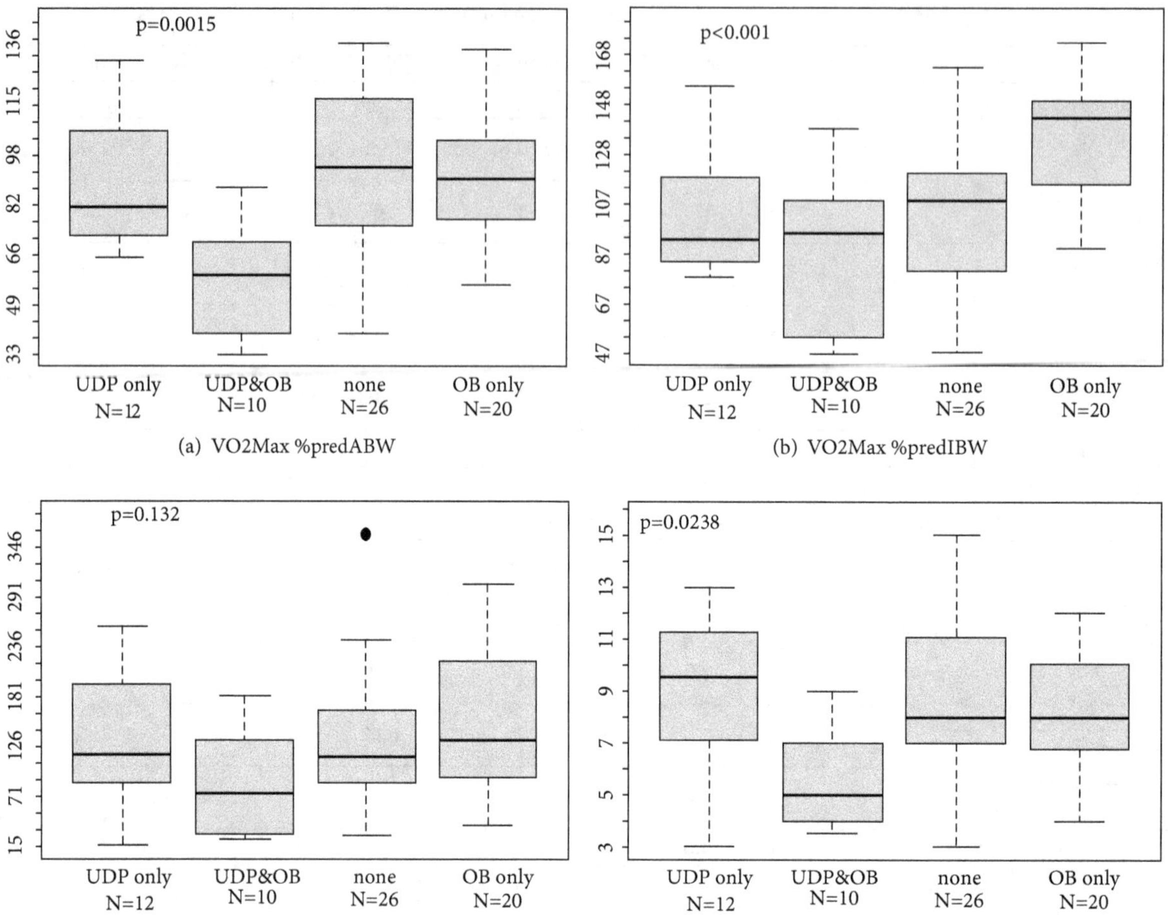

(a) VO2Max %predABW

(b) VO2Max %predIBW

(c) Estimated peak work rate

(d) Exercise time

FIGURE 2: CPET parameters in matched UDP and non-UDP subjects, with and without obesity. Box plot showing the interquartile range, median, min, max, and possible outliers. UDP= unilateral diaphragm paralysis; OB= obesity. Outliers are indicated as dots on the figure. p-values based on stratified linear regression. Panel (a): VO2 at peak exercise, as percent predicted referenced to *actual* body weight. Panel (b): VO2 at peak exercise, as percent predicted referenced to *ideal* body weight. Panel (c): (PWR, watts) = 9.81(m∗v∗i)/100, where m is mass (kg); v is velocity (m/sec); i is treadmill %incline. Panel (d): total exercise time, minutes.

chest wall. To our knowledge this is the first study to quantify their interactive effect on exercise performance, though there is a large body of prior related research.

4.1. Effect of Obesity Alone on Exercise Performance. It is well demonstrated that during cycle ergometry, obese subjects compared to lean ones have a higher VO2 at each incremental work rate, even though the slope of the VO2/WR curve is normal, indicating reduced mechanical exercise efficiency [10, 18, 19]. At any given level of submaximal exercise, minute ventilation is also higher among obese compared to lean individuals, indicating a normal ventilatory response to the high metabolic demand of exercising with a heavy body [20, 21]. At peak exercise, multiple studies have shown that healthy obese subjects achieve maximal work rates that are 9%-28% lower than lean controls, due to the excessive metabolic demand of moving heavy limbs [10, 19, 21–23] and ventilating a heavy chest wall [13, 21]. These same studies have also shown overall equivalent values for VO2 at peak exercise (approximately 2.3 L/min) as well as equal VO2 at the ventilatory threshold, in both obese and lean subjects. These numerical data are derived from healthy individuals with moderate-to-severe obesity (BMI ~40) and indicate preserved aerobic function of the cardiorespiratory system in obesity with normal supply of O2 to the exercising muscles and normal ventilatory drive, even though peak external work capacity is reduced. This differs somewhat from the findings in our subjects, most of whom had concurrent cardiopulmonary disease and were less obese: our obese subjects without UDP had BMI ranging from 31 to 38 and exercised to PWR values that were actually a bit higher than nonobese subjects, though they achieved this PWR at a value of peak VO2 that was substantially higher than that of nonobese subjects, when indexed to ideal body weight. This implies aerobic "conditioning" was greater in the obese compared to nonobese subjects, most likely a training effect induced by the high energy-cost of daily activities [22, 24, 25]. The relatively milder obesity in our subjects may account for this discrepancy between our study and other published work, since the degree of obesity is known to affect exercise capacity, fitness, and work efficiency.

4.2. Effect of Combined Obesity and UDP on Exercise Performance. Both groups of UDP subjects (obese and nonobese) had low values for FVC and peak minute ventilation and essentially had no ventilatory reserve. Sixteen of the 22 UDP subjects (73%) adopted a rapid, shallow breathing pattern at peak exercise and thus a high dead-space fraction that may have reduced alveolar ventilation even further. This ventilatory limitation did not reduce the peak work rate or exercise time among nonobese subjects. Obese subjects, however, also breathe with lower tidal volume and higher frequency during exercise, most likely to reduce elastic work of breathing [26]. When this effect is superimposed on the rapid-shallow respiratory pattern of UDP, it is reasonable to infer that the work of breathing become intolerable. In this case, the obese subject with UDP reaches a ventilatory limitation to exercise that imposes a "ceiling" limit on the supranormal level of VO2 that is required to sustain the high metabolic cost of moving heavy limbs and ventilating a heavy chest wall. Thus, in our study, while neither obesity nor UDP alone reduced peak work rate, the combined effect of high metabolic burden due to obesity and ventilatory limitation due to UDP was associated with a substantial reduction in peak work rate and exercise time on an incremental protocol. Notably, the normalization of VO2 to actual body weight (not ideal body weight) was a good indicator of reduced exercise capacity due to the interaction of UDP and obesity (Figure 2(a)). Conversely the normalization of peak VO2 relative to ideal body weight was a better indicator of the "conditioning" effect of obesity (Figure 2(b)).

Small declines in SpO2 at peak exercise were seen equally in all groups, generally in those with underlying cardiac disease. Its severity was not associated with obesity or UDP.

4.3. Methodologic Limitations of the Study. First, this is a retrospective study; a substantial number of potential subjects were rejected due to missing clinical data. Second, half our subjects had concurrent cardiorespiratory disease. This potentially confounds our observations on the effects of obesity and UDP on exercise capacity, despite the matching process. However, our findings are relevant to the real-world clinical situation, where obesity coexists with cardiopulmonary comorbidities. Third, among the *non*obese groups, mean BMI was 25.8, slightly above normal (i.e., roughly half were overweight, though not obese), reducing the BMI-separation between groups. These two factors may account for our finding that PWR in our nonobese subjects was approximately 25% lower than the values reported by others in lean healthy subjects. Nonetheless we demonstrated a difference in exercise performance related to obesity. The use of BMI to describe obesity is itself problematic. Individuals with identical BMI have differing amounts and/or distribution of body fat, resulting in variable mechanical loads on the respiratory muscles. In this retrospective analysis we did not quantify body fat or truncal obesity, variables known to determine how obesity impacts respiratory function [27]. Fourth, calculating peak work rate on treadmill testing by a standard formula is controversial, since it does not fully account for the energy expended accelerating and decelerating the limbs. The metabolic cost of exercise in obesity is magnified in weight-bearing (treadmill) protocols compared to cycle ergometry, though treadmill testing tends to elicit higher PWR and peak VO2 values [18, 28, 29]. These studies, which used the same equation to calculate treadmill PWR, found that at comparable work rates, treadmill and cycle modalities yield similar data for exercise time, dyspnea scores, lung mechanics, and ventilatory equivalents, supporting use of this equation. In this regard, the calculated peak work rates in our non-UDP subjects were almost identical to the mean published values of PWR by cycle ergometry (149.1 W versus 148.8 W). Finally, fluoroscopic sniff testing was used to document UDP in our cohort. Its accuracy in diagnosing UDP has been questioned, with reports of false-negatives and false-positives [14, 30]. When correctly performed, however, fluoroscopy demonstrates paradoxical inspiratory elevation in >90% of cases with phrenic nerve paralysis [7]. It has shown 81% concordance with ultrasonic assessment of diaphragm function, another widely used method [31, 32].

4.4. Conclusion and Clinical Implications. Normal-weight patients with UDP have a mildly reduced peak minute ventilation but normal exercise capacity. Moderate obesity alone does not significantly reduce exercise performance. Superimposed UDP and obesity create a substantial ventilatory limitation to exercise, with reductions in peak-VO2 and peak work rate. Patients who are dyspneic in association with UDP should be cautioned against gaining weight. In already obese UDP patients, the effect of weight reduction or surgical treatment of diaphragm dysfunction deserves further study.

Abbreviations

BMI:	Body mass index
CPET:	Cardiopulmonary exercise testing
OB:	Obese
PWR:	Peak work rate
UDP:	Unilateral diaphragm paralysis
VE:	Minute ventilation
VO2peak:	Oxygen uptake at peak exercise
VO2Max% ABW:	Maximal oxygen uptake as a percent predicted for actual body weight
VO2Max% IBW:	Maximal oxygen uptake as a percent predicted for ideal body weight.

Disclosure

No funding or other external support was provided for any aspect of the study. The study was performed as part of the employment of the authors at the Stony Brook University Medical Center.

Acknowledgments

We acknowledge the biostatistics consultation and support of Dr. Jiawen Zhu, Ph.D., and Lijuan Kang, M.S., and the Biostatistics Consulting Core at the School of Medicine, Stony

Brook University. We also acknowledge the professional work of the Stony Brook Exercise Physiology Lab in caring for the study subjects and providing the data files.

References

[1] J. Elefteriades, M. Singh, P. Tang et al., "Unilateral diaphragm paralysis: etiology, impact, and natural history," *Journal of Cardiovascular Surgery*, vol. 49, no. 2, pp. 289–295, 2008.

[2] N. Hart, A. H. Nickol, D. Cramer et al., "Effect of severe isolated unilateral and bilateral diaphragm weakness on exercise performance," *American Journal of Respiratory and Critical Care Medicine*, vol. 165, no. 9, pp. 1265–1270, 2002.

[3] A. Qureshi, "Diaphragm paralysis," *Seminars in Respiratory and Critical Care Medicine*, vol. 30, no. 3, pp. 315–320, 2009.

[4] M.-L. Chuang, D. C. C. Chuang, I.-F. Lin, J. R. E. Vintch, J. J. W. Ker, and T. C. Y. Tsao, "Ventilation and exercise performance after phrenic nerve and multiple intercostal nerve transfers for avulsed brachial plexus injury," *CHEST*, vol. 128, no. 5, pp. 3434–3439, 2005.

[5] C. M. Laroche, N. Carroll, J. Moxham, and M. Green, "Clinical significance of severe isolated diaphragm weakness," *American Review of Respiratory Disease*, vol. 138, no. 4, pp. 862–866, 1988.

[6] R. K. Freeman, J. Van Woerkom, A. Vyverberg, and A. J. Ascioti, "Long-term follow-up of the functional and physiologic results of diaphragm plication in adults with unilateral diaphragm paralysis," *The Annals of Thoracic Surgery*, vol. 88, no. 4, pp. 1112–1117, 2009.

[7] J. M. Piehler, P. C. Pairolero, D. R. Gracey, and P. E. Bernatz, "Unexplained diaphragmatic paralysis: a harbinger of malignant disease?" *The Journal of Thoracic and Cardiovascular Surgery*, vol. 84, no. 6, pp. 861–864, 1982.

[8] D. M. Bhammar, J. L. Stickford, V. Bernhardt, and T. G. Babb, "Effect of weight loss on operational lung volumes and oxygen cost of breathing in obese women," *International Journal of Obesity*, vol. 40, no. 6, pp. 998–1004, 2016.

[9] A. Cortés-Télles, L. Torre-Bouscoulet, M. Silva-Cerón et al., "Combined effects of mild-to-moderate obesity and asthma on physiological and sensory responses to exercise," *Respiratory Medicine*, vol. 109, no. 11, pp. 1397–1403, 2015.

[10] J. A. Dempsey, W. Reddan, B. Balke, and J. Rankin, "Work capacity determinants and physiologic cost of weight-supported work in obesity," *Journal of Applied Physiology*, vol. 21, no. 6, pp. 1815–1820, 1966.

[11] K. Wasserman and B. J. Whipp, "Exercise physiology in health and disease," *American Review of Respiratory Disease*, vol. 112, no. 2, pp. 219–249, 1975.

[12] B. J. Whipp and J. A. Davis, "The ventilatory stress of exercise in obesity," *American Review of Respiratory Disease*, vol. 129, no. 2, pp. S90–S92, 1984.

[13] J. Kress, A. Pohlman, J. Alverdy, and J. Hall, "The impact of morbid obesity on oxygen cost of breathing ($V^{\bullet}o_{2RESP}$) at rest," *American Journal of Respiratory and Critical Care Medicine*, vol. 160, no. 3, pp. 883–886, 1999.

[14] R. D. Tarver, D. J. Conces, D. A. Cory, and V. A. Vix, "Imaging the diaphragm and its disorders," *Journal of Thoracic Imaging*, vol. 4, no. 1, pp. 1–18, 1989.

[15] M. R. Miller, J. Hankinson, V. Brusasco et al., "Standardisation of spirometry," *European Respiratory Journal*, vol. 26, no. 2, pp. 319–338, 2005.

[16] J. L. Hankinson, J. R. Odencrantz, and K. B. Fedan, "Spirometric reference values from a sample of the general U.S. population," *American Journal of Respiratory and Critical Care Medicine*, vol. 159, no. 1, pp. 179–187, 1999.

[17] N. L. Jones, *Clinical Exercise Testing*, W.B. Saunders Company, Philadelphia, Pa, USA, 4th edition, 1997.

[18] C. L. Lafortuna, F. Agosti, R. Galli, C. Busti, S. Lazzer, and A. Sartorio, "The energetic and cardiovascular response to treadmill walking and cycle ergometer exercise in obese women," *European Journal of Applied Physiology*, vol. 103, no. 6, pp. 707–717, 2008.

[19] A. Salvadori, P. Fanari, P. Mazza, R. Agosti, and E. Longhini, "Work capacity and cardiopulmonary adaptation of the obese subject during exercise testing," *CHEST*, vol. 101, no. 3, pp. 674–679, 1992.

[20] T. G. Babb, D. Korzick, M. Meador, J. L. Hodgson, and E. R. Buskirk, "Ventilatory response of moderately obese women to submaximal exercise," *International Journal of Obesity*, vol. 15, no. 1, pp. 59–65, 1991.

[21] D. Ofir, P. Laveneziana, K. A. Webb, and D. E. O'Donnell, "Ventilatory and perceptual responses to cycle exercise in obese women," *Journal of Applied Physiology*, vol. 102, no. 6, pp. 2217–2226, 2007.

[22] American Thoracic Society and American College of Chest Physicians, "ATS/ACCP statement on cardiopulmonary exercise testing," *American Journal of Respiratory and Critical Care Medicine*, vol. 167, no. 2, pp. 211–277, 2003.

[23] D. S. DeLorey, B. L. Wyrick, and T. G. Babb, "Mild-to-moderate obesity: Implications for respiratory mechanics at rest and during exercise in young men," *International Journal of Obesity*, vol. 29, no. 9, pp. 1039–1047, 2005.

[24] L. Laviolette, F. Sava, D. E. O'Donnell et al., "Effect of obesity on constant workrate exercise in hyperinflated men with COPD," *BMC Pulmonary Medicine*, vol. 10, no. 1, p. 33, 2010.

[25] D. E. O'Donnell, C. D. J. O'Donnell, K. A. Webb, and J. A. Guenette, "Respiratory consequences of mild-to-moderate obesity: impact on exercise performance in health and in chronic obstructive pulmonary disease," *Pulmonary Medicine*, vol. 2012, Article ID 818925, 12 pages, 2012.

[26] T. G. Babb, "Obesity: challenges to ventilatory control during exercise—a brief review," *Respiratory Physiology & Neurobiology*, vol. 189, no. 2, pp. 364–370, 2013.

[27] C. M. Salome, G. G. King, and N. Berend, "Physiology of obesity and effects on lung function," *Journal of Applied Physiology*, vol. 108, no. 1, pp. 206–211, 2010.

[28] C. E. Ciavaglia, J. A. Guenette, J. Ora, K. A. Webb, J. A. Neder, and D. E. O'Donnell, "Does exercise test modality influence dyspnoea perception in obese patients with COPD?" *European Respiratory Journal*, vol. 43, no. 6, pp. 1621–1630, 2014.

[29] S. M. Holm, W. Rodgers, R. G. Haennel et al., "Effect of modality on cardiopulmonary exercise testing in male and female COPD patients," *Respiratory Physiology & Neurobiology*, vol. 192, no. 1, pp. 30–38, 2014.

[30] D. S. Gierada, R. M. Slone, and M. J. Fleishman, "Imaging evaluation of the diaphragm," *Chest Surgery Clinics of North America*, vol. 8, no. 2, pp. 237–280, 1998.

[31] M. Epelman, O. M. Navarro, A. Daneman, and S. F. Miller, "M-mode sonography of diaphragmatic motion: Description of technique and experience in 278 pediatric patients," *Pediatric Radiology*, vol. 35, no. 7, pp. 661–667, 2005.

[32] J. G. Houston, M. Fleet, M. D. Cowan, and N. C. McMillan, "Comparison of ultrasound with fluoroscopy in the Assessment of suspected hemidiaphragmatic movement abnormality," *Clinical Radiology*, vol. 50, no. 2, pp. 95–98, 1995.

32

Tracheobronchoplasty and Diaphragmatic Plication under VV ECMO for Combined ECAC and Diaphragmatic Paralysis

Mehmet M. Tatari,[1] David Abia-Trujillo,[1] Mathew Thomas,[2] Neal M. Patel,[1] Sebastian Fernandez-Bussy,[1] Britney N. Hazelett,[1] and Margaret M. Johnson[1]

[1]*Division of Pulmonary Medicine, Mayo Clinic, Jacksonville, FL. 4500 San Pablo Road, Jacksonville, FL 32224, USA*
[2]*Department of Cardiothoracic Surgery, Mayo Clinic, Jacksonville, FL. 4500 San Pablo Road, Jacksonville, FL 32224, USA*

Correspondence should be addressed to Mehmet M. Tatari; tatari.mehmet@mayo.edu

Academic Editor: Akif Turna

The coexistence of expiratory central airway collapse and diaphragmatic paralysis presents a diagnostic and treatment challenge. Both entities are underrecognized causes of dyspnea, cough, sputum production, and orthopnea. Optimal treatment must be individualized and is best achieved by a multidisciplinary team. We present a case of a patient with profound functional impairment from dyspnea and hypoxemia due to expiratory central airway collapse, complicated by bronchiectasis from recurrent respiratory infections, and diaphragmatic paralysis.

1. Introduction

There are a myriad of causes of dyspnea, hypoxemia, and excessive sputum production. Identifying the relevant contributors to patient's presenting concerns is critical for appropriate management. Expiratory central airway collapse (ECAC) involving either the cartilaginous tracheal wall or the posterior membranous portion may be suggested by computed tomography imaging of the chest obtained during forced expiration and confirmed by dynamic bronchoscopy. Fluoroscopy and diaphragm ultrasound are used to diagnose diaphragmatic paralysis. Surgical management includes tracheobronchoplasty and diaphragmatic plication. ECAC and diaphragm paralysis both compromise gas exchange during surgery but the effect can be mitigated by the use of intraoperative extracorporeal membrane oxygenation (ECMO).

2. Case Presentation

A 54-year-old man presented with progressive shortness of breath, cough, and recurrent pneumonia. Chest examination was notable for reduced bilateral lung excursion, coarse breath sounds diffusely, and paradoxical breathing in the supine position. Pulmonary function testing suggested severe restriction with FVC of 27% predicted, FEV 1 28% predicted, normal FEV1/FVC ratio, and respiratory muscle strength < 10% predicted.

Computed tomography (CT) of the chest revealed basilar bronchiectasis and bilateral diaphragmatic elevation with associated atelectasis. Dynamic CT showed anterior displacement of the posterior tracheal wall at the distal trachea, bilateral main stem bronchi, and bronchus intermedius. Electromyogram demonstrated bilateral phrenic neuropathy and left brachial plexus neuropathy. Ultrasound confirmed the absence of diaphragm movement bilaterally. He had progressive clinical decline requiring near constant noninvasive positive pressure ventilation (NPPV). Dynamic bronchoscopy showed severe expiratory central airway collapse (ECAC) with >90% collapse of the trachea, main stem bronchi, and bronchus intermedius (Figure 1(a)). A stent trial (Figure 1(b)) was performed with placement of three uncovered self-expandable metallic stents in the left mainstem bronchus, distal and mid trachea and right mainstem bronchus and bronchus intermedius. This resulted in measurable improvements in the quality of life by validated

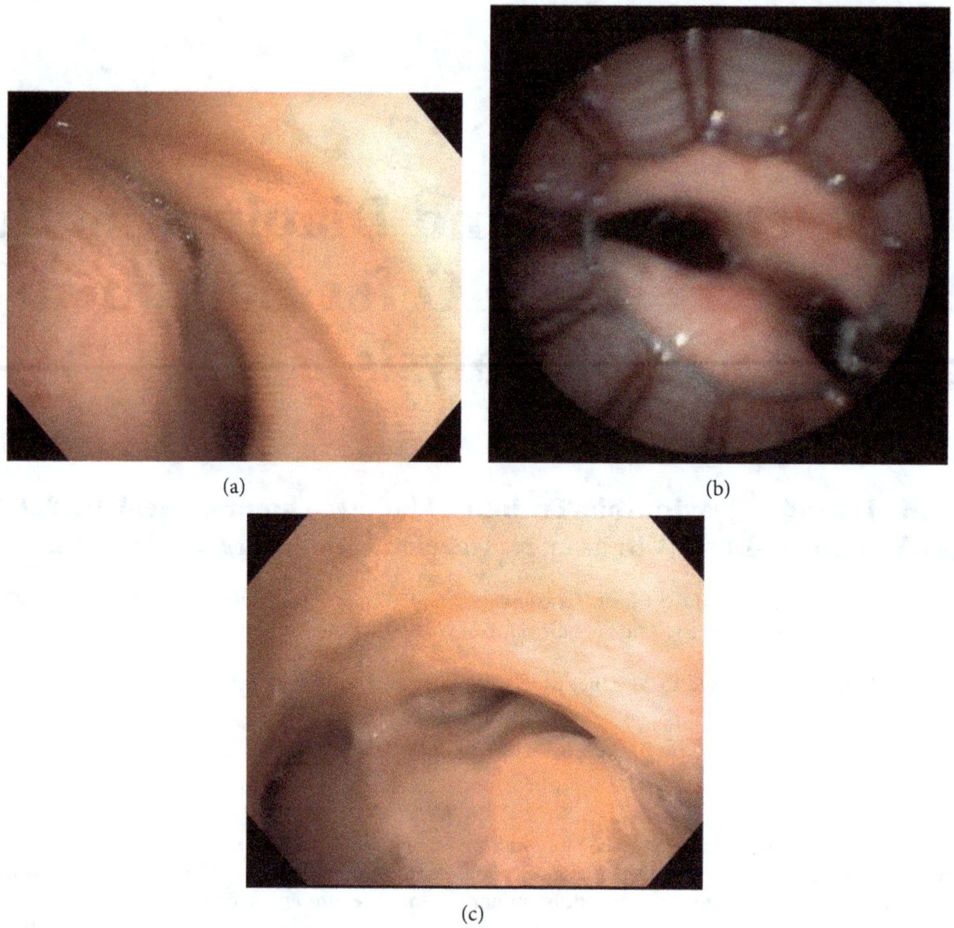

FIGURE 1: (a) Dynamic bronchoscopy showing severe expiratory central airway collapse of the distal trachea, left main stem bronchus, and right main bronchus. (b) Self-expandable metallic stents deployed in the airway during stent trial. (c) Dynamic bronchoscopy showing <70% collapse of the distal trachea, left main stem bronchus, and right main bronchus.

questionnaires at two weeks and the stents were removed. He was recommended to undergo combined tracheobronchoplasty and right diaphragmatic plication.

The initial surgery was aborted due to the inability to maintain adequate oxygenation during single lung ventilation. One week later, the procedure was successfully completed through right thoracotomy under venous-venous extra-corporeal membrane oxygenation (VV ECMO) support. Central airway stabilization was achieved by suturing a knitted polypropylene mesh to the posterior membrane of the trachea and bilateral main bronchi. Due to persistent ventilator dependency, left diaphragm plication through a left thoracotomy was performed 5 days postoperatively. He was discharged home on postoperative day #23.

At follow-up evaluation, he no longer required NPPV and regained independence in activities of daily living. Pulmonary function testing showed improvement with FVC of 53% predicted, FEV1 42% predicted, and respiratory muscle strength 13% predicted. CT of the chest demonstrated improved lung volumes (Figure 2). Dynamic bronchoscopy showed improvement in the degree of ECAC (Figure 1(c)).

3. Discussion

Although diagnostic parsimony encourages identifying a single unifying explanation for one's symptoms, this case illustrates the veracity of Hickam's dictum: "A man may have as many diseases as he damn well pleases [1]." We hypothesized that both ECAC and diaphragmatic paralysis (DP) were major contributors to his clinical presentation, and thus, therapy directed at each was mandated. Bronchiectasis was exacerbated by both conditions and the airway clearance therapy needed for bronchiectasis was precluded by the physiologic limitations imposed by coexistent ECAC and DP (Figure 3).

3.1. Diaphragm Dysfunction. Unilateral or bilateral dysfunction of the diaphragm can result from phrenic nerve dysfunction, neuromuscular junction disease, or myopathy. Paradoxical respiratory efforts and decline in FVC while supine suggest DP with confirmation achieved with fluoroscopy, ultrasound, or phrenic nerve EMG. Symptomatic unilateral disease that cannot be explained by another underlying disease process may be amenable to plication.

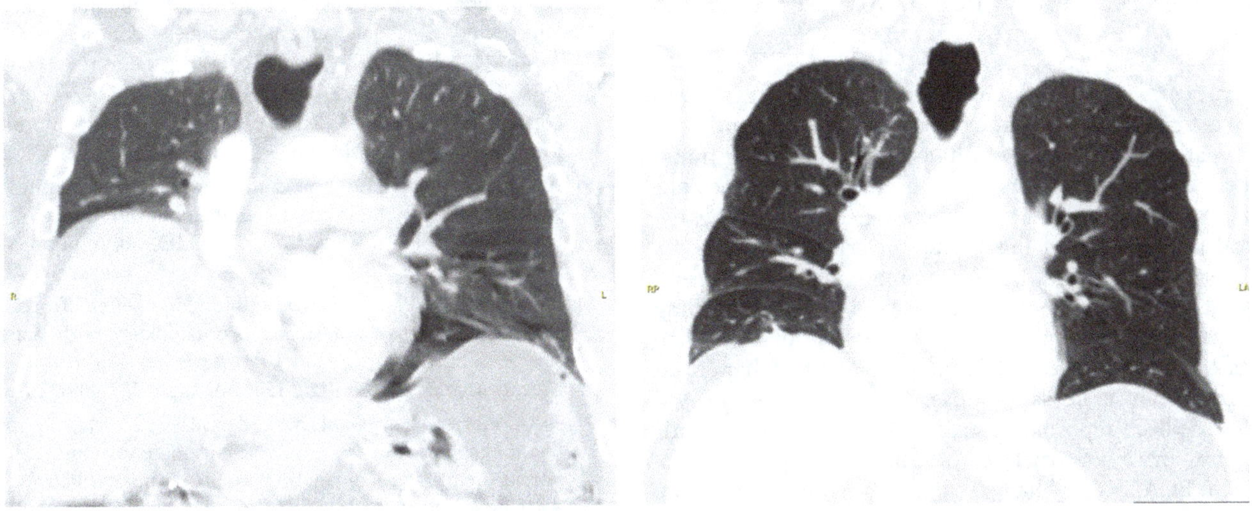

(a) (b)

FIGURE 2: Coronal reconstruction of chest computed tomography (a) pre- and (b) postdiaphragmatic plication with noted improved lung expansion.

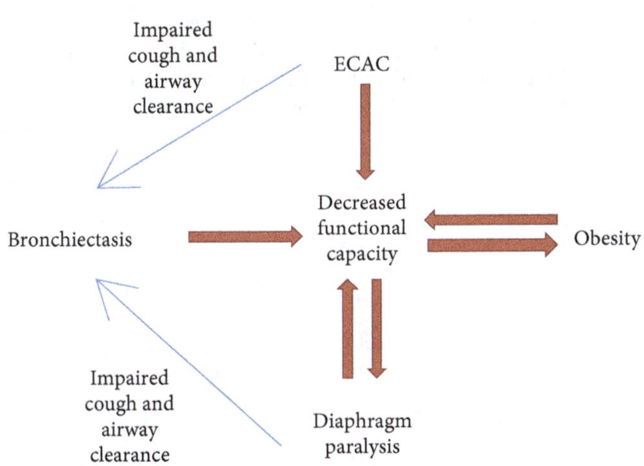

FIGURE 3: Interplay between conditions.

Bilateral DP can be managed by noninvasive positive-pressure ventilation and treatment, if available, of the underlying cause. Diaphragmatic pacing may be beneficial if phrenic nerve function is intact. The goal of plication is at eliminating the paradoxical upward motion of the paralyzed diaphragm and decreasing the basilar parenchymal compression. Although historically performed via a thoracotomy, plication can also be performed effectively with minimally invasive robotic, thoracoscopic, or laparoscopic techniques [2]. Surgical plication of the diaphragm has shown a sustained improvement in FVC of 20% at 48 months [2, 3].

3.2. Expiratory Central Airway Collapse (ECAC). Recognition of large airway dysfunction during expiration as a cause of chronic respiratory symptoms is gradually increasing. Two patterns have been described in ECAC: (1) tracheobronchomalacia (TBM) in which the cartilaginous component of the anterolateral tracheal wall collapses on forced expiration and (2) excessive dynamic airway collapse (EDAC) in which there is anterior displacement of the posterior (membranous) tracheal wall during expiration [4]. When clinically suspected, dynamic images of the chest obtained during forced expiration can suggest ECAC. Dynamic bronchoscopy during which the degree of expiratory compromise is estimated during spontaneous awake breathing remains the diagnostic gold standard. Nonsevere disease can be treated conservatively with measures to improve bronchial hygiene, weight loss, treatment of coexisting diseases, and intermittent use of positive airway pressure.

When the degree of airway collapse is severe, surgical repair should be considered. A preoperative stent trial with uncovered self-expandable metallic stents is strongly advised to estimate the potential surgical benefit prior to surgical intervention [4]. In our patient, we used three uncovered stents to preserve mucociliary function and prevent the mucus plugging seen with silicone stents. Also, self-expandable metallic stents adapt better than silicone stents to any airway irregularity. Since these uncovered stents are removed 7–10 days later, they are not embedded into the airway mucosa [5].

Our technique for tracheobronchoplasty involves plication of the redundant posterior membrane of the trachea and mainstem bronchi and fixation to a semirigid permanent (polypropylene) permeable mesh. The standard approach is through a right thoracotomy, although minimally invasive robotic and thoracoscopic approaches have also been reported to be feasible but with unknown long-term results [6].

3.3. Bronchiectasis. We hypothesize that basilar bronchiectasis in this patient was due to inadequate airway clearance from both ECAC and DP resulting in recurrent lower respiratory infections. Medical management of bronchiectasis to improve airway mucous clearance was limited due to compromised large airways from ECAC and weak cough from DP.

3.4. Extracorporeal Membrane Oxygenation. VV ECMO is used most commonly in acute respiratory distress syndrome and in patients with advanced lung disease requiring transplant either intraoperatively or as a bridge to lung transplantation. As the use of ECMO increases, understanding the surgical implications of this therapy is critical. In a review of 563 patients on ECMO, 269 required noncardiac surgery. There was no difference in outcomes between those needing or not needing surgery [7]. Anticipatory use of ECMO to facilitate intraoperative support for a patient with pulmonary compromise holds promise. Preemptive use of VV ECMO has been reported to support surgical repair of critical central airway obstruction and tumors [8, 9].

Both ECAC and bilateral diaphragmatic dysfunction, with associated bronchiectasis, synergistically lead to dyspnea, cough, respiratory infections, and severe functional impairment in this patient. Demonstration of the improvement in clinical outcomes with an airway stent trial before entertaining surgical correction of ECAC is critical to optimize patient selection. As demonstrated, surgical intervention for both ECAC and diaphragm paralysis can dramatically improve the quality of life and functional capability. Intraoperative ECMO may permit definitive surgical treatment of ECAC in patients with gas exchange abnormalities that would otherwise preclude surgery.

This case elucidates three critical concepts to comprehensive patient-centered care. The importance of thoroughly investigating all the relevant contributors to a patient's symptoms, with specific attention to those for which therapy can be offered, is illustrated. Additionally, the novel use of ECMO demonstrates the need to embrace unconventional surgical approaches as mandated by the patient's clinical scenario. Finally, it was only the multidisciplinary team-based approach to care, involving pulmonologists, interventionalists, thoracic surgeons, anesthesiologists, and intensivists that allowed successful management of this patient's complex presentation.

Disclosure

An abstract for this case report titled "Tracheobronchoplasty and Diaphragmatic Plication under VV ECMO for combined ECAC and Diaphragmatic Paralysis" was presented at American Association for Bronchology and Interventional Pulmonology 2020 conference.

References

[1] A. A. Hilliard, S. E. Weinberger, L. M. Tierney Jr., D. E. Midthun, and S. Saint, "Occam's razor versus Saint's triad," *The New England Journal of Medicine*, vol. 350, no. 6, pp. 599–603, 2004.

[2] E. Podgaetz, R. Garza-Castillon, and R. Andrade, "Best approach and benefit of plication for paralyzed diaphragm," *The Annals of Thoracic Surgery*, vol. 26, no. 3, pp. 333–346, 2016.

[3] B. P. Dube and M. Dres, "Diaphragm dysfunction: diagnostic approaches and management strategies," *Journal of Clinical Medicine*, vol. 5, no. 12, p. 113, 2016.

[4] D. Abia-Trujillo, A. Majid, M. Johnson et al., "Central airway collapse, an underappreciated cause of respiratory morbidity," *Mayo Clinic Proceedings*, vol. 95, no. 12, pp. 2747–2754, 2020.

[5] A. Majid, D. Alape, F. Kheir et al., "Short-term use of uncovered self-expanding metallic airway stents for severe expiratory central airway collapse," *Respiration*, vol. 92, no. 6, pp. 389–396, 2016.

[6] R. Lazzaro, B. Patton, P. Lee et al., "First series of minimally invasive, robot-assisted tracheobronchoplasty with mesh for severe tracheobronchomalacia," *The Journal of Thoracic and Cardiovascular Surgery*, vol. 157, no. 2, pp. 791–800, 2019.

[7] M. A. Fierro, M. A. Daneshmand, and R. R. Bartz, "Perioperative management of the adult patient on venovenous extracorporeal membrane oxygenation requiring noncardiac surgery," *Anesthesiology*, vol. 128, no. 1, pp. 181–201, 2018.

[8] W. J. Dunkman, A. Nicoara, J. Schroder et al., "Elective venovenous extracorporeal membrane oxygenation for resection of endotracheal tumor: a case report," *A&A Case Reports.*, vol. 9, no. 4, pp. 97–100, 2017.

[9] Y. Hong, K. Jo, J. Lyu et al., "Use of venovenous extracorporeal membrane oxygenation in central airway obstruction to facilitate interventions leading to definitive airway security," *Journal of Critical Care*, vol. 28, no. 5, pp. 669–674, 2013.

33

Impact of Moderate Sedation versus Monitored Anesthesia Care on Outcomes and Cost of Endobronchial Ultrasound Transbronchial Needle Aspiration

Ziad Boujaoude,[1] **Rohan Arya**,[2] **Aseem Shrivastava**,[3] **Melvin Pratter**,[1] **and Wissam Abouzgheib**[1]

[1]*Division of Pulmonary and Critical Care Medicine, Cooper Medical School of Rowan University, Camden, NJ 08103, USA*
[2]*Division of Pulmonary and Critical Care Medicine, University of South Carolina School of Medicine, Columbia, SC 29203, USA*
[3]*WellStar Pulmonary Medicine, Marietta, GA, USA*

Correspondence should be addressed to Ziad Boujaoude; boujaoude-ziad@cooperhealth.edu

Academic Editor: Kazuyoshi Kuwano

Background and Objectives. The ideal type of sedation for endobronchial ultrasound transbronchial needle aspiration (EBUS-TBNA) is not known. Two previous studies comparing the diagnostic yield between moderate sedation (MS) and deep sedation/general anesthesia (DS/GA) had provided conflicting results with one study clearly favoring the latter. No study had addressed cost. This is concerning for pulmonologists without routine access to anesthesia services. Our objective was to assess the impact of MS and Monitored Anesthesia Care (sedation administered and monitored by an anesthesiologist) on the outcomes and cost of EBUS-TBNA. *Materials and Methods.* We performed a retrospective review of prospectively collected data on consecutive EBUS-TBNA performed under two different types of sedation in a single academic center. A diagnostic TBNA was defined as an aspirate yielding any specific diagnosis or if subsequent surgery or follow-up of nondiagnostic/normal aspirates showed no pathology. Current Medicare time-based allowances were used for professional charges calculation. *Results.* There was no difference observed between MS and MAC in regards of the diagnostic yield (92.9% versus 91.9%), procedure duration, number, location, and size of lymph node (LN) sampled, but there were more passes per LN with MAC. The average charges were 74.30 USD for MS and 319.91 for MAC. There were more hypotensive and desaturations episodes with MAC but none required escalation of care. *Conclusions.* When performed under MS, EBUS-TBNA has similar diagnostic yield as under MAC but may be associated with less side effects. The difference in sedation cost is modest; however, an additional 245$ for each EBUS done under MAC would have significant cost implications on the health system. These findings are of critical importance for bronchoscopists without routine access to anesthesia services and for optimization of healthcare cost and resource utilization.

1. Introduction

Bronchoscopy is one of the most common procedures performed by chest physicians. It is generally an uncomfortable procedure and the use of analgesia and sedation is recommended to enhance patient satisfaction and achieve optimal procedural conditions for physicians. Sedation technique varies among practitioners, institutions, and locations with a continuum ranging from minimal sedation to general anesthesia (GA). The majority of bronchoscopies in the United States are performed under either moderate or deep sedation. Moderate sedation (MS) is defined as a drug-induced depression of consciousness during which patient maintains spontaneous ventilation, cardiovascular function, and responsiveness to verbal or light tactile stimulus and no interventions are required to maintain a patent airway. During MS, the responsible physician typically assumes the dual role of performing the procedure and supervising the sedation. In contrast to MS, higher level of depression of consciousness is achieved during deep sedation (DS) and the ability to independently maintain ventilatory function and patent airway may be impaired. DS should be always administered by an anesthesiologist (American Society of Anesthesiologists advisory regarding privilege to nonanesthesiologist to perform procedures under deep sedation published in October 2017) and it is referred to as Monitored Anesthesia Care or MAC. During MAC, an anesthesia clinician continuously monitors and supports the patient's vital functiolns, administers sedative drugs and analgesics as needed, diagnoses and treats clinical problems that occur, and converts to GA if required [1].

Since its introduction in 2004, endobronchial ultrasound-guided transbronchial needle aspiration (EBUS-TBNA) has become one of the most important diagnostic tools available to chest physicians for the diagnosis of mediastinal and hilar lymphadenopathy, parabronchial structures, and lung cancer staging [2, 3]. It is associated with an overall median sensitivity of 89% and it is recommended as a first step sampling technique by the American College of Chest Physicians 2013 evidence-based practice guidelines [4]. The EBUS bronchoscope has a larger diameter than the regular bronchoscope and the staging procedure typically requires more time for complete sampling of the mediastinum. The choice of sedation in EBUS procedures is an important question for bronchoscopists as they seek the best conditions to optimize their diagnostic yield, enhance patient's satisfaction, and minimize complications. Sedation also represents a significant element in the economics of EBUS-TBNA as it relates to cost of care, work flow, and healthcare resources utilization.

The ideal type of sedation for EBUS has not been determined yet. The data is limited to three studies that compared MS and GA during EBUS [5–7]. Two of the three studies reported on diagnostic yield but had conflicting results with one study clearly favoring GA over MS [5, 6]. None of the studies reported on cost. These findings had generated great concerns for bronchoscopists who do not have routine access to General Anesthesia and Operating Rooms. EBUS procedures are performed in our institution in the bronchoscopy suite under either MS or MAC, depending on the availability of the anesthesiologist. An artificial airway (AA) is not used with MAC. This study's purpose was to assess the effect of all these variables on the diagnostic yield and complications rate from the perspective of a single center. We also attempted to determine the differences in cost associated with the use of the different sedation techniques.

2. Methods

The study protocol was approved by the Institutional Review Board at Cooper University Hospital, Cooper Medical School of Rowan University, Camden, New Jersey.

We performed a retrospective chart review of inpatients and outpatients who underwent EBUS-TBNA for evaluation of mediastinal and hilar lymphadenopathy from January 2012 to December 2013. Chart review continued until 100 consecutive cases were identified and included in each group. Only Patients who had cytopathology data were included. We excluded patients if an additional procedure was performed (radial EBUS, electromagnetic navigation, transbronchial biopsies, or therapeutic intervention). At our institution, and during that period of time, anesthesia services were only available on specific days. Patients scheduled on days when anesthesia was available received MAC, while those who had their procedures done on other days received MS. MAC sedation was administered by a certified registered nurse anesthetist (CRNA) under the supervision of a board-certified anesthesiologist. A combination of propofol, ketamine, midazolam, and fentanyl was used with no AA. MS was induced by boluses of midazolam and fentanyl administered by a registered nurse and managed by the operating physician. During both types of sedation, continuous electrocardiographic, pulse oximetry, respiratory rate, and intermittent blood pressure monitoring was provided. All procedures were performed in the bronchoscopy suite by an interventional pulmonologist and assisted by an interventional pulmonary fellow. EBUS-TBNA was performed with a real-time ultrasound bronchoscope (BF-UC-180F; Olympus Ltd., Tokyo, Japan) using a dedicated 22-gauge needle (NA-201SX; Olympus Ltd. All cases had rapid on-site cytological evaluation (ROSE)). Data collected included demographics, procedure duration (measured from the initial bronchoscope introduction until last bronchoscope removal), number, location, and size of lymph nodes (LN) stations sampled, number of passes per LN, postprocedure cytopathologic diagnosis, and complications related to procedure. Complications noted were hypotension (decrease in systolic BP below 90 requiring intervention), desaturations below 90% requiring intervention beyond the increase of FIO2 and jaw thrust maneuver, and escalation of care. A diagnostic TBNA was defined as an aspirate showing any specific diagnosis or if subsequent surgery or at least six months' imaging follow-up of nondiagnostic/normal aspirates showed no pathology. The diagnostic yield was defined as the percentage of subjects in whom EBUS-TBNA provided any specific definitive diagnosis. The professional cost for the administration of the sedation was calculated based on the current time-based Medicare allowances. This is separate from the professional cost for bronchoscopy, which is similar regardless of the type of sedation [8]. For the initial 15 minutes of MS services, the allowances are 57.93$. Thereafter, the services are billed in 15 minutes' increment, and the allowances are 12.47$ for every 15 minutes. MAC charges have a base unit of 6 for the first 15 minutes and then time is charged in 15 minutes' increments. The Medicare allowances for 6 units are 225.14$ and 75.05$ for every 15 minutes' increment. If there is a CRNA, the service is charged twice, but Medicare splits the bills and pays half of each bill.

For statistical analysis, independent t-tests were used to compare between the study groups for normally distributed continuous variables and Mann-Whitney tests were used to compare rank data for variables that were not normally distributed. We used chi-square tests for analysis of categorical data.

3. Results

Ninety-Nine patients were included in the analysis in each group as the follow-up data were not complete for one patient in each group. Baseline age and gender were similar. In the

TABLE 1: Patients and procedure characteristics.

	MS	MAC	P Value
Number of patients	**99**	**99**	
Age (Mean/SD)	62.45 (14.43)	60.38 (18.81)	0.387
Sex - Male (n/%)	46 (46.5%)	44 (44.4%)	0.775
EBUS-TBNA diagnosis (n/%)			
Adenocarcinoma	29 (29.3%)	24 (24.2%)	
Squamous Cell Carcinoma	9 (9.1%)	15 (15.2%)	
Sarcoid	11(11.1%)	8 (8.1%)	0.536
Lymphoma	5 (5.1%)	8 (8.1%)	
Small Cell Carcinoma	10(10.1%)	5 (5.1%)	
*Other**	6 (6.1%)	6 (6.1%)	
Nondiagnostic/normal	29 (29.3%)	33 (33.3%)	
Procedure Time in minutes (Median/IQR)	30 (23 – 40)	30 (22 – 38)	0.630
Sedative dose			
Fentanyl (Median/IQR)	100 (100 – 125)	50 (8 - 60)	< 0.001
Midazolam (Mean/SD)	4.84 (1.97)	1.25 (0.92)	<0.001
Lymph node station sampled			
Total Lymph nodes (n/%)	**226**	**204**	
2R	2 (0.9%)	3 (1.5%)	
2L	0 (0%)	1 (0.5%)	
3P	0 (0%)	1 (0.5%)	
4R	57 (25.2%)	42 (20.6%)	
4L	16 (7.1%)	11 (5.4%)	
7	74 (32.7%)	66 (32.4%)	
8	0 (0%)	2 (1%)	
10R	10 (4.4%)	9 (4.4%)	
10L	1 (0.4%)	2 (1%)	
11R	41 (18.1%)	31 (15.2%)	
11L	20 (8.8%)	32 (15.7%)	
12R	5 (2.2%)	4 (2%)	
Number of LN sampled/patient (Mean/SD)	2.29 (0.87)	2.06 (0.77)	0.048
Size of LN (Mean/SD)	18.88 (7.41)	18.03 (7.82)	0.440
Number of passes per LN	1.6 (0.6)	2.24 (0.91)	<0.001

*The diagnoses that were included in "Other" were 6 breast cancers, 2 esophageal cancers, and one of each of the following: CLL, colon cancer, large cell carcinoma, or mesothelioma.
MS: moderate sedation; MAC: monitored anesthesia care; LN: lymph node.

univariate analysis, and as expected, the dose of fentanyl was significantly higher in MS (median 100 (IQR 100-125) than MAC (median 50, IQR 8-60) (p<0.001)). There was also a significant difference between the use of medazolam with MAC (mean 1.25 (SD 0.92)) versus MS (mean 4.84 (SD1.97)). These are consistent with prior reports of mean dose to achieve MS [9]. There was no difference in the number, location, the average size, and the distribution of the diagnostic categories of the LN sampled. However, there were a higher number of passes per LN in MAC group. The average procedure duration was 30 minutes in both groups. The procedure and LN characteristics are shown in Table 1.

There was no significant difference in the diagnostic yield between the two groups (92.9% MS versus 91.9% MAC, p = 0.788) (Figure 1). The diagnostic sensitivity and negative predictive values were comparable as well: sensitivity of 90% and 87.9% (p=0.693) and NPV of 80.6% and 80.5% (p=0.994) for MS and MAC, respectively (Figure 2).

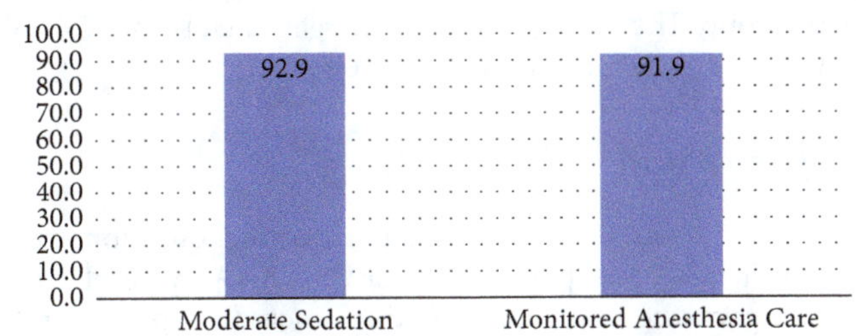

FIGURE 1: EBUS-TBNA diagnostic yield %.

There were 15 patients who had relative hypotension in MAC group and none reported in the MS group. These

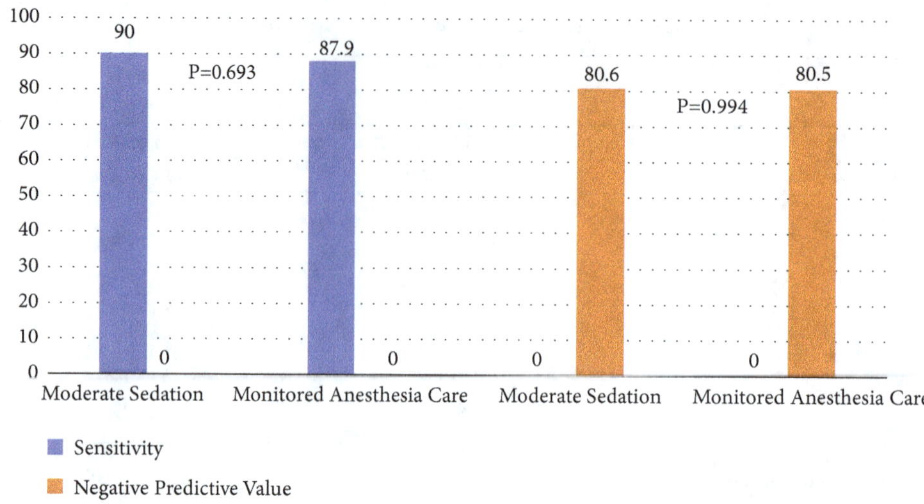

FIGURE 2: EBUS-TBNA sensitivity and negative predictive value.

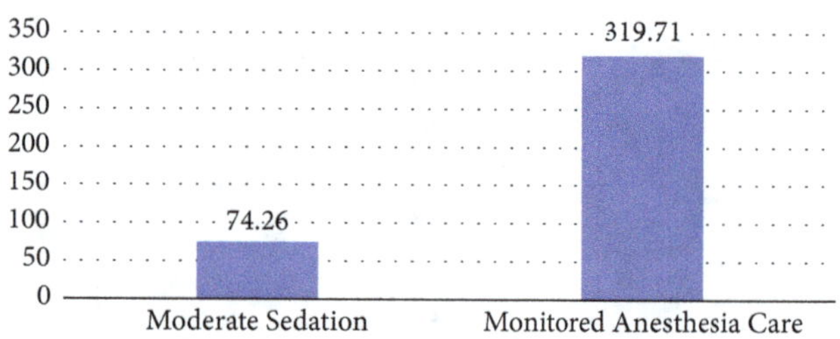

FIGURE 3: Average patient professional sedation charges in US dollars.

hypotensive episodes were treated with boluses of phenylephrine as per the judgement of the anesthesiologist/CRNA. Outside of expected procedural desaturation easily corrected by minor interventions (9 patients requiring increasing FIO2 in MS group and 17 patients requiring Increasing FIO2 with or without jaw thrust in MAC group), none of the patients from either group developed significant hypoxemia that required escalation of care. In addition to baseline sedation charges and the first 15 minutes' increment, 31 patients had a second 15 minutes' increment charge in MS group and 26 in MAC group. The average sedation charges in USD were 74.26 and 319.71 per patient, respectively (Figure 3).

4. Discussion

The type of sedation remains an important question facing bronchoscopist performing EBUS-TBNA. Several factors impact the choice of sedation, including procedural outcomes, patient satisfaction, and cost. Unfortunately, the available data that attempted to answer this question is very limited, has shown conflicting results, and does not address differences in cost. This has led to a grade 2C recommendation by the ACCP 2016 guidelines on sedation aspects of EBUS-TBNA. The recommendation suggests that either moderate or deep sedation is an acceptable approach [10]. Furthermore, DS is performed with an AA and this requires the use of operating room (OR) in most instances as the majority of the bronchoscopy suites are not equipped for GA. This by itself generates concern among many pulmonologists in nontertiary settings where access to GA is limited or not available, and this without mentioning the significant implications on cost, work flow, and healthcare utilization.

To our knowledge, this is the first study that provides a direct comparison between EBUS-TBNA performed under MS or MAC in the bronchoscopy suite, without AA. This is also the first study that attempts to report on cost. We found that EBUS-TBNA is equally effective and safe when performed under either MS or MAC, with MAC associated with higher sedation professional cost.

Methods of sedation for EBUS-TBNA have been studied since its introduction in 2004, but most studies focused on safety and sedation tolerance [11–13]. Steinfort et al. concluded that EBUS-TBNA may safely be performed under conscious sedation and is associated with very high patient satisfaction. Ando et al. reported that EBUS-TBNA under the intravenous sedation by meperidine was as feasible and safe as that under GA. Sarkiss and coworkers described the performance of EBUS-TBNA under the use of propofol. They had no major complications but there was no data regarding diagnostic yield.

Similarly, the impact of various factors on EBUS-TBNA success rate and diagnostic yield has been extensively studied; however, only three studies reported on the impact of type of sedation on the diagnostic yield [5, 6, 14]. In Kennedy's study, factors such as lymph node size and location influenced the result but the procedure was performed under one type of sedation and the effect on the yield was not reported [14]. The two studies that provided a direct comparison of the effect of sedation on the yield between two groups were a retrospective study by Yarmus et al. and a randomized trial by Casal et al. [5, 6]. Both studies compared the diagnostic yield under MS and GA. These two studies reported conflicting results. Yarmus et al. reported a greater diagnostic yield when EBUS was performed under GA. This study was performed in two different centers, one performing all cases under MS and the other performing all cases under GA. This was the main limitation that was acknowledged by the authors. Performing the procedure in two different institutions can potentially lead to multiple confounding factors (different population, operators, and pathologist) that can influence the results. They also speculate that GA allows sampling of more LN and more needle passes per site leading to higher yield. In contrast to these findings, Casal and coworkers found no significant differences in diagnostic yield between the two groups. Also they found no difference in the number, size, and number of passes per LN. Our findings were more aligned with the findings of Casal's study in regards of the diagnostic yield and the number of LN stations sampled; however, there were more passes per LN in our MAC group.

Interestingly, the number of LN stations involved per patient has recently gained more attention with the publication of the Eighth Edition of Lung Cancer Stage Classification [15]. Subgroup analyses revealed separation in survival based on the number of unique LN involved in N1 and N2 stations [16]. The eighth edition makes a recommendation to quantify nodal disease by the number of involved nodal stations. This potentially will lead some bronchoscopist to favor deep sedation if they believe it will allow for more lymph node station sampling; however, the recommendation was clear in regards of the purpose, which is not to determine treatment options but rather should be considered together with patient-specific factors in clinical decision-making.

Another interesting finding in our study that could have potential effect on bronchoscopist decision is the higher number of passes per LN with MAC, a similar finding reported in the Yarmus study with GA. The number of passes per sampling site has potential implications on procedural efficiency, diagnostic yield, and sample adequacy for molecular testing. The ACCP 2016 guidelines suggest that a minimum of 3 separate needle passes be performed per sampling site to maximize diagnostic yield; however, this weak recommendation was based on only one study by Lee et al. [4]. In his study sample, adequacy was 90.1% after the first pass and 98.1% after two passes and reached 100% after three passes [17].

EBUS has been shown to have a very high adequacy rate for obtaining enough tissue to test for mutational markers [18], but only one retrospective study addressed the number of passes required [19]. A median of four passes, in conjunction with ROSE, was needed to establish an adequacy rate of 93.5% in this study. This data, as stated by ACCP 2016 guidelines, is insufficient to identify the number of passes needed to obtain adequate tissue for molecular marker testing. The higher number of passes with MAC should not be considered an argument for the routine use of MAC for EBUS.

None of the two studies by Yarmus and Casal reported on cost. This is an important factor to take into consideration when making choices for sedation technique. Our analysis shows that professional sedation charges are approximately 4 times higher with MAC. While the cost of MAC compared to MS may not be much different for a given case, a 245$ additional cost for each EBUS done under MAC would have significant cost implications for the US health system. A major advantage for the cost of MAC in our study is the absence of use of an artificial airway (whether a laryngeal mask airway or endotracheal tube). The artificial airway requires the use of the OR in most instances as the majority of the bronchoscopy suites are not equipped for GA, and this might increase significantly the cost and affect the availability and the work flow. The cost of EBUS in OR is comparable to mediastinoscopy [20].

Finally, we found no significant difference in the major complications rate associated with the two types of sedation; however, MS may potentially have less side effects (hypotension and desaturations).

This is in agreement with the majority of the published studies but is not aligned with the Quality Improvement Registry, Evaluation, and Education (AQuIRE) Data Registry finding of an association between GA and greater need for postprocedure escalation of care [21].

There are limitations to this study mainly related to the retrospective design; however, the study compared two similar groups during the same time period and was performed with same operators. Some bias concerning patient allocation is inevitable, although the decision to choose MAC versus MS was most often made by chance, mainly depending on whether the patient was scheduled on a day when anesthesia is available or not. This fact may have led to a pseudorandomization to this study.

Patient satisfaction was not addressed in the study; however, equal satsisfaction with both types of sedation has been repetitively shown in multiple studies as discussed earlier. Last, we could not report the rate of patients that could not tolerate or complete the procedure due to exclusion criteria.

In summary, EBUS-TBNA may be performed under moderate sedation without compromising the diagnostic yield and may potentially have less side effects. It is associated with less impact on the cost for the health system. This is of critical importance in this era where reducing expenses and optimizing resource utilization are becoming more and more essential.

MAC may have a potential to be superior in lung cancer staging and when more tissues are needed for molecular testing (sampling more LN stations and more passes per LN); however, the data is not sufficient to clearly favor this approach for these purposes and future research examining this effect will be valuable.

Acknowledgments

The authors gratefully thank Krystal Hunter, Department of Biostatistics, for her contribution to the statistical analysis.

References

[1] "Practice guidelines for moderate procedural sedation and analgesia 2018: a report by the american society of anesthesiologists task force on moderate procedural sedation and analgesia, the american association of oral and maxillofacial surgeons, american college of radiology, american dental association, american society of dentist anesthesiologists, and society of interventional radiology," *Anesthesiology*, vol. 128, no. 3, pp. 437–479, 2018.

[2] I. S. Sehgal, S. Dhooria, A. N. Aggarwal, D. Behera, and R. Agarwal, "Endosonography versus mediastinoscopy in mediastinal staging of lung cancer: systematic review and meta-analysis," *Annals of Thoracic Surgery*, vol. 102, no. 5, pp. 1747–1755, 2016.

[3] P. Gu, Y.-Z. Zhao, L.-Y. Jiang, W. Zhang, Y. Xin, and B.-H. Han, "Endobronchial ultrasound-guided transbronchial needle aspiration for staging of lung cancer: a systematic review and meta-analysis," *European Journal of Cancer*, vol. 45, no. 8, pp. 1389–1396, 2009.

[4] G. A. Silvestri, A. V. Gonzalez, M. A. Jantz et al., "Methods for staging non-small cell lung cancer: diagnosis and management of lung cancer, 3rd ed: american college of chest physicians evidence based clinical practice guidelines," *Chest*, vol. 143, supplement 5, pp. e211S–e250S, 2013.

[5] R. F. Casal, D. R. Lazarus, K. Kuhl et al., "Randomized trial of endobronchial ultrasound-guided transbronchial needle aspiration under general anesthesia versus moderate sedation," *American Journal of Respiratory and Critical Care Medicine*, vol. 191, no. 7, pp. 796–803, 2015.

[6] L. B. Yarmus, J. A. Akulian, C. Gilbert et al., "Comparison of moderate versus deep sedation for endobronchial ultrasound transbronchial needle aspiration," *Annals of the American Thoracic Society*, vol. 10, no. 2, pp. 121–126, 2013.

[7] T. Dal, H. Sazak, M. Tunç, Ş. Şahin, and A. Yilmaz, "A comparison of ketamine-midazolam and ketamine-propofol combinations used for sedation in the endobronchial ultrasoundguided transbronchial needle aspiration: a prospective, singleblind, randomized study," *Journal of Thoracic Disease*, vol. 6, no. 6, pp. 742–751, 2014.

[8] T. R. Gildea and K. Nicolacakis, "Endobronchial ultrasound: clinical uses and professional reimbursements," *Chest*, vol. 150, no. 6, pp. 1387–1393, 2016.

[9] G. Clark, M. Licker, A. B. Younossian et al., "Titrated sedation with propofol or midazolam for flexible bronchoscopy: a randomised trial," *European Respiratory Journal*, vol. 34, no. 6, pp. 1277–1283, 2009.

[10] M. M. Wahidi, F. Herth, K. Yasufuku et al., "Technical aspects of endobronchial ultrasound-guided transbronchial needle aspiration: chest guideline and expert panel report," *Chest*, vol. 149, no. 3, pp. 816–835, 2016 (Arabic).

[11] D. P. Steinfort and L. B. Irving, "Patient satisfaction during endobronchial ultrasound-guided transbronchial needle aspiration performed under conscious sedation," *Respiratory Care*, vol. 55, no. 6, pp. 702–706, 2010.

[12] K. Ando, Y. Ohkuni, M. Fukazawa, M. Abe, A. Takeshi, and N. Kaneko, "Sedation with meperidine for endobronchial ultrasound-guided transbronchial needle aspiration," *Journal of Bronchology & Interventional Pulmonology*, vol. 17, no. 4, pp. 329–333, 2010.

[13] M. Sarkiss, M. Kennedy, B. Riedel et al., "Anesthesia technique for endobronchial ultrasound-guided fine needle aspiration of mediastinal lymph node," *Journal of Cardiothoracic and Vascular Anesthesia*, vol. 21, no. 6, pp. 892–896, 2007.

[14] M. P. Kennedy, C. A. Jimenez, R. C. Morice et al., "Factors influencing the diagnostic yield of endobronchial ultrasound-guided transbronchial needle aspiration," *Journal of Bronchology & Interventional Pulmonology*, vol. 17, no. 3, pp. 202–208, 2010.

[15] F. C. Detterbeck, D. J. Boffa, A. W. Kim, and L. T. Tanoue, "The eighth edition lung cancer stage classification," *Chest*, vol. 151, no. 1, pp. 193–203, 2017.

[16] H. Asamura, K. Chansky, J. Crowley et al., "International association for the study of lung cancer lung cancer staging project: proposals for the revision of the N descriptors in the forthcoming 8th edition of the TNM classification for lung cancer," *Journal of Thoracic Oncology*, vol. 10, no. 12, pp. 1675–1684, 2015.

[17] H. S. Lee, G. K. Lee, H.-S. Lee et al., "Real-time endobronchial ultrasound-guided transbronchial needle aspiration in mediastinal staging of non-small cell lung cancer: how many aspirations per target lymph node station?" *Chest*, vol. 134, no. 2, pp. 368–374, 2008.

[18] R. Lee, D. J. Cousins, E. Ortiz-Zapater, R. Breen, E. Mclean, and G. Santis, "Gene expression profiling of endobronchial ultrasound (EBUS)-derived cytological fine needle aspirates from hilar and mediastinal lymph nodes in non-small cell lung cancer," *Cytopathology*, vol. 24, no. 6, pp. 351–355, 2013.

[19] L. Yarmus, J. Akulian, C. Gilbert et al., "Optimizing endobronchial ultrasound for molecular analysis how many passes are needed?" *Annals of the American Thoracic Society*, vol. 10, no. 6, pp. 636–643, 2013.

[20] R. S. Andrade, E. Podgaetz, N. M. Rueth et al., "Endobronchial ultrasonography versus mediastinoscopy: a single-institution cost analysis and waste comparison," *The Annals of Thoracic Surgery*, vol. 98, no. 3, pp. 1003–1007, 2014.

[21] G. A. Eapen, A. M. Shah, X. Lei et al., "American college of chest physicians quality improvement registry, education, and evaluation (AQuIRE) participants. complications, consequences, and practice patterns of endobronchial ultrasound-guided transbronchial needle aspiration: results of the AQuIRE registry," *Chest*, vol. 143, no. 4, pp. 1044–1053, 2013.

34

Uniportal Subcostal Video-Assisted Thoracoscopic Surgery: A Feasible Approach for a Challenging Middle Lobectomy in an Obese Patient

Samer Al Sawalhi, Deping Zhao, Haomin Cai, and Yuxing Jin

Department of Thoracic Surgery, Shanghai Pulmonary Hospital, Tongji University, Shanghai, China

Correspondence should be addressed to Deping Zhao; zdp1992@163.com

Academic Editor: Akif Turna

Subcostal access is a novel approach for anatomical lung resection. To perform surgery via this access, specially designed long instruments are required. Subcostal access provides excellent visualization of the mediastinum and anterior lung hilum. We exhibit here a subcostal middle lobectomy with systematic en-block mediastinal lymphadenectomy in an obese 52-year-old male patient with body mass index (BMI=37.7) performed via this single incision. The operation was completed efficiently within 30 minutes with negligible postoperative pain.

1. Introduction

Thoracic surgical access has moved towards minimally invasive methods. The presumed advantages of this are lesser tissue trauma, swift recovery, minor wound infection, lower pain scores, and reduced hospital stay. However, there are also reports of prolonged port-site pain with single or multiple video-assisted thoracoscopic surgery (VATS) [1]. Moreover, single-port thoracoscopic surgery could also cause a similar problem. Liu et al. [2] reported first subxiphoid uniportal VATS left upper lobectomy on 2014 and hence subcostal is proposed as an alternative access to dwindling intercostal pain and neuralgia by avoidance damage of the intercostal nerve. This technique is more challenging due to the instruments-fighting problem. That is why it required long, curved, and articulated instruments to deal with upper, lower lung hilum and mediastinum. The mean BMI reported in the literature for the subxiphoid technique is around (22.0±0.83) [3]. This case is unique due to the high BMI and we propose that it is a safe technique in expert hands. We discuss the pros and cons of this approach for the first time in an obese patient.

2. Case Report

We report a 52-year-old gentleman, asymptomatic, and nonsmoker, without comorbidities but with class II obesity BMI of 37.7. He was referred from the lung cancer screening program as the high-resolution chest computed tomography (CT) scan delineated a 1.5 cm mixed ground glass opacity (GGO) with a larger solid component in the right middle lobe (RML) (Figure 1(a)). This nodule increased in size at the follow-up CT scan; therefore we decided to resect the middle lobe anatomically using subcostal access.

2.1. Procedure. The patient was given general anesthesia with double lumen endotracheal intubation and placed in a lateral decubitus position (dorsal decubitus 40 degrees) (Figure 1(b)). A 5 cm oblique incision parallel to the costal arch was made. Then the subcutaneous tissue and rectus abdominis were dissected along the subcostal margin; xiphoid process and pericardiophrenic fatty tissue were detached. A subcostal tunnel was bluntly dissected using finger until the mediastinal pleura was opened at the cardiophrenic angle. Lastly, covidien wound protector (WPLGR914) was placed (Figure 1(c)). A thoracoscopic lens with a 30° angle (Olympus,

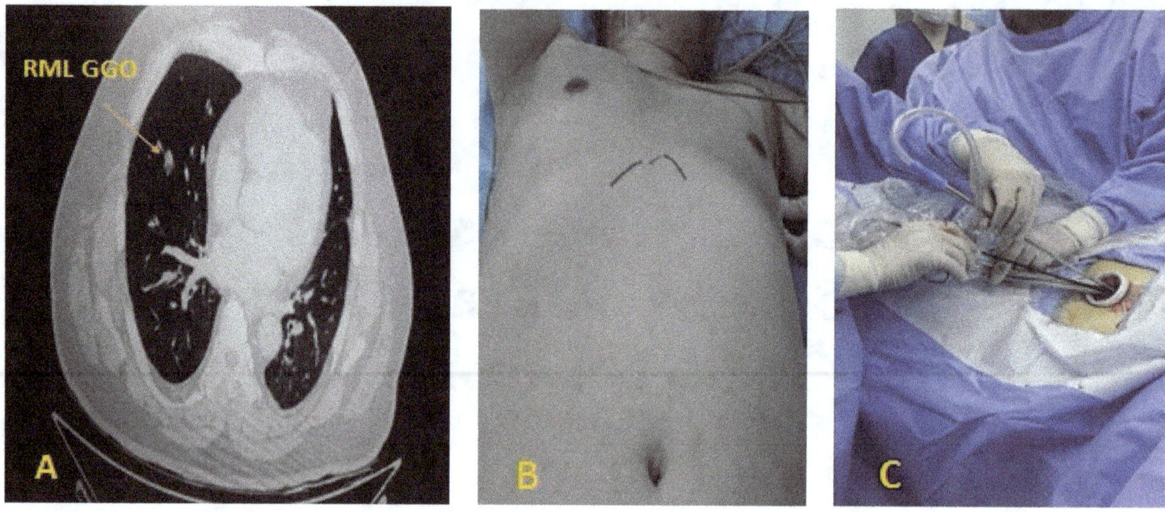

(a) (b) (c)

FIGURE 1: (a) Chest C-T scan delineates the right lung middle lobe with a solid GGO measuring 1.5 cm in size. (b) Dorsal decubitus patient position with 40° angle during subcostal approach for right middle lobe lung lobectomy. (c) Subcostal oblique incision (5 cm) parallel to right costal arc and covidien wound protector with arrangement of instruments through the port.

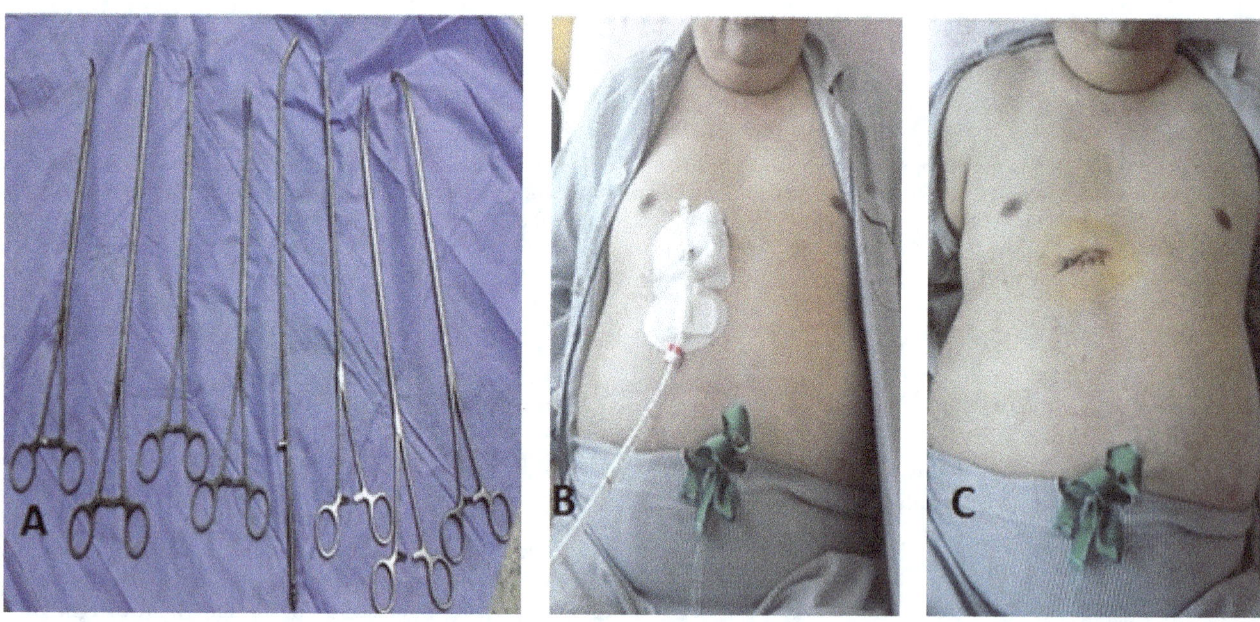

(a) (b) (c)

FIGURE 2: (a) Long curved instruments were recommended to use in subcostal approach. (b) First postoperative day in an obese class II patient with chest tube inserting through subcostal wound. (c) 5 cm subcostal incision after removing chest tube.

Melville, NY) was used and interlobar fissure was examined. Lobectomy was performed as in the video [subcostal right middle lobe lobectomy video] (available here). Systematic mediastinal lymph nodes dissection includes stations 2,4 right paratracheal, 9,10,11,12 and subcarinal lymph nodes. Long and sturdier VATS instruments were used. Also, curved tip stapler technology aids to allow passage around the vascular structures (Figure 2(a)). We did not put any extra ports and the operative time was 30 minutes.

After completing the procedure, a 28 F chest tube (Figure 2(b)) was inserted through the same subcostal wound. The patient was given routine venous thromboembolism prophylaxis (6000 i.u UFH) 12 hours after operation. No postoperative arrhythmia or air leak was detected. The patient was discharged on the third postoperative day with an uneventful recovery (Figure 2(c)). Postoperative pain score (Wong-Baker FACES) on 1, 2, 3,7,15 days was evaluated. It was (4-2-0-0-0) consecutively. During the follow-up, no incisional hernia was detected. The pathology results delineated a (1x 0.8) cm invasive infiltrating adenocarcinoma [80% ductal/20% papillary] without lymphovascular, neural, or pleural invasion (T1aN0M0), stage I A1 according to the non-small-cell lung carcinoma (NCCN) guidelines version 4.2018-8th edition]. Five lymph nodes were harvested, and all were negative for metastasis (0/5).

3. Discussion

Nowadays, we noticed that surgery has moved towards gentleness for more than a century, with minimally invasive surgery instructing us to treat tissue gently. The subcostal uniportal VATS lobectomy is an innovative modification of VATS. Several studies and meta-analyses have suggested a long-term oncological benefit of VATS lobectomy in the radical treatment of patients with NSCLC in the early stages of the disease [4]. The indications for using the uniportal subcostal approach included the presence of early stage T1 or T2 tumor (<5 cm), N0 status, and thymectomy. Furthermore, it is a good option to deal with bilateral metastasectomies, bilateral lung lesions, and bilateral lung bulla resection in bilateral pneumothorax.

Those patients who are vulnerable for subcostal approach should be selected carefully, especially those having a tumor, or GGO (solid, pure, or mixed) less than 2 cm in maximum diameter and they do not have suspicious of mediastinal lymph nodes metastasis. Moon Y et al. [5] delineated in his study that mediastinal lymph nodes evaluation is not mandatory for clinical N0 NSCLC presenting as a 3 cm or smaller GGO-predominant.

Exclusion criteria for using the uniportal subcostal approach were chest wall tumor involvement, central masses, previous thoracic surgery, adhesion, body mass index BMI>30 kg/m^2 [3, 6, 7], cardiomegaly, cardiac comorbidities due to compression on the heart specially on the left side, and enlarged lymph nodes with confirmed N1 or N2 disease [7].

We concluded from our previous research which included 77 patients with lung cancer who underwent mediastinal lymph nodes sampling or dissection that there were no significant differences in lymph node dissection between subxiphoid and intercostal groups [8]. We chose subcostal access in this patient due to the following reasons:

(1) In obese patients uniportal VATS lung resection may be arduous, as the thickness of the subcutaneous fat in the chest wall makes the manipulation of instruments through the port much more difficult.

(2) Narrow intercostal spaces in obese people will exacerbate more entrapment of intercostal neurovascular bundle which leads more postoperative neuropathic pain.

(3) Subcostal incision is a "true" thoracic wound; i.e., the surgical wound is below the sternocostal triangle and above the diaphragm; therefore, herniation of viscera through the incision is rare.

The advantages of this approach for anatomical lobectomies or segmentectomies are shortening the operation time and blood loss especially in patients who got bilateral lung lesions at the same time. Moreover, no need to change the patient position during the surgical operation.

As the subcostal incision is away from the breast, it is cosmetically more acceptable for women. The presence of excessive fatty tissue, like in our patient, may pose a burden to this procedure (Figure 2(b)). Furthermore, chronic postoperative intercostal pain and neuralgia were significantly lower in the subcostal approach [2]. Upon our experience and our previous research [8] within this approach, we found that oblique incision is much better regarding field exposure and instruments manipulation. Therefore, we suggest an oblique incision for unilateral operations and transverse incisions for bilateral operations in the subxiphoid uniportal VATS.

It was reported that patients with obesity are not good candidate for subcostal approach [7]; therefore the challenging point also in obese patients is high location of the diagram, because of the abdominal pressure effect; therefore we compromise that, by resection both xiphoid process, mediastinal and pericardial fatty tissue, these steps allow enlarging the space for instruments manipulation.

For a routine lung cancer resection, a minimum of three N2 mediastinal lymph node stations should be sampled or complete dissection, based on the NCCN Guidelines version 4.2018 non-small-cell lung cancer 8th edition. Liu et al. [2] reported that systemic lymph nodes dissection through the xiphoid incision was difficult. Systematic lymph nodes dissection including the lymph nodes of the left group 4L,5,6,7,8,9,10,11 and the right group 2,3a,4R,7,8,9,10,11 should be carried on by an expert surgeon with a subcostal approach to avoid complications through traction of the lung and the coordinated reversal of the operation table [8].

Tips, tricks, and recommendations for mediastinal lymph nodes dissection are as follows:

(1) Using subcostal oblique incision facilitates access to subcarinal lymph nodes [8].

(2) Using thoracoscopic lens with a 30° angle or articulated lens gives good visualization for subcarinal space.

(3) Releasing inferior pulmonary ligament enables easy access to subcarinal space.

(4) Energy devices like Harmonic Scalpel (Ethicon, Inc.) can be used for dissection and maintaining hemostasis at the same time [7].

(5) Proper traction of the lung anteriorly and medially facilitates exposure subcarinal space.

(6) Superior vena cava was retracted and the azygos vein was pulled up using a suction device to harvest paratracheal lymph nodes.

The instrument-fighting problem during the subcostal single-port surgery would be even more challenging than the transthoracic approach since the mediastinum occupies the lower part of the working tunnel, which reduces the working space. We used a small tidal volume to let the mediastinum drop into the dependent nonoperative side. The surgeon practicing subcostal uniportal VATS needs previous experience in uniportal VATS lobectomy and skilled assistant [6].

The drawback of subcostal approach is difficult to control bleeding, once it happens because you are working from a small window; therefore our advice in such situation is to compress the bleeding site by pillar gauze and convert to thoracotomy immediately. Furthermore, this approach required specific designed long instruments like curved ring forceps, Harmonic Scalpel, curved long suction, long DeBakey forceps, and long electrocautery hook, in addition to long, curved articulated stapler technology to enable passage around the vessels and bronchus smoothly.

Subcostal approach is easier on the right side than on the left side, because of the presence of beating heart and incidence of arrhythmia while compressing the heart by instruments manipulation. Expert thoracic surgeons with a skilled assistant allow performing more sophisticated kinds of challenging operations using a subcostal approach like [9]; lobectomy in an obese patient, calcified lymph nodes, and fissure less lobe.

The cornerstone of choosing the surgical approach is the achievement of complete radical resection (R0) and efficient mediastinal lymph nodes dissection.

It is worth considering the subcostal approach in patients who are a candidate for it, taking into consideration the safety and the oncological principles.

Finally, in an era of robotic surgery, using uniportal subcostal access is promising in such cases, once articulated instruments will add more help in the procedure and lymph node dissection.

Supplementary Materials

Uniportal subcostal video-assisted thoracoscopic surgery, a feasible approach for a challenging middle lobectomy in an obese patient. Subcostal approach is proposed as an alternative access due to avoidance of damage intercostal nerves. The cornerstone of choosing the surgical approach is the achievement of complete radical resection (R0). The patient was given general anesthesia with double lumen endotracheal intubation and placed in a lateral decubitus position (dorsal decubitus 40°). A 4 cm oblique incision parallel to the costal arch was made; then the subcutaneous tissue and rectus abdominis were dissected along the subcostal margin. A subcostal tunnel was bluntly dissected using finger until the mediastinal pleura was opened at the cardiophrenic angle. We used electrocautery to dissect the mediastinal pleura to get access to the chest cavity; covidien wound protector (WPLGR914) was placed. A thoracoscopic lens with a 30° angle was used and interlobar fissure was examined. Interlobar vein was cut after applying hemlock clip using (Harmonic Scalpel (Ethicon, Inc.)) knife. Long and sturdier VATS instruments were used. Also curved tip stapler technology aids to allow passage around the vascular structures. We started dissection of middle lobe vein and stapling using endovascular vascular cartridge [Medtronic, Minneapolis, MN, USA]. Middle lobe bronchus was dissected with endoscopic green stapler. Peribronchial lymph nodes were harvested. Two middle lobe arteries were stapled by endovascular vascular cartridge. Finally, the fissure was stapled and the lobe was harvested by endobag TKBAG HSD-130 (Guangzhou T.K Medical Instrument Co., Ltd.). Systematic mediastinal lymph nodes dissection including stations 2,4 right paratracheal and subcarinal lymph nodes after releasing the inferior pulmonary ligament and traction of the lung anteriorly and medially facilitates exposure subcarinal space. *(Supplementary Materials)*

References

[1] M. Rogers and J. P. Duffy, "Surgical aspects of chronic post-thoracotomy pain," *European Journal of Cardio-Thoracic Surgery*, vol. 18, no. 6, pp. 711–716, 2000.

[2] C. Liu, B. Wang, C. Shih, Y. Liu et al., "Subxiphoid single-incision thoracoscopic left upper lobectomy," *The Journal of Thoracic and Cardiovascular Surgery*, vol. 148, no. 6, pp. 3250-3251, 2014.

[3] L. A. Hernandez-Arenas, L. Lin, Y. Yang et al., "Initial experience in uniportal subxiphoid video-assisted thoracoscopic surgery for major lung resections," *European Journal of Cardio-Thoracic Surgery*, vol. 50, no. 6, pp. 1060–1066, 2016.

[4] W. C. Hanna, M. de Valence, E. G. Atenafu et al., "Is video-assisted lobectomy for non-small-cell lung cancer oncologically equivalent to open lobectomy?" *European Journal of Cardio-Thoracic Surgery*, vol. 43, no. 6, pp. 1121–1125, 2013.

[5] Y. Moon, S. W. Sung, M. Namkoong, and J. K. Park, "The effectiveness of mediastinal lymph node evaluation in a patient with ground glass opacity tumor," *Journal of Thoracic Disease*, vol. 8, no. 9, pp. 2617–2625, 2016.

[6] L. A. Hernandez-Arenas, W. Guido, and L. Jiang, "Learning curve and subxiphoid lung resections most common technical issues," *Journal of Visualized Surgery*, vol. 2, p. 117, 2016.

[7] W. Guido Guerrero, L. A. Arenas, G. Jiang, Y. Yang, D. Gonzalez-Rivas, and L. Jiang, "Subxiphoid mediastinal lymphadenectomy," *Journal of Visualized Surgery*, vol. 7, no. 2, p. 105, 2016.

[8] N. Song, D.-P. Zhao, L. Jiang et al., "Subxiphoid uniportal video-assisted thoracoscopic surgery (VATS) for lobectomy: A report of 105 cases," *Journal of Thoracic Disease*, vol. 8, Supplement 3, pp. S251–S257, 2016.

[9] D. Gonzalez-Rivas, F. Lirio, J. Sesma, and F. Abu Akar, "Subxiphoid complex uniportal video-assisted major pulmonary resections," *Journal of Visualized Surgery*, vol. 3, p. 93, 2017.

35

Nasal Provocation Test with Cat and Dog Extracts: Results according to Molecular Components

Andres Sánchez,[1,2,3] Ricardo Cardona,[1] Marlon Munera,[2] Victor Calvo,[1] Manuela Tejada-Giraldo,[1] and Jorge Sánchez[1,3]

[1]*Group of Clinical and Experimental Allergy, Clinic "IPS Universitaria", University of Antioquia, Medellín, Colombia*
[2]*Medicine Department, University Corporation, Rafael Nuñez, Cartagena, Colombia*
[3]*Foundation for the Development of Medical and Biological Sciences, Cartagena, Colombia*

Correspondence should be addressed to Jorge Sánchez; jotamsc@yahoo.com

Academic Editor: Kazuyoshi Kuwano

Background. IgE sensitization (atopy) to pets is commonly evaluated using pet dander extracts. However, the diagnosis by components seems to be more adequate to evaluate the clinical relevance (allergy) of sIgE sensitization. *Objective.* To study the association between IgE sensitization to pet allergen components and clinical symptoms. *Methodology.* Dander extracts and sIgE levels to pet components (Can f 1, Can f 2, Can f 3, Can f 5, Fel d 1, Fel 2, and Fel 4) were measured in a rhinitis group ($n = 101$) and a control group ($n = 68$). Nasal provocation tests with pet extract were done in patients with atopy to pets. *Results.* Dog (34.6% vs. 23.5%) and cat dander (26.7% vs. 8.8%, $p = 0.05$) IgE sensitization was frequent among rhinitis and no-rhinitis subjects, and it was similar to dog (29.7% vs. 20.5%) and cat (18.8% vs. 8.8%) components. Polysensitization for dog (3.1, 95% CI: 1.5 to 6.1, $p < 0.001$) or cat (2.5, 95% CI: 0.8 to 8.0, $p = 0.01$) components was the principal risk factor for a positive nasal provocation test. Additionally, positive nasal provocation test with one animal increased the risk of atopy and positive nasal provocation test to others animals. Pet ownership or asthma was not associated with increased risk of atopy or positive nasal provocation test. *Conclusions.* Sensitization to pet dander extract identifies atopic patients, but its utility to predict clinical relevance is poor. Allergenic components could help to define the clinical relevance of sensitization to furry animals and could reduce the need for provocation test.

1. Introduction

Atopy to pets is considered an important risk factor for respiratory allergic diseases [1, 2]. According to GA^{2}LEN [3], sIgE sensitization to pets, especially cats (24.8% to 27.9%) and dogs (25.6% to 28.8%), is very common among rhinitis patients in Europe, North America, and South America [4, 5]. The high sIgE sensitization to pets could be explained by the increasing exposure to cats and dogs in homes especially in urban cities [6, 7], but other investigations suggest that close contact with some pets prevents the development of allergy diseases [8].

Although there is extensive information about the prevalence of atopy to pet dander, there are still questions that merits particular analysis. Similar to what happens with allergy to food or pollen grains [9, 10], several studies based in patient's self-report suggest a relationship between furry animal allergen components and the risk of asthma, rhinitis, and the severity of these allergic diseases [11–13], but few studies verify this association with objective measures. The aim of this study was to evaluate pet dander extract and molecular components from cats and dogs, as specific markers of clinical response according to the results of nasal provocation test (NPT). Additionally, we evaluated if other factors like being in contact with pets could be associated with pet sensitization and respiratory symptoms.

2. Methodology

2.1. Study Design. This is a cross-sectional study of cases and controls, with two principal aims. The first one is to compare the frequency of sIgE sensitization to different dander extracts and pet's allergens between a group of patients with rhinitis and a control group; the second one is to evaluate the clinical relevance of pet sensitization according to NPT.

2.2. Study Population. Informed consent for children and adults were approved by the institutional and ethics committees of the University of Antioquia and "IPS Universitaria" Clinic (Medellín, Colombia). Patients over six years old were selected from a population of individuals who were diagnosed with rhinitis and attended to the allergy service for skin prick test (SPT). Disease diagnosis for rhinitis and asthma was established according to ARIA guidelines [14, 15] and GINA recommendations (https://www.ginasthma.org). Control subjects were recruited from the University of Antioquia staff and from patient companions that attended the university clinic. The control group consisted of healthy subjects without rhinitis or any other allergy diseases.

2.3. IgE Sensitization to Pet Dander and to Other Allergenic Sources. Pet dander sensitization was evaluated according to SPT and serum levels for cat and dog dander extracts. The extracts for SPT were provided by Inmunotek Laboratory (Madrid, Spain). We followed the international recommendations for the SPT [3, 16] and a wheal ≥ 3 mm was considered as positive compared to the negative control.

Serum levels of sIgE for the different molecular components from *Canis familiaris* (Can f 1, Can f 2, Can f 3, and Can f 5) and *Felis domesticus* (Fel d 1, Fel d 2, and Fel d 4) were measured using fluorescence-enzyme immunoassay (Phadia ImmunoCap System, Uppsala, Sweden). The results of serum sIgE were analyzed as a continuum variable (quantitative analysis) and as a categorical variable (qualitative analysis); values equal or above 0.35 KUA/L were considered positive (+) and the ones below that (<0.35 KUA/L) were considered negative (−) as recommended by the manufacturer.

To evaluate atopy with other allergenic sources, according to the prevalence of them in the region, SPT to mites, fungus, insects, and grass was done [1, 17].

2.4. Nasal Provocation Test (NPT). All subjects in both groups with a positive atopy test SPT/sIgE (either to pet dander or molecular components) were called to perform a NPT with pet extract, to confirm the clinical relevance of sIgE sensitization. Patients with sIgE sensitization to more than one animal have two or more provocation tests. NPT was done according to international recommendations [18, 19]. We used subjective (symptoms scale) and objective (acoustic rhinometry) parameters to evaluated nasal provocations tests before and after allergen exposition. Baseline conditions of the nose before performing nasal provocation test was recorded to evaluate if the patients were in optimal conditions to the test and the changes that occurred after the exposure. Standardized extracts were used for nasal provocation (Inmunotek Laboratory), and any medication that could alter the provocation was suspended before the test for at least one week. Fifty microliters of saline solution was applied in each of the patient's nostril using a spray, and the evaluation of nonspecific reactions was done after 30 minutes. Afterwards, the same procedure was done using the extract to be tested, following the manufacturer recommendations, and the patient was kept in observation for one hour. Finally, if the patient did not present any reaction, a tenfold higher concentration was applied and the patient was left under observation for another hour. A positive result was considered according rhinoscopy and clinical evaluation [18].

Prior to use, the presence in the extracts of each of the allergens studied in the serum was evaluated and its concentration measured. Although the concentration of some allergens was variable among the extracts, the concentration was always higher than 2.2 μg/ml and remained in a range between 2.4 and 3.2 μg/ml, which ensures a good representativeness and potency of these allergens for the nasal challenge.

2.5. Statistical Analyses. Analyses were performed with IBM SPSS®, version 21, for Windows. For the descriptive analysis of the sociodemographic and clinical aspects of the patients, absolute, relative distributions, and summary indicators were used, such as median, quartiles, interquartile range (IQR), maximum values, and minimum values. The criterion of normality of some clinical variables was established by means of the Shapiro-Wilk test. We used the interquartile range because the variables did not show normal behavior. To establish the relationship between the study groups (rhinitis vs. control) with the characteristics of sensitization to pets, nonparametric tests were applied such as Pearson's chi-squared test of independence, exact Fisher's, or Mann–Whitney U test; similarly, the strength of association was evaluated by means of the proportion ratio (PR) with their respective 95% confidence intervals. A p value of <0.05 was considered statistically significant.

The same protocol used for dogs and cats was applied in both groups with horse dander, horse serum, and horse allergen molecular components (Equ c 1); however, horse IgE sensitization was low (5 patients, 4.9%) and we were unable to perform additional analyses.

3. Results

3.1. Population Characteristics. A total of 101 patients with rhinitis and 68 control subjects were included in the study (Table 1). Thirty-five patients with rhinitis also had asthma. Atopy to cat dander but not dog dander was higher in the rhinitis group according to serum sIgE ($p = 0.05$) and SPT ($p = 0.002$).

Dog and cat ownerships were similar between rhinitis and control group (Table 1). In the rhinitis group, 41 (40.5%) patients had a self-report of respiratory exacerbation with dog contact and 20 (29.4%) with cats; when focusing on pet ownership patients, 32% (8 of 25 patients) had a self-report of symptoms with dog ($p = 0.2$) and 40% (6 of 15 patients) with cat ($p = 0.2$), without significant differences with control group. IgE sensitization to other allergenic sources especially mites was common among the rhinitis group (84%) and lower in the control group (18%); 64% of patients with pet sensitization had also mite sensitization.

Table 1: Population characteristics.

Characteristics	Rhinitis group ($n = 101$)	Control group ($n = 68$)	p
Mean age in years	20 (median: 17, IQR: 5 to 60)	18 (median: 12, IQR: 6 to 54)	>0.05
Sex: female, n (%)	46 (45%)	34 (50%)	>0.05
Asthma, n (%)	35 (34%)	0	<0.001
Dog ownership	25 (24.8%)	24 (35.3%)	>0.05
Cat ownership	15 (14.9%)	12 (17.6%)	>0.05
Positive SPT to any animal	33 (32.7%)	14 (20.6%)	>0.05
Positive SPT dog dander (%)	32 (31%)	14 (20%)	>0.05
Positive SPT cat dander (%)	17 (16.8%)	1 (1.5%)	0.002
(+) IgE dog dander, n (%)	$n = 30$ (29.7%)	$n = 16$ (23.5%)	>0.05
(+) IgE cat dander, n (%)	$n = 19$ (18.8%)	$n = 6$ (8.8%)	0.05
(+) IgE levels to dog dander, median	5.5 (IQR: 11.7)	1.1 (IQR: 1)	0.02
(+) IgE levels to cat dander, median	4 (IQR: 10)	0.8 (IQR: 0.6)	0.001

Population characteristics and sensitization to pet dander according skin prick test (SPT) and serum IgE. IQR: interquartile range.

3.2. Sensitization to Dog Dander and Molecular Components. Between patients and healthy subjects, there was not a significant difference in the frequency of atopy to dog dander according to SPT, sIgE to dog dander (Table 1), or dog components (Figure 1(a)). Patients with sIgE to dog components were all of them positive to sIgE to dog dander, and most of them had a positive SPT with dog dander extract (Figure 1(a)). Sensitization to at least one molecular component of dog was present in 30 (29.7%) patients and 14 (20.5%) healthy subjects ($p = 0.12$) (Figure 1(a)). Sensitization to Can f 1 and Can f 2 was higher in the rhinitis group, but without statistically significant difference when compared with the control group (Figure 1(a)). Only the rhinitis group had sIgE sensitization to Can f 3 and Can f 5.

The concentration of sIgE to Can f 1 among the (+) sIgE subjects was higher in the rhinitis group ($p = 0.05$) (Figure 2). Polysensitization to two or more dog components was more frequent in the rhinitis group than in the control group (15 of 30 patients (50%) vs. 3 of 14 healthy subjects (21.4%), $p = 0.05$) (Figure 3(a)).

Dog ownership was similar in the rhinitis and control groups (Table 1), but rhinitis subjects with dog ownership had a higher concentration levels of sIgE to Can f 1 ($p = 0.03$) and Can f 2 ($p = 0.04$) (data not shown). The frequency of dog ownership among patients with (+) sIgE to Can f 3 was 66%, the same as that for patients with (+) sIgE to Can f 5.

In the rhinitis group, patients with asthma had a higher sensitization to Can f 1 (54.2% vs. 15.1%, $p < 0.001$), Can f 2 (22.8% vs. 7.5%, $p = 0.05$), Can f 3 (11.4% vs. 3%, $p = 0.01$), and Can f 5 (11.4% vs. 3%, $p = 0.01$) than patients without asthma. There was a strong relationship among SPT and sIgE results.

3.3. Sensitization to Cat Dander and Molecular Components. The number of patients with cat dander atopy was higher in the rhinitis group than in the control group according to SPT or sIgE (Table 1). Sensitization to at least one cat component was present in 19 (18.8%) patients from the rhinitis group and 6 (8.8%) in the control group ($p = 0.05$). Positive sIgE to Fel d 1 but not to Fel d 2 and Fel d 4 was significantly higher in the rhinitis group (Figure 1(b)). From both groups, rhinitis patients with (+) sIgE to Fel d 1 had higher concentration levels than control subjects (Figure 2). Polysensitization to cat components was higher in the rhinitis group (Figure 3(b)).

Cat ownership was similar in rhinitis and control groups ($n = 15$, 14.9% vs. $n = 12$, 17.6%, respectively). Among ownership subjects, levels of Fel d 1 were higher in patients with cat ownership than that in the control group (data not shown). In the rhinitis group, patients with asthma had a higher sensitization to cat components than in patients without asthma; Fel d 1 (31.4% vs. 10.6%, $p = 0.009$), Fel d 2 (11.4% vs. 1.5%, $p = 0.04$), and Fel d 4 (25.7% vs. 6%, $p = 0.01$).

Fourteen of the nineteen (73.6%) patients with sensitization to at least one cat allergen had cosensitization with dog allergens (Figure 3(c)). From the lipocalin components, thirteen of the fourteen (92.8%) patients with cosensitization were sensitize to Fel d 4; all of them had (+) sIgE to Can f 2 and 12 (85.7%) to Can f 1. From the albumin components, four of the fourteen (28.5%) patients with cosensitization had (+) sIgE to Fel d 2 and three of them (75%) to Can f 3.

3.4. Evaluation of the Clinical Relevance of IgE Sensitization to Dog. Subjects with atopy to dog dander or any dog component underwent NPT with dog extract (thirty-five patients and sixteen control subjects; two control subjects did not accept NPT). Positive NPT was higher in the rhinitis group than in the control group ($p = 0.01$). In the control group, two subjects had a (+) NPT with dog extract (Figure 4(a)); both subjects were sensitized to Can f 1 and one of them also to Can f 2.

Sensitization to pet dander ($p = 0.12$), or with Can f 1 ($p = 0.06$), had no significant association with (+) NPT but there was a higher concentration of sIgE to Can f 1 among patients with (+) NPT (median: 4.9, IQR: 7 vs. 0.39, IQR: 0.05, $p < 0.001$). Among the rhinitis group, polysensitization with Can f 1 and any additional dog components had a

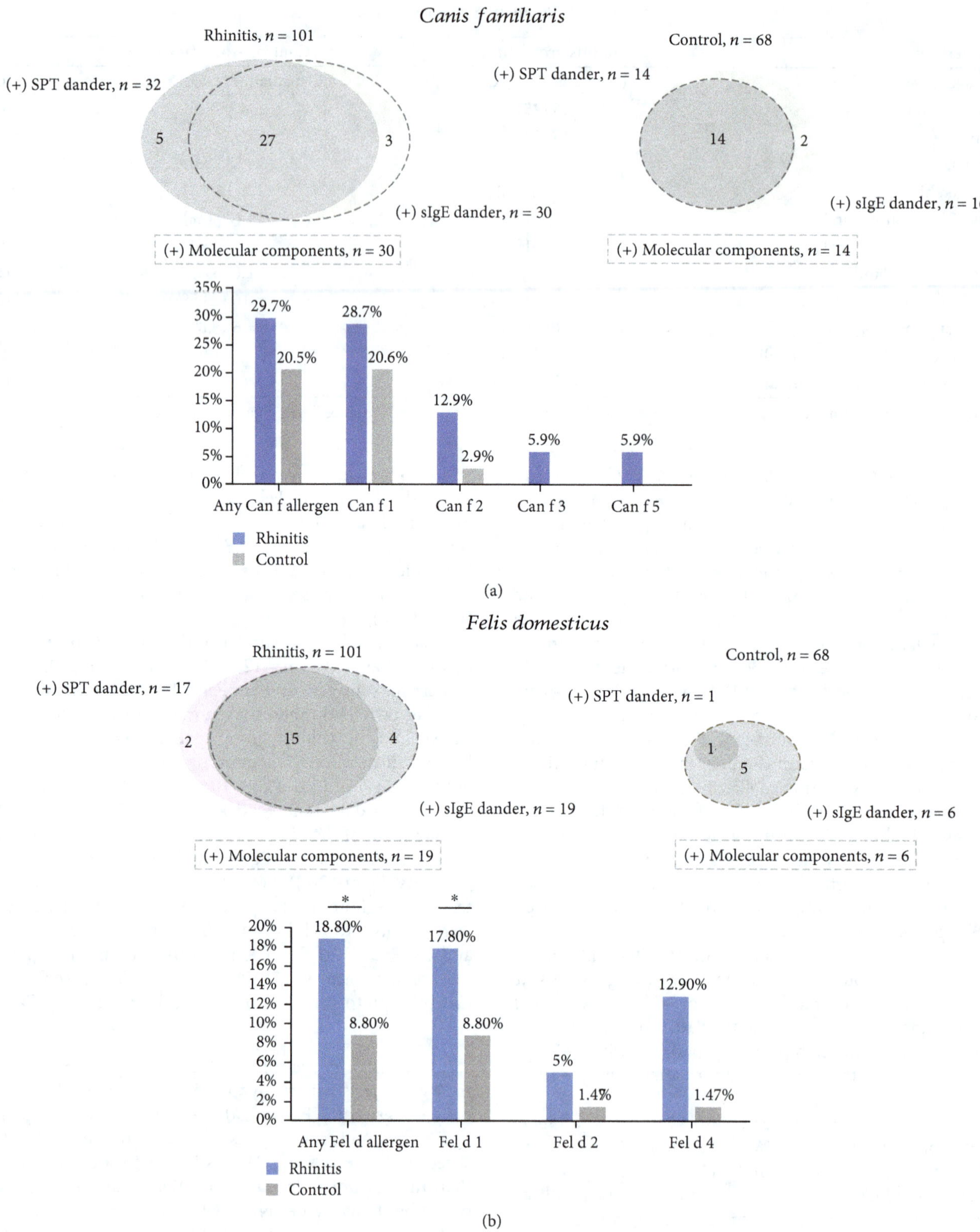

Figure 1: Prevalence of IgE sensitization to cat and dog dander. Concordance of IgE sensitization with dander extract and molecular components are represent in circles. Prevalence of patients with sIgE over 0.35 kUA/L to allergenic components for dog (a) and cat (b) is represented in columns. $^*p \leq 0.05$.

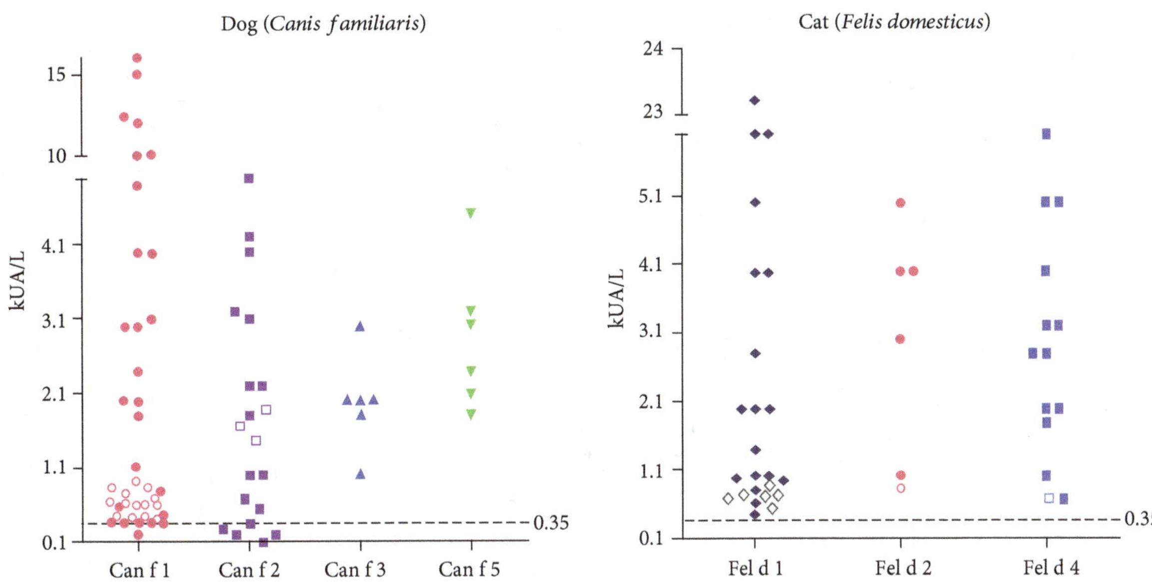

Characteristics	Rhinitis group ($n = 101$)	Control group ($n = 68$)	p
Can f 1	3 kUA/L (IR 6.1), $n = 29$	0.8 kUA/L (IR 0.46), $n = 14$	0.05
Can f 2	3.1 kUA/L (IR 3.29), $n = 13$	1.6 kUA/L (IR n.a), $n = 3$	0.09
Can f 3	2 kUA/L (IR 0.7), $n = 6$	0	n.a
Can f 5	2.7 kUA/L (IR 1.5), $n = 6$	0	n.a
Fel d 1	2.9 kUA/L (IR 4.7), $n = 18$	0.57 kUA/L (IR 0.51), $n = 6$	>0.001
Fel d 2	4 kUA/L (IR 2.5), $n = 5$	0.68 kUA/L, $n = 1$	n.a
Fel d 4	3.2 kUA/L (IR 3) $n = 13$	0.58 kUA/L, $n = 1$	n.a

FIGURE 2: Concentration of dog and cat allergenic components. Patients from the rhinitis group (stuffed) and control group (empty) with sIgE to molecular components. The median and interquartile range (IQR) for each allergenic component among subjects with (+) sIgE over 0.35 kUA/L. n.a: not applicable.

significant association with (+) NPT (Figures 4(b) and 4(c)). The ration of proportion for polysensitization as a risk factor to (+) NPT was 3.1 (95% CI: 1.5 to 6.1, $p < 0.001$).

Dog ownership (Figure 4(d)) or asthma was not associated with (+) NPT in the rhinitis or control group.

3.5. Evaluation of the Clinical Relevance of IgE Sensitization to Cat. Patients ($n = 21$) or control subjects ($n = 6$) with a positive test to cat dander (SPT or serum test) or any cat component underwent NPT with cat extract. Positive NPT was higher in the rhinitis group than in the control group ($p = 0.01$) (Figure 5(a)).

Sensitization to pet dander ($p = 0.07$) had no significant association with (+) NPT. Patients with sIgE to Fel d 1, especially those with high concentrations (three quartile), had a higher probability to have a (+) NPT (Figure 5(b)) (median: 4.0, IQR: 5 vs. 1.4, IQR: 1.8, $p = 0.026$). This probability was higher when the patient had sIgE sensitization to Fel d 1 and any other additional cat components (Fel d 1 and others) (Figures 5(b) and 5(c)). The ration of proportion for polysensitization as a risk factor to (+) NPT was 2.5 (95% CI: 0.8 to 8.0, $p = 0.01$).

Cat ownership was not associated with NPT results in any group (Figure 5(d)). Eight of thirteen patients with (+) NPT had asthma, but it was not a statistically significant factor for a (+) NPT ($p = 0.3$).

4. Discussion

Allergies to furry animals affect the population worldwide and is a growing public health concern [20]. The highest densities of pets are found in metropolitan areas [21], and allergens from furry animals are encountered widely in public places [22]. Indeed, the presence of pet allergens has been demonstrated in schools, in day-care centers, on public transport, and in households of non-pet owners [23, 24]. Prevalence of sIgE sensitization to dogs and cats changes according to the evaluated population [20] but also according to the diagnostic technique used to evaluate atopy [25]. We observed that evaluation of cat and dog atopy, using pet dander extracts in SPT and serum test, was similar than molecular components in the rhinitis and control groups, but dander extracts were not specific enough to predict positive NPT to dog or cat adequately. Therefore, additional

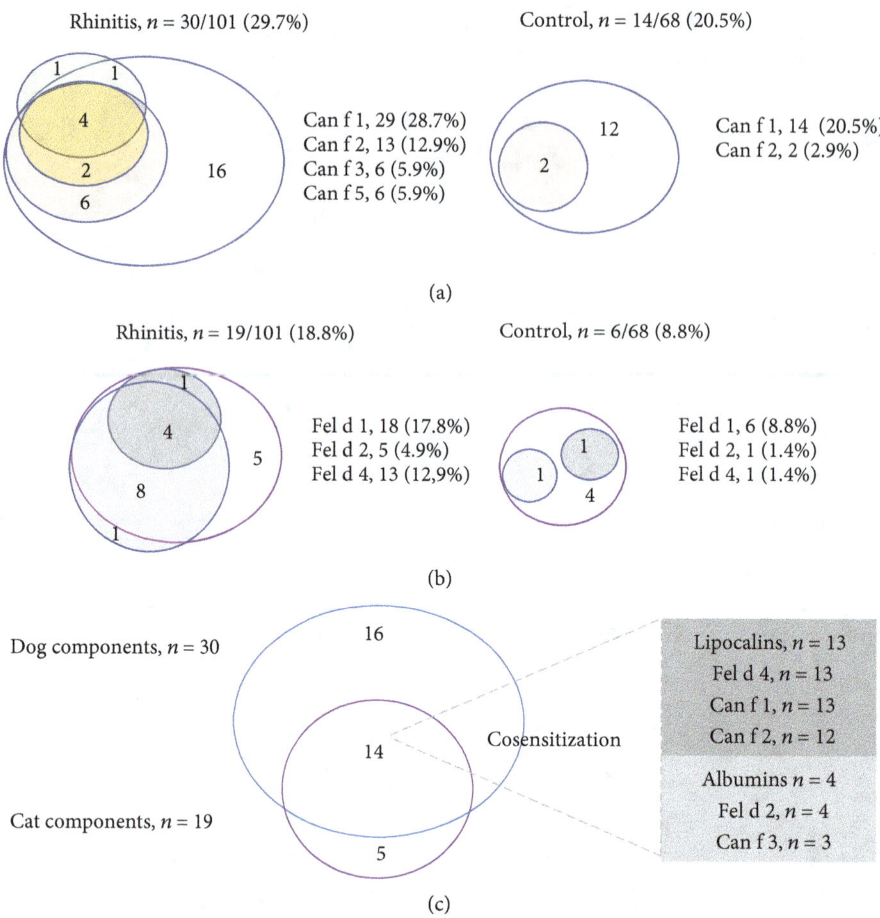

FIGURE 3: Interaction of cat and dog components. The number of patients or control subjects with (+) IgE (≥0.35 kUA/L) to each component from dogs (a) and cats (b) is represented in circles with different sizes. Cosensitization of cat and dog components is presented in (c).

tools are required to identify patients with clinically relevant atopy to furry animals.

Stokholm et al. [8] noted that extreme exposure to cats (but not dogs) could protect against the development of respiratory symptoms. However, Collin et al. [26] found that pets including cats and dogs could be a risk factor for a non-atopic asthma. According to our results, having a cat or dog was not a significant risk factor of atopy or positive NPT; perhaps because even in subjects without pets in homes, indirect contact with pet allergens is high. These apparently contradictory results indicate that each population have specific factors [22], which may influence the onset of atopy, and if it is clinically relevant. Horseback riding in some populations is a common leisure activity [27], but contact with horse in our population was low, which could explain the low frequency of sensitization (data not shown).

Similar to previous studies, we observed that Can f 1 and Fel d 1 are the most prevalent allergens from dogs and cats in the rhinitis group and in healthy population. The high sensitization to Can f 1 and Fel d 1 can be explained by the fact that these are proteins abundantly produced by pets and their contact with humans is facilitated by their ability to move in the air [6, 28].

We observed a high cosensitization between Can f 1 and Can f 2 in the rhinitis group. Likewise, the cross-reactivity with lipocalins and albumins from different species could explain the high frequency of atopy to dogs among patients with cat sensitization, but cross-reactivity does not explain the high cosensitization among Can f 1 (lipocalin) and other dog allergens like Can f 3 (albumin protein) and Can f 5 (prostatic kallikrein). Also, most patients sensitized to Fel d 2 (albumin) and Fel d 4 (lipocalin) were sensitized to Fel d 1 (uteroglobin), being the three components from different protein families. We believe that in allergic patients, due to their proinflammatory state and/or the lack of counter-regulatory mechanisms, the initial sIgE sensitization to Can f 1 and Fel d 1 (the most frequently found and in higher concentration levels) favors IgE sensitization to other molecular components; this hypothesis is supported by the observation that sensitization to Can f 3 and Can f 5 was exclusive in the rhinitis group, and they had a higher frequency of sensitization to Fel d 2 and Fel d 4. In addition, mechanisms not associated with cross-reactivity, like tissue damage and enzymatic activity, may contribute with increasing inflammation [29–34].

The association of a particular molecular component from furry animals with specific clinical conditions seems to change between populations [35, 36]. In a Spain population, Can f 3 and Can f 5 had a low prevalence of 9.3% and 33%, respectively, but it was associated with self-report of

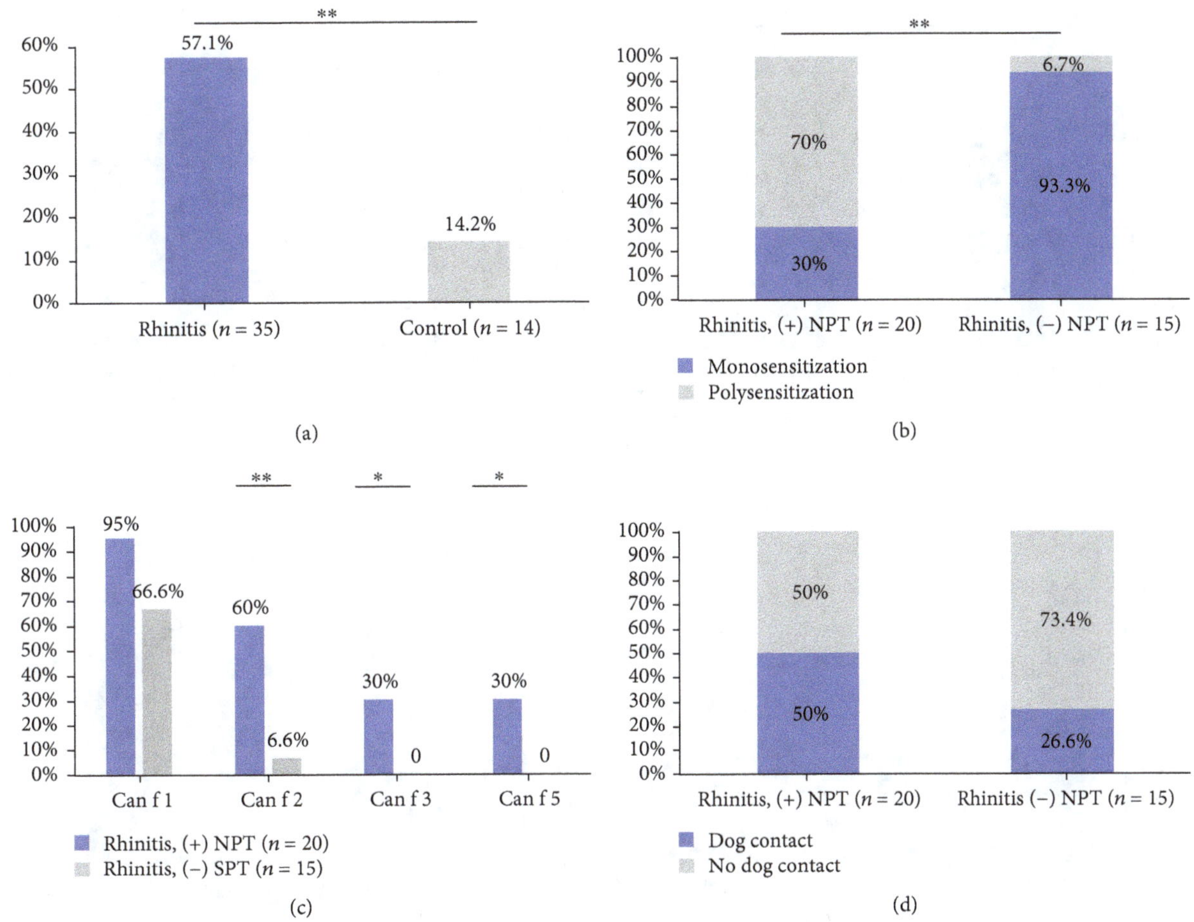

FIGURE 4: Nasal provocation test with dog components. Positive nasal provocation test (NPT) results were higher in the rhinitis group (a). Patients sensitized with Can f 2, Can f 3, or Can f 5 and (+) NPT had cosensitization with Can f 1 (b). Poly and monosensitization according NPT results are represented in (c). Panel (d) represents the NPT results according dog contact. $^{*}p \leq 0.05$, $^{**}p \leq 0.01$.

moderate/severe rhinitis [11]; in a Sweden population, sensitization to Can f 5 was high (61%), but it was not associated with nasal symptoms [37]. The divergent results about the clinical relevance of sensitization to dog or cat components might be explained, in part, by the lack of objective evaluations like provocation test in most of the studies. Käck et al. [37] observed that Can f 5 could be regarded differently in the contexts of monosensitization (low risk for (+) NPT) and polysensitization (high risk for (+) NPT) and other studies perceived a relationship among Can f 5 and Can f 3's monosensitization and respiratory symptoms [11, 12, 38].

We could not explore the clinical relevance of monosensitization to Can f 2, Can f 3, Can f 5, Fel d 2, and Fel d 4 because in our population, almost all patients sensitized to these molecular components were also sensitized to Can f 1 and Fel d 1, respectively. Nevertheless, we found a significant association between (+) NPT and polysensitization. Polysensitization to Can f 1 and any other dog component (Can f 2, Can f 3, or Can f 5) increases the probability for a (+) NPT. In a similar way, polysensitization of Fel d 1 with Fel d 2 or Fel d 4 have a better prognostic index than Fel d 1 alone. Additionally, polysensitization to several components from different animals was a risk factor to have multiple positive nasal provocations; patients with (+) NPT to cat had sensitization to dogs and most of them also have a (+) NPT with dogs. In this scenario, the cross-reactivity to lipocalins and albumins seems to be important, and the fact that the dog was the animal with the highest prevalence of sensitization suggests that it is the primary sensitizer in most of the cases, maybe due to its greater distribution. In the five patients with horse sensitization, the two patients with positive NPT had a positive provocation test with dog and one with cat, but we do not present these results due to the small number of sensitized subjects.

Our study has some limitations. The sample size was calculated according to the frequency of occurrence of the event (people with specific IgE to an allergen) reported in other studies. Interestingly, our population had a much lower sensitization for some allergens, which limited the extent of our analyses. However, the calculated power for the available sample was greater than 80% despite the lower incidence of the study event. Only 35 patients with varying sensitization patterns to both cats and dogs are the main drawback and limit the possibility to subgroup analysis. Nevertheless, the source population was large ($n = 101$), so the low number of patients sensitized to several sources adequately reflects

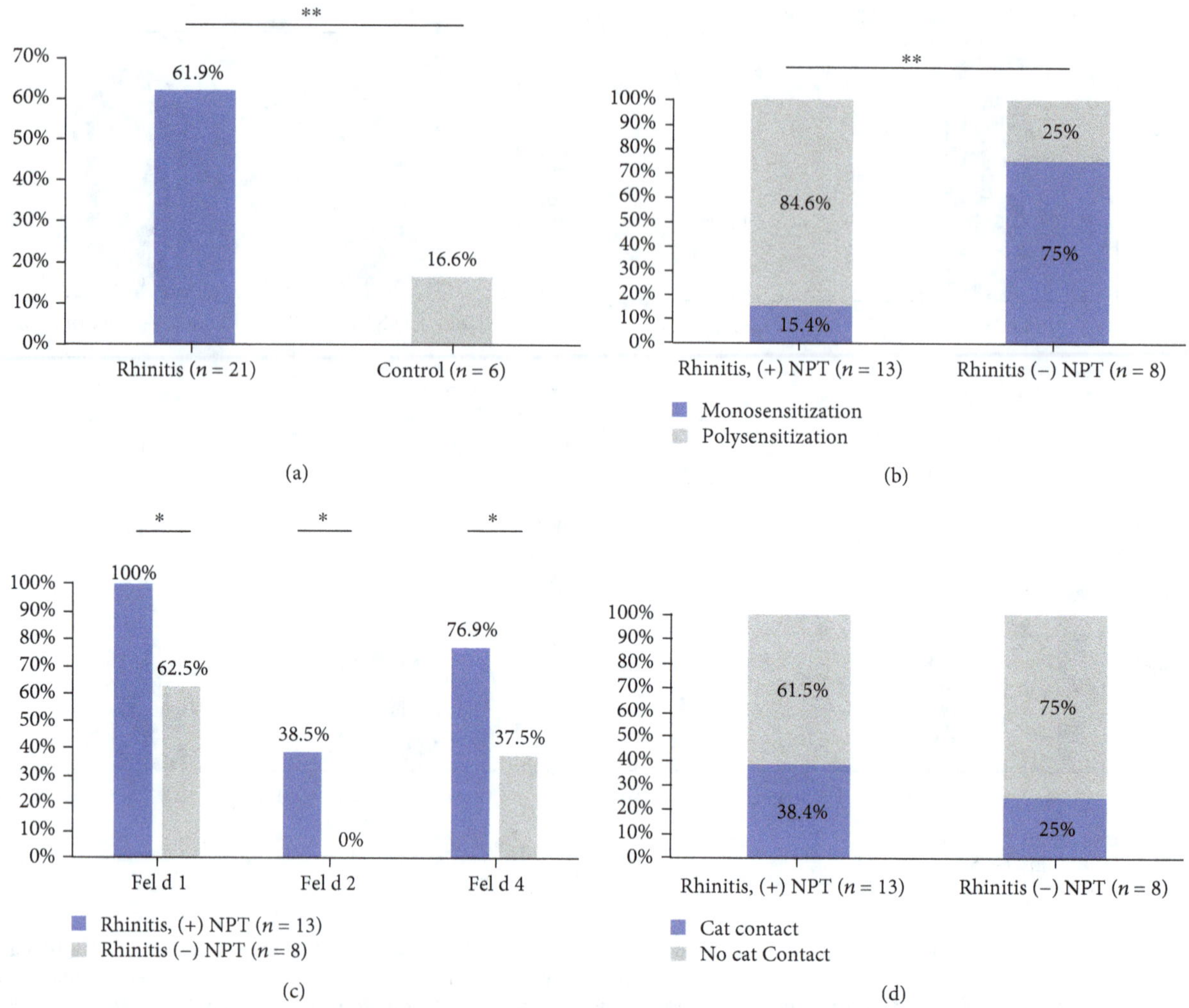

FIGURE 5: Nasal provocation test with cat components. Positive nasal provocation test (NPT) results were higher in the rhinitis group (a). Patients sensitized with Fel d 2 and Fel d 4 and (+) NPT (b) had cosensitization with Fel d 1. Poly and monosensitization according NPT results are represented in (c). Panel (d) represents the NPT results according cat contact. $^{*}p \leq 0.05$, $^{**}p \leq 0.01$.

the sensitization pattern of this population. Extracts for nasal provocation tests and SPT could differ significantly in the content of allergenic proteins, and such a difference for instance could induce information bias. To ensure the relevance of each component, it would be necessary to perform an individual nasal test with each one, which was not possible for us and is usually not practical in the clinic. However, in the extracts used in the provocation test, the minimum concentration of each component studied was 2.2 μg/ml, and it remained in a range between 2.4 and 3.2 μg/ml, which ensures a good representativeness and potency of these allergens for nasal challenge. Additionally, all tested molecular components of both cats and dogs have expression in the epithelium of pets which decreases the probability that it is not found in the extract used.

We observed differences in the pattern of sensitization between patients with rhinitis only and rhinitis with asthma, but the presence or absence of asthma does not seem to be an additional risk factor for a (+) NPT to cats or dogs. Additional studies comparing the pattern of patients with only asthma could clarify if these differences in allergen sensitization have a clinical relevance or not.

In conclusion, we observed that sIgE sensitization to pet dander identifies most atopic patients, but its utility to predict clinical relevance is unclear. Diagnosis of polysensitization to pet components is a useful tool to predict clinical relevance in rhinitis patients. The sIgE cross-reactivity to lipocalins and albumins seems to explain the high cosensitization to dogs among patients sensitized to cat and horse, but it is necessary to perform studies with a larger sample size of patients, additional animals, and include other allergens to confirm these results. The clinical implications of the different patterns of sensitization in immunomodulatory treatment should also be studied.

Disclosure

The abstract of this article was presented in the EAACI Congress 2019 (European Academy of Allergy and Clinical Immunology). The base data used to support the findings of this study are available from the corresponding author upon request.

Acknowledgments

We thank the corporation "IPS Universitaria" and the University of Antioquia for the technical and economic support (interinstitutional grant year: 2015-2016). We also thank Drs. Glora Gil, Catalina Lopez, and Steven Fuentes for reviewing the discussion of this article.

References

[1] L. Caraballo, J. Zakzuk, B. W. Lee et al., "Particularities of allergy in the tropics," *World Allergy Organization Journal*, vol. 9, p. 20, 2016.

[2] A. Bjerg, A. Winberg, M. Berthold, L. Mattsson, M. P. Borres, and E. Rönmark, "A population-based study of animal component sensitization, asthma, and rhinitis in schoolchildren," *Pediatric Allergy and Immunology*, vol. 26, no. 6, pp. 557–563, 2015.

[3] L. M. Heinzerling, G. J. Burbach, G. Edenharter et al., "GA(2)LEN skin test study I: GA(2)LEN harmonization of skin prick testing: novel sensitization patterns for inhalant allergens in Europe," *Allergy*, vol. 64, no. 10, pp. 1498–1506, 2009.

[4] J. Sánchez, S. Diez, and R. Cardona, "Frequency of sensitization to animals in a tropical area," *Revista Alergia México*, vol. 61, no. 2, pp. 81–89, 2014.

[5] P. J. Mandhane, M. R. Sears, R. Poulton et al., "Cats and dogs and the risk of atopy in childhood and adulthood," *Journal of Allergy and Clinical Immunology*, vol. 124, no. 4, pp. 745–750.e4, 2009.

[6] J. Sánchez, S. Díez, and R. Cardona, "Pet avoidance in allergy cases: is it possible to implement it?," *Biomédica*, vol. 35, no. 3, pp. 357–362, 2015.

[7] C. Pelucchi, C. Galeone, J. F. Bach, C. La Vecchia, and L. Chatenoud, "Pet exposure and risk of atopic dermatitis at the pediatric age: A meta- analysis of birth cohort studies," *Journal of Allergy and Clinical Immunology*, vol. 132, no. 3, pp. 616–622.e7, 2013.

[8] J. Stokholm, B. L. Chawes, N. Vissing, K. Bønnelykke, and H. Bisgaard, "Cat exposure in early life decreases asthma risk from the 17q21 high-risk variant," *The Journal of Allergy and Clinical Immunology*, vol. 141, no. 5, pp. 1598–1606, 2018.

[9] M. A. López-Matas, R. Moya, V. Cardona et al., "Relevance of allergenic sensitization to Cynodon dactylon and Phragmites communis: cross-reactivity with Pooideae grasses," *Journal of Investigational Allergology & Clinical Immunology*, vol. 26, no. 5, pp. 295–303, 2016.

[10] P. M. Gamboa, M. L. Sanz, M. Lombardero et al., "Component-resolved in vitro diagnosis in peach-allergic patients," *Journal of Investigational Allergology & Clinical Immunology*, vol. 19, no. 1, pp. 13–20, 2009.

[11] S. A. Uriarte and J. Sastre, "Clinical relevance of molecular diagnosis in pet allergy," *Allergy*, vol. 71, no. 7, pp. 1066–1068, 2016.

[12] A. Asarnoj, C. Hamsten, K. Wadén et al., "Sensitization to cat and dog allergen molecules in childhood and prediction of symptoms of cat and dog allergy in adolescence: a BAMSE/-MeDALL study," *Journal of Allergy and Clinical Immunology*, vol. 137, no. 3, pp. 813–821.e7, 2016.

[13] B. I. Nwaru, S. Suzuki, L. Ekerljung et al., "Furry animal allergen component sensitization and clinical outcomes in adult asthma and rhinitis," *The Journal of Allergy and Clinical Immunology. In Practice*, vol. 7, no. 4, pp. 1230–1238.e4, 2019.

[14] J. Bousquet, N. Khaltaev, A. A. Cruz et al., "Allergic rhinitis and its impact on asthma (ARIA) 2008 update (in collaboration with the World Health Organization, GA(2)LEN and Allergen)," *Allergy*, vol. 63, Supplement 86, pp. 8–160, 2008.

[15] J. L. Brożek, J. Bousquet, I. Agache et al., "Allergic Rhinitis and its Impact on Asthma (ARIA) guidelines–2016 revision," *The Journal of Allergy and Clinical Immunology*, vol. 140, no. 4, pp. 950–958, 2017.

[16] J. Bousquet, L. Heinzerling, C. Bachert et al., "Practical guide to skin prick tests in allergy to aeroallergens," *Allergy*, vol. 67, no. 1, pp. 18–24, 2012.

[17] J. Sanchez, S. Diez, and R. Cardona, "Sensibilización a aeroalergenos en pacientes alérgicos de Medellín, Colombia," *Revista Alergia México*, vol. 59, no. 3, pp. 139–147, 2012.

[18] M. T. Dordal, M. Lluch-Bernal, M. C. Sánchez et al., "Allergen-specific nasal provocation testing: review by the rhinoconjunctivitis committee of the Spanish Society of Allergy and Clinical Immunology," *Journal of Investigational Allergology and Clinical Immunology*, vol. 21, no. 1, pp. 1–12, 2011.

[19] J. Gosepath, R. G. Amedee, and W. J. Mann, "Nasal provocation testing as an international standard for evaluation of allergic and nonallergic rhinitis," *The Laryngoscope*, vol. 115, no. 3, pp. 512–516, 2005.

[20] S. K. Chan and D. Y. M. Leung, "Dog and cat allergies: current state of diagnostic approaches and challenges," *Allergy, Asthma & Immunology Research*, vol. 10, no. 2, pp. 97–105, 2018.

[21] J. Aegerter, D. Fouracre, and G. C. Smith, "A first estimate of the structure and density of the populations of pet cats and dogs across Great Britain," *PLoS One*, vol. 12, no. 4, article e0174709, 2017.

[22] A. Mendy, J. Wilkerson, P. M. Salo, R. D. Cohn, D. C. Zeldin, and P. S. Thorne, "Exposure and sensitization to pets modify endotoxin association with asthma and wheeze," *The Journal of Allergy and Clinical Immunology: In Practice*, vol. 6, no. 6, pp. 2006–2013.e4, 2018.

[23] E. Zahradnik and M. Raulf, "Animal allergens and their presence in the environment," *Frontiers in Immunology*, vol. 5, p. 76, 2014.

[24] J. Shargorodsky, E. Garcia-Esquinas, R. Umanskiy, A. Navas-Acien, and S. Y. Lin, "Household pet exposure, allergic sensitization, and rhinitis in the U.S. population," *International Forum of Allergy & Rhinology*, vol. 7, no. 7, pp. 645–651, 2017.

[25] M. Al Ahmad, N. Arifhodzic, J. Nurkic, E. Jusufovic, A. L. Hanoun, and T. Rodriguez, "Role of nasal challenge and local eosinophilia in indirect exposure to cat in allergic rhinitis patients," *European Annals of Allergy and Clinical Immunology*, vol. 50, no. 3, pp. 125–131, 2018.

[26] S. M. Collin, R. Granell, C. Westgarth et al., "Pet ownership is associated with increased risk of non-atopic asthma and reduced risk of atopy in childhood: findings from a UK birth cohort," *Clinical and Experimental Allergy*, vol. 45, no. 1, pp. 200 210, 2015.

[27] G. Liccardi, G. Emenius, A. S. Merritt, A. Salzillo, M. D'Amato, and G. D'Amato, "Direct and indirect exposure to horse: risk for sensitization and asthma," *Current Allergy and Asthma Reports*, vol. 12, no. 5, pp. 429–437, 2012.

[28] G. Liccardi, A. Salzillo, B. Dente et al., "Horse allergens: an underestimated risk for allergic sensitization in an urban atopic population without occupational exposure," *Respiratory Medicine*, vol. 103, no. 3, pp. 414–420, 2009.

[29] N. Ukleja-Sokołowska, E. Gawrońska-Ukleja, M. Żbikowska-Gotz et al., "Analysis of feline and canine allergen components in patients sensitized to pets," *Allergy, Asthma and Clinical Immunology*, vol. 12, no. 1, p. 61, 2016.

[30] M. Sánchez-Borges, E. Fernández-Caldas, A. Capriles-Hulett, and F. Caballero-Fonseca, "Mite-induced inflammation: more than allergy," *Allergy & Rhinology*, vol. 3, no. 1, pp. e25–e29, 2012.

[31] M. Wills-Karp, A. Nathan, K. Page, and C. L. Karp, "New insights into innate immune mechanisms underlying allergenicity," *Mucosal Immunology*, vol. 3, no. 2, pp. 104–110, 2010.

[32] F. Shakib, A. M. Ghaemmaghami, and H. F. Sewell, "The molecular basis of allergenicity," *Trends in Immunology*, vol. 29, no. 12, pp. 633–642, 2008.

[33] W. R. Thomas, "Molecular mimicry as the key to the dominance of the house dust mite allergen Der p 2," *Expert Review of Clinical Immunology*, vol. 5, no. 3, pp. 233–237, 2009.

[34] A. Trompette, S. Divanovic, A. Visintin et al., "Allergenicity resulting from functional mimicry of a toll-like receptor complex protein," *Nature*, vol. 457, no. 7229, pp. 585–588, 2009.

[35] B. Nordlund, J. R. Konradsen, I. Kull et al., "IgE antibodies to animal-derived lipocalin, kallikrein and secretoglobin are markers of bronchial inflammation in severe childhood asthma," *Allergy*, vol. 67, no. 5, pp. 661–669, 2012.

[36] J. A. Wisniewski, R. Agrawal, S. Minnicozzi et al., "Sensitization to food and inhalant allergens in relation to age and wheeze among children with atopic dermatitis," *Clinical and Experimental Allergy*, vol. 43, no. 10, pp. 1160–1170, 2013.

[37] U. Käck, A. Asarnoj, H. Grönlund et al., "Molecular allergy diagnostics refine characterization of children sensitized to dog dander," *The Journal of Allergy and Clinical Immunology*, vol. 142, no. 4, pp. 1113–1120.e9, 2018.

[38] L. Mattsson, T. Lundgren, H. Everberg, H. Larsson, and J. Lidholm, "Prostatic kallikrein: a new major dog allergen," *The Journal of Allergy and Clinical Immunology*, vol. 123, no. 2, pp. 362–368, 2009.

Correlation between Reduced FEF25-75% and a Positive Methacholine Challenge Test in Adults with Nonobstructive Baseline Spirometry

Irfan Shafiq, Mateen Haider Uzbeck, Zaid Zoumot, Mohamed Abuzakouk, Niyas Parappurath, and Ali Saeed Wahla

Respiratory and Allergy Institute, Cleveland Clinic Abu Dhabi, Abu Dhabi, UAE

Correspondence should be addressed to Irfan Shafiq; irfanshafiq@gmail.com

Academic Editor: Zsofia Lazar

Rationale. FEF25-75% is routinely reported on spirometry and is thought to be a marker of small airway obstruction. It is reduced in children with asthma, but its significance in adults and especially those without asthma diagnosis remains unclear. *Objective.* To clarify whether in adults with a nonobstructive spirometry a reduced FEF25-75% is associated with a positive methacholine challenge test (MCT). *Methods.* Data was collected for all the patients who had a MCT done between April 2014 and January 2020 but had nonobstructive baseline spirometry. Logistic regression was utilized to estimate the log odds of a positive methacholine test as a function of FEF25-75% and also for age, gender, BMI, FEV1, and FEV1/FVC. *Results.* Out of 496 patients, 187 (38%) had a positive MCT. Baseline characteristics in two groups were similar except that patients with positive MCT were younger (32 ± 11.57 vs. 38 ± 13.25 years, respectively, $p < 0.001$). Mean FEF25-75% was lower in MCT positive (3.12 ± 0.99 L/s) vs. MCT negative (3.39 ± 0.97 L/s) patients, $p = 0.003$. Logistic regression results suggest that MCT outcome is inversely related to FEF25-75%, age, and gender. Specifically, as FEF25-75% percentage of predicted value increases, the log odds of a positive MCT decrease (odds ratio (OR) = 0.90, 95% confidence intervals (CI) = 0.84-0.96, $p = 0.002$). Also, as age increases, the log odds of a positive MCT decrease (OR = 0.95, 95%CI = 0.94-0.97, $p < 0.001$). *Conclusions.* Reduced FEF25-75% in adults with nonobstructive spirometry can predict a positive response to MCT in younger patients. However, this relationship becomes weaker with increasing age.

1. Introduction

Asthma remains one of the most prevalent chronic respiratory illnesses and carries a high clinical and socioeconomic burden [1]. An accurate diagnosis of asthma is of paramount importance as it can avoid unnecessary investigations and costly treatments for patients [2]. However, at the milder end of the spectrum, the diagnosis can be difficult to establish as the baseline spirometry in this group of patients is often normal while the symptoms are in remission. Airway hyperresponsiveness is a key component of bronchial asthma [3], and demonstrating its presence or absence can greatly help in establishing a diagnosis and guiding treatment. Bronchial challenge tests are commonly utilized in the secondary and tertiary care setting to look for airway hyperresponsiveness and can be performed using inhaled methacholine, histamine, and mannitol or by exercise or eucapnic hyperventilation as provocative stimulus. These tests have high sensitivity but low specificity for diagnosis of asthma [4, 5]. The methacholine challenge test (MCT) is one of the commonest tests used in clinical practice to elicit airway hyperresponsiveness and is the test we use at our institution.

The majority of mild asthma patients are managed in primary care facilities where bronchial challenge testing is not readily available, and simple spirometry is the only diagnostic tool at hand. This raises the question of whether other spirometry-derived parameters can help identify patients who could have airway hyperresponsiveness and would benefit from either further testing to confirm the diagnosis of asthma, or in whom a trial of treatment with inhaled corticosteroids is warranted.

Forced expiratory volume in 1 second (FEV1), forced vital capacity (FVC), and FEV1/FVC are the usual measurements of interest in patients with obstructive airway disease. Forced expiratory flow 25–75 (FEF25-75%) is also routinely measured and reported on spirometry. It is defined as "forced expiratory flow over the middle one-half of the FVC; the average flow from the point at which 25% of the FVC has been exhaled to the point at which 75% of the FVC has been exhaled." A reduced FEF25-75% is thought to be a marker of small airway obstruction [6], and there is now ample evidence of small airway obstruction in asthma [2, 7]. FEF25-75% has been reported to be reduced in children with asthma [8], associated with increased asthma severity in adults [9], and also correlates well with both a raised fractional exhaled nitric oxide (FeNO) and a raised peripheral blood eosinophil count [10]. Some authors have suggested that FEF25-75% can be used as an early marker of airway hyperreactivity in mild asthma [11]; however, its clinical significance especially in adults without a prior diagnosis of asthma and a nonobstructive spirogram remains unclear.

Our study is aimed at investigating whether a reduced FEF25-75% is associated with increased airway hyperresponsiveness as demonstrated by a positive methacholine challenge test, in adults with asthma-like symptoms and a nonobstructive spirogram (Normal FEV1 and FEV1/FVC).

2. Methods

2.1. Subjects. In this retrospective observational study, we identified and reviewed the electronic medical records of all adult patients who underwent a methacholine challenge test between April 2014 and January 2020, having presented to our respiratory clinic with asthma-like symptoms (i.e., a chronic cough, SOB, or intermittent wheeze), and had at least one baseline spirometry assessment which ruled out airflow obstruction. Patients with a prior confirmed diagnosis of asthma and those with alternate diagnoses that could explain their symptoms were excluded from the study.

2.2. Study Variables. We recorded absolute values as well as % predicted values for FEV1, FEV1/FVC, and FEF25-75% for all participants. Only the tests that met the American Thoracic Society (ATS) criteria for spirometry were included in the study, and Global Lung Function Initiative (GLI) reference values were used to determine the % predicted values. The results of methacholine challenge results were recorded as positive or negative. As per the ATS guidelines [5], a PC20 (provocative concentration causing a 20% fall in FEV1) of more than 16 mg/mL was recorded as a negative MCT. Demographic data including gender, age, and BMI was also collected for all participants.

2.3. Statistical Analysis. Logistic regression was utilized to estimate the log odds of a positive methacholine test as a function of patient age, gender, BMI, FEF25-75%, FEV1, and FEV1/FVC. As a first step in the model building process, main effects, two-way interactions between clinical variables, and 2nd and 3rd degree polynomial terms for continuous variables were all examined. Model reduction was performed in a stepwise fashion by removing interaction and higher-order polynomial terms that failed to reach statistical significant at the 0.05 level. Main effects were retained in the final model in all instances; however, all nonsignificant ($p > 0.05$) main effects were grand-mean centered to facilitate model interpretation. Proportions were used as descriptive statistics for categorical variables, and data are expressed as the mean ± standard deviation (SD). Comparisons of values between groups were performed by using Student's t-test, and $p < 0.05$ was considered statistically significant.

3. Results

Four hundred and ninety-six patients had a methacholine challenge test between April 2014 and January 2020 and met the inclusion criteria for the study including 186 (37.5%) men and 310 (62.5%) women. MCT was positive in 187 (38%) and negative in 309 (62%) patients. Mean age of the study subjects was 36 ± 12.97 years. Patients with positive MCT were significantly younger, mean age 32 ± 11.57 vs. 38 ± 13.25 years, respectively, $p < 0.001$. There was no significant difference between the two groups in terms of BMI. Mean FEF25-75% was significantly lower in MCT positive (3.12 ± 0.99 L/s) vs. MCT negative (3.39 ± 0.97 L/s) patients, $p = 0.003$. This effect was more pronounced on comparison of FEF25-75% percentage of predicted values, 88.29 ± 22.05% for MCT positive vs. 100.13 ± 22.85% for negative patients, $p < 0.001$. Prebronchodilator FEV1 and FEV1% predicted values were not significantly different between the two patient groups. Baseline characteristics and outcomes are listed in Table 1.

The final logistic regression model along with odds ratio point estimate results is provided in Table 2. Logistic regression results suggest that the MCT outcome is related to patient's FEF25-75%% predicted, age, and gender. Specifically, as FEF25-75% percentage of predicted value increases, the log odds of a positive MCT decrease (OR = 0.90, 95% CI = 0.84-0.96, $p = 0.002$), though the associated 2nd degree polynomial term indicates that the rate of this decrease lessens as FEF25-75% predicted values increase (coef = 0.0003, OR = 1, $p = 0.028$). Similarly, as age increases, the log odds of a positive MCT also decrease (OR = 0.95, 95%CI = 0.94-0.97, $p < 0.001$). Finally, we found that males have lower odds of a positive MCT relative to females (OR = 0.56, 95%CI = 0.37-0.85, $p = 0.006$).

Next, the estimated log odds based on age and FEF25-75%% predicted values were transformed into probabilities. A contour graph was then constructed to show how the probability of a positive MCT changes as a function of age and FEF25-75% percentage of predicted values—see Figure 1. Here, the x-axis and y-axis represent FEF25-75% percentage of predicted value and age, respectively, while the contour lines represent the probability of a positive test.

The Receiver Operating Characteristic (ROC) curve resulting from the final model is shown in Figure 2. Overall, the area under the ROC curve is approximately 0.69 suggesting that over the full range of probability thresholds for classification, the model has low to moderate predictive value.

Table 1: Baseline characteristics and results.

	Total	Positive	Negative	p value
n	496	187 (38%)	309 (62%)	
Male	186	58 (31%)	128 (69%)	
Female	310	129 (42%)	181 (58%)	
Age	36 ± 12.97	32 ± 11.57	38 ± 13.25	<0.001
BMI	28.27 ± 6.28	27.76 ± 6.72	28.58 ± 5.99	0.169
FEF25-75% (L/s)	3.29 ± 0.98	3.12 ± 0.99	3.39 ± 0.97	0.003
FEF25-75% (percentage of predicted)	95.67 ± 23.25	88.29 ± 22.05	100.13 ± 22.85	<0.001
FEV1/FVC	83.43 ± 5.91	83.94 ± 6.53	82.59 ± 5.45	0.019
Prebronchodilator FEV1	3.00 ± 0.72	2.96 ± 0.69	3.02 ± 0.74	0.367
FEV1% predicted	90.32 ± 11.14	89.13 ± 11.01	91.04 ± 11.18	0.064

Results shown as n (%) and means ± SD.

Table 2: Logistic regression results.

Predictors	p value	Odds ratio (95% CI)
Age	0.000	0.95 (0.94-0.97)
Male (vs. female)	0.006	0.56 (0.37-0.85)
BMI	0.839	1.00 (0.97-1.04)
FEV1 (% of predicted)	0.169	1.02 (0.99-1.04)
FEF25-75% (% of predicted)	0.002	0.90 (0.84-0.96)

Outcome = methacholine test result; negative = 0; positive =1.

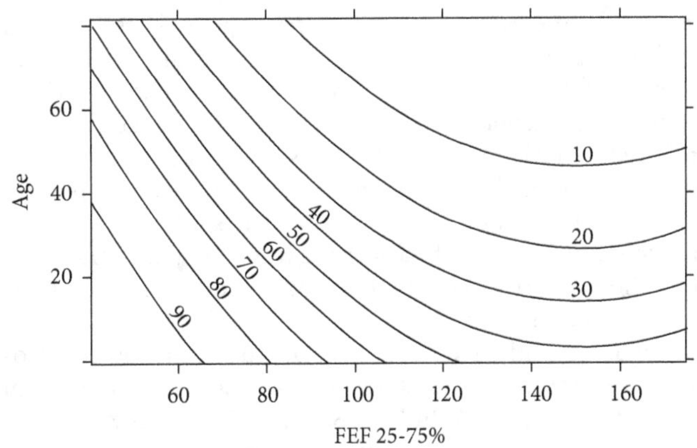

Figure 1: Probability of positive methacholine test contour graph: age by FEF% predicted value.

4. Discussion

Our study shows reduced midexpiratory flow rates as evidenced by a low FEF25-75% in patients with nonobstructive spirometry, but asthma-like symptoms can predict a positive response to MCT in younger patients. However, this relationship becomes weaker with increasing age. Hence, it is perhaps unsurprising that the association between FEF25-75% and asthma has been more established in pediatric than the adult populations.

Boggs et al. were one of the earliest groups to look at FEF25-75% in asthmatics [12]. In 1982, they evaluated the clinical significance of FEF25-75% among 167 known asthmatics and its utility in predicting airway responsiveness to inhaled bronchodilators and noted that FEF25-75% provided no benefit over FEV1 in predicting response to bronchodilation. Subsequently, in the 2005 American Thoracic Society (ATS) guidelines [13], it was observed that although the earliest change associated with airflow obstruction is a reduction in midflow (FEF25-75%) and terminal flow; however, these midflow measurements are not specific for small airway disease in individual patients.

The Severe Asthma Research Program (SARP) looked at 829 severe adult asthmatics and noted that FEF25-75% was an independent predictor of severe asthma symptoms after controlling for FEV1, FEV1/FVC, and demographic variables [14]. Their results were similar to those of Rao and colleagues who looked at 744 children diagnosed with asthma and noted that among those patients who had a normal FEV1, a reduced FEF25-75% was associated with increased asthma severity, exacerbations, and need for systemic steroids [15].

Malerba et al. looked at the association between impairment in FEF25-75% and bronchial hyperresponsiveness through methacholine challenge testing in adults [11]. They followed 400 consecutive patients aged 17.8-41.4 years who had normal FEV1, FVC, and FEV1/FVC but presented with asthma-like symptoms; FEF25-75% was abnormal in 27.5% of these patients. Two hundred and twenty-four had a positive methacholine challenge test (defined as $PD_{20} < 16$ mg/mL). A significant moderate positive correlation between bronchial hyperresponsiveness and FEF25-75% (Spearman's coefficient 0.339, $p < 0.001$) was noted. However, the authors did not look at differences in bronchial hyperresponsiveness based upon the age of patients. Additionally, patients with lower FEF25-75% were noted to have higher fractional exhaled nitric oxide (FeNO) levels and sputum eosinophils. In a separate study, Raji and colleagues also looked at FEF25-75% values in 234 patients with normal FEV1 and FEV1/FVC ratios with asthma-like symptoms who went for bronchial hyperresponsiveness testing [16]. They observed that mean FEF25-75% was 70.9 ± 19.2% for patients with a positive methacholine test versus 84.2 ± 22.7% for those with a negative methacholine test ($p < 0.001$). However, they were unable to determine an optimal

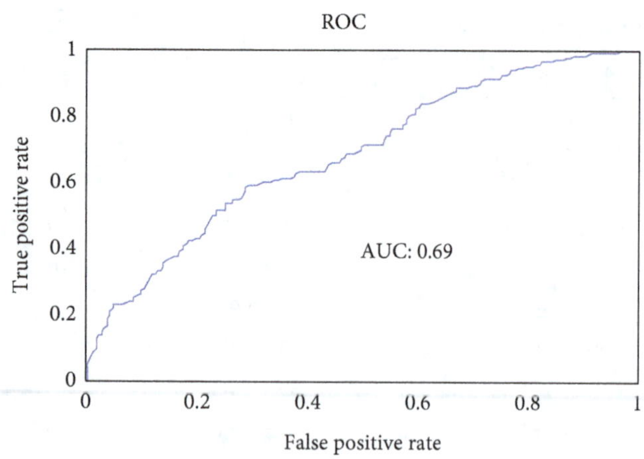

FIGURE 2: Receiver operating characteristic curve.

discrimination threshold of FEF25-75% that could be used as a cut-off for predicting bronchial hyperresponsiveness. Drewek and colleagues also looked at a pediatric population of 532 children aged 4-18 years and observed that those patients with a positive methacholine challenge test were more likely to have reduced FEF25-75% [17]. They also suggested that FEF25-75% may be used as an adjunct to FEV1 to define a positive methacholine study. Similarly, another study also showed reduced FEF25-75% to be associated with long-term persistence of asthma and risk of poor asthma outcomes, even after adjustment for FEV1 [18].

Most recently, Hou et al. performed a multicenter retrospective cross-sectional study of 846 Chinese adults with suspected asthma and FEV1 $\geq$ 80% predicted and found that FEF25-75% values were significantly lower and FENO values significantly higher in patients with a positive methacholine challenge test. Combining these two values gave an area under the curve (AUC) of 0.865 (95% CI: 0.833-0.893). They observed that the optimal cut-off for predicting a positive methacholine results to be FEF25-75% of less than 74.9% predicted in patients younger than 55 years of age and less than 62.9% in patients > 55 years of age [19].

FEF25-75% also has certain limitations due to the fact that it is directly dependent on FVC maneuver. Hence, if the FVC is reduced due to the patient effort during the test, then the FEF25-75% will also be reduced. This error can be minimized by making sure that the patient understands the test instructions and that the ATS criteria for spirometry performance are followed and met. Secondly, the FVC and can also be reduced due to a disease process which in turn will affect the FEF25-75%. For this reason, we only included the patients without preexisting lung disease in our study [20].

Our study is unique as it demonstrates a variable relationship between FEF25-75% and a positive MCT depending on the age of the subjects as it shows that younger patients with a reduced FEF25-75% were more likely to have a positive MCT as compared to an older patient with the same degree of midrange airflow limitation. The use of Figure 1 allows a clinician to decide the probability of a positive methacholine tested based upon a patient's age. For example, a 20-year-old patient with FEF25-75% 60% of predicted would have a greater than 90% chance of having a positive methacholine test; however, a 40-year-old patient with the same FEF25-75% would have a greater than 60% chance of a positive methacholine test and this would reduce further to 40% for a 60-year-old patient. Hence, our experience shows that the cut-off threshold for predicting a positive response to bronchial hyperresponsiveness testing varies with the age of the patient.

The limitations of our study include the fact that it is a retrospective one and most of the patients were of a single (Arab) ethnic group; hence, there is a need to validate our age-based threshold cut-off findings in a prospective manner and test these thresholds cut-offs in different ethnicities. Also, since most of the MCTs and the data collection was done prior to the European Respiratory Society's guidance on technical standards for bronchial challenge testing [21], the MCTs were performed and interpreted using PC20 rather than PD20. Lastly, the appropriate cut-offs for defining an abnormal FEF25-75% have not been defined properly especially in adults. A cut-off value of 65% has been suggested as abnormal by Ciprandi et al. [8] based on their observation of this parameter in children with an established diagnosis of asthma; however, the appropriate reference range in adults and in those without a preexisting asthma diagnosis is not really known.

In conclusion, this study shows an age-related correlation between the midrange flow limitation and presence of bronchial hyperresponsiveness in adult patients, meaning that younger patients had a much higher likelihood of a positive MCT if they had reduced FEF25-75% which in turn could be a marker of undiagnosed asthma and a predictor of BHR positivity in a select group of younger patients.

Authors' Contributions

I confirm that all the listed authors meet the ICMJE rules for authorship as they meet all of the following 4 criteria: substantial contributions to the conception or design of the work or the acquisition, analysis, or interpretation of data for the work; AND drafting the work or revising it critically for important intellectual content; AND final approval of the version to be published; AND agreement to be accountable for all aspects of the work in ensuring that questions related to the accuracy or integrity of any part of the work are appropriately investigated and resolved.

References

[1] M. Mukherjee, A. Stoddart, R. P. Gupta et al., "The epidemiology, healthcare and societal burden and costs of asthma in the UK and its member nations: analyses of standalone and linked national databases," *BMC Medicine*, vol. 14, no. 1, p. 113, 2016.

[2] S. D. Aaron, K. L. Vandemheen, J. M. FitzGerald et al., "Reevaluation of diagnosis in adults with physician-diagnosed asthma," *Journal of the American Medical Association*, vol. 317, no. 3, pp. 269–279, 2017.

[3] P. K. Pattemore, M. I. Asher, A. C. Harrison, E. A. Mitchell, H. H. Rea, and A. W. Stewart, "The interrelationship among bronchial hyperresponsiveness, the diagnosis of asthma, and asthma symptoms," *The American Review of Respiratory Disease*, vol. 142, no. 3, pp. 549–554, 1990.

[4] G. F. Joos and B. O'Connor, "Indirect airway challenges," *The European Respiratory Journal*, vol. 21, no. 6, pp. 1050–1068, 2003.

[5] R. O. Crapo, R. Casaburi, A. L. Coates, P. L. Enright, J. L. Hankinson, and C. G. Irvin, "Guidelines for methacholine and exercise challenge testing-1999. This official statement of the American Thoracic Society was adopted by the ATS Board of Directors, July 1999," *American Journal of Respiratory and Critical Care Medicine*, vol. 161, no. 1, pp. 309–329, 2000.

[6] M. Terra Filho, F. S. Vargas, A. Cukier, E. Fiss, M. Romeiro Neto, and J. Croce, "Forced mid-expiratory flow rate (FEF 25-75%): a critical analysis of its value in recognizing diseases of the small airways," *Allergologia et immunopathologia*, vol. 14, no. 3, pp. 199–203, 1986.

[7] M. Contoli, P. Santus, and A. Papi, "Small airway disease in asthma," *Current Opinion in Pulmonary Medicine*, vol. 21, no. 1, pp. 68–73, 2015.

[8] G. Ciprandi, M. Capasso, M. Tosca et al., "A forced expiratory flow at 25-75% value <65% of predicted should be considered abnormal: a real-world, cross-sectional study," *Allergy and Asthma Proceedings*, vol. 33, no. 1, pp. e5–e8, 2012.

[9] C. M. Riley, S. E. Wenzel, M. Castro et al., "Clinical implications of having reduced mid forced expiratory flow rates (FEF25-75), independently of FEV1, in adult patients with asthma," *PLoS One*, vol. 10, no. 12, article e0145476, 2015.

[10] M. A. Tosca, M. Silvestri, N. Solari, G. A. Rossi, and G. Ciprandi, "Inflammation markers and FEF25-75: a relevant link in children with asthma," *Allergy, Asthma & Immunology Research*, vol. 8, no. 1, pp. 84-85, 2016.

[11] M. Malerba, A. Radaeli, A. Olivini et al., "Association of FEF25-75% impairment with bronchial hyperresponsiveness and airway inflammation in subjects with asthma-like symptoms," *Respiration*, vol. 91, no. 3, pp. 206–214, 2016.

[12] P. B. Boggs, K. D. Bhat, W. A. Vekovius, and M. S. Debo, "The clinical significance of volume-adjusted maximal mid-expiratory flow (Iso-volume FEF25-75%) in assessing airway responsiveness to inhaled bronchodilator in asthmatics," *Annals of Allergy*, vol. 48, no. 3, pp. 139–142, 1982.

[13] R. Pellegrino, "Interpretative strategies for lung function tests," *The European Respiratory Journal*, vol. 26, no. 5, pp. 948–968, 2005.

[14] C. Riley, S. E. Wenzel, E. R. Bleecker, W. W. Busse, M. Castro, and S. C. Erzurum, "The association between reduced mid-forced expiratory flow rates (FEF25-75) with clinical outcomes in patients with asthma participating in the severe asthma research program (SARP). In: C32 CLINICAL ASTHMA II," *American Journal of Respiratory and Critical Care Medicine*, vol. 191, article A4188, 2015.

[15] D. R. Rao, J. M. Gaffin, S. N. Baxi, W. J. Sheehan, E. B. Hoffman, and W. Phipatanakul, "The utility of forced expiratory flow between 25% and 75% of vital capacity in predicting childhood asthma morbidity and severity," *Journal of Asthma*, vol. 49, no. 6, pp. 586–592, 2012.

[16] H. Raji, M. Haddadzadeh Shoushtari, E. Idani, H. Tavakol, S. Afrakhteh, and M. Dastoorpoor, "Forced expiratory flow at 25-75% as a marker for airway hyper responsiveness in adult patients with asthma-like symptoms," *Tanaffos*, vol. 17, no. 2, pp. 90–95, 2018.

[17] R. Drewek, E. Garber, S. Stanclik, P. Simpson, M. Nugent, and W. Gershan, "The FEF25-75 and its decline as a predictor of methacholine responsiveness in children," *Journal of Asthma*, vol. 46, no. 4, pp. 375–381, 2009.

[18] V. Siroux, A. Boudier, M. Dolgopoloff et al., "Forced midexpiratory flow between 25% and 75% of forced vital capacity is associated with long-term persistence of asthma and poor asthma outcomes," *The Journal of Allergy and Clinical Immunology*, vol. 137, no. 6, pp. 1709–1716.e6, 2016.

[19] L. Hou, H. Hao, G. Huang et al., "The value of small airway function parameters and fractional exhaled nitric oxide for predicting positive methacholine challenge test in asthmatics of different ages with FEV $1 \geq 80\%$ predicted," *Clinical and Translational Allergy*, vol. 11, no. 1, article e12007, 2021.

[20] P. H. Quanjer, D. J. Weiner, J. J. Pretto, D. J. Brazzale, and P. W. Boros, "Measurement of FEF25–75% and FEF75% does not contribute to clinical decision making," *The European Respiratory Journal*, vol. 43, no. 4, pp. 1051–1058, 2014.

[21] A. L. Coates, J. Wanger, D. W. Cockcroft et al., "ERS technical standard on bronchial challenge testing: general considerations and performance of methacholine challenge tests," *European Respiratory Journal*, vol. 49, no. 5, article 1601526, 2017.

Covered Stent of the Left Common Carotid and Subclavian Arteries Assist the Invasive Tumor Resection

Yo Tsukamoto,[1] Takeo Nakada,[1] Soichiro Fukushima,[1] Mitsuo Yabe,[1] Naoki Toya,[1] Tadashi Akiba,[1] Takashi Ohtsuka,[2] and Takao Ohki[2]

[1]*Department of Surgery, Jikei University Kashiwa Hospital, 163-1 Kashiwashita, Kashiwa, Chiba 277-8567, Japan*
[2]*Department of Surgery, The Jikei University School of Medicine, Nishishinbashi 3-19-18, Minatoku, Tokyo 105-8471, Japan*

Correspondence should be addressed to Yo Tsukamoto; young1017@triton.ocn.ne.jp

Academic Editor: Inger F. Oey

Background. Some recent reports have described the usefulness of thoracic aortic stent grafts to facilitate en bloc resection of tumors invading the aortic wall. We report on malignant peripheral nerve sheath tumor resection in the left superior mediastinum of a 16-year-old man with neurofibromatosis type 1. The pathological margin was positive at the time of the first tumor resection, and radiation therapy was added to the same site. After that, a local recurrence occurred. The tumor was in wide contact with the left common carotid and subclavian arteries and was suspected of infiltration. After stent graft placement of these arteries to avoid fatal bleeding and cerebral ischemia by clamping these arteries and bypass procedure, we successfully resected the tumor without any complications. *Conclusions.* Here, we report the usefulness of the prior covered stent placement to aortic branch vessels for the resection of invasive tumor.

1. Background

Some recent reports have described the usefulness of thoracic aortic stent graft placement for the en bloc resection of malignant tumors that had invaded the thoracic aortic wall [1–4]. In this report, we could resect a superior mediastinal recurrent malignant tumor successfully, which was earlier irradiated with total of 60 Gy, using the covered stents in the left common carotid artery (LCCA) and the left subclavian artery (LSA). Covered stent placement in the aortic branch vessels was extremely useful in this case to avert catastrophic intraoperative bleeding. Herein, we describe an effectiveness of the prior stent graft placement to the aortic branch vessels as a new surgical indication. We propose a stent graft-assisted thoracic surgery, because it may help expand operative indications for patients who are otherwise deemed as unsuited to undergo surgical replacement of major arteries.

2. Case Presentation

A 16-year-old male with neurofibromatosis type 1 was referred to our hospital for management of left superior mediastinal tumor. The surgery in this case reports is for the patient at the time of the fourth surgery for malignant peripheral nerve sheath tumor (MPNST). For the first surgery, owing to the rapid growth of the tumor and presence of dyspnea, he underwent an emergent operation through trap door thoracotomy (Figures 1(a) and 1(b)). The tumor was 123 × 120 × 88 mm in size and was originated from the left thoracic vagal nerve distal to the bifurcation of the recurrent laryngeal nerve. We could barely exfoliate the tumor from the LCCA and LSA, and it was diagnosed as MPNST with 56 mitosis cells per 20 high-power fields. Radiotherapy of total dose 60 Gy was administered to the mediastinum owing to pathologically positive margins. In the second operation, a hook approach was used to

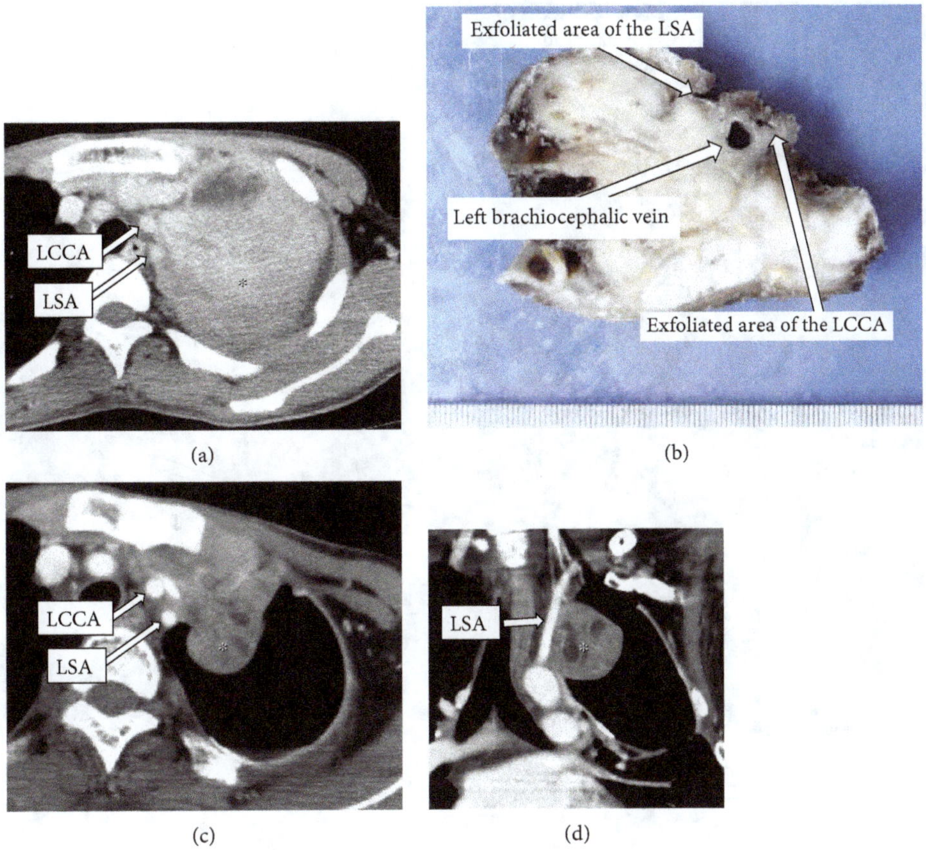

Figure 1: Before initial operation: (a) horizontal view, (b) frontal view. Chest computed tomography (CT) radiograph showing a left superior mediastinal tumor (*) measuring 123 × 120 × 88 mm in size with massive pleural effusion. Before third operation: (c) horizontal view, (d) frontal view. Follow-up chest CT revealing local recurrence with rapid growth in the left superior mediastinum. The tumor had attached to the left common carotid artery (LCCA) and the left subclavian artery (LSA).

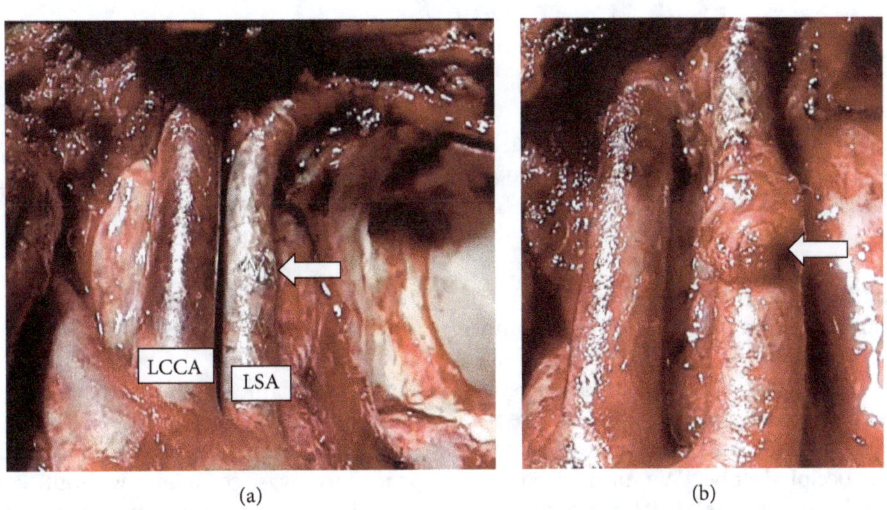

Figure 2: Intraoperative view. (a) Resected wall of the left subclavian artery (LSA), one-third of the circumference, causing no bleeding (arrow). (b) The resected portion was covered with a pericardial patch (arrow).

perform combined resection of the left chest wall including the 2nd-4th ribs for locally recurrent tumor. In the third operation, a distal pancreatectomy was performed for metastasis to the pancreas. Ten months after the first operation, we observed rapid growing local recurrence in the left superior mediastinum. The recurrent tumor was

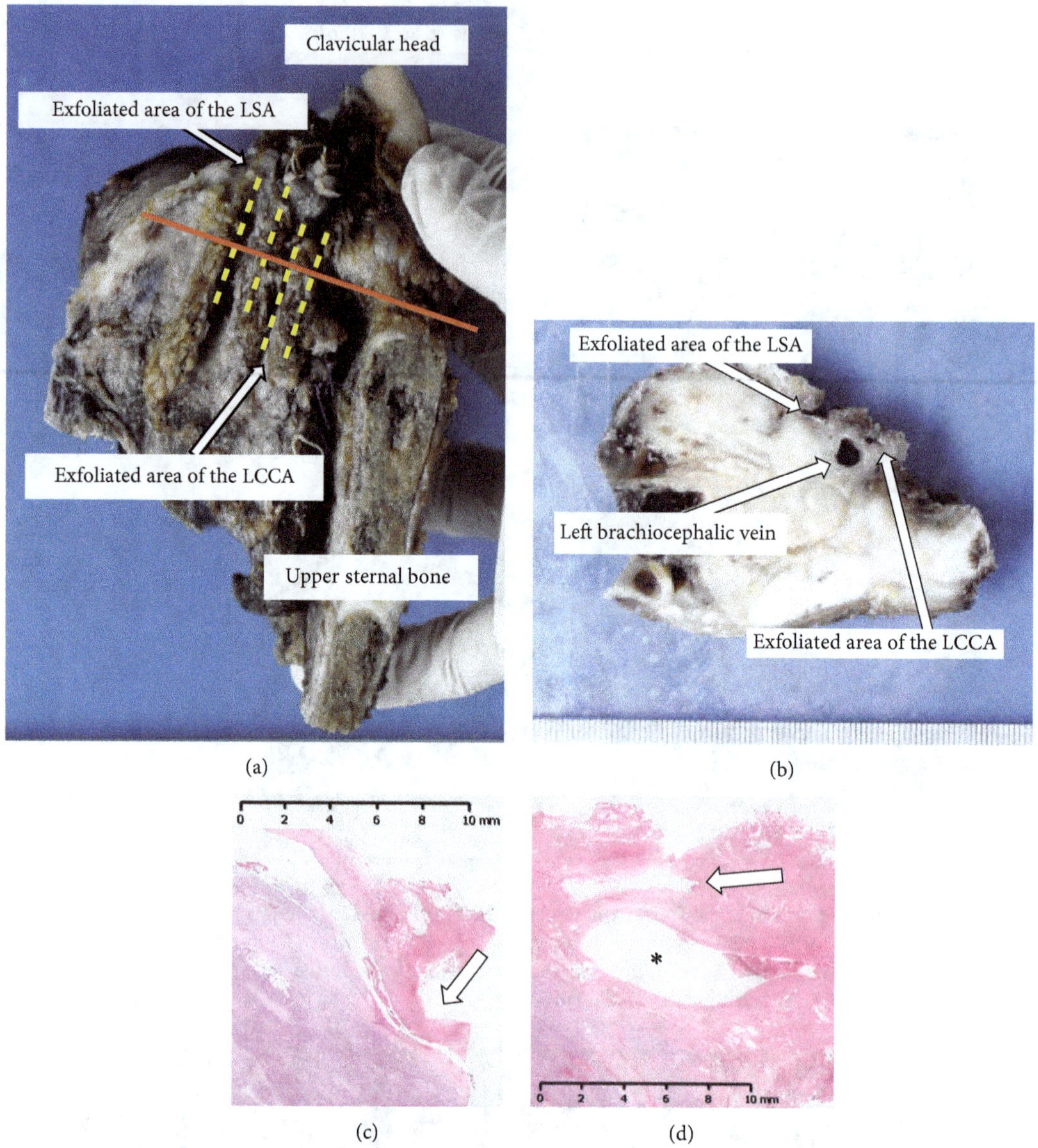

FIGURE 3: (a) The resected specimen (mediastinal view); (b) the cut surface on the red line of (a). (c) Microscopically, the fibrotic tissue surrounding the left subclavian artery (LSA) was free of malignancy (arrow). (d) Microscopically, the fibrosis surrounding the left common carotid artery (LCCA: arrow) was free from malignancy, but the tumor had infiltrated the left brachiocephalic vein (*).

not found on examination a month ago. Chest computed tomography (CT) showed that the recurrent tumor attached the left clavicular head, the first rib, upper sternal bone, the LCCA, and LSA (Figures 1(c) and 1(d)). Preoperative cranial magnetic resonance angiography showed a normal vertebral-basilar system, and a tumor measured 35 mm in size in the occipital lobe. We prioritized the operation of the thoracic tumor due to its rapid growth, and we planned an endovascular technique to avoid intraoperative fatal bleeding. We obtained written informed consent from his parents for the off-label use. An 8 mm in diameter and 60 mm in length polytetrafluoroethylene-covered stent (PTFE-CS) for biliary tract (Fluency®; Bard, Karlsruhe, Germany) was inserted in the area where the tumor was sufficiently covered from the LCCA bifurcation by cutting down at the left neck, and postdilatation was performed with a 6 mm balloon dilatation catheter. Then, other PTFE-CS, 8 mm in diameter and 60 mm in length, was inserted from LSA bifurcation. Another PTFE-CS, 8 mm in diameter and 40 mm in length, was further inserted peripherally to cover the left vertebral artery to cover the tumor, and postdilatation was performed. The procedure was complete without complications. On the next day, we performed tumor resection, combined resection of the left brachiocephalic vein and pericardium and partial resection of the left upper lobe and chest wall (from the first to third ribs, the left clavicular head, and the upper left half of the sternum). Because the tumor was firmly fixed in the left upper mediastinum due to the effect of past radiotherapy, the tumor could be barely exfoliated from the both arteries. In spite of resecting the wall of the LSA during the operation, there was no bleeding from the defect of the LSA with one-third of the circumference, and it was covered with a pericardial patch. Subsequently, the thoracic wall was reconstructed with Gore-Tex® dual mesh (Figures 2(a) and 2(b)). Pathologically, the tumor had not infiltrated into LCCA and LSA, and the surgical margin was negative (Figure 3). He was discharged on postoperative day 19 without any complication. Subsequently, cranial surgery was performed 3 months after the thoracic surgery. Six months after the operation, a local recurrence occurred in the left thoracic cavity. Pazopanib was administered, but the tumor grew. At 10 months postoperatively, tracheal stenosis due to tumor growth occurred, and a tracheal stent was placed. He was treated with trabectedin but was unsuccessful and died 11 months after the surgery.

3. Discussion and Conclusions

Surgical resection of a thoracic tumor near major vessels, including aorta, aortic branch vessels, and other major veins, in patients with poor general conditions is inherently challenging due to the difficulty in determining the optimal approach and the extent of surgery. Recently, stent graft-assisted thoracic surgery has expanded operative indications as a minimally invasive surgery which precludes the need for a biventricular assist device or aortic arch replacement. This is the first report of stent graft placement to the LCCA and LSA prior to the invasive tumor resection. In this case, we opted for the use of covered stent due to the following considerations. First, chest CT showed fixation of the LCCA and LSA to the tumor without obvious intravenous infiltration. This region had been irradiated with a total dose of 60 Gy. There would be a high risk of fatal intraoperative bleeding from these arteries during exfoliation of the tumor. If the tumor infiltrated these arteries, we intended to perform combined resection of the tumor with partial artery. Similar cases where partial resection of the aorta was safely performed have been reported [1, 2, 5]. Second, the patient had undergone multiple invasive surgeries over a short period of time, and his physical tolerance was decreased. Further, we had planned brain tumor resection as soon as possible after this surgery. In the present case, although we injured the LSA, the operation was successful without any bleeding complication. He safely underwent brain surgery after thoracic surgery owing to the minimal physical damage.

Covered stents for the branch vessels of the thoracic aorta have already been developed. Their authority or import depends on each country, so these could not be used in emergency. We opted for prompt surgery with use of a readily available biliary stent, because the properties of the biliary stents were considered to be similar to that of covered stents for the LCCA and LSA. We chose biliary stents for the following reasons: Being a covered stent, the specifications (blood vessel diameter/length) conforming to the target blood vessel, it has been reported to be used in endovascular treatment [6, 7], and it has already been used in endovascular treatment of other patients at our hospital. Nonetheless, we needed informed consent of the patient given the off-label use. Furthermore, risk of delayed complications such as stenosis, aneurysm formation, and thrombosis is not clear. In this case, he died 11 months after the time of fourth operation due to the progression of the primary disease, but there were no stent complications during that time. The recurrent tumor including chest wall and lung were resected immediately after stent placement, and no antiplatelet drug or anticoagulant was used. Since we planned a surgery for metastatic brain tumors, we did not use antiplatelet and anticoagulants because of the risk of bleeding. In the case which the urgency is low and a long-term prognosis is expected, it is preferable to use an indicated intravascular stent and to use antiplatelets and anticoagulants in combination considering the risk of bleeding. As the reports on long-term follow-up are few, the accumulation of future cases is necessary.

Abbreviations

LCCA:	Left common carotid artery
LSA:	Left subclavian artery
MPNST:	Malignant peripheral nerve sheath tumor
CT:	Computed tomography
PTFE-CS:	Polytetrafluoroethylene-covered stent.

Acknowledgments

We are grateful to Dr. Haruka Mastuzawa for useful pathorogical discussions.

References

[1] S. Collaud, T. K. Waddell, K. Yasufuku et al., "Thoracic aortic endografting facilitates the resection of tumors infiltrating the aorta," *The Journal of Thoracic and Cardiovascular Surgery*, vol. 147, no. 4, pp. 1178–1182, 2014.

[2] G. Marulli, S. Lepidi, P. Frigatti, M. Antonello, F. Grego, and F. Rea, "Thoracic aorta endograft as an adjunct to resection of a locally invasive tumor: a new indication to endograft," *Journal of Vascular Surgery*, vol. 47, no. 4, pp. 868–870, 2008.

[3] P. Berna, P. Bagan, F. De Dominicis, C. Dayen, Y. Douadi, and M. Riquet, "Aortic endostent followed by extended pneumonectomy for T4 lung cancer," *The Annals of Thoracic Surgery*, vol. 91, no. 2, pp. 591–593, 2011.

[4] G. N. Mody, M. Janko, V. Vasudeva, J. H. Chi, M. J. Davidson, and S. Swanson, "Thoracic endovascular aortic stent graft to facilitate aortic resection during pneumonectomy and vertebrectomy for locally invasive lung cancer," *The Annals of Thoracic Surgery*, vol. 101, no. 4, pp. 1587–1589, 2016.

[5] H. Sasahara, S. Sueyoshi, T. Tanaka, H. Fujita, and K. Shirouzu, "Evaluation of an aortic stent graft for use in surgery on esophageal cancer involving the thoracic aorta," *The Japanese Journal of Thoracic and Cardiovascular Surgery*, vol. 52, no. 5, pp. 231–239, 2004.

[6] R. W. Franz, "Delayed treatment of a Traumatic left subclavian artery pseudoaneurysm," *Vascular and Endovascular Surgery*, vol. 42, no. 5, pp. 482–485, 2008.

[7] J. Nazil, A. Ammar, L. G. Alexandros, F. K. Jawad, and I. Q. Adnan, "Covered stent graft for treatment of a psudoaneurysm and carotid blowout syndrome," *Journal of Vascular and Interventional Neurology*, vol. 1, pp. 5–8, 2008.

Noninvasive Neurally Adjusted Ventilator Assist Ventilation in the Postoperative Period Produces Better Patient-Ventilator Synchrony but Not Comfort

L. O. Harnisch,[1] U. Olgemoeller,[2] J. Mann,[1] M. Quintel,[1] and O. Moerer[1]

[1]*Department of Anaesthesiology, University Medical Centre Göttingen, Germany Robert-Koch-Str. 40 D-37099 Göttingen*
[2]*Department of Cardiology and Pulmonology, University Medical Centre Göttingen, Robert-Koch-Str. 40 D-37099 Göttingen, Germany*

Correspondence should be addressed to L. O. Harnisch; lars-olav.harnisch@med.uni-goettingen.de

Academic Editor: Akio Niimi

Background. Noninvasive neurally adjusted ventilatory assist (NAVA) has been shown to improve patient-ventilator interaction in many settings. There is still scarce data with regard to postoperative patients indicated for noninvasive ventilation (NIV) which this study elates. The purpose of this trial was to evaluate postoperative patients for synchrony and comfort in noninvasive pressure support ventilation (NIV-PSV) vs. NIV-NAVA. *Methods.* Twenty-two subjects received either NIV-NAVA or NIV-PSV in an object-blind, prospective, randomized, crossover fashion (observational trial). We evaluated blood gases and ventilator tracings throughout as well as comfort of ventilation at the end of each ventilation phase. *Results.* There was an effective reduction in ventilator delays ($p < 0.001$) and negative pressure duration in NIV-NAVA as compared to NIV-PSV ($p < 0.001$). Although we used optimized settings in NIV-PSV, explaining the overall low incidence of asynchrony, NIV-NAVA led to reductions in the NeuroSync-index ($p < 0.001$) and all types of asynchrony except for double triggering that was significantly more frequent in NIV-NAVA vs. NIV-PSV ($p = 0.02$); ineffective efforts were reduced to zero by use of NIV-NAVA. In our population of previously lung-healthy subjects, we did not find differences in blood gases and patient comfort between the two modes. *Conclusion.* In the postoperative setting, NIV-NAVA is well suitable for use and effective in reducing asynchronies as well as a surrogate for work of breathing. Although increased synchrony was not transferred into an increased comfort, there was an advantage with regard to patient-ventilator interaction. The trial was registered at the German clinical Trials Register (DRKS no.: DRKS00005408).

1. Introduction

Noninvasive ventilation (NIV) is increasingly used for COPD (chronic obstructive pulmonary disease) and acute respiratory insufficiency [1], in home mechanical ventilation [2], and postextubation care [3]. However, several mechanisms like poor tolerance, mask-related complications, severity of the underlying disease, but also poor patient-ventilator interaction can lead to NIV failure [4, 5].

Asynchrony between patient and ventilator is a common finding and underestimated problem [6] being an important cause for NIV failure [7], since it might actually increase work of breathing [8]. Signs of impaired patient-ventilator interaction are ineffective triggering and double-triggering where the ventilator either does not support a breath at all or one inspiratory effort is sensed as two and supported by the ventilator as such, resulting in hyperinflation of the lung, respectively.

During neurally adjusted ventilatory assist (NAVA), an adaptive ventilator mode, the ventilator respiratory cycle and a proportional ventilatory assist are based on the electrical activity of the diaphragm (EAdi) detected via an oesophageal catheter ([9]). Thus, during NAVA airway pressure, ventilator system flow, intrinsic PEEP (positive endexpiratory pressure), lung volume, and airleaks only marginally influence ventilator cycling [10]. NAVA is able to significantly reduce respiratory workload and asynchrony during invasive as well as noninvasive ventilation [11–13]. Furthermore, by way of proportionally assisting a patient's breath rather than assisting it in a not-changing manner for each breath, NAVA also exercises lung-protective ventilation. A recent meta-analysis revealed that NIV-NAVA significantly enhances patient-ventilator interaction and lowers severe asynchrony compared to NIV-PSV[14]. However, the effects on synchrony and patient comfort in previously lung-healthy patients needing NIV for postextubation care have not been evaluated. NIV-NAVA in these subjects is of special interest in some regards: first, reduced asynchrony may accelerate the improvement of gas exchange and reduce ICU- and hospital length-of-stay. Second, NIV-NAVA is an elegant way to ensure lung-protective ventilation [15], which may often not be thought of in these subjects or is admittedly often difficult to follow due to the dynamic situation of postoperative respiratory failure. Therefore, we decided to target postoperative subjects, because lung-protective ventilation is critical in these patients as well and increased synchrony with accelerated improvement in gas exchange may reduce the length of ICU- and hospital stay.

The objective of this trial was to evaluate if NIV-NAVA would improve patient-ventilator synchrony measured by NeuroSync-index [16] (primary outcome) as well as perceived patient comfort (secondary outcome) compared to NIV-PSV. We conducted a prospective randomized crossover observational trial and assessed differences in patient comfort and patient-ventilator interaction between noninvasive pressure support ventilation (NIV-PSV) and NIV-NAVA in previously lung-healthy adult subjects in the postoperative period.

2. Material and Methodes

The study was conducted in an adult surgical ICU (intensive care unit) of a tertiary medical centre in 2012/13 and 2016 and designed as a single-blind prospective randomized crossover observational trial. This study was approved by the Research Ethics Board of Georg-August University Goettingen (#19/1/12), and written informed consent was obtained from all subjects participating in the trial prior to data acquisition. The trial was registered at the German Trials Register (http://www.drks.de; DRKS00005408, date of registration: 30.10.2013).

Subjects were eligible if attending physicians indicated postextubation noninvasive ventilation. After informed consent, the EAdi-catheter was placed as described elsewhere [17], and the facemask was tightly strapped to the subject's face (AcuCare™ F1-0 Hospital NV Full Face Mask, ResMed, Martinsried, Germany). Subjects received both ventilation modes successively but were randomized to the initial mode and were kept unaware of the actual mode. We used the Servo-I ventilator (Maquet, Getinge Group; Rastatt, Germany) as the only ventilation device throughout the whole trial. Before ventilation was started, RASS Score (Richmond Agitation and Sedation Scale) was documented and correct catheter position was verified using the EAdi positioning tool [17]. Ventilator settings were at the discretion of the attending physician with respect to the subject's clinical status; PEEP was set according to the low PEEP/FiO_2 table as proposed by the ARDS Network.

Measurements were started after stable conditions were achieved. We recorded a total of 20 minutes for each ventilation mode, every five minutes clinical parameters (heart rate, blood pressure, respiratory rate) as well as ventilation parameters (fraction of inspired oxygen, tidal volume, PEEP, maximum inspiratory pressure, NAVA-level/pressure support, EAdi-peak) were documented (ESM figure 1). Ventilator parameters as well as flow and pressure curves were extracted through an interface at a sampling rate of 100 Hz using a dedicated software (Servo-Tracker V4.1, Maquet, Getinge Group, Solna, Sweden). Acquired data were transferred to a dedicated software (NeuroVent Analysis Software, Research Inc., Toronto, ON, Canada) measuring in- (TI) and expiratory time (TE), trigger and off-cycling delays, and negative pressure duration (defined as the time from the pressure drop below PEEP level up to the moment when PEEP level is reached again by pressure support) by placing cursors in the ventilator tracings and calculating differences between them during six continuous minutes of the recording (ESM table 1, ESM figure 2 and "cursor placement"). Ventilator tracings were also assessed for ineffective efforts, double-triggering, and autotriggering [16].

Based on the assessed variables, asynchrony-index [16] (asynchrony – index [%] = number of asynchrony events/ total respiratory rate [ventilator cycles + wasted efforts] × 100) and NeuroSync-index ([18]) (average of all absolute values for the errors [both-sided trigger-on and cycle-off errors] for all events) were calculated manually. Classification of asynchrony was used as defined before: asynchrony index >10%; NeuroSync-index >33% = dysynchrony, 100% = asynchrony.

After fifteen minutes of ventilation, an arterial blood gas was drawn and subjects were questioned about comfort and quality of ventilatory support. The questionnaire consisted of five closed-ended questions and two open-ended questions about the general experience of ventilation, where a visual analogue scale (VAS), was used for each ventilation mode received. The VAS was charted in centimetres starting from the left side (low values, very bad comfort) (ESM figures 3 and 4).

Questions to the subjects at the end of each session:

(i) Does the ventilation via facemask facilitate your breathing? Yes; no

(ii) Do you feel your exhalation is impaired? Yes; no

(iii) Does the ventilator react too fast/too slow? (Does the ventilator adapt to your breathing?) Yes; no

(iv) Do you get too much/too little air? Yes; no

(v) Do you feel the mask does not seal properly/too much air leaks? Yes; no

(vi) How comfortable do you feel? VAS-scale (one for each ventilation mode)

2.1. Statistical Analysis. Statistical analysis was performed using SPSS 25.0 (Statistical Package for Social Sciences, International Business Machines Corporated [IBM], Armonk, New York, USA). Data were tested for normal distribution using Shapiro-Wilk test. Parametric variables were analysed by paired t-test, nonparametric variables were analysed by Wilcoxon signed-rank test. Variables were further analysed by two-way-repeated-measure ANOVA (analysis of variance) with Bonferroni post hoc correction with respect to the subject "mode" to account for the cross-over design. Quantitative parameters were transformed onto a nominal scale (yes = 1, no = 0) and analysed using Fishers exact-test. Results are presented as mean and standard deviation (SD) for parametric and median and interquartile range (IQR) for nonparametric variables; level of significance was assumed at $p < 0.05$.

This manuscript adheres to the applicable CONSORT guidelines.

3. Results

All subjects had a RASS Score of zero and did not receive sedation/analgesia throughout the study period; subject characteristics and ventilator settings are shown in Tables 1 and 2, respectively. Blood gas parameters did not differ between modes (ESM table 2).

NIV-NAVA led to shorter inspiratory delay (NIV-PSV 186 ± 81 ms vs. NIV-NAVA 50 ± 36 ms; $p < 0.001$) as well as expiratory delay (NIV-PSV −48 ± 85 ms vs. NIV-NAVA 10 ± 14 ms; $p = 0.003$).

Inspiratory and expiratory time did not differ (TI: NIV-PSV 1171 ± 314 ms vs. NIV-NAVA 1138 ± 383 ms; $p = 0.564$; TE: NIV-PSV 2268 ± 800 ms vs. NIV-NAVA 2074 ± 770 ms, $p = 0.130$; TTOT NIV-PSV 3429 ± 1076 ms vs. NIV-NAVA 3222 ± 1094 ms; $p = 0.353$). Negative pressure duration showed statistical significance favouring NIV-NAVA (NIV-PSV 253 ± 55 ms vs. NIV-NAVA 108 ± 58 ms; $p < 0.001$) (Figure 1, Table 3).

Double triggering was more frequent in NIV-NAVA (NIV-PSV 0.06 ± 0.08/min vs. NIV-NAVA 0.16 ± 0.18/min ; $p = 0.02$). While auto triggering was the same in both modes (NIV-PSV 0.15 ± 0.43/min vs. NIV-NAVA 0.13 ± 0.24/min; $p = 0.584$), ineffective efforts did not appear in NIV-NAVA but in NIV-PSV (NIV-PSV 0.26 ± 0.62/min vs. NIV-NAVA 0 ± 0/min; $p = 0.001$) (Figure 2). Asynchrony-index was not different in NIV-NAVA vs. NIV-PSV (NIV-PSV 2.43 ± 3.12% vs. NIV-NAVA 1.58 ± 1.89%; $p = 0.258$), whereas NeuroSync-index was significantly less in NIV-NAVA compared to NIV-PSV (NIV-PSV 18.22 ± 8.19% vs. NIV-NAVA 9.21 ± 5.85%; $p = 0.001$).

Two-way-repeated-measure ANOVA revealed no significant interaction regarding the order in which the modes were used ($p = 0.06$) (ESM table 3).

Questionnaires were analysed regarding comfort of NIV-NAVA vs. NIV-PSV. Most subjects found NIV helpful, (question one) (NIV-NAVA 70%, NIV-PSV 68%, $p = 0.293$) and about half of the subjects denied impeded expiration (question two) (NIV-NAVA 53%, NIV-PSV 53%, $p = 0.351$). Asked for the subjective feeling of premature or delayed cycling most subjects answered "no" (NIV-NAVA 57%, NIV-PSV 73%, $p = 0.192$) and most subjects did not feel the flow to be insufficient (NIV-NAVA 61%, NIV-PSV 71%; $p = 0.325$). The general impression of the ventilation mode did not differ between modes (VAS: NIV-PSV 5.31 ± 2.36 cm, NIV-NAVA 5.41 ± 2.31 cm; $p = 0.907$).

4. Discussion

Our results concur with most recent studies in that NIV-NAVA improves patient-ventilator interaction compared to pressure support ventilation in all measures of asynchrony except for double triggering [12, 19–25].

During NIV, the ventilator is triggered by electromyographic signals, this is advantageous because it antagonizes the devastating effect of leakage. In an early study in healthy volunteers receiving NIV-NAVA via a helmet interface, the advantages of a neural trigger were revealed [26] . Our data, in concert with recent studies [22], confirm this effect showing an inspiratory delay decidedly shorter for NIV-NAVA than for NIV-PSV.

Expiratory delay was also reduced during NIV-NAVA compared to NIV-PSV as reported before ([11, 22, 24]); although, the delays we found were substantially shorter than previously reported. The most prevalent difference is the set off-cycling value during NIV-PSV (our trial 40 ± 7.32%, Schmidt et al. 30%, Ducharme-Crevier not given, probably default 30%, Longhini 35%), whereas during NIV-NAVA the ventilator cycles off at 70% EAdi-peak as fixed by the manufacturer. Our data support evidence that synchrony can be improved in NIV-PSV by meticulous adjustments of ventilator settings, although with a limited effect [27].

Double triggering was more prevalent in NIV-NAVA than in NIV-PSV [21, 25]. Other investigators report double-triggering to be caused by an EAdi wave most likely due to sighs or periodic neural respiratory hyperactivity [12, 21] which can be confirmed from our tracings. One might explain these sighs to be due to relative insufficient inspiratory flow. Since the inspiratory flow in NIV-NAVA is proportional to EAdi-slope, the subject might augment a relative too small inspiratory flow due to normal respiratory variability by a consecutive sigh. This phenomenon is less likely in NIV-PSV because the inspiratory flow is usually high, sometimes even too high [28]. Moreover, we also found a lesser rate of double triggering in NIV-PSV than shown before [16].

Ineffective efforts are usually very frequent in PSV which is most likely due to the fact that they are the common final path of a lot of suboptimal ventilator settings (inspiratory trigger too high or too low, pressure support too high or too low) [16, 19, 21, 29]. Fifty percent of our subjects experienced ineffective efforts in NIV-PSV, which is less than described by others [30] but still unacceptably high. With NIV-NAVA, ineffective efforts can be avoided completely as has consistently been shown [11, 19, 30, 31].

To globally evaluate for asynchronies during ventilator assisted breathing indices such as asynchrony-index and

Table 1: Individual patient characteristics including age, diagnosis ICU admission, type of surgery, and SAPS II on admission.

Included patient	Sex	Age (years)	Diagnosis (admission)	Type of surgery	SAPS II
1	Male	75	Endocarditis	SVR	66
2	Female	69	Aortic ulceration	Aortic arch replacement	41
3	Male	83	Combined aortic vitium, endocarditis	SVR	67
4	Male	60	Decompensated congestive heart failure	CABG	47
5	Female	71	Aortic and mitral valve stenosis	SVR	64
6	Male	74	Postoperative pneumonia	CABG	40
7	Male	76	Hemorrhagic shock	CABG	28
8	Male	74	Coronary artery disease	CABG	60
9	Male	41	Hemorrhagic shock	CABG	45
10	Male	67	NSTEMI	CABG	37
11	Male	68	Tricuspid valve insufficiency	SVR	44
12	Male	45	Multiple extremity fractures	Surgical bone repair	34
13	Male	51	Aortic dissection	Aortic arch replacement	66
14	Male	44	Aortic valve insufficiency	SVR	36
15	Female	57	Postoperative respiratory failure	CABG	42
16	Female	74	Coronary artery disease	CABG	39
17	Female	75	NSTEMI	CABG	35
18	Male	46	Aortic valve stenosis	SVR	29
19	Male	65	Coronary artery disease	CABG	39
20	Male	74	Coronary artery disease	CABG	46
21	Male	84	Lung mass	Diagnostic VATS	47
22	Female	73	Coronary artery disease	CABG	34

Table 2: Respiratory characteristics displayed as mean and standard deviation.

Parameter	Mean (SD)
Age (years)	65.7 ± 12.25
SAPS II on admission	44.82 ± 11.90
Ratio female: male	1:2.7
Catheter depth (cm)	64.29 ± 6.15
Pre-NIV pH	7.44 ± 0.04
Pre-NIV paO_2 (mmHg)	88.70 ± 24.89
Pre-NIV $paCO_2$ (mmHg)	41.55 ± 4.80
PEEP (cmH_2O)	6.23 ± 1.07
F_iO_2	40.54 ± 4.54
Horowitz-index	170.99 ± 95.89
NAVA level ($cmH_2O/\mu V$)	0.77 ± 0.45
P_{insp} (cmH_2O)	13.64 ± 2.46
Pressure support (cmH_2O)	6.25 ± 2.29
Expiratory trigger NIV-PSV (%)	40 ± 7.32
Tidal volume (ml/kg IBW)	8.30 ± 1.86
Respiratory rate (bpm)	20.75 ± 6.74

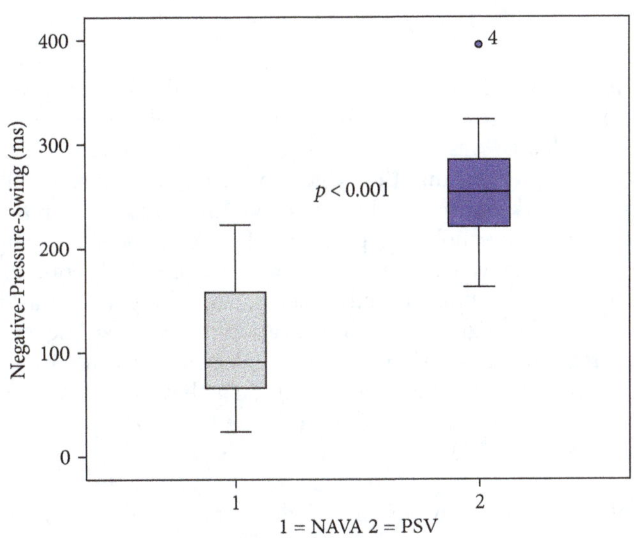

Figure 1: Whiskers-boxplots of negative pressure swing as a surrogate for work-of-breathing.

NeuroSync-index have been proposed ([16], [18]). Compared to others, we found lower indices [14, 24] most likely due to our study population which was previously lung healthy.

A successful (i.e., synchronous) patient-ventilator interaction leads to on-time triggering and adequate ventilatory support and is therefore effective in unloading respiratory muscles. Respiratory muscle workload is often measured as (inspiratory) pressure-time-product (PTP), by oesophageal pressure or as P0.1 (airway occlusion pressure 0.1 seconds after the start of inspiratory flow). All of these methods have

TABLE 3: Presented are the mean respiratory times for NIV-NAVA and NIV-PSV, (SD), median (IQR), respectively; ∗significant difference.

	NIV-PSV	NIV-NAVA	
Inspiratory time (ms)	1171 ± 314	1138 ± 383	$p = 0.564$
Expiratory time (ms)	2267 ± 800	2074 ± 770	$p = 0.130$
Total respiratory time (TTOT) (ms)	3180 (3071-4047)	3289 (2832-3843)	$p = 0.353$
Negative pressure duration (ms)∗	253 ± 55	108 ± 58	$p < 0.001$ ∗

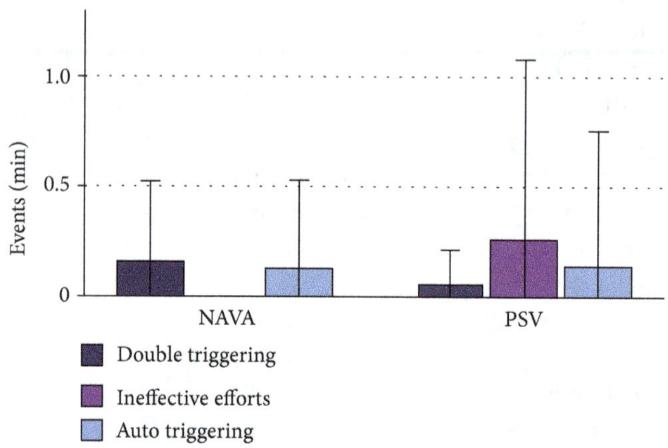

FIGURE 2: Frequency of asynchrony sorted by type; modes contrasted. Differences showed statistical significance for double triggering ($p = 0.02$) and ineffective efforts ($p = 0.001$), but not for auto triggering ($p = 0.584$).

their drawbacks [32–34]. Due to the clinical situation, being limited to assess work of breathing invasively during NIV, we evaluated respiratory muscle workload by calculating negative pressure duration which corresponds approximately to the work performed by the respiratory muscles to reach the trigger threshold (purple area in Figure 3). Ideally, during NAVA, this value would be zero, because the ventilator should start support exactly when the diaphragm contracts. We found a negative pressure duration that was significantly shorter for NIV-NAVA than for NIV-PSV which resembles results those of other trials concluding that NIV-NAVA is more effective with regard to unloading respiratory muscles than NIV-PSV [31].

NAVA mode has a pneumatic trigger safety back-up intended for situations of catheter-failure or displacement following the "first-come-first-serve" principle. In other trials, one-fifth to one-third of breaths in NAVA was triggered pneumatically [13, 31] (our trial: 29.7%). Possible explanations are displaced catheters or a modified activation of respiratory muscles, yet another explanation seldomly addressed is the ECG-filter of the NAVA mode [18]. By means of proximity of the catheter to the heart, ECG signals are part of the electrical recording and are actually used in the catheter positioning tool [17]. Since ECG amplitude might be high in relation to the electromyographic signals, a complex filtering algorithm has been developed [35]. While filtering during the rise in the EAdi signal can be compensated, a filtered signal during the triggering phase might cause (negative) trigger delays specifically related to the NAVA mode [18] (Figure 3).

To account for this systematic failure, we placed the "EAdi-true" cursor; we are aware that the name of this cursor suggests an absoluteness that it might not have. However, the assumption of ECG interference might be false if accessory ventilatory muscles generate an inspiratory pressure earlier than the diaphragm, for example, in case of ICU acquired weakness syndrome. In our study, the value for the inspiratory delay without EAdi-true would be 50 ms which is more than half that of what we tend to call the true delay (111 ms). Clinical usefulness of this corrected inspiratory trigger can be questioned because no measure can be taken to account for it. However, studies on NAVA with regard to patient-ventilator interaction should report this value, as well as the amount of pneumatically triggered breaths.

Our study has some limitations: we studied a small group of previously healthy subjects being clinically indicated by attending physicians to receive postextubation NIV. Probably most of these subjects would have done well without NIV, and therefore, they might not have experienced the need for ventilatory support. None of our subjects had experience with NIV, so other than subjects receiving NIV regularly like patients suffering from COPD our subjects might not have felt subtle differences a more experienced NIV-receiver might have recognized. Furthermore, we did not measure leakage during the study period. We only clinically minimized leak by tight mask fitting and checked and adjusted mask fitting with regard to leak due to our standard-of-care which includes keeping leakage below 30%.

We hypothesized that patient comfort would be higher during NIV-NAVA. This effect has been shown in children [12] and in adults at risk for extubation failure ventilated via helmets [20], as well as in healthy subject by [36]. In agreement with two other studies [19, 22], we were not able to show a difference in comfort between NIV-PSV and NIV-NAVA. One possible explanation is the difference in need for NIV, where a subject with a high demand for ventilatory assist will probably directly estimate the benefit of improved synchronization, whereas a subject that might also benefit from simple NIV-CPAP (continuous positive airway pressure) might not. Especially in case of subjects not used to NIV, felt differences between the modes are minute and might easily be overshadowed by environmental factors. Another possible explanation is the short time of application to compare the two modes; with longer application time, a positive effect of improved synchrony on comfort might have become evident.

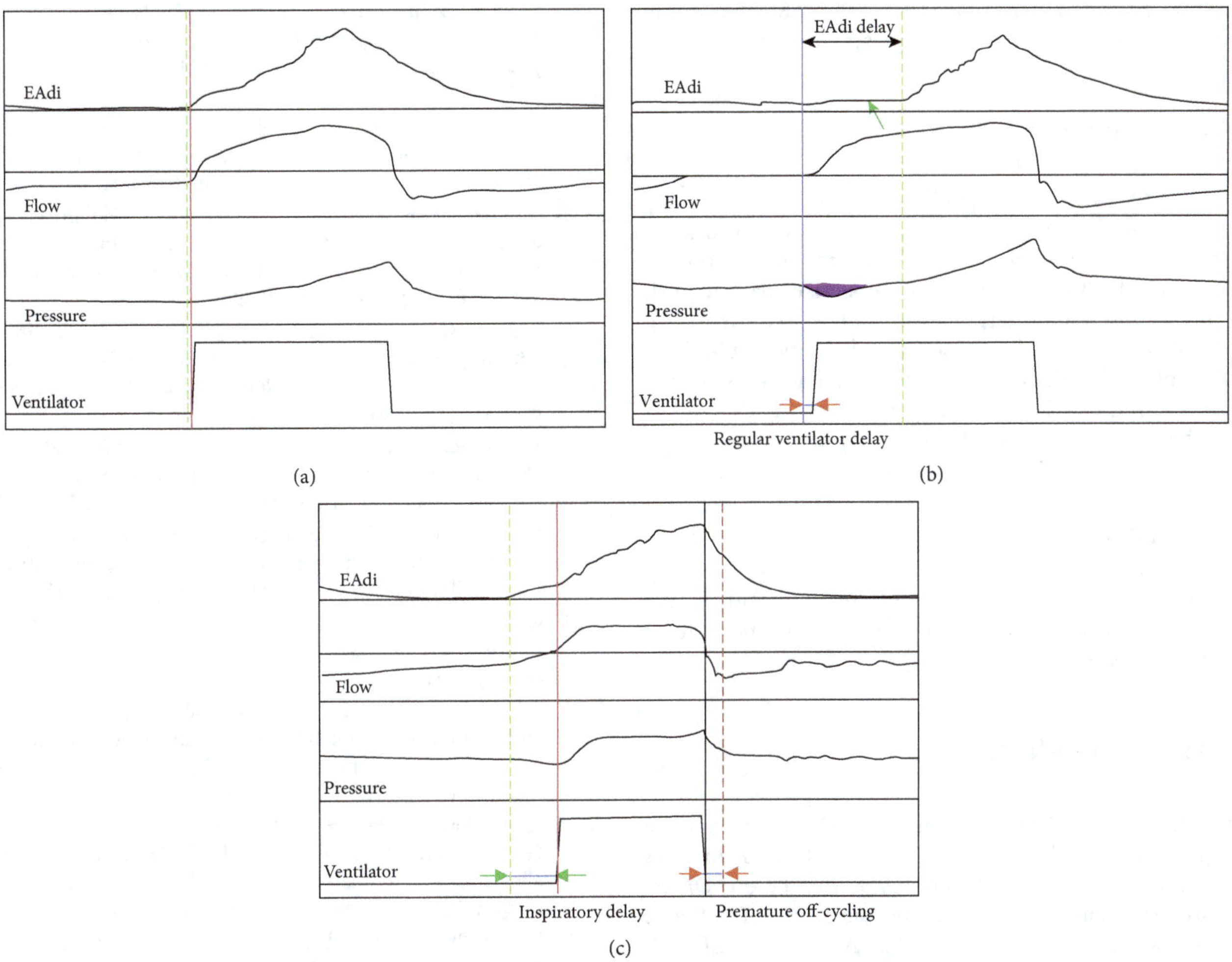

Figure 3: Presented are three different screenshots of ventilator tracings; tracing on top always EAdi, second tracing flow, third tracing pressure, fourth tracing ventilator signal. The axes are as follows: EAdi in microvolt, flow in liters per minute, pressure in mbar, ventilator dichotomous off/on, y-axes: time in milliseconds. Values are spared intentionally because this figure should be seen as a schematic rather than a visual representation of study data. (a) Perfect neuronal triggering, the ventilator cycles on (red vertical line) at exactly the same time as the increase in EAdi signal tracing (green broken vertical line) happens; times not marked because in this perfectly triggered breath there is no delay. (b) Visual presentation of the concept of "EAdi true". The time point marked with the black double-arrow is the moment when a decrease in pressure happens but the EAdi tracing does not show an increase, rather does it show the plateau mentioned in the text, representing a blacked out ECG signal (green arrow). During the plateau inspiratory activity of the diaphragm cannot be detected. The start of inspiration is therefore not where the EAdi tracing starts to rise, but rather where a drop in pressure tracing during the EAdi-plateau is detected. This is where the EAdi-signal would rise, if ECG "disturbance" had not happened. EAdi-delay: black double-arrow; regular ventilator delay: red arrows; purple area: negative pressure swing. (c) Pneumatically triggered breath during PSV, visual presentation of inspiratory and expiratory delay. The beginning of the EAdi tracing representing the start of inspiration is marked by the vertical broken green line. The start of ventilator activity (red vertical line) happens belated relative to EAdi but perfectly in time in regard to PSV criteria. Without the EAdi tracing this inspiratory delay cannot be detected. The end of ventilator activity (black vertical line) happens before EAdi tracing has reached the off-cycling criterion (vertical broken red line, 70% EAdi-peak); at this moment, the patient's diaphragm was still activated denoting that inspiration was still ongoing. Expiratory delay is marked by red arrowhead.

A strength of our study is that we used the same ventilator for both modes; nevertheless, our results may not be automatically applied to other ventilators.

5. Conclusion

NAVA used in noninvasive ventilation is able to safely increase its efficiency in postoperative, previously lung-healthy subjects. Our postoperative subjects did not experience improved comfort with NIV-NAVA vs. NIV-PSV. However, the reduction of asynchrony is an argument to use NAVA in noninvasive ventilation; although, a larger randomized controlled trial that targets intubation rates and outcome with NIV-NAVA compared to conventional NIV-PSV is needed.

Additional Points

Take-home message: NAVA used during NIV for postoperative respiratory support in lung-healthy patients effectively reduces asynchrony. NIV-NAVA actually reduces ineffective respiratory efforts to zero compared to NIV-PSV. Nevertheless, this does not translate into increased comfort.

Authors' Contributions

LOH and UO contributed equally and share first-authorship equally. LOH supervised and helped with data acquisition, analysed and interpreted the data, and drafted and revised the manuscript. UO helped with and supervised data acquisition, helped with data interpretation, and revised the manuscript. JM acquired and analysed the data and revised the manuscript. MQ helped interpreting the data and revised the manuscript. OM initiated and supervised the trial, interpreted the data, and revised the manuscript.

Acknowledgments

The study was fully financed by departmental funding. We acknowledge support by the Open Access Publication Funds of the Göttingen University.

Supplementary Materials

ESM table 1: used delays and their calculation formula from the placed cursors. ESM table 2: results of ABG analyses (mean and SD) after fifteen minutes of ventilation. Differences are marginal and statistically not significant. ESM table 3: results of repeated measures ANOVA for main effect of "mode" and the interaction between mode and order, significance is marked∗. ESM figure 1: study design. ESM figure 2: tracings and cursors used in the study. For cursor description please refer to "cursor placement", for definition of times and delays please refer to ESM table 1. ESM figure 3: questionnaire to assess patient comfort for each ventilation mode; original sheet for the first mode; for the second mode, the sheet is headlined, mode 2 "but otherwise just the same". ESM figure 4: visual analog scale to evaluate overall impression of the ventilation mode, each mode was evaluated separately. The patient was given a pen and asked to draw a vertical line at the place where they feel their comfort level is. Translation: headline "noninvasive ventilation mode 1/ 2"; left means "very uncomfortable, wearing", right means a very pleasant experience. These explanations were also given to the patient during the trial. *(Supplementary Materials)*

References

[1] A. Demoule, E. Girou, J. C. Richard, S. Taillé, and L. Brochard, "Increased use of noninvasive ventilation in French intensive care units," *Intensive Care Medicine*, vol. 32, no. 11, pp. 1747–1755, 2006.

[2] W. Windisch, "Impact of home mechanical ventilation on health-related quality of life," *The European Respiratory Journal*, vol. 32, no. 5, pp. 1328–1336, 2008.

[3] S. Nava, C. Gregoretti, F. Fanfulla et al., "Noninvasive ventilation to prevent respiratory failure after extubation in high-risk patients," *Critical Care Medicine*, vol. 33, no. 11, pp. 2465–2470, 2005.

[4] L. Blanch, A. Villagra, B. Sales et al., "Asynchronies during mechanical ventilation are associated with mortality," *Intensive Care Medicine*, vol. 41, no. 4, pp. 633–641, 2015.

[5] L. Vignaux, F. Vargas, J. Roeseler et al., "Patient-ventilator asynchrony during non-invasive ventilation for acute respiratory failure: a multicenter study," *Intensive Care Medicine*, vol. 35, no. 5, pp. 840–846, 2009.

[6] J. Beck, M. Tucci, G. Emeriaud, J. Lacroix, and C. Sinderby, "Prolonged neural expiratory time induced by mechanical ventilation in infants," *Pediatric Research*, vol. 55, no. 5, pp. 747–754, 2004.

[7] A. Carlucci, L. Pisani, P. Ceriana, A. Malovini, and S. Nava, "Patient-ventilator asynchronies: may the respiratory mechanics play a role?," *Critical Care*, vol. 17, no. 2, p. R54, 2013.

[8] D. C. Chao, D. J. Scheinhorn, and M. Stearn-Hassenpflug, "Patient-ventilator trigger asynchrony in prolonged mechanical ventilation," *Chest*, vol. 112, no. 6, pp. 1592–1599, 1997.

[9] C. Sinderby and J. Beck, "Neurally adjusted ventilatory assist in non-invasive ventilation," *Minerva Anestesiologica*, vol. 79, no. 8, pp. 915–925, 2013.

[10] J. Beck, F. Campoccia, J. C. Allo et al., "Improved synchrony and respiratory unloading by neurally adjusted ventilatory assist (NAVA) in lung-injured rabbits," *Pediatric Research*, vol. 61, no. 3, pp. 289–294, 2007.

[11] L. Ducharme-Crevier, J. Beck, S. Essouri, P. Jouvet, and G. Emeriaud, "Neurally adjusted ventilatory assist (NAVA) allows patient-ventilator synchrony during pediatric noninvasive ventilation: a crossover physiological study," *Critical Care*, vol. 19, no. 1, p. 44, 2015.

[12] P. de la Oliva, C. Schuffelmann, A. Gomez-Zamora, J. Villar, and R. M. Kacmarek, "Asynchrony, neural drive, ventilatory variability and COMFORT: NAVA versus pressure support in pediatric patients. A non-randomized crossover trial," *Intensive Care Medicine*, vol. 38, no. 5, pp. 838–846, 2012.

[13] L. Piquilloud, L. Vignaux, E. Bialais et al., "Neurally adjusted ventilatory assist improves patient-ventilator interaction," *Intensive Care Medicine*, vol. 37, no. 2, pp. 263–271, 2011.

[14] I. S. Sehgal, S. Dhooria, A. N. Aggarwal, D. Behera, and R. Agarwal, "Asynchrony index in pressure support ventilation (PSV) versus neurally adjusted ventilator assist (NAVA) during non-invasive ventilation (NIV) for respiratory failure: systematic review and meta-analysis," *Intensive Care Medicine*, vol. 42, no. 11, pp. 1813–1815, 2016.

[15] L. Brander, O. Moerer, G. Hedenstierna et al., "Neural control of ventilation prevents both over-distension and de-recruitment of experimentally injured lungs," *Respiratory Physiology & Neurobiology*, vol. 237, pp. 57–67, 2017.

[16] A. W. Thille, P. Rodriguez, B. Cabello, F. Lellouche, and L. Brochard, "Patient-ventilator asynchrony during assisted mechanical ventilation," *Intensive Care Medicine*, vol. 32, no. 10, pp. 1515–1522, 2006.

[17] J. Barwing, M. Ambold, N. Linden, M. Quintel, and O. Moerer, "Evaluation of the catheter positioning for neurally adjusted ventilatory assist," *Intensive Care Medicine*, vol. 35, no. 10, pp. 1809–1814, 2009.

[18] C. Sinderby, S. Liu, D. Colombo et al., "An automated and

standardized neural index to quantify patient-ventilator interaction," *Critical Care*, vol. 17, no. 5, p. R239, 2013.

[19] P. M. Bertrand, E. Futier, Y. Coisel, S. Matecki, S. Jaber, and J. M. Constantin, "Neurally adjusted ventilatory assist vs pressure support ventilation for noninvasive ventilation during acute respiratory failure: a crossover physiologic study," *Chest*, vol. 143, no. 1, pp. 30–36, 2013.

[20] G. Cammarota, F. Longhini, R. Perucca et al., "New setting of neurally adjusted ventilatory assist during noninvasive ventilation through a helmet," *Anesthesiology*, vol. 125, no. 6, pp. 1181–1189, 2016.

[21] G. Carteaux, A. Córdoba-Izquierdo, A. Lyazidi, L. Heunks, A. W. Thille, and L. Brochard, "Comparison between neurally adjusted ventilatory assist and pressure support ventilation levels in terms of respiratory effort," *Critical Care Medicine*, vol. 44, no. 3, pp. 503–511, 2016.

[22] F. Longhini, C. Pan, J. Xie et al., "New setting of neurally adjusted ventilatory assist for noninvasive ventilation by facial mask: a physiologic study," *Critical Care*, vol. 21, no. 1, p. 170, 2017.

[23] S. Nava and L. Pisani, "Neurally adjusted non-invasive ventilation in patients with chronic obstructive pulmonary disease: does patient-ventilator synchrony matter?," *Critical Care*, vol. 18, no. 6, p. 670, 2014.

[24] M. Schmidt, M. Dres, M. Raux et al., "Neurally adjusted ventilatory assist improves patient-ventilator interaction during postextubation prophylactic noninvasive ventilation," *Critical Care Medicine*, vol. 40, no. 6, pp. 1738–1744, 2012.

[25] L. Vignaux, S. Grazioli, L. Piquilloud et al., "Patient-ventilator asynchrony during noninvasive pressure support ventilation and neurally adjusted ventilatory assist in infants and children," *Pediatric Critical Care Medicine*, vol. 14, no. 8, pp. e357–e364, 2013.

[26] O. Moerer, J. Beck, L. Brander et al., "Subject-ventilator synchrony during neural versus pneumatically triggered noninvasive helmet ventilation," *Intensive Care Medicine*, vol. 34, no. 9, pp. 1615–1623, 2008.

[27] L. O. Harnisch and O. Moerer, "Off-cycling during NIV in chronic obstructive pulmonary disease: clinical implications," in *Noninvasive Mechanical Ventilation*, A. M. Esquinas, Ed., pp. 153–159, Springer, 2016.

[28] D. Colombo, G. Cammarota, V. Bergamaschi, M. de Lucia, F. D. Corte, and P. Navalesi, "Physiologic response to varying levels of pressure support and neurally adjusted ventilatory assist in patients with acute respiratory failure," *Intensive Care Medicine*, vol. 34, no. 11, 2008.

[29] A. W. Thille, B. Cabello, F. Galia, A. Lyazidi, and L. Brochard, "Reduction of patient-ventilator asynchrony by reducing tidal volume during pressure-support ventilation," *Intensive Care Medicine*, vol. 34, no. 8, pp. 1477–1486, 2008.

[30] L. Piquilloud, D. Tassaux, E. Bialais et al., "Neurally adjusted ventilatory assist (NAVA) improves patient-ventilator interaction during non-invasive ventilation delivered by face mask," *Intensive Care Medicine*, vol. 38, no. 10, pp. 1624–1631, 2012.

[31] M. J. Heulitt, K. C. Clement, S. J. Holt, T. L. Thurman, and C. H. Jo, "Neurally triggered breaths have reduced response time, work of breathing, and asynchrony compared with pneumatically triggered breaths in a recovering animal model of lung injury," *Pediatric Critical Care Medicine*, vol. 13, no. 3, pp. e195 e203, 2012.

[32] G. Hedenstierna, "Esophageal pressure: benefit and limitations," *Minerva Anestesiologica*, vol. 78, no. 8, pp. 959–966, 2012.

[33] T. Kera, A. Aihara, and T. Inomata, "Reliability of airway occlusion pressure as an index of respiratory motor output," *Respiratory Care*, vol. 58, no. 5, pp. 845–849, 2012.

[34] G. Natalini, M. Marchesini, A. Tessadrelli, A. Rosano, A. Candiani, and A. Bernardini, "Effect of breathing pattern on the pressure-time product calculation," *Acta Anaesthesiologica Scandinavica*, vol. 48, no. 5, pp. 642–647, 2004.

[35] C. A. Sinderby, J. C. Beck, L. H. Lindström, and A. E. Grassino, "Enhancement of signal quality in esophageal recordings of diaphragm EMG," *Journal of Applied Physiology (Bethesda, MD: 1985)*, vol. 82, no. 4, pp. 1370–1377, 1997.

[36] O. Moerer, J. Barwing, and M. Quintel, "Neurally adjusted ventilatory assist (NAVA). A new mode of assisted mechanical ventilation," *Anaesthesist*, vol. 57, no. 10, pp. 998–1005, 2008.

Permissions

All chapters in this book were first published by Hindawi Publishing Corporation; hereby published with permission under the Creative Commons Attribution License or equivalent. Every chapter published in this book has been scrutinized by our experts. Their significance has been extensively debated. The topics covered herein carry significant findings which will fuel the growth of the discipline. They may even be implemented as practical applications or may be referred to as a beginning point for another development.

The contributors of this book come from diverse backgrounds, making this book a truly international effort. This book will bring forth new frontiers with its revolutionizing research information and detailed analysis of the nascent developments around the world.

We would like to thank all the contributing authors for lending their expertise to make the book truly unique. They have played a crucial role in the development of this book. Without their invaluable contributions this book wouldn't have been possible. They have made vital efforts to compile up to date information on the varied aspects of this subject to make this book a valuable addition to the collection of many professionals and students.

This book was conceptualized with the vision of imparting up-to-date information and advanced data in this field. To ensure the same, a matchless editorial board was set up. Every individual on the board went through rigorous rounds of assessment to prove their worth. After which they invested a large part of their time researching and compiling the most relevant data for our readers.

The editorial board has been involved in producing this book since its inception. They have spent rigorous hours researching and exploring the diverse topics which have resulted in the successful publishing of this book. They have passed on their knowledge of decades through this book. To expedite this challenging task, the publisher supported the team at every step. A small team of assistant editors was also appointed to further simplify the editing procedure and attain best results for the readers.

Apart from the editorial board, the designing team has also invested a significant amount of their time in understanding the subject and creating the most relevant covers. They scrutinized every image to scout for the most suitable representation of the subject and create an appropriate cover for the book.

The publishing team has been an ardent support to the editorial, designing and production team. Their endless efforts to recruit the best for this project, has resulted in the accomplishment of this book. They are a veteran in the field of academics and their pool of knowledge is as vast as their experience in printing. Their expertise and guidance has proved useful at every step. Their uncompromising quality standards have made this book an exceptional effort. Their encouragement from time to time has been an inspiration for everyone.

The publisher and the editorial board hope that this book will prove to be a valuable piece of knowledge for researchers, students, practitioners and scholars across the globe.

List of Contributors

Jason S. Oh
Wellstar Health System, Wellstar Pulmonary and Critical Care Medicine, Medical College of Georgia at Augusta University, Department of Medicine, Augusta, GA, USA

Uni Wong
Department of Medicine, Division of Gastroenterology, University of Maryland School of Medicine, Baltimore, MD, USA

Divyansh Bajaj
Department of Internal Medicine, Quinnipiac University Frank H. Netter MD School of Medicine/ St. Vincent's Medical Center, Bridgeport, CT, USA

Stella E. Hines
Department of Medicine, Division of Occupational and Environmental Medicine and Division of Pulmonary & Critical Care Medicine, University of Maryland School of Medicine, Baltimore, MD, USA

Husain Kadhem and Naser Naser
Department of Internal Medicine, Salmaniya Medical Complex, Manama, Bahrain

Kannan Sridharan
Department of Pharmacology & Therapeutics, College of Medicine & Medical Sciences, Arabian Gulf University, Manama, Bahrain

Athanasios Voulgaris and Paschalis Steiropoulos
MSc Program in Sleep Medicine, Medical School, Democritus University of Thrace, Alexandroupolis, Greece
Department of Pneumonology, Medical School, Democritus University of Thrace, Alexandroupolis, Greece

Maria Antoniadou and Michalis Agrafiotis
MSc Program in Sleep Medicine, Medical School, Democritus University of Thrace, Alexandroupolis, Greece
Department of Pneumonology, General Hospital "G. Papanikolaou", Thessaloniki, Greece

Jarmanjeet Singh
Internal Medicine Residency Program,The Cleveland Clinic Foundation, Cleveland, OH, USA

Hanine Inaty and Atul C. Mehta
Respiratory Institute, The Cleveland Clinic Foundation, Cleveland, OH, USA

Sanjay Mukhopadhyay
Department of Pathology, The Cleveland Clinic Foundation, Cleveland, OH, USA

Isaac Biney, Tina Dudney and Elise Schriver
Department of Medicine, Division of Pulmonary Disease and Critical Care Medicine, University of Tennessee Graduate School of Medicine, Knoxville, TN, USA

Mitchell Goldman and Lee Carder
Department of Surgery, University of Tennessee Graduate School of Medicine, Knoxville, TN, USA

Jaskaran K. Purewal, N. F. N. Sakul, Nikhita R. Balabbigari and Alberto Nenninger
Department of Medicine, Overlook Medical Center, Summit, NJ 07901, USA

Nisha Kotecha
Department of Pulmonary Critical Care, Overlook Medical Center, Summit, NJ 07901, USA

Nevenka Piskac Zivkovic and Nina Petra Novak
University Hospital Dubrava, Zagreb, Croatia

Igor Cikara
University Hospital Dubrava, Zagreb, Croatia
Faculty of Medicine Osijek, University Josip Juraj Strossmayer Osijek, Croatia

Boris Brkljacic and Neven Tudoric
University Hospital Dubrava, Zagreb, Croatia
School of Medicine, University of Zagreb, Zagreb, Croatia

Olivier Taton, Benjamin Bondue and Dimitri Leduc
Department of Pneumology, Hôpital Erasme, Université Libre de Bruxelles, 808 Route de Lennik, 1070 Brussels, Belgium

Pierre Alain Gevenois
Department of Radiology, Hôpital Erasme, Université Libre de Bruxelles, 808 Route de Lennik, 1070 Brussels, Belgium

Myriam Remmelink
Department of Pathology, Hôpital Erasme, Université Libre de Bruxelles, 808 Route de Lennik, 1070 Brussels, Belgium

Aram Barbaryan, Yonatan Gizaw and Stefania Bailuc
Division of General, Geriatric & Hospital Medicine, University of Kansas Health System, Kansas City, KS, USA

Travis Abicht
Department of Cardiothoracic Surgery, University of Kansas Health System, Kansas City, KS, USA

Sergey Barsamyan
Department of Cardiology, John Radcliffe Hospital, Oxford University Hospitals NHS Trust, Oxford, UK

Aibek E.Mirrakhimov
Division of Pulmonary and Critical Care Medicine, University of New Mexico, Albuquerque, USA

Muhammad Imtiaz
Division of Pulmonary and Critical Care Medicine, Conemaugh Memorial Medical Center, Johnstown, Pennsylvania, USA
Department of Internal Medicine, Conemaugh Medical Memorial Center, Johnstown, PA, USA

Biplab Saha
Division of Pulmonary and Critical Care Medicine, Albany Medical Center, Albany, New York, USA

Uzma Sana Ullah
Department of Medicine, Conemaugh Memorial Medical Center, Johnstown, Pennsylvania, USA

Aditi Saha
Department of Medicine, Saint Barnabas Medical Center, Livingston, New Jersey, USA

Anshika Singh, Qiuxue Tan, Nicole M. Saccone and David H. Lindner
NCH Healthcare System, Naples, FL 34102, USA

Hassan Baig and Jorge Mallea
Department of Pulmonary and Critical Care Medicine, Mayo Clinic Florida, 4500 San Pablo Road, Jacksonville, FL 32224, USA

Sushilkumar Sonavane
Department of Diagnostic Radiology, Mayo Clinic Florida, 4500 San Pablo Road, Jacksonville, FL 32224, USA

Ian Makey
Department of Thoracic Surgery, Mayo Clinic Florida, 4500 San Pablo Road, Jacksonville, FL 32224, USA

Andras Khoor
Department of Anatomic and Clinical Pathology, Mayo Clinic Florida, 4500 San Pablo Road, Jacksonville, FL 32224, USA

Kartikeya Rajdev, Susanna G. Von Essen, Peter J. Murphy and Sabin Bista
Department of Internal Medicine, Division of Pulmonary, Critical Care & Sleep Medicine, University of Nebraska Medical Center, 42nd and Emile St., Omaha, Nebraska 68198-7400, USA

Pretty Sara Idiculla
Sree Gokulam Medical College & Research Foundation, Kerala, India

Shubham Sharma
University College of Medical Sciences & GTB Hospital, New Delhi, India

Michael A. Simon, Christopher Tan, Lyle Gesner and Barry Julius
Department of Radiology, RWJBH–Saint Barnabas Medical Center, Livingston, New Jersey, USA

Patrick Hilden
Department of Biostatistics, RWJBH–Saint Barnabas Medical Center, Livingston, New Jersey, USA

Dessalegn Demeke
Bahir Dar University College of Medicine and Health Sciences, Department of Physiology, Bahir Dar, Ethiopia

Diresibachew W. Haile
Addis Ababa University College of Medicine and Health Sciences, Department of Physiology, Addis Ababa, Ethiopia

Or Inbar, Hayit Greenspan and Mickey Scheinowitz
Department of Biomedical Engineering, Tel-Aviv University, Israel

Omri Inbar
The Edmond and Lily Safra Children's Hospital, Sheba Medical Center, Tel Hashomer, Israel

Ronen Reuveny
Pulmonary Institute, Sheba Medical Center Tel-Hashomer, Israel

Michael J. Segel
Pulmonary Institute, Sheba Medical Center Tel-Hashomer, Israel
Sackler School of Medicine, Tel-Aviv University, Tel-Aviv, Israel

Mathanki Sooriyakanthan and Sivapalan Kanagasabai
Department of Physiology, Faculty of Medicine, University of Jaffna, Jaffna, Sri Lanka

Savithri Wimalasekera
Department Physiology, Faculty of Medical Sciences, University of Sri Jayewardenepura, Nugegoda, Sri Lanka

Carla Máximo Prado
Department of Bioscience, Federal University of Sao Paulo, Santos, Rua Silva Jardim 136, 11015-020 Santos, SP, Brazil

Fernanda Degobbi Tenorio Quirino dos Santos Lopes, Edna Aparecida Leick, Fernanda Magalhães Arantes-Costa, Francine Maria de Almeida, Paulo Hilário Nascimento Saldiva, Thais Mauad, Iolanda de Fátima Lopes Calvo Tibério and M-lton de Arruda Martins
Faculdade de Medicina FMUSP, Universidade de São Paulo, Av. Dr. Arnaldo 455, Sala 1210, 01246-903 São Paulo, SP, Brazil

Renato Fraga Righetti
Faculdade de Medicina FMUSP, Universidade de São Paulo, Av. Dr. Arnaldo 455, Sala 1210, 01246-903 São Paulo, SP, Brazil
Hospital Sírio-Libanês, Rua Adma Jafet 115, 01308-060 São Paulo, SP, Brazil

Julyan Al Fori, Maryam Al Belushi, Mohammed Al Shuraiqi and Nasser Al Busaidi
Department of Chest Medicine, The Royal Hospital, Muscat, Oman

Ghalia Al Mohanny
Department of Cardiology, The Royal Hospital, Muscat, Oman

Rashid Al Umairi
Department of Radiology, The Royal Hospital, Muscat, Oman

Shahab Rezvani, Marie Tominna and Sayf Al-Katib
Beaumont Health, Oakland University William Beaumont School of Medicine, Department of Diagnostic Radiology and Molecular Imaging, 3601W13 Mile Rd, Royal Oak, MI 48073, USA

Marc D. Smith and Craig Cousineau
Beaumont Health, Oakland University William Beaumont School of Medicine, Department of Clinical Pathology, 3601W13 Mile Rd, Royal Oak, MI 48073, USA

Ayad Al-Katib
Wayne State University School of Medicine, Lymphoma Research Laboratory, 540 E Canfield Room No. 8829, Detroit, MI 48202, USA

Fatima Alhamed Alduihi
Department of Internal Medicine, Aleppo University, Aleppo, Syria

Linda P. Vien
Department of Medicine, Temple University Hospital, 3401 North Broad Street, Philadelphia, PA 19140, USA

Robert M. Marron and James C. Brown
Department of Thoracic Medicine and Surgery, Temple University Hospital, 3401 North Broad Street, Philadelphia, PA 19140, USA

Abbas Charlie and Maruti Kumaran
Department of Radiology, Temple University Hospital, 3401 North Broad Street, Philadelphia, PA 19140, USA

Veena Dronamraju, Navneet Singh and Justin Poon
Department of Internal Medicine, SUNY Downstate Medical Center, USA

Sachi Shah
Department of Infectious Disease, Montefiore Medical Center, USA

Joseph Gorga
Division of Pulmonary and Critical Care Medicine, New York Health and Hospitals Corporation, Kings County Hospital Center, USA

Hector Ojeda-Martinez
Department of Infectious Disease, SUNY Downstate Medical Center, USA

Samy McFarlane
Department of Internal Medicine, SUNY Downstate Medical Center, USA
Department of Endocrinology, SUNY Downstate Medical Center, USA

Mohammed Ali, Mihir Buch, Manuel Ramos-Ramirez, Munish Sharma, Humayun Anjum and Alamgir Khan
Department of Pulmonary Medicine, Corpus Christi Medical Center, Texas, USA

Kashmala Khan, Seema Patel and Saiara Choudhury
Department of Internal Medicine, Corpus Christi Medical Center, Texas, USA

Salim Surani
Department of Pulmonary Medicine, Corpus Christi Medical Center, Texas, USA
Department of Pulmonary, Critical Care & Sleep Medicine, Texas A&M University, Health Science Center, Texas, USA

Md Didar Ul Alam and Khandakar Hussain
Department of Internal Medicine, Conemaugh Medical Memorial Center, Johnstown, PA, USA
Department of Hospital Medicine, Conemaugh Medical Memorial Center, Johnstown, PA, USA

Samsone Garedew
Department of Hospital Medicine, Conemaugh Medical Memorial Center, Johnstown, PA, USA

Bryno Gay, Zachary Field and Mario Madruga
Department of Medicine, Orlando Regional Healthcare, Orlando, Florida, USA

Sachin Patel and Wael Nasser
Department of Pulmonary, Critical Care and Sleep Medicine, Orlando Regional Healthcare, Orlando, USA

Rodrigo Murillo Alvarez
Department of Pathology, Orlando Regional Healthcare, Orlando, USA

S. J. Carlan
Division of Academic Affairs and Research, Orlando Regional Healthcare, Orlando, USA

Daniel Temas and Armin Meyer
University of South Carolina School of Medicine-Greenville/Prisma Health-Upstate, 701 Grove Rd., Greenville, SC 29605, USA

Amr Essa, Saboor Randhawa and Carrie Valenta
Creighton University School of Medicine, Department of Internal Medicine, Omaha, USA

Jeffrey Macaraeg, Nikhil Jagan, Stanley Thomas, Shraddha Narechania, Michael Kaster, Venketraman Sahasranaman and Douglas Moore
Creighton University School of Medicine, Department of Pulmonary, Critical Care, and Sleep Medicine, Omaha, USA

Daniel Kwon
Creighton University School of Medicine, Department of Pathology, Omaha, USA

Matthew Kruse
Creighton University School of Medicine, Department of Radiology, Omaha, USA

Manasa Velagapudi and John Horne
Creighton University School of Medicine, Department of Infectious Diseases, Omaha, USA

Kimberly E. Foil, M. Gwen Blanton, Haitham S. Al Ashry, Suchit Kumbhare and Charlie Strange
Division of Pulmonary, Critical Care, Allergy and Sleep Medicine, Medical University of South Carolina, Charleston, SC, USA

Chris Sanders and Joannah Kim
Biocerna LLC, Gaithersburg, MD, USA

Bruno Max Borguezan
Post-graduate Programme in Medical Sciences, School of Medical Sciences, State University of Rio de Janeiro, Rio de Janeiro, Brazil

Agnaldo José Lopes
Post-graduate Programme in Medical Sciences, School of Medical Sciences, State University of Rio de Janeiro, Rio de Janeiro, Brazil
Rehabilitation Sciences Post-graduate Programme, Augusto Motta University Centre (UNISUAM), Rio de Janeiro, Brazil

Eduardo Haruo Saito
Post-graduate Programme in Medical Sciences, School of Medical Sciences, State University of Rio de Janeiro, Rio de Janeiro, Brazil
Division of Thoracic Surgery, Pedro Ernesto University Hospital, State University of Rio de Janeiro, Rio de Janeiro, Brazil

Claudio Higa
Division of Thoracic Surgery, Pedro Ernesto University Hospital, State University of Rio de Janeiro, Rio de Janeiro, Brazil

Aristófanes Corrêa Silva
Technology Centre, Federal University of Maranhão, São Luis, Brazil

Rodolfo Acatauassú Nunes
Post-graduate Programme in Medical Sciences, School of Medical Sciences, State University of Rio de Janeiro, Rio de Janeiro, Brazil
Division of Thoracic Surgery, Pedro Ernesto University Hospital, State University of Rio de Janeiro, Rio de Janeiro, Brazil
University Centre for Cancer Control, State University of Rio de Janeiro, Rio de Janeiro, RJ, Brazil

Paul S. Richman
Pulmonary and Critical Care Division, Stony Brook University Health Sciences Center, Stony Brook, NY 11794-8172, USA

Pomin Yeung
Weill Cornell University Medical Center, 1300 York Ave, New York, NY, USA

Thomas V. Bilfinger
Cardiothoracic Surgery Division, Stony Brook University Health Sciences Center, Stony Brook, NY 1174-8172, USA

Jie Yang
Department of Family, Population & Preventive Medicine, Stony Brook University Health Sciences Center, Stony Brook, NY 11794-8172, USA

William W. Stringer
Los Angeles Biomedical Institute (LABIOMED) at Harbor-UCLA Medical Center, 1000 West Carson St, Torrance, CA 90509, USA

Mehmet M. Tatari, David Abia-Trujillo, Neal M. Patel, Sebastian Fernandez-Bussy, Britney N. Hazelett and Margaret M. Johnson
Division of Pulmonary Medicine, Mayo Clinic, Jacksonville, FL. 4500 San Pablo Road, Jacksonville, FL 32224, USA

Mathew Thomas
Department of Cardiothoracic Surgery, Mayo Clinic, Jacksonville, FL. 4500 San Pablo Road, Jacksonville, FL 32224, USA

Ziad Boujaoude, Melvin Pratter and Wissam Abouzgheib
Division of Pulmonary and Critical Care Medicine, Cooper Medical School of Rowan University, Camden, NJ 08103, USA

Rohan Arya
Division of Pulmonary and Critical Care Medicine, University of South Carolina School of Medicine, Columbia, SC 29203, USA

Aseem Shrivastava
WellStar Pulmonary Medicine, Marietta, GA, USA

Samer Al Sawalhi, Deping Zhao, Haomin Cai and Yuxing Jin
Department of Thoracic Surgery, Shanghai Pulmonary Hospital, Tongji University, Shanghai, China

Victor Calvo, Manuela Tejada-Giraldo and Ricardo Cardona
Group of Clinical and Experimental Allergy, Clinic "IPS Universitaria", University of Antioquia, Medellín, Colombia

Marlon Munera
Medicine Department, University Corporation, Rafael Nuñez, Cartagena, Colombia

Andres Sánchez
Group of Clinical and Experimental Allergy, Clinic "IPS Universitaria", University of Antioquia, Medellín, Colombia
Medicine Department, University Corporation, Rafael Nuñez, Cartagena, Colombia
Foundation for the Development of Medical and Biological Sciences, Cartagena, Colombia

Jorge Sánchez
Group of Clinical and Experimental Allergy, Clinic "IPS Universitaria", University of Antioquia, Medellín, Colombia
Foundation for the Development of Medical and Biological Sciences, Cartagena, Colombia

Irfan Shafiq, Mateen Haider Uzbeck, Zaid Zoumot, Mohamed Abuzakouk, Niyas Parappurath and Ali Saeed Wahla
Respiratory and Allergy Institute, Cleveland Clinic Abu Dhabi, Abu Dhabi, UAE

Yo Tsukamoto, Takeo Nakada, Soichiro Fukushima, Mitsuo Yabe, Naoki Toya and Tadashi Akiba
Department of Surgery, Jikei University Kashiwa Hospital, 163-1 Kashiwashita, Kashiwa, Chiba 277-8567, Japan

Takashi Ohtsuka and Takao Ohki
Department of Surgery, The Jikei University School of Medicine, Nishishinbashi 3-19-18, Minatoku, Tokyo 105-8471, Japan

L. O. Harnisch, J. Mann, M. Quintel and O. Moerer
Department of Anaesthesiology, University Medical Centre Göttingen, Germany Robert-Koch-Str. 40 D-37099 Göttingen

U. Olgemoeller
Department of Cardiology and Pulmonology, University Medical Centre Göttingen, Robert-Koch-Str. 40 D-37099 Göttingen, Germany

Index

www.ingramcontent.com/pod-product-compliance
Lightning Source LLC
LaVergne TN
LVHW060057220926
848484LV00008BA/2122